DUTCH POST-WAR FICTION FILM
THROUGH A LENS OF PSYCHOANALYSIS

PETER VERSTRATEN

DUTCH POST-WAR FICTION FILM THROUGH A LENS OF PSYCHOANALYSIS

Routledge
Taylor & Francis Group
LONDON AND NEW YORK

This publication is made possible by grants from the Nederlands Filmfonds, the Netherlands Society of Cinematographers, and Leiden University Centre for the Arts in Society.

Published by Eye Filmmuseum

First published in 2021 by Amsterdam University Press Ltd.

Published 2025 by Routledge
4 Park Square, Milton Park, Abingdon, Oxon OX14 4RN
605 Third Avenue, New York, NY 10158

Routledge is an imprint of the Taylor & Francis Group, an informa business

ISBN: 9789463725330 (hbk)
ISBN: 9781041178354 (pbk)
ISBN: 9781003694250 (ebk)
NUR 674

Cover illustration: *Van God los* [Tygo Gernandt, Egbert Jan Weeber, Mads Wittermans]
© Rinkel Film BV. Photo: Bas Losekoot
Cover design: Magenta Xtra, Bussum

DOI 10.5117/9789463725330

TABLE OF CONTENTS

Preface

Verstraten, P., *Dutch Post-War Fiction Film Through a Lens of Psychoanalysis.* Taylor & Francis Group, 2021
DOI 10.5117/9789463725330_PREF

ABSTRACT

In the preface I explain why this study, a sequel to the *Humour and Irony* book, should not be taken as a scholarly survey of 'national cinema' issues. Owing to the many influences from foreign pictures, Dutch fiction films are best read against the background of an international cinematic context. It is an oft-voiced claim that Dutch cinema is rooted in realism, but I employ a version of psychoanalysis 'lite' in order to explore the imaginative potential of Dutch cinema. Moreover, the advantage of reading the films through the prism of psychoanalysis is that it enables me to structure this study as a 'database': surprising associations between films are favoured over chronological accounts.

KEYWORDS
Psychoanalysis 'lite' – imaginative potential – database structure – surprising associations

Hopefully, this study is to my previous book *Humour and Irony in Dutch Post-war Fiction Film* what MAD MAX: THE ROAD WARRIOR (George Miller, 1981) is to Miller's MAD MAX (1979): the sequel is even better than the original. The study from 2016 covered a great many titles, but still some of the very best Dutch films were missing: the theatrical DE DANS VAN DE REIGER (Fons Rademakers, 1966), the adventurous SOLDAAT VAN ORANJE (Paul Verhoeven, 1977), the nail-biting SPOORLOOS (George Sluizer, 1988), the painfully intimate LEEDVERMAAK (Frans Weisz, 1989), the merciless VAN GOD LOS (Pieter Kuijpers, 2003), to name just a few. This study is intended to make up for this lack, but despite the term 'Dutch' as the first word of the title, the reader should not take this as a scholarly survey of 'national cinema' issues nor as a study of new directions in national cinema. This book contains hardly any discussions of production histories, of industrial forces, or reception by critics and/or audiences (but I cordially invite scholars to use this book to contribute to such discussions). This study does not even address Dutch cinema as a national cultural practice. I could have selected only those films that have a common style or have similar dramatic themes in order to agree on some national specificities or cultural curiosities. But to be frank, after watching many Dutch films, my notion of '*oer-Hollands*' (typically Dutch) is hardly more profound than the comic observations made in such popular books you find at newsstands in airports and stations. I hesitate to qualify 'Dutchness', since I simply have no real answer to the question what is identifiably Dutch about such films as AMNESIA (Martin Koolhoven, 2001), BLUEBIRD (Mijke de Jong, 2003), CHARLOTTE (Frans Weisz, 1981), et cetera.

In my previous study *Humour and Irony*, I note that Dutch culture is rooted in a Calvinist tradition of austerity, which is at odds with the exuberance and vivid imagination of Catholicism, exemplified by the cinema of Federico Fellini. Calvinism aims to remove the possible ambiguity of images or text by boiling it down to only one preferably rational meaning. According to Calvinists, one can be pretty accurate about one's intentions with words, but visual representations are by definition too indeterminate. Given the Calvinist distrust of cinema, several Dutch filmmakers like to quote Wim Verstappen's dictum that 'film is a Catholic medium' (Verstraten *Humour and Irony*, 233) to argue that the Netherlands does not really have a cinematic culture. Paradoxically, however, I would suggest that insofar as a certain 'Dutchness' in

Dutch cinema can be articulated at all, this might be discerned in the kinds of (black) humour and irony that satirizes the puritanism of Calvinism. Against that background, I discussed in my previous study such films as DE MANTEL DER LIEFDE (Adriaan Ditvoorst, 1978), DE VIERDE MAN (Paul Verhoeven, 1983), SCHATJES! (Ruud van Hemert, 1984), FLODDER (Dick Maas, 1986), DE WISSELWACHTER (Jos Stelling, 1986), DE NOORDERLINGEN (Alex van Warmerdam, 1992), SIMON (Eddy Terstall, 2004), whose comic and ironic sensibility one also sees in several critically acclaimed satirical television programmes—VAN KOOTEN EN DE BIE (working as a duo from 1974-1998), KREATIEF MET KURK (1993-1994), JISKEFET (1990-2005)—and successful comedians such as Freek de Jonge, Theo Maassen, Hans Teeuwen. Their jokes (sometimes crude) and satirical irony are meant to put prevailing opinions into perspective, aiming to underscore the idea of the Netherlands as a country with a 'live and let live' mentality to oppose the supposed strictness of the Calvinist tradition. It could be wishful thinking on my part, tinged with a degree of nostalgia, but I have the hunch that a certain tendency of self-relativism characterized the Dutch in the second half of the twentieth century in the less politically charged times preceding the murder of filmmaker Theo van Gogh in November 2004. Since then, humour and irony have not lost their impact, but they have too often been misused as a stopgap to legitimize narrow-minded ideas.

There is, however, one particular hypothesis about the Dutch that is at the heart of my entire project. The Dutch are 'not lacking in self-esteem' (White and Boucke, 4), for they have their pride, but this pride is restricted to domains that are outside the scope (and sound) of their language. When it comes to sports (ice skating, hockey, cycling, the national soccer team), the Dutch usually tend to think they are 'naturally' world class. The building of the Delta Works to protect the flat country from the sea is officially acknowledged as one of the greatest civil engineering achievements of the twentieth century. The artists the Netherlands are most famous for date from an era without audio: think of Rembrandt van Rijn, Johannes Vermeer, Vincent van Gogh, and other painters from previous centuries. In current times, the Netherlands has a number of pre-eminent DJs (Martin Garrix, Armin van Buuren, Hardwell, Tiësto), but it is striking that their music evades the discomfort of language—and the same could be said of the architectural projects of Rem Koolhaas, the photography of Anton Corbijn and of Rineke Dijkstra, and the fashion designs by Viktor and Rolf. Moreover, every foreigner who has visited the Netherlands knows that as soon as the Dutch note that you are not a native speaker, they immediately switch to English. For foreigners, it is difficult to 'master' the language, for they rarely get the chance to put the command of Dutch into practice. Or in the words of Colin White and Laurie Boucke in their *The Undutchables*: 'The more you try to learn Dutch, the more the Dutch refuse to speak Dutch to you and the more they complain that you haven't learned it' (193). The Dutch language has easily adopted loanwords, from the English in particular, and in this era of digitization, worldwide communication, and the gradual decline of academic studies taught in Dutch, this development has only accelerated. If you want to make a Dutch person happy, all you have to do is tell that person: 'Your proficiency in English is above average.'

If the Dutch are slightly embarrassed by the acoustics of their language, it should not surprise us that they are indifferent to their cinema. The three times a Dutch picture actually won an Academy Award for Best Foreign Language Film—DE AANSLAG (Fons Rademakers, 1986); ANTONIA (Marleen Gorris, 1995), and KARAKTER (Mike van Diem, 1997)—it caught the Dutch by surprise. The awards were considered chance occurrences rather than indications that the overall quality of Dutch cinema is on a par with that of other small nations in Europe. If Dutch films are that good, critics wondered, how come they have been so rarely selected for the main competitions of prestigious film festivals in the last 40 years? These critics have a point here, and Dutch sceptics have used this poor statistic to wallow in a Calimero complex (based on the Italian cartoon figure with an egghead who is always complaining 'They are big and I am little, but it is an injustice, it is!'). To all the Dutch film lovers who suffer from such an inferiority complex, I offer this book as a cure.

In the introduction to this book, I will address several prejudices against Dutch cinema, but the most seminal one for a start is the idea that Dutch cinema is rooted in realism. According to film director Martin Koolhoven, 'we Dutch are so Calvinist that we can only bear realist acting'. If a scene is too dramatic or too compelling, the Dutch tend to disqualify it as exaggerated, for they live by an adage that promotes sobriety: 'Just act normal, that's already crazy enough.' The assumption that the Dutch prefer films with a likeness to the 'real world' over fancy and/or overtly dramatic stuff is regarded by some filmmakers and critics as an unwanted limitation. In 1999, the so-called Fantasts wrote a manifesto—signed by Dutch directors, screenwriters, directors of photography, editors, and actors—that made a plea for the 'power of imagination', claiming that a fantasy film or a sci-fi thriller can be serious, too. Probably propelled by 'our great documentary tradition', they argued, it has become habitual—and therefore 'so average'—to reproduce reality, but imagination has the advantage that it increases the opportunity to create 'new realities' and to entice 'philosophical problems'. Even when I acknowledge that there is much truth in Koolhoven's claim and in the complaint by the Fantasts, my main rhetorical move is to read against the grain. I will put forward that, on closer examination, many of these films have more imaginative potential than has been attributed to them. In order to disclose this potential, I will use textual analysis as a method in combination with theories of psychoanalysis, owing to the latter's focus on imaginary scenarios. A caveat is in order here, for I employ a 'lite' version of psychoanalysis, meaning that the theory is subservient to the films and will function as a stepping stone to a textual analysis. Ideally, my recourse to psychoanalysis will help to explain why there is reason to derive more pleasure from the selected films than we might have realized so far.

One advantage of reading the films through the prism of psychoanalysis is that it enables me to structure this study according to a method I already tried in *Humour and Irony*: deliberate anachronism can lead to surprising associations. One could try to figure out analogies among Dutch films made in 2016, but I think a picture such as Martin Koolhoven's BRIMSTONE has much more in common with Paul Verhoeven's FLESH + BLOOD (1985) than with any other title in this book, let alone with any other title from 2016, such as Boudewijn Koole's BEYOND SLEEP or Mijke de Jong's LAYLA M., to mention some of the better ones. In a slight variant upon a phrase from the preface of my previous study, I want to state that I am much more interested in detecting affinities between films on the basis of shared preoccupations than in sticking to chronological accounts or in reconstructions of historical contexts.

Additionally, by exploring an imaginative potential, I intend to put the notion of Dutch fiction cinema as such into perspective. Rather than responding to developments in Dutch society, the Film Academy generation of the 1960s (Adriaan Ditvoorst, Nikolai van der Heyde, Frans Weisz, Pim de la Parra) had an eye for cinematic tendencies in France and Italy. The most intriguing directors of later generations also clearly drew on foreign sources of inspiration who either favour fantasy over reality or take an askance look at reality: Alex van Warmerdam was inspired by Luis Buñuel and Roy Andersson (see my previous study); Marleen Gorris by Chantal Akerman and the Taviani brothers; Orlow Seunke by David Lean and Buster Keaton; Nanouk Leopold by Michelangelo Antonioni and Bruno Dumont; Martin Koolhoven by Sergio Leone and John Carpenter; Boudewijn Koole by Gus van Sant and Ingmar Bergman; and Jim Taihuttu by Martin Scorsese and Mathieu Kassovitz.

This quite random list is meant to suggest, first, that Dutch post-war fiction film is too heterogeneous to draw reductive conclusions about national cinema or cultural identity. This study does not amount to an overall argument, and I have decided to order the chapters according to the logic of a database, offering the reader a sampling of case studies. Second, the list of foreign influences also begs the question whether we can speak of 'Dutch cinema' at all. On the one hand, it is a fairly arbitrary term, since I use it in a broad sense. It covers not only homegrown pictures but can also include Flemish-Dutch co-productions, even when the director is Flemish (in the case of Harry Kümel and Hugo Claus); international co-productions (such as the English-spoken films Shock Head Soul and Brimstone); and films that Paul Verhoeven made abroad (such as RoboCop and Elle). On the other hand, as I will address in both the introduction and the epilogue, is it not the best option to read films from a small nation like the Netherlands against the background of an international cinematic context?

The great majority of films discussed here is Dutch-spoken, obviously. This means, as I also mentioned in my previous study, that 'when I use quotation marks to indicate the words of a character, the quotation is not exact. The translation is either provided by me or it comes from the English-language subtitles from the DVD. In situations where characters use English terms, as they do occasionally, I have italicized the quotation or part of the statement.'

This study was made possible with the generous financial support of Het Nederlands Filmfonds, the N.S.C. (Netherlands Society of Cinematography), and LUCAS (Leiden University Centre for the Arts in Society). I am grateful for the confidence they had in this project. Abundant thanks for my proofreaders: Ernst van Alphen, professor of Literary Studies at Leiden University, who has a keen eye, as ever, for the fine-tuning of theory and textual analysis; Yasco Horsman, Assistant Professor of Film and Literary Studies, whose broad interest in culture not only covers cinema, comic books, and cycling races but psychoanalysis as well. Film and media scholar Gertjan Willems alerted me to the remarkable dynamic of Flemish-Dutch co-productions, such as the films made by Hugo Claus, Harry Kümel, and Fons Rademakers' Mira. Ernest Mathijs, a respected cinephilic professor of Film Studies at the University of British Columbia in Vancouver, pointed out some pitfalls which I hope I have been able to avoid (and if not, the mistakes are mine). Rommy Albers and Leo van Hee, both from Eye Filmmusuem, were always helpful in sharing their knowledge of Dutch cinema as well as cinema in general.

If this were a movie, the 'special thanks' in the end credits would include: my mother Lenie, my late father Theo, my brother Marcel, Marjon, Julia, Mika, my sister Sandra, Obinze, River, Hero, my colleagues at Leiden University, the film students in Leiden (special mention of Vincent, Jop, Michel, Constantijn), Maryse, Chantal, Mike, and Gioia. Even though a film lover likes to sit in a darkened auditorium, I would not be able to function without some lights of my life. I restrict myself to mentioning only the three brightest ones: Fatma as well as my daughters Febe and Bodil.

Parts of this book have been previously published as excerpts (sometimes very brief) in these articles:

In chapter two: 'Theatrical Films and Cinematic Novels: De dans van de reiger and L'Année dernière à Marienbad', *Image [&] Narrative* 17, 2 (2016), 61-73.

In chapter nine: 'A French Connection: Paul Verhoeven's ELLE in Tandem with Jean Renoir's THE RULES OF THE GAME', *Senses of Cinema* 81 (2016).

In chapters two and nine: 'Fortunate Sinners: Martin Koolhoven's BRIMSTONE as an "Edam" Western', *Senses of Cinema* 83 (2017).

In the introduction and chapter three: '"My Very Own CITIZEN KANE," Inspired by Godard and Fellini: Frans Weisz's Adaptation of Remco Campert's *Het gangstermeisje*', *Journal of Dutch Literature* 8, 1 (2017), 60-74.

A few paragraphs in chapter seven correspond to passages from 'The Freedom to Make Racial Jokes: Satires on Nationalism and Multicultural Comedies in Dutch Cinema', ed. by James Harvey, *Nationalism in Contemporary Western European Cinema* (Cham, Schwitzerland: Palgrave Macmillan, 2018), 125-143.

NOTES

1 In those books, 'Dutchness' is pinpointed according to the most general assumptions, such as the Dutch have a tendency to be 'moralizing', and are 'bursting with dikes, liberalism, independence, equality and global beliefs' (White and Boucke, 4) or the Dutch 'always ask for a receipt & double-check if everything is correct', for they are 'thrifty' (Geske, 45).

2 The Oscar-winning directors did not prosper after receiving the awards. Rademakers made only one more picture, and he himself did not count it among his best work. Gorris had the opportunity to make some feature films in English, but adaptations such as MRS. DALLOWAY (1997) and THE LUZHIN DEFENCE (2000) did not become as famous as the novels they were based upon, by Virginia Woolf and Vladimir Nabokov respectively. When working on a project in 2015, Gorris suffered from a burnout, and Mike van Diem took over, which resulted in TULIPANI: LIEFDE, EER EN EEN FIETS (2017). Almost 20 years after his Academy Award, this was only Van Diem's second feature since KARAKTER. DE SURPRISE (2015) was his first feature after a time gap of 18 years.

3 Koolhoven said in an interview on the extras of the 3-Disc Special Edition of OORLOGSWINTER: 'Wij zijn zo calvinistisch, dat we qua acteren alleen maar realistisch spel verdragen.'

4 In *Humour and Irony*, I discussed DE MINDER GELUKKIGE TERUGKEER VAN JOSZEF KATÚS NAAR HET LAND VAN REMBRANDT (Wim Verstappen, 1966), which is an early example of a Dutch 'nouvelle vague' film but one that also reacts to contemporary developments in society, best proven by the dominant presence in Amsterdam of the so-called Provos, a pacifist countercultural movement.

BIBLIOGRAPHY

De Fantasten, 'Manifest voor de Verbeelding / Manifesto for the Imagination', https://dht.home.xs4all.nl/fantasten/manifesto.html [Accessed 10 May 2020].

Geske, Colleen, *You Know That You're Dutch When ...* (Amsterdam, Edenfrost VOF, 2017).

Verstraten, Peter, *Humour and Irony in Dutch Post-war Fiction Film* (Amsterdam: Amsterdam University Press, 2016).

White, Colin and Laurie Boucke, *The UnDutchables: An Observation of the Netherlands, Its Culture, and Its Inhabitants*, 8th edition (Lafayette, Colo.: White Boucke Pub., 2017).

Introduction

Verstraten, P., *Dutch Post-War Fiction Film Through a Lens of Psycho-analysis*. Taylor & Francis Group, 2021
DOI 10.5117/9789463725330_INTRO

ABSTRACT

The introduction addresses why the unfortunate history of the war picture ALS TWEE DRUPPELS WATER (Rademakers, 1963) was a bad omen for attempts to establish an 'art cinema' in the late 1960s. Whereas pictures with artistic and international ambitions failed to attract viewers, Dutch cinema began to enjoy increasing popular success at home in the early 1970s largely due to a 'hyper-realistic' depiction of sex scenes. Rather than confirm the assumption that Dutch cinema has a realist orientation, I propose—inspired by the work of Slavoj Žižek—to explore the domain of desire and fantasy. By adopting the perspective of a cinephile, I aim to highlight on what grounds we can learn to reconsider—or even to appreciate—the many underrated Dutch films.

KEYWORDS
Repressed key film – 'failure' of Dutch art cinema in the 1960s – The Imaginary, the Symbolic, the Real – three cameos by Rademakers – cinephilia

When Fons Rademakers decided to adapt *De donkere kamer van Damokles* [*The Darkroom of Damocles*], the critically acclaimed novel by Willem Frederik Hermans published in 1958, for the screen, the signs were favourable. Within the span of only a few years—between 1958 and 1961—Rademakers had directed three little gems, each quite unlike the other,[1] and an adaptation of Hermans' book set in World War II about a mysterious secret agent and his doppelgänger promised to be something else again. In fact, by 1962, when he started preparing the shooting of this film, he was the one-eyed man in the country of the blind who is king in the domain of Dutch fiction feature films, for that other household name, Bert Haanstra, had returned to making documentary films. Haanstra was disappointed that his film DE ZAAK M.P. [THE MANNEKEN PIS CASE] (1960) did not come close to the success of his comic debut fiction film FANFARE (1958). The press had been less positive about DE ZAAK M.P., and it attracted 'only' 746,302 viewers versus the more than 2.6 million for its predecessor.

Initially, Hermans had been very supportive of Rademakers' project, and they agreed that a few changes were required for the screen version, such as a different ending. Moreover, they thought it was a safe bet to alter the title and the name of the protagonist, for Hermans had had a quarrel with his publisher. During a stay in Norway in the summer of 1961, however, Hermans turned his own book into a complete first draft of the screenplay and did not accept any of the critical remarks that Rademakers made. The two exchanged a number of letters and had several arguments by telephone, but the net result was that Hermans wanted to end the collaboration. He insisted on breaking the contract because, according to unsubstantiated rumours, someone else—probably an American—was interested in adapting the book but only on the condition that no other film version was already in pre-production (Bernink, 51).[2]

When Rademakers went on to make his adaptation of *De donkere kamer van Damokles*, which he gave the title ALS TWEE DRUPPELS WATER [LIKE TWO DROPS OF WATER] (1963), Hermans critized it a few months after its premiere in an article for the magazine *Podium*. His main critique was that the film had what he called 'witte paters' [white priests], the term he used to qualify Dutch cinema as amateurish. Hermans felt strongly that all details in a book or film had to be functional and relevant. In Rademakers' previous film HET MES [THE KNIFE] (1961), however, Hermans had observed that there was a white missionary who was talking about Congo in Africa while standing next to a map of Indonesia. Referring to this error, Hermans pointed out some 'white priests' in ALS TWEE DRUPPELS WATER as well. While the book emphasizes the fact that Osewoudt could not grow a beard, which Hermans explains was used as a recurring motif to indicate Osewoudt's lack of manliness, in the film the protagonist mentions his own beardless chin only once,[3] and for no particular reason. On top of that, Hermans noticed some stubbles on the actor's face in a close-up (41).[4] The remark about his beardlessness was isolated and hence non-functional, he concluded, and the close-up illustrated the director's inattention to details.

Apart from Hermans' disdain, the fact that former resistance fighters were angered by ALS TWEE DRUPPELS WATER did put a dent in the film's reception. One of them, Jef Last, wrote letters to journals to complain that the collaborators were represented by prettier girls than the ones in the resistance, and he considered it an insult that the protagonist was ruthlessly shot in the back by the Dutch police (Bernink, 55). At the time the movie came out, hardly any war pictures had been produced in the Netherlands. A few were made in the immediate post-war years,[5] but there was a remarkable hiatus in the 1950s, as Wendy Burke notes (53), until the release of DE OVERVAL [THE SILENT RAID] (Paul Rotha, 1962). Rotha's film had been a well-attended resistance thriller with a clear distinction between good and evil, and Last had expected a similar film.[6] But Rademakers' film was, to quote Burke, 'something of an "art" film, with its modern-looking monochrome cinematography and jazz-influenced soundtrack'. Because of its blurred lines between hero and traitor, ALS TWEE DRUPPELS WATER appeared 'slightly out of place for the time it was made' (87). Although the presentation of moral ambiguity in a war picture was deemed too delicate by the resistance in the early 1960s, most critics were enthusiastic about the film. Moreover, ALS TWEE DRUPPELS WATER attracted 473,162 paying viewers. This is a considerable achievement for a controversial picture, even when the uncontroversial DE OVERVAL which had premiered two months earlier, had more than three times this number (1,474,000 viewers, still number fourteen on the list of best attended Dutch movies of all times).

The selection of ALS TWEE DRUPPELS WATER as the Dutch entry for the competition of the Cannes Film Festival in 1963 was the icing on the cake, and the beer tycoon Freddy Heineken organized a big party in the South of France to celebrate its nomination. Back when Rademakers had been searching for backers of his new production company Cineurope to raise money for the film, Heineken had made him a generous offer. Little did Rademakers know that it would turn out to be a poisoned chalice. Heineken had stipulated that he would guarantee a sufficient budget for the film on the condition that Rademakers cancelled the other donors. Rademakers complied, for believed he had a true patron of culture on his side. After the screening at the Cannes Film Festival, the foreign press was most generous, so Rademakers seemed to have more than consolidated his reputation, despite the negative comments by Hermans and Last. To his disappointment, however, when Rademakers then asked Heineken to finance another film, the latter replied that he makes much more money with beer (Bernink, 56).

Their one-time collaboration took a turn for the worse when Heineken, who held the rights to ALS TWEE DRUPPELS WATER, soon thereafter obstructed any further screening of the film except for rare and special events.[7] An official reason was not given, but a persistent rumour has it that Heineken took revenge for the fact that his mistress Nan Los, who played the female lead, had ended their affair. When Dutch television wanted to broadcast the film in 1983, Heineken refused permission because, as his lawyer wrote, he feared that people would make video copies of it. When the Nederlandse Filmdagen—an annual festival established in 1981 to celebrate Dutch cinema—organized a retrospective of Dutch war pictures in 1984, Heineken's answer was 'no' yet again. Moreover, his lawyer wrote a letter to the Filmmuseum, the Dutch film archive and museum, demanding that it hand over the one existing copy of the film. Rademakers started an arbitration case to acquire the rights to the film himself, but the Bioscoopbond (the Dutch association of movie theatres, producers and distributors) postponed a judgement time and again. The story making the rounds was that the Bioscoopbond feared that a decision on the case would push up prices for beer (Bernink, 58). When Heineken died in 2002, his family lifted the ban, allowing ALS TWEE DRUPPELS WATER to be seen again almost 40 years after its release. It soon appeared on DVD, first as part of a Rademakers box, and then also in the 'Quality Film Collection'. Moreover, it was one of only five post-war narrative fiction features selected for the official Dutch film canon (in 2007).

This thumbnail sketch of these disputes is presented here for two reasons. First, the critiques by both Hermans and Last were in fact improper arguments that only indirectly relate to the quality of Rademakers' film. Hermans' comments were unduly hair-splitting and were probably made out of a certain degree of annoyance: it could be because his screenplay had been criticized or because he had wanted to make a different deal. Jef Last was irritated by the ambiguity of the film: he had wanted a heroic depiction of the resistance and a clear condemnation of those who sympathized with the German cause. Second, and what was more damaging, the film was withheld from view due to Heineken's caprices for about four decades, and thus only a contemporary audience had been able to appreciate ALS TWEE DRUPPELS WATER for the admirable achievement it was. One such enthusiast was Adriaan Ditvoorst, who sent Rademakers a friendly note to congratulate him on a magnificent film. Young film students like Ditvoorst were particularly impressed by the film's exquisite cinematography. The black-and-white film was shot in Francscope widescreen format, which Rademakers had seen in LOLA (Jacques Demy, 1961) and in JULES ET JIM (François Truffaut, 1962). Thanks to his friend Truffaut, Rademakers was able to hire the director of photography of these films, Raoul Coutard, who had also shot some Jean-Luc Godard pictures—À BOUT DE SOUFFLE [BREATHLESS] (1960), UNE FEMME EST UNE FEMME [A WOMAN IS A WOMAN] (1961), VIVRE SA VIE [MY LIFE TO LIVE] (1962). Since he had worked with Godard, Coutard was acquainted with improvised shooting conditions. In addition to the superb lighting, his camerawork brought a great dynamism to the usually fairly static approach in Rademakers' previous films, which had often relied heavily on the acting performances.

Ditvoorst wrote in his letter: 'GREAT FONS! ... a Dutchman who walks the high road ... at last'.[8] In the same vein, I will entertain the claim that ALS TWEE DRUPPELS WATER is the repressed key film of Dutch cinema. By 'repressed', I am not merely referring to the fact that the film had been hidden from sight for such a long time. As Sigmund Freud argued, one of the main characteristics of the repressed is that it always returns, albeit in a different guise. With hindsight, as Lili Rademakers remarks in an episode of the television programme *Andere tijden* broadcast on 3 November 2012, we can say that the enigmatic ban was also to the benefit of the film's reputation, for ALS TWEE DRUPPELS WATER is still talked about because of its curious history. But it is also talked about because a ban is usually instituted against films that are provocative, morally repellent, and/or aesthetically poor, but in this case the prohibition was targeted against 'perhaps the best Dutch film from the previous century' according to the narrator of *Andere tijden*.[9] And indeed, precisely because one is aware of the many years of neglect, one is inclined to eulogize the film. But there is a more serious point to be made, for as I will try to suggest, ALS TWEE DRUPPELS WATER initiated a tendency in Dutch cinema that was only too short-lived. In retrospect, one can say that the repression of Rademakers' war picture was a bad omen for cautious attempts to establish an 'art cinema' in the Netherlands in the second half of the 1960s. And this failed attempt, I hope to explain in this introduction, was to have its repercussions for both the development and the perception of Dutch fiction films.[10]

THE UNREALIZED POTENTIAL OF DUTCH 'ART' CINEMA

The idea that cinema could be artistic was firmly embedded in countries like Italy and above all France, but it was rather alien in the 1960s to a Dutch audience in terms of fiction features. For viewers in the Netherlands, cinema was first and foremost entertainment, confirmed by the all-time box-office records for THE SOUND OF MUSIC (Robert Wise, 1965) and IRMA LA DOUCE (Billy Wilder, 1963), respectively number one and number two with 3.99 million and 3.62 million cinemagoers. Dutch audiences were used to the idea that avant-garde and experimental films were artistic, as this had been enthusiastically acclaimed by De Nederlandsche Filmliga whose ideas had been influential for a much longer period than the actual lifespan of this collective of filmmakers and cinephiles (1927-1933). In the Netherlands, documentaries were traditionally linked to visual art rather than cinema, and this connection ensured that documentaries were held in high critical esteem (Hofstede, 75). Herman van der Horst, Joris Ivens, and Johan van der Keuken built themselves a more than respectable reputation, whereas the documentaries that Haanstra made in the mid-sixties, such as ALLEMAN [EVERYMAN] (1964) and DE STEM VAN HET WATER [THE VOICE OF THE WATER] (1966), were immensely popular.[11] These titles confirmed Haanstra's reputation as the filmmaker laureate (Schoots *Bert Haanstra*, 150).

Dutch drama, Rademakers himself realized, was best regarded as an oxymoron. When he had requested Jan Blokker to write an essay on the occasion of the release of his fifth feature film DE DANS VAN DE REIGER [THE DANCE OF THE HERON] (1966), Blokker commented with gusto that the Dutch landscape is so 'undramatically flat' that it should not surprise us that 'no great conflict can arise from such flatness'. The Dutch may fear God, but they consider themselves 'sober, tolerant, cautious and confident—and these features do not quickly trigger conflicts' (Blokker, qtd. in Bernink, 142, my translation).[12] Since the Dutch are more inclined towards 'observation than towards exploration' (ibid.), there is a tendency to favour a documentary school of 'wheat waving in the wind' over a depiction of human tragedies, Rademakers noted.[13] He wondered how it was possible to create drama with a language that is 'sharp and empty', for the 'monotonous' Dutch pales in comparison to the 'masculine Swedish', the 'wonderful French', the 'fast and fluent Italian', and the 'tough American' languages (qtd. in Bernink, 142, my translation).[14]

It is no coincidence that Rademakers liked to cooperate with the Flemish writer-poet Hugo Claus, who had written the screenplays of five of his first seven features (out of a total of 11).[15] Claus used the Dutch-Flemish language in an unconventional and rhythmic fashion. As an experimental poet, he was interested in the acoustic quality of language. The partnership between Claus and Rademakers that started with the latter's debut feature DORP AAN DE RIVIER [VILLAGE BY THE RIVER] (1958) foreshadows what I described in my earlier book (referring to Hans Schoots' study *Van Fanfare to Spetters*) as the key tendency of Dutch cinema in the 1960s: the rebellious stance taken by some Dutch filmmakers in this decade is in fact a belated aping of the mentality of an artistic avant-garde from the 1950s (Verstraten *Humour and Irony*, 262). A cross-fertilization between this avant-garde and cinema started in the early 1960s with documentaries on the Cobra painter Karel Appel (by Jan Vrijman) and on the Vijftiger poet-painter Lucebert (by Johan van der Keuken) who were both, like Claus, interested in primitive painting styles and associative linguistic expressions. In the aftermath of the release of ALS TWEE DRUPPELS WATER with its superb cinematography, Dutch fiction film underwent an unprecedented sea change in the second half of the 1960s.

Ditvoorst received accolades from Godard and Bernardo Bertolucci at international film festivals for his *nouvelle vague*-inspired short film IK KOM WAT LATER NAAR MADRA [THAT WAY TO MADRA] (1965). The soundtrack, celebrated by Godard, contains few spoken words but mostly asynchronous background noise and even total silence. Ditvoorst's first feature was the bleak but aesthetically pleasing PARANOIA (1967) based upon a story by the same Hermans who had written *De donkere kamer van Damokles*. In the playful short film AAH … TAMARA (1965), made by former film student Pim de la Parra who later teamed up with Wim Verstappen for some fifteen years, there were cameo appearances by three generations of directors: Joris Ivens (b. 1898), Rademakers (b. 1920), and Frans Weisz (b. 1938). Weisz, who was the very first student at the Nederlandse Filmacademie (the Dutch Film Academy) when it was founded in 1958, continued his studies in Rome at the Centro Sperimentale di Cinematografia, and his graduation silent comic short, PING PONG E POI (1962) was clearly a tribute to Agnès Varda's CLÉO, DE 5 À 7 [CLÉO FROM 5 TO 7] (1962). He then made, as part of an Italian omnibus film,[16] the 30-minute-long HELDEN IN EEN SCHOMMELSTOEL [HEROES IN A ROCKING CHAIR] (1963), which can best be described as 'JOHNNY GUITAR (Nicholas Ray, 1954) in Rome' and was an unwitting prelude to the spaghetti western craze that was to dominate Italian cinema for some ten years after the release of PER UN PUGNO DI DOLLARI [A FISTFUL OF DOLLARS] (Sergio Leone, 1964).

Back in the Netherlands, Weisz made the short commissioned film EEN ZONDAG OP HET EILAND VAN DE GRANDE JATTE [A SUNDAY ON THE ISLAND OF THE GRANDE JATTE] for a special occasion: the so-called Boekenbal [Book Ball] on 13 May 1965. It has a playful tone and rhythmic editing, and it is littered with a variety of highbrow references. An establishing shot in the beginning is an imitation of the painting *Un dimanche après-midi à l'Île de la Grande Jatte* (1886) by French post-Impressionist Georges Seurat: it shows shiny, happy people in a park, until heavy rain makes them take shelter in a castle. In the film, writers clad in black are passive onlookers who see how the people in the castle misuse books as material objects: books are used for some sort of hopscotch, jumping from one to the other, or as a wedge to keep a sash window open; children even throw books at each other for fun in a reference to a slow-motion pillow fight in ZÉRO DE CONDUITE [ZERO FOR CONDUCT] (Jean Vigo, 1933). There is a transition to the writers in a library, where they start to write feverishly on typewriters. The sound of their typing changes into a melody, and as the rhythm increases, the editing accelerates, showing us pictures of a great number of writers. In some subsequent scenes, we see how people are reading books in the most unlikely of situations, such as a window cleaner on a stepladder and a woman jumping from a diving board. Towards the end of EEN ZONDAG OP HET EILAND VAN DE GRANDE JATTE, there is a return to the very same set-up of Seurat's painting.

In a longer analysis of this 20-minute short (Verstraten, 'My Very Own', 62-64), I have pointed out the playful irony of this film, which has neither voice-over nor dialogues even though it is about writers and had writers as its primary audience. The only way the authors can make contact with the readers is not by starting a conversation with them but simply through the melodic sounds of their typewriters. The actual content of their texts seems irrelevant; they are only capable of mesmerizing people through the rhythmic but apparently meaningless playing of typewriter keys. Most important to my aim here is that Weisz's short is the best example of how filmmakers were starting to explore the connections between cinema and an artistic undercurrent in art and literature, underscored by the cameo appearances of a great number of prominent Dutch authors in the vanguard such as Gerard van 't Reve, Cees Nooteboom, Ed Hoornik, Adriaan Morriën, Jan Cremer, Belcampo, and Remco Campert.

Weisz's next film project, his ambitious debut feature HET GANGSTERMEISJE [ILLUSION IS A GANGSTER GIRL] (1966), is an even better case of the cross-fertilization between cinema and literature. Campert had written the screenplay for HELDEN IN EEN SCHOMMELSTOEL, and Weisz wanted to adapt Campert's 1961 novel *Het leven is vurrukkulluk* [*Life is Wonderful*].[17] The production was aborted, but then Weisz read the first fourteen pages of an as yet unfinished manuscript by Campert, intrigued by the title *Het gangstermeisje*. They decided to embark on a dialogic co-creation, which meant that they held a number of meetings to discuss the characters and the narrative developments. Weisz already started shooting his adaptation of the still incomplete book, while Campert worked on both the novel and the scenario. Since dialogues were often not perfectly lip-synched in Italian cinema, Weisz did not bother to do so in his Dutch film either. The film first had to be dubbed in Dutch anyway, since two of his main actors—Paolo Graziosi and Gian Maria Volontè—were Italian and did not speak the language. Second, Campert kept on sending new lines during filming, even of scenes that had already been shot, so lip synchronicity was an illusion anyway.

In my article on Weisz's debut feature, I have pointed out that HET GANG-

STERMEISJE has parallels with both Godard's LE MÉPRIS [CONTEMPT] (1963) and Federico Fellini's OTTO E MEZZO [8½] (1963) in terms of narrative, for all three films are about the problems in writing a screenplay. Stylistically, the film comes close to Godard's À BOUT DE SOUFFLE with its frontally staged shots, brief inserts, unorthodox framing, relatively fast zooms, out-of-focus shots, and swish pans. Godard had tried to transgress cinematic rules in 1960, and Weisz had aimed to do this with his grandiose ambitious undertaking in 1966. Initially, HET GANGSTERMEISJE did well at the box office, but after six fairly successful weeks in Amsterdam, the movie theatres were practically empty. Weisz concluded from this decline in movie attendance that while a considerable number of cinephiles had come to see the film, there had been no word-of-mouth advertising for his film. This kind of 'art cinema' was apparently doomed to fall flat in a country with an as yet immature fiction film tradition.

Like Weisz, Rademakers made a feature film in 1966 in the Dutch language, with an international orientation. For Weisz, Godard and Fellini had been key references, whereas for Rademakers' new film the work of French director Alain Resnais was a prominent source of inspiration.[18] Based upon a 1962 theatre play by Claus, Rademakers' adaptation DE DANS VAN DE REIGER bears comparison to Resnais's L'ANNÉE DERNIÈRE À MARIENBAD [LAST YEAR IN MARIENBAD] (1961): there are suspicions of female adultery; the acting is quite inexpressive; the continuity of space is unexpectedly disrupted, creating jarring jump cuts; the present can be suddenly interrupted with scenes from a past, but we are never sure whether this past is hallucinated. To underscore this indebtedness to L'ANNÉE DERNIÈRE À MARIENBAD, Rademakers hired Sacha Vierny, who had been the director of photography on four films by Resnais.

It would have made sense for Rademakers to cast the original actors from De Nederlandse Comedie—a prominent theatre company between 1950 and 1971. Apart from the fact that Ellen Vogel and Paul Cammermans had performed Claus's play on stage, Rademakers had already worked with these two actors for his third movie HET MES.[19] Instead, Rademakers recruited three main actors with significant reputations among cinephiles: Jean Desailly had already starred in Jean-Pierre Melville's LE DOULOS [THE FINGER MAN] (1962) and in Truffaut's LA PEAU DOUCE [THE SOFT SKIN] (1964); Gunnel Lindblom in a few Ingmar Bergman films; and Van Doude in Billy Wilder's LOVE IN THE AFTERNOON (1957) and Eric Rohmer's LE SIGNE DU LION [SIGN OF THE LION] (1962) in addition to having a brief part in À BOUT DE SOUFFLE.[20] Art cinema was particularly versatile in the 1960s, given the critical acclaim for films by Bergman, Godard, Truffaut, Fellini, Varda, Luis Buñuel, and others. And with his 'mimicry' of Resnais's film, one of the quintessential titles of European art cinema, Rademakers was apparently betting on an international breakthrough. The stars seemed to be properly aligned for him, since DE DANS VAN DE REIGER was selected for competition in the Cannes Film Festival 1966. According to the existing regulations, the film could count as a Dutch submission only if the film's dialogue was spoken in Dutch. Since his own company was co-producing the film, Rademakers spent considerable money to have the voices of his three main actors dubbed in Dutch, and he himself spoke Jean Desailly's lines. While a screening of the film at Cannes was being prepared, festival director Robert Favre le Bret blocked its showing, arguing that the largely French public would not accept Desailly speaking not in his native tongue but in a peculiar language that sounded like he had a throat ailment (Bernink, 75).

If the quite successful ALS TWEE DRUPPELS WATER had seemed to announce the advent of 'Dutch quality film' or rather 'Dutch art cinema', then its sudden disappearance from the public arena was symptomatic of the fate of the films that followed in its aftermath. A film like DE DANS VAN DE REIGER was too austere and cerebral to attract more than a handful of Dutch cinephiles. At the same time, the lack of airplay at Cannes obviously crippled Rademakers' hopes of achieving international recognition with this picture. 1966 and 1967 were perhaps the golden years of 'Dutch art cinema' that saw the release of not only the aforementioned titles (PARANOIA; HET GANGSTERMEISJE; DE DANS VAN DE REIGER) but also Nikolai van der Heyde's enjoyable EEN OCHTEND VAN ZES WEKEN [A MORNING OF SIX WEEKS] (1966), which had a similar plot as a French film that had been released a few months later, Claude Lelouch's UN HOMME ET UNE FEMME [A MAN AND A WOMAN]. In both films, a racing driver embarks on a romantic liaison with a woman. Chapter three discusses several resemblances between the two films, but there is a crucial difference to be noted here as well: whereas the French picture was thrust into the limelight when it won a Golden Palm at Cannes and an Academy Award for Best Foreign Language Picture, the Dutch version remained under the radar.

Films like HET GANGSTERMEISJE, EEN OCHTEND VAN ZES WEKEN, PARANOIA, the playful low-budget DE MINDER GELUKKIGE TERUGKEER VAN JOSZEF KATÚS NAAR HET LAND VAN REMBRANDT [THE NOT SO FORTUNATE RETURN OF JOSZEF KATÚS TO THE COUNTRY OF REMBRANDT] (Wim Verstappen, 1966),[21] and the equally *nouvelle vague*-inspired LIEFDESBEKENTENISSEN [CONFESSIONS OF LOVING COUPLES] (Verstappen, 1967) were not flawless, but they were nonetheless highly interesting first or second attempts at feature filmmaking. While the audience of Dutch lovers for art cinema was quite small, acknowledgement abroad for Dutch films was quite problematic, for the bar of quality had been lifted to unprecedented heights. In his study *Screening Modernism*, András Bálint Kovács dedicated an entire chapter to the year 1966 because he considers it the most memorable year in European art cinema, as illustrated by the release of three phenomenal feature films: ANDREI RUBLEV by Andrei Tarkovski, PERSONA by Ingmar Bergman, and BLOW-UP by Michelangelo Antonioni. Given that art cinema had reached its peak in quality in 1966, it was no surprise that the Dutch features failed to raise sufficient interest abroad. Praise from foreign critics seemed to be a prerequisite for visibility in one's own country, as the case of the Flemish surrealist film DE MAN DIE ZIJN HAAR KORT LIET KNIPPEN [THE MAN WHO HAD HIS HAIR CUT SHORT] (1965), the debut feature by André Delvaux, had shown. It received a lukewarm response in Belgium at its original release, but thanks to appreciative reviews from mainly French critics, it was rereleased in 1967 in Belgium and grew into a preeminent Flemish art film classic (Mosley, 79). None of the Dutch art films in the second half of the 1960s, despite their international orientation, had the luck of receiving a step up in the form of such a positive reception abroad that would have convinced a national public to embrace it as one of 'their' fine pictures.

THE GARGLING SOUNDS OF DUTCH

In the preface to this book, I mentioned that the Dutch feel uncomfortable about their national cinema because they have a slight aversion to the language they speak. To recall the words of Rademakers: Dutch is 'empty' and 'monotonous'. To foreigners, it sounds as if the Dutch are gargling all the time. Some of the 'art' films from the 1960s, especially the shorter ones, have few spoken words if any: take for example IK KOM WAT LATER NAAR MADRA; PING PONG E POI; EEN ZONDAG OP HET EILAND VAN DE GRANDE JATTE; or the astonishing 20-minute short BIG CITY BLUES (Charles Huguenot van der Linden, 1962).[22] Some films were shot in English such as the voice-over texts in René Daalder's magnificent short BODY AND SOUL (1967) or the dialogue in OBSESSIONS (1969), De la Parra's debut feature as director. Some films use a mixture of languages, as in EEN OCHTEND VAN ZES WEKEN, or a protagonist will speak Dutch with a thick German accent, almost to comic effect, as in DE BLANKE SLAVIN [THE WHITE SLAVE] (René Daalder, 1969). One of the very few Dutch 'art films' in the early 1970s is George Sluizer's debut fiction feature JOÃO EN HET MES [JOÃO AND THE KNIFE] (1972), and it is spoken entirely in Portuguese, shot in Brazil with Brazilian actors and a largely Dutch crew. Its poor box-office showing in Holland contrasted with the fact that it was the Brazilian submission for the Academy Awards. If the unfortunate invisibility of ALS TWEE DRUPPELS WATER was a foreshadowing of the fact that no true film culture would blossom in the Netherlands, then the poor box-office results in Holland for the amazing JOÃO EN HET MES proved the point.

Most striking, however, is the nonchalance that comes with the practice of dubbing: DE DANS VAN DE REIGER was in Dutch because the rules and regulations of Cannes required it to be. In HET GANGSTERMEISJE, the apparent indifference to the matter of lip synchronization makes it seem as though the film could have been screened in any language. It was as though the director had said, 'If the public wants a version in French or one in Italian, let's give it to them.' All these titles, which I have categorized for the sake of convenience under the umbrella term of 'Dutch art cinema', treat spoken Dutch as if it is a necessary evil. It is strictly hypothetical, but this attitude of insouciance towards the Dutch language could be born from the fact that the words in Dutch films, among others in ALS TWEE DRUPPELS WATER, voiced by non-experienced film actors (Lex Schoorel and Nan Los) in the main roles, are sort of a tin-eared tune. To film viewers of today, accustomed as they are to hyper-modern audio design, the dialogues and the dubbing sound tinny. That can also have its charm, especially when the idea is that it is meant to be that way. But ALS TWEE DRUPPELS WATER is not such a film because it does not aim to violate the conventions of psychological realism. Maybe Rademakers had his own film in mind when in 1966 he compared the Dutch language unfavourably to Swedish, Italian, and English. The fact is that for MIRA (1971), the film he made after the disappointing experience that DE DANS VAN DE REIGER turned out to be, the dialogue written by Claus was couched in an invented dialect. Hence, the stylized language contrasted with the presumed naturalism of the small rural community depicted in MIRA.

By 1971, the year MIRA was released, most of the fiction feature directors from the 1960s began to change course, since their films had resonated more poorly than they had expected. In the early 1970s, they sacrificed their artistic ambitions for 'national cinema' as a model. According to Bart Hofstede in his study *Nederlandse cinema wereldwijd*, this category of 'national cinema' includes humorous pictures and genre films, which proved to be a profitable strategy, as I indicated in my previous study on humour and irony in which many of these popular films were examined. In this period, Dutch filmmakers introduced the profitability of sex as a theme, implying that protagonists could benefit from a licentious lifestyle. Moreover, the sexual display in Dutch films was also profitable in another respect, for it resulted in astonishing box-office results.

The downside of the enormous commercial successes at home was that these films were conspicuously absent at international film festivals, as Hofstede notes.[23] Thanks to its sexually tantalising trailer, Rademakers' MIRA attracted large audiences in the Netherlands (and Belgium). It was the same with Verstappen and the erotic display in BLUE MOVIE (1971), Weisz with the crime action in DE INBREKER [THE BURGLAR] (1972), and Van der Heyde with the humour and sexual innuendo in HELP! DE DOKTER VERZUIPT [HELP! THE DOCTOR IS DROWNING] (1974). And the shift in focus from the international to the national market not only implied that the promise of Dutch art cinema was squandered in the early 1970s;[24] it also meant that the language was no longer considered an obstacle or a nuisance, since these films were only meant for the Dutch. Hence Dutch expressions were used bluntly, including profanities being shouted out, with 'godverdomme' [Goddamn it] as a favourite curse word.[25]

This national orientation went hand in hand with the advent of a 'sex wave' in Dutch cinema, which was a blessing in the 1970s from a commercial perspective but which became quite a burden thereafter from a more artistic angle, for Dutch cinema became too often associated with nude actors. This shift from blessing to burden, I will claim, had to do with a changed context for sexual display in cinema. In the 1970s, sex scenes were embedded in an often playful atmosphere of tolerance and liberation, mindful of the hippie slogan 'make love, not war'. From the more cynical decade of the 1980s onwards, however, sex was increasingly deployed in a context of manipulation and cunning strategies.

SEX SELLS, TO SOME EXTENT

The films Paul Verhoeven made in the early 1970s are helpful in understanding the dominant approach towards the representation of sex as liberating and proudly provocative. His debut feature WAT ZIEN IK!? (1971) helped to create the image of the 'happy hooker'. Greet's male clients are pathetic types, and all of them are weird in comparison to the 'normal' Greet, our point of identification throughout the film. She joyfully participates in the sorts of theatre play that the odd whoremongers have invented for her, except when the man who wants her to walk and chuck like a chicken transgresses a limit for her. 'Business is business', according to one of the English titles in use for the film, but a comic tone towards sex prevails.

Verhoeven's TURKS FRUIT (1973) became a landmark film about an *amour fou*. Inspired by Jan Wolkers' eponymous novel, TURKS FRUIT depicts the impassionate liaison between the bohemian artist Erik and the red-haired Olga. In an episodic sequence at the beginning of the film, we see that Erik has some quick sexual adventures with several anonymous girls. These first ten minutes may give the impression that TURKS FRUIT is a licentious picture, but this obfuscates the fact that these flings do not satisfy Erik. He suffers from such lovesickness that he can only enjoy sex with Olga, the one woman who had left him and had soon thereafter contracted an incurable disease, as a lengthy flashback will reveal. The merit of TURKS FRUIT resides in its ability to keep a balance between ever-changing moods: it was free-spirited and funny, romantic and macabre. This 'porn-chic' production exceeded all box-office expectations and became the all-time number one in the Netherlands with over 3.3 million viewers. The frank depiction of sex is obviously a provocative gesture, for in this period preceding the popular soft eroticism of the EMMANUELLE films, sex was associated with liberal and open minds rather than with commercialism, and the notorious case of BLUE MOVIE, two years earlier, clearly undergirds this argument. With its sex-addicted housewives who help a former jailbird to reintegrate into society, the film was initiated by the director—Wim Verstappen—as a challenge to the film censorship board in the Netherlands. It was thanks to Verstappen's enthusiastic reply to the board's critique that an uncut version of the film was released in theatres.[26]

Verhoeven's next film KEETJE TIPPEL [KATIE TIPPEL] (1975) offers a slightly bleaker depiction of sex, even though the film ends with a favourable prospect for the title heroine, much like Mira in Rademakers' film. By seducing the engineer Maurice Rondeau, Mira can turn her back on the small community of Waterhoek, although she considers him only a 'dopey kind of a lover'. Keetje Tippel is a young, working-class woman whose first sexual experience is disconcerting: she loses her virginity when her employer rapes her. Initially naïve, she comes to realize, encouraged by her mother, that prostitution can be an escape from hunger and misery. It was better to use the laws of capitalism—sell your body as a scarce commodity—and rise above poverty. While her first client—a cameo by Fons Rademakers (!)—thinks she is an amateur, another client named George picks her up from the street but pays her to be a model. Thanks to her good looks, she climbs up the social ladder and finds herself among the upper echelon of society. George and two of his friends take her to dinner, and while André obviously fancies her, she starts an affair with Hugo. She distances herself from her family, but the banker Hugo also lives according to the laws of capitalism: when he has the opportunity to marry a woman from an affluent background, Keetje leaves him. 'Money turns people into bastards', she concludes. She joins a socialist demonstration where she meets André again. When the police intervene, André gets injured and she sees to it that he is brought home. His mother dismissively remarks that her son has taken her out of the gutter, but her meeting with the filthy rich André means she can finally enjoy the '*heady delights of high society*', as the final text before the end credits tells us.[27]

The main reason why Verhoeven's SPETTERS, released in 1980, had such a hostile reception from both the press and a group called the Nederlandse Anti Spetters Aktie (NASA, the Dutch anti-Spetters movement) consisting of feminists and homosexuals is that the film's detractors were not prepared for a cynical depiction of sex.[28] The film was such an affront to them, I would suggest, because SPETTERS presents sex scenes that are joylessly at odds with any notion of 'free love'. Whereas the sex in the 1970s still had an odour of progressive rebellion, this aura was increasingly shattered in SPETTERS and in many Dutch films thereafter. One could argue that some of the most annoying pictures in Dutch cinema are those post-1980 titles that ignored this shift and seemed to aspire to become a new TURKS FRUIT (without coming close, I might add). To name just a few, BRANDENDE LIEFDE [BURNING LOVE] (Ate de Jong, 1983); DE GULLE MINNAAR [THE GENEROUS LOVER] (Mady Saks, 1990); and ZOMERHITTE [SUMMER HEAT] (Monique van de Ven, 2008) all rightfully received a poor reception. Reinout Oerlemans's KOMT EEN VROUW BIJ DE DOKTER [STRICKEN] (2009) was an exception in terms of box-office results with its 1.1 million viewers, but the way the sex has been embedded has given the sceptics of Dutch cinema an opportunity to make their case.

The advertising executive Stijn van Diepen introduces himself in KOMT EEN VROUW BIJ DE DOKTER as a 'major-league hedonist'. He marries the 'most beautiful woman in the Western hemisphere', he says in one of his many voice-overs, but this Carmen has to 'tolerate his cheating as a bad habit'. When she gets cancer, he accompanies her on her hospital visits, but he also goes out to meet other women, as crosscutting scenes in discos and nightclubs show us. He starts a serious affair with the visual artist Roos, 'my surrogate queen', who gives Stijn a renewed 'lust for life'. When Carmen is cured from her disease, he promises to be faithful, but when her recovery is only temporary, he breaks the promise, for 'love has its own rules in times of cancer'. The combination of sex and decay that worked so well in TURKS FRUIT is here presented as an annoying split: whereas his wife is deadly sick, he has sex with his mistress to whom he is 'even more addicted' than in their previous period together. Since he has to divide his time between two women—or actually three, for Stijn is also the father of a young daughter—he complains: 'My diary suffered from inhuman time management.' Sex functions here as an escape from sorrow, and he gets seriously hooked to Roos; in TURKS FRUIT, sex is an outlet for Erik's lovesickness, and it reminds him that there is no one like Olga. Verhoeven's film can be regarded as an ode to love, which makes it all the more ironic that the subtitle EEN ODE AAN DE LIEFDE (an ode to love) was added to the film title KOMT EEN VROUW BIJ DE DOKTER whereas, as some critics have noted, 'an ode to adultery' would have been more fitting. Oerlemans' film only deserves its actual subtitle on the basis of the last twenty-five minutes when Stijn ultimately returns to Carmen's deathbed. But once she is dead, he phones Roos to invite her to the funeral. In contrast to the rebellious potential of the representation of sex in the early 1970s, sex and nudity have been gradually turned into a commodity or, as in KOMT EEN VROUW BIJ DE DOKTER, a hedonistic practice. Its suggestion that sleeping around has the odour of freedom and independence is one thing, but the all too decent style of the film makes it worse. Either Oerlemans' film should have been shot in a deliberately sleazy style to indicate its objection to the protagonist's behaviour, or it should have exaggerated its slickness to the point of ridicule of Stijn's adultery. But instead, KOMT EEN VROUW BIJ DE DOKTER is just a 'slick' movie in both content and form, having missed the opportunity to give a provocative edge to the display of sex.

Unlike KOMT EEN VROUW BIJ DE DOKTER, THE PARADISE SUITE (Joost van Ginkel, 2015) acknowledges that its modern-day characters practice sex in times of cynicism. The two films are opposites not only in terms of their attitude towards sex but also in terms of their box-office success. Van Ginkel's arthouse film received only about one per cent of the 1.1 million viewers for Oerlemans' movie. Moreover, KOMT EEN VROUW BIJ DE DOKTER won a number of Rembrandt Awards, which are awarded on the basis of public votes, and one Golden Calf for main actor Barry Atsma; THE PARADISE SUITE won three Golden Calves, including a well-deserved one for Best Picture, and was the Dutch entry for the Academy Awards. THE PARADISE SUITE is a so-called mosaic film, depicting six immigrant residents in Amsterdam whose jarring lives intersect, sometimes only for a fleeting moment. Seka, a woman from former Yugoslavia, is keen on exacting revenge on Ivica who has committed war crimes against her relatives. Ivica has started a family in Holland and is proud of his baby Mateja. He has built himself a fortune in the red light district: he asks women from abroad to come over for a visit to do a photo shoot, but once in Amsterdam, they are brutally raped by his minions and forced to prostitute themselves. A key character is the young Jenya from Bulgaria who, like her two girlfriends, does not want to participate in Ivica's scheme but has no choice but to do so. She turns out to be very popular among whoremongers, so Ivica proposes that she do a show in a night club: Ivica promises her that she will have sex with only one guy a day, in front of paying customers. During her first show, this man is the African Yaya. He is new in the business, for he is in such desperate need of money that he accepts the job, though it embarrasses him greatly. Earlier we are shown how Yaya sends a young girl away who offered him sexual favours. Moreover, he is trying, unselfishly, to help a black family with young kids to pay their rent arrears .

Yaya's ultimate act of altruism will be fatal to him. When Jenya is forced to please a customer in the so-called Paradise Suite, she objects, pointing out that Ivica is breaking his promise. But eventually she gives in, fearing that further resistance would cost her dearly. This customer is the sixth of the immigrant protagonists in the film, the famous Swedish conductor Stig Lindh, whose face is on a huge banner next to Mozart's. His encounter with Jenya is a gift given out of gratitude after Stig's orchestra had given a magnificent performance. Stig leaves after only three minutes, however, because he receives news that his son Lukas is not at home. Lukas is being bullied at school, and while his mother is on a concert tour in Japan, his father has been harsh on him. The boy cannot take it anymore and is drifting around Amsterdam on his mountain bike. This builds up to the film's most memorable scene, for Seka has stolen baby Mateja in one of Ivica's off-guard moments. She wants to abandon the baby by stowing him in a baby car seat behind bin bags near a canal at night. At that moment, Lukas passes by and stops his bike. There is an intense exchange of looks between the boy and Seka. Whatever it is that she reads in Lukas' eyes—his unhappiness, his helplessness—it prompts her to take Mateja with her and to make sure the baby is reunited with his parents after all. Meanwhile, Ivica presumes that Jenya is to blame for Stig's instant departure from the Paradise Suite, and he orders Milijan, one of his minions, to make her pay. Then, out of nowhere, Yaya intervenes and hits Milijan to the ground. He steals a huge amount of money Milijan was carrying with him and also takes his car. Through this act, Yaya is able to pay the black family's debts. After Jenya has recovered, he encourages her to drive back with the pimp's car to her mother in Bulgaria. But Milijan tracks down Yaya, and instead of betraying Jenya's whereabouts, the African man only says in French: 'Father, forgive him.' He is shot instantly.

The Paradise Suite is such a sombre picture because it identifies sex exclusively with exploitation and violence, both of a physical and mental nature. When Yaya asks Jenya how she feels, the only thing that comes to her mind is 'dirty'. And from Yaya's body language, we can conclude that he feels humiliated as well, which is possibly the main reason he helps her out. In Van Ginkel's mosaic film, sex is no fun and it only offers gain to those who force others to practice it. When journalist Henk Bovekerk went to see this 'cocktail of misery and woe',[29] he noted that viewers were complaining after the screening about the choice they had made, for the nasty scenes had spoilt their evening. It was no surprise that there was no word of mouth on this film, which explains the limited attendance for this award-winning picture.

Here we arrive at what I would hypothesize is the ambiguous split regarding the persistent prejudices of Dutch cinema. Watching scenes of sexual excitement and nudity in a context of humour and/or liberation usually produces mixed feelings: it is easy to be attracted by such scenes, but it is more problematic to admit that they give one visual pleasure. The way out of this slight embarrassment caused by the enjoyment is to sneer at the display of sex and nudity: the typical reaction is to laugh furtively while calling it 'functional'. The problem with the representation of graphic sex in a film is that it threatens to derail the story. Inserting a steaming love scene of only a few minutes in Out of Africa (Sidney Pollack, 1985), Slavoj Žižek has postulated, would bring the entire romantic drama out of balance (*Looking Awry*, 111). The sentimental or lyrical tone of a film can only be guaranteed by turning sex into a narrative ellipsis, but Dutch films have too often violated this. The prejudice is that it is used for sensational purposes and not on narrative grounds. At the risk of superfluity, this means that those critical viewers who categorize the sexual display 'functional' do so ironically.[30] The resulting bias is only perpetuated when films such as KOMT EEN VROUW BIJ DE DOKTER – with its cleanly cut camerawork, nothing gritty about it – become box-office successes. And in case a Dutch film such as THE PARADISE SUITE undermines the prejudice from within by linking sex with unpleasant subjects – trafficking in women, humiliation, rape – it brings together the words 'Dutch' and 'art film', and this combination, albeit critically acclaimed, seems a misnomer in the public eye.

In an interview with Gerhard Busch for cinema.nl, Martin Koolhoven argued that the Netherlands does not really have a 'true film culture' and never has. A self-declared aficionado of genre cinema, Koolhoven regrets that Dutch cinema has always been ruled by 'realism as a guiding principle', and it is always a risk for a filmmaker in the Netherlands to deviate from this principle.[31] Koolhoven appreciates films such as ANGEL HEART (Alan Parker, 1987) and MILLER'S CROSSING (Joel Coen, 1990) tremendously, but if their dialogues were translated to Dutch, he argues, many viewers would unjustly consider them ludicrous because they are too unrealistic. With this tradition in the back of his mind, Mike van Diem made KARAKTER [CHARACTER] in 1997 (discussed in chapter two) as a deliberately theatrical film in which the characters speak a very formal and archaic Dutch. The film is, so to speak, 'Catholic' rather than 'Calvinist', and especially Victor Löw's over-the-top performance as the lawyer De Gankelaar is much appreciated by Koolhoven as an 'un-Dutch' exception to the rule of 'realism'.

Throughout his career, Rademakers also regularly complained that the Dutch have a fear of coming across as affected and anti-naturalistic (Bernink, 42). A Dutch actor is required to perform his role as naturally as possible to avoid the charge of theatricality. Rademakers himself was fond of stylized dialogues, but to his dismay, many Dutch are uncomfortable when introduced to a different reality than they are acquainted with (see Bernink, 42). This suggests that Dutch film viewers prefer to see on screen what they know from daily life. In fact, popular films such as BLUE MOVIE and TURKS FRUIT could be called hyper-realistic: their frank depiction of sexual acts was much more 'true to nature' than American box-office hits with their vague hints of sensuality.

To stress his point of 'realistic' and 'un-cinematic' tendencies in the Netherlands, Koolhoven mentions that the only tradition that can be found in Dutch cinema is not one of the classical genres such as horror, science fiction, or action thriller but instead an atypical category: World War II films.[32]

Since these war pictures are usually embedded in 'realist' narrative dramas, this underscores Koolhoven's argument that a preference for lifelikeness is prioritized over cinematic considerations.

Even though Dutch cinema is not entirely steeped in exaggerated adherence to realism, I would agree with Koolhoven that Dutch cinema may in general be more oriented towards realism in comparison to other national cinemas. That being said, this book tries to answer the question whether Dutch cinema is perhaps not more imaginative than our initial assumptions imply. To examine this question, I take psychoanalysis as an approach, for it offers a set of theories related to the unconscious and desire, to fantasy and imagination. Even though desire and fantasy can be well-embedded in a realist depiction of diegetic worlds, I hope that my angle de-emphasizes any concerns about realism.

SCENES FROM A MARRIAGE: PSYCHOANALYSIS AND CINEMA

Neither Sigmund Freud nor Jacques Lacan were known as film aficionados, but both psychiatrists' work has been employed for many a film analysis. In the 1970s in particular, when film scholars were going to great lengths to legitimize film as an object of academic study, psychoanalysis was a source of inspiration for Jean-Louis Baudry and his apparatus theory, for Laura Mulvey and her concept of the male gaze, for Christian Metz and his 'imaginary signifier', for Raymond Bellour and his writings on 'symbolic blockage' (including more than 100 pages on one film alone—Hitchcock's NORTH BY NORTHWEST). The idea was to use theoretical tools to expose gender inequalities, Oedipal scenarios, and/or ideological mechanisms. The most serious backlash against this approach, which suspicious minds pejoratively termed 'theoretical excess', was perhaps the volume *Post-Theory* (1996), edited by David Bordwell and Noël Carroll, which made a claim for empirical and cognitive research instead.

However, as Žižek has argued, once the theory of the unconscious is 'invented', it cannot be negated anymore, despite post-theoretical efforts to discard it in the false hope of a magical return to some kind of naiveté before Freud's insights (*The Fright*, 14). Ever since the late 1980s, with the publication of his *The Sublime Object of Ideology*, Žižek has consistently attempted to claim the relevance of Lacan's thinking for mass culture in general and cinema in particular. The attraction of Žižek's output rests in his relentless efforts to explain difficult theory via well-known examples (Alfred Hitchcock, film noir, the ALIEN franchise). If there is no popular example at hand to support the theoretical ideas, we can only come to the conclusion that these ideas happen to be built upon quicksand. Moreover, as Žižek adds in brackets, if his book *Looking Awry* now and then mentions 'great' names like Shakespeare and Kafka, 'the reader need not be uneasy: they are read strictly as kitsch authors' on the same level as Stephen King or Patricia Highsmith (vii). Over the years, psychoanalysis has run the risk of becoming marginalized both in and outside of film studies, but thanks to a prominent scholar like Žižek, one can say—in a nod to his fascination with horror—that the 'living dead' has returned after all.

Even though I pay tribute to Žižek's illuminating approach, the reader must understand that there is a slight difference that separates us. His main concern, especially in his early studies, was to acquaint the reader with Lacan—who is interpreted through the philosophical tradition of German idealism—by using film examples as illustration for theory, for cinema, as Žižek asserts frequently, 'teaches us how to desire'. To be honest, I have to say to his credit that several of his film analyses are so subtle and smart that 'illustration' is too modest a term for his accurate eyes and sharp-witted comments. Further, over the years his interests have extended into various fields that can be subsumed under his ambition to be a guide to ideology in an attempt to reload Marxism. This does not, however, alter the fact that, originally, one of his major goals was to introduce Lacan through popular culture by using cinema (or literature or opera) as a means to explicate psychoanalytic concepts. My approach slightly diverges from Žižek, for I will be reading Dutch films through the prism of psychoanalytic concepts to shed a light on a great number of the very best titles in Dutch cinema.

In *Looking Awry*, Žižek points to specific motifs, such as the 'empty place' or the 'maternal superego', in a series of films by Hitchcock in order to argue that they illustrate the Lacanian triad of the Imaginary, the Symbolic, and the Real. In the Imaginary, a child lives in a symbiosis with the mother and derives a sense of identity from seeing itself in the mirror. It may think, 'That's me', but that would be incorrect, for the mirror is only an external image. Deceptive appearances are at stake in Hitchcock's VERTIGO (1958) because the main protagonist, Scottie, is obsessed with Madeleine who turns out to be a false creation, designed to take the place of a dead woman. In the Symbolic, signifiers and names determine a subject's place in a social circuit. In NORTH BY NORTHWEST (1959), Roger O. Thornhill desperately searches for the secret agent 'Kaplan' only to find out that he is a decoy, for the name is no more than an 'empty signifier' to lead the Russians astray. The Real concerns that which resists symbolization and refers to a realm beyond that is 'evidence of a psychotic state' (Žižek, 99). In his mad moments, Norman Bates in PSYCHO (1960) identifies with his already dead mother, and in taking her place, he dresses in his mother's clothes and acts on behalf of her.

As regards the 'maternal superego', Žižek notes that the male protagonists in the three successive films NORTH BY NORTHWEST, PSYCHO, and THE BIRDS

(1963) are fatherless, and the mothers are so possessive that there is hardly any room for a woman in these men's lives. The mother in NORTH BY NORTHWEST is constantly mocking her 40-something son Roger. When he is running away from the men whom he has called his kidnappers, his mother shouts after him: '*Roger, will you be home for dinner?*' to the delight of the crowd. With a mother like that, whom Roger sees on a regular basis, it is no wonder that he has been divorced twice, since he is still 'mama's boy' who has never developed a proper distance from his own scornful mother (the Imaginary). Norman attacks Marion in PSYCHO as a result of his identification with his dead mother whom he imagines would be torn apart by jealousy: he keeps on hearing her commanding voice in his head and acts according to 'her' instructions (the Symbolic). The seagulls in THE BIRDS fill the vacuum left by the father's absence and terrorize Melanie on behalf of a mother who wants to block any interest a woman might have in her son of nubile age (Žižek *Looking Awry*, 99). The most logical answer to the question 'Why do the birds attack?' is that they materialize to prevent Melanie from 'snatching' the son away from his mother (the Real).[33] I refer to this Hitchcockian triad because I cannot resist the hypothesis that the three highly remarkable minor roles that Rademakers played in feature films between 1968 and 1971, following upon the financial disaster of his film DE DANS VAN DE REIGER, conform to the triad of the Imaginary, the Symbolic, and the Real, albeit in reverse chronology.

THE IMAGINARY, THE SYMBOLIC, THE REAL: THREE CAMEOS BY FONS RADEMAKERS

Rademakers' most noteworthy cameo is unequivocally his role as the mother in the Belgian-French-Italian-German-American co-production LES LÈVRES ROUGES [DAUGHTERS OF DARKNESS] (Harry Kümel, 1971), advertised as a stylish adult vampire movie.[34] Despite the fact that he is only in one scene that lasts no more than two-and-a-half minutes, the performance, exactly halfway into the film, is memorable. Due to a delay by train, a newly-wed couple misses the boat to England. In a series of close-ups and two-shots, they discuss their options: Valerie considers the 3 o'clock boat a good idea, but Stefan wants to spend the night in a hotel in Ostend. It turns out that they have been married only a couple of hours ago in secret, but Stefan's mother, who has a 'heart condition' does not know about it yet. Valerie insists that her husband inform his mother. She is already aware that the lady will not approve of her type of girl, but she adds: '*She can't be that aristocratic.*' Stefan laughs and says: '*For years she has been telling me: Stefan, we are different, that's God's gift to us. We must never debase it.*' If Stefan then denies that he is '*ashamed*' of his wife, as Valerie supposes, she asks him about his mother: '*You're not afraid of her, are you?*' He keeps silent, and after scrutinizing his face, Valerie says: '*Stefan, you are afraid!*' '*Me afraid?*' he replies calmly. '*When we arrive in Ostend, I will phone her.*'

After checking in, Valerie encourages Stefan to ask the hotel porter to call his mother in England. Unnoticed by his wife, Stefan gives him some money and a small letter, which reads: '*Say there is no reply.*' It is clear that Stefan is trying to find reasons to postpone any contact with his mother, and the arrival of an enigmatic Hungarian countess and her female secretary is much to his advantage. The porter tells them that the ravishing countess still looks exactly the same as she did 40 years ago. Stefan comes under her spell once he realizes that drinking human blood is the elixir of her youth. Valerie is deeply worried by Stefan's strange attraction to this Countess Bathory.

Because his wife does not tire of asking Stefan to contact his mother, there is finally a telephone call after a brief dissolve in which the audience sees an entirely red screen. The butler of the manor picks up the phone and brings it to a sort of greenhouse where the mother is having her breakfast. The butler says: '*It's master Stefan*' and kneels down. We do not see the mother, only a hand that touches the butler's balding head. When we see her after some time, the mother turns out to be a decadent figure with a whitened face. Speaking with his characteristic bass voice at a slow pace, Rademakers/mother asks whether Stefan has not been doing foolish things. When Stefan has difficulty expressing himself, the mother immediately guesses: '*You did do foolish things.*' When he says he cannot explain, Valerie grabs him and he pushes her away, whereupon the mother guesses correctly: '*You are not alone. There is someone with you.*' Stefan's reply is inaudible, for we still see mother in close-up and then, in an apparent repeat of what Stefan says, mother says the name '*Valerie*'. Stefan then tells that they were married three days ago in Switzerland, and when we see mother again, she keeps silent for a while and then replies: '*What a nice surprise.*' But then she continues to say that this was not foolish but merely '*unrealistic*'. What shall we do with that '*poor, little uh, Valerie*', she wonders. '*The day she hears about us, I hate to think of that.*' After she has disqualified her son's action as an '*ungrateful thing*', we see a purple orchid in close-up as mother says: '*I can't wait for you to see our newest laeliocattleya Valencia* (she smells the flower which she is now holding in her hand). *And by the way, Stefan, be sure to tell the young woman that mother sends regards.*'

Watching Rademakers in this small part, which he plays 'with visible pleasure' (103), as Ernest Mathijs observes, it is obvious why Stefan hesitated to contact his mother. She still treats him as 'mama's boy', and he has not sufficiently liberated himself from her influence. For that reason, he could only marry Valerie in utmost secrecy, for his domineering mother would have prevented him from doing such a '*foolish thing*'.

Elements of a suffocating mother-son relationship are not only condensed in the interaction between the mother and Stefan in LES LÈVRES ROUGES—the mockery, the hostile attitude towards the blonde Valerie—but are also exaggerated. *'The day she hears about us, I hate to think of that'* has an undeniable ring of a perverse relationship between mother and son, and this possible perversion is even reinforced by the image of a male actor playing the mother. His clothing, gestures, and red lips may recall femininity, but the character is recognizably male given his voice, the absence of a wig, and his facial features. If the paternal function in the Hitchcock films is suspended, as Žižek mentions, here we have a mother with fatherly characteristics, which puts further emphasis on her/his possessive qualities over the son. Moreover, for a Flemish director like Kümel, twenty years younger than Rademakers, the Dutch filmmaker could indeed be regarded as a representative of 'Daddy's cinema', in a positive sense of the term.

The suggestion of extravagance was also stylistically underscored. As Mathijs explains, it was a deliberate strategy on Kümel's part to disrupt the clear split in Belgian cinema between state-funded artistic/auteurist films and non-subsidized commercial pulp. In the 1960s, Kümel had a reputation of belonging to a cultural elite, and his output until then had earned him the honorary label of 'auteur'. He had made some promising shorts, one of them based on a play by Franz Kafka; and he also wrote for film magazines and made television portraits of people such as John Huston, Roman Polanski and Vincente Minnelli for the public broadcast service in Belgium. Due to the troubled reception of his first feature-length production, MONSIEUR HAWARDEN (1968), however, Kümel was so angered that he decided to do 'something nasty' (quoted in Mathijs, 100). He did not apply for state support, for his second feature had to become 'undignified trash' (quoted in Mathijs, 101). In terms of genre, LES LÈVRES ROUGES is a lesbian vampire film and thus a so-called exploitation picture, but at the same time, Kümel's movie is littered with highbrow references. Apart from the mother played by Rademakers, the role of the countess was performed by none other than Delphine Seyrig, who had starred as the female protagonist in L'ANNÉE DERNIÈRE À MARIENBAD. According to Mathijs, the surreal settings and the superb cinematography by Eduard van der Enden—who had been director of photography of four films by Rademakers[35]—turned the shots into 'postcards of paintings, inviting not only evident comparisons with René Magritte and Paul Delvaux, but also with James Ensor and Léon Spilliaert, both resident artists in Ostend' (Mathijs, 103). Thus, LES LÈVRES ROUGES was remarkable for radically cutting through the categories of lowbrow and highbrow.

Rademakers' DE DANS VAN DE REIGER and Kümel's LES LÈVRES ROUGES can be regarded as two sides of the same coin: the first was a mild parody of psychoanalysis couched in the format of an art film (see chapter two); the second incorporated highbrow references into the format of an exploitation genre, exploring the combination of sexual desire and gruesome violence. The first was a box-office failure, but the second was quite a commercial success, also internationally. And the fact that LES LÈVRES ROUGES was considered 'too raunchy to be art, too chic to be exploitation' ultimately assured its status as an 'underground cult hit' (Mathijs, 104).

Nowadays, De la Parra's OBSESSIONS can be regarded as the Dutch equivalent of LES LÈVRES ROUGES. This 'artsploitation' has become one of the Dutch 'cult epics', to quote from the label of the DVD/Blu-ray release of this film in 2017. Rademakers had a cameo in the film as the rich and biggest '*skirt-chaser*' Raoul Orlov who near the end of the film organizes a fancy party in Bloemendaal. The two protagonists, the doctoral student of medicine Nils Janssen and his girlfriend, the journalist Marina, come to the party, for they got a call that the model Stella Olsen would be attending. For days, Marina had been trying to contact this old girlfriend of hers, for she is investigating the death of the American soldier Joseph Petrucci. Marina knows that Stella used to date a guy by that name, but that was before Stella became hooked to drugs and served six months in prison. At the party, Marina learns that Raoul keeps Stella in hiding, and, as it turns out, he does so to protect her: Petrucci had made it look like he was the dead soldier, but since Stella knew that Petrucci was actually the man's killer, she was now being pursued by Petrucci. Marina also finds out Petrucci's address: he is the mysterious man living next door to Nils. She calls a colleague to alarm the police and she goes back with Nils to his apartment.

The couple does not know, however, that while they were away, Petrucci has discovered the small hole in the wall, which was caused when a painting that was too heavy—a reproduction of a Van Gogh—had fallen from the wall in Nils' room. From the very beginning of the film, Nils had been secretly spying on the 'strange' activities of his neighbour whose name he did not know then: there are always attractive women around and the neighbour regularly makes love to them, shown to us via peephole shots. Marina is irritated by Nils '*playing peeping Tom all day*'. Nils is amazed that the girls at his neighbour's place are often sound asleep, and he occasionally enters the room with a false key when Petrucci is absent. Twice he finds a drugged woman tied to the bathtub. Moreover, he lifts another drugged woman from the bed and when she regains consciousness, she goes away without saying a word. Nils follows her into her house and they start kissing, still not exchanging a word. He meets her again at the party at Raoul's place, where they kiss once more and remain silent. After her conversation with Stella, Marina returns with Nils to his apartment. And as the proverb goes, curiosity kills the cat: Nils is about to close the hole in the wall, but he decides to peep through it one last time. At that very moment, Petrucci fires his gun and kills the protagonist. Petrucci runs away, but outside the police arrest him.

When De la Parra was preparing to make OBSESSIONS, he received some support from unexpected sources. Kümel had taken Truffaut in 1967 to Amsterdam to see the Dutch film LIEFDESBEKENTENISSEN, directed by Verstappen and produced by De la Parra. Truffaut wrote three pages of critical notes, but he was sufficiently impressed to help De la Parra and Verstappen (known as Pim & Wim), who had their own production company Scorpio Films since 1965. Thanks to Truffaut, they became acquainted with Bernard Herrmann who had made a great number of musical scores, including for some key films by Hitchcock. Herrmann gave De la Parra permission to work with an unused score, and thus OBSESSIONS had an immediately recognisable 'Hitchcock sound'. The role of Marina was performed by French-Canadian actress Alexandra Stewart, who had played in LE FEU FOLLET [THE FIRE WITHIN] (Louis Malle, 1963), MICKEY ONE (Arthur Penn, 1965), and in Truffaut's LA MARIÉE ÉTAIT EN NOIR [THE BRIDE WORE BLACK] (1968). With hindsight, the film's biggest claim to fame was that a young Martin Scorsese had worked on the script. De la Parra had met him after the two of them had each presented a short film at the Knokke Experimental Film Festival in Belgium. Since De la Parra's command of English was not that good, Scorsese was prepared to help him with the scenario for his feature film.

The fact that the story of OBSESSIONS was explicitly inspired by Hitchcock's REAR WINDOW (1954) was impossible to miss, but there are many more references to American movies, in particular to films by the master of suspense. For example, Nils visits a shop that is reminiscent of Pop Leibel's bookshop in VERTIGO; Nils sees a stuffed owl in there, which could have been part of Norman's collection in PSYCHO. There is a narratively redundant scene in which Marina takes a shower and Nils makes her scream by approaching her from behind—not to kill her as Norman did, dressed as mother, but for fun. Moreover, the peeping hole in OBSESSIONS is a copy of the hole covered by the reproduction of a Willem van Mieris painting in the Bates motel from PSYCHO. Frequently, Nils puts on a cowboy hat, a gift from his mother, and says ironically that it makes him look like '*John Wayne*'. Finally, the credits mention that OBSESSIONS is '*dedicated to and in memory of Republic Pictures*', the studio of many B-movies that had ended its activities in 1959 after producing such films as THE QUIET MAN (John Ford, 1952) featuring John Wayne and the western JOHNNY GUITAR (Nicholas Ray, 1954). De la Parra called his film a 'sex psycho suspense murder mystery', and the sheer number of terms he uses to describe his feature already indicates that he is more interested in showing off his influences than presenting an original angle. Because of the nudity in the film, OBSESSIONS can be called a sensational variant of a suspense thriller, with the male protagonist posing as a tougher guy than the typical male lead in a Hitchcock film. In the end, the Dutch-German co-production OBSESSIONS did relatively well in the Netherlands (184,000 viewers), but it was a much bigger success in Germany. Moreover, it was distributed to about 65 countries, so it did not go unnoticed.

Whereas LES LÈVRES ROUGES put its emphasis on an imaginary level with a 'mother' who wants to keep her boy under her wings, OBSESSIONS is embedded in a symbolic circuit. Lacan explains that the close bond between mother and child is disrupted by the intrusion of language upon the subject: once we learn to speak, our name pins down our position in a social network. We are dictated by signifiers: 'who we are' is determined by calling ourselves by our name. Recall that in OBSESSIONS, Marina is investigating what has happened to the dead 'Petrucci', but then she learns that the name of the victim is not right. The victim was an anonymous blackmailer, whereas the neighbour-with-no-name turns out to be Petrucci.

Moreover, as the symbolic order is built upon lack-in-being, desire is set in motion; and OBSESSIONS makes it adamantly clear that desire is triggered by obsessive looking. Halfway through De la Parra's movie, we suddenly see a sequence of brief shots, presented in disarray. After the fast sequence ends, we see Nils, eyes closed, on his bed, so the brusqueness of the series is apparently the result of a dream. We recognize a great many shots from the first half, and most striking is the big close-up of Nils's right eye, peeping at the spectacle in the room of his neighbour. Nils is irresistibly drawn to this hole because the presence of naked women is on the one hand an enigma to him but on the other hand offers him visual pleasure. His desire also induces anxiety, but this anxiety also fuels his desire. His fear of what might happen is also included in the series of brief shots. Most poignant is the frontally staged shot, shown twice, of the gun the neighbour holds very close to the camera, pointed right at Nils himself and the spectator.

While the hole was caused by the Van Gogh reproduction having fallen from the wall, this painting was, significantly, a gift to Nils by his mother. Hence, one can say that the mother in De la Parra's film inadvertently introduces the son to the domain of sexual desire, to the annoyance of his steady girlfriend. This is in striking contrast to LES LÈVRES ROUGES, for 'Rademakers as mother' in Kümel's film had tried to usurp the place of her son's desire, leaving no room for competitors. But the son's attempt to escape the mother's influence had made him stay in the hotel in Ostend, with lethal consequences.

In comparison to his cameos in the films by Kümel and De la Parra, Rademakers had a much more substantial role as the bulky Kraut Willy in the darkly humorous black-and-white picture DE VIJANDEN [THE ENEMIES] (Hugo Claus,

1968). During World War II, Richard, an eighteen-year-old guy from Antwerp, is drifting around in snow-frost Belgium when he meets the American GI Mike who is searching for his squad. When they shoot a German truck driver, they chase down the victim's co-driver, but instead of killing him, this Willy becomes their travelling companion.[36] The German soldier is not a brute but a sad and forlorn man. At one point, the American and the Belgian tie Willy to a tree with a rope, for he is slowing their pace. Many hours later they release him from his unfortunate position, but Willy suffers from cold feet, no matter how much the American and the Belgian encourage him to keep on walking. We follow them on their survival trip in the frosty landscape until at the end of Claus's debut feature, this unlikely bunch of comrades become enmeshed in a firefight and they are all killed by the American troops they had been searching for all the time.

Visually, DE VIJANDEN is a schizophrenic movie. Claus had wanted to convey the grim banality and the arbitrariness of life and death in times of war, and 16mm images would have been good enough for that purpose. However, the director of photography, Herman Wuyts, insisted on shooting on 35mm film so he could create 'poetic' shots. In the end, in Claus's opinion the beauty of the cinematography clashed with the sloppy aesthetics of newsreel journalism that he originally had in mind (Willems 'Hugo Claus', 80). Especially due to its morbid ending, DE VIJANDEN is closest to the level of the Real: according to the rules of war, the three are supposed to act as enemies, but in the lawless landscape in which hierarchies and authorities are sidelined, pragmatics reign over any rule. No organization is as hierarchically structured as the army, but the one scene with a general in DE VIJANDEN is a hilarious one. He arrives in a jeep, gives both Richard and Mike a Cuban cigar and poses with them for a photograph before moving on. This general behaves like a clown rather than a commander-in-chief.

Since death lurks around the corner or behind every tree, the three protagonists have created an inconceivable friendship that lasts till death strikes them after all. Claus's film seems to depict a universe with orphaned souls in which symbolically articulated desires have given way to basic instincts and random violence. Moreover, the film stands out for its mismatch of languages. Richard meets a group of soldiers in German uniforms, and because he is hungry he asks them in German whether they have food. They reply in Ukrainian and then force him to run. The characters predominantly speak English, French, and German, whereas the Flemish in this Belgian-Dutch co-production is restricted to a silly children's song and terms of abuse. The most tragic-comic scene is Richard's death. He walks towards two American soldiers and says that he is their buddy, for he is an American. The one then asks him: '*What's the capital of Nevada?*' The other joins in: '*Who's the girl-*

friend of Popeye?' In desperation, Richard replies: *'I am not a German. Okay? Okay?'* whereupon a third soldier shoots him instantly. This final scene illustrates once again that the chaotic universe depicted in DE VIJANDEN is rooted in a confusion of tongues, as if language is short-circuited.

As Žižek did with Hitchcock films, I have chosen a series of three films in which Rademakers played a minor role to examine whether they complied with Lacan's triad of the Imaginary, the Symbolic, and the Real. For Žižek, Hitchcock functions as a director who has unwittingly put Lacan's theory in practice. An early volume in English edited by Žižek happened to be called *Everything You Always Wanted to Know about Lacan (But Were Afraid to Ask Hitchcock)*. This could sound like a pretentious title if one failed to see the punning reference to Woody Allen's hilarious comedy EVERYTHING YOU ALWAYS WANTED TO KNOW ABOUT SEX * BUT WERE AFRAID TO ASK (1972). Along the same lines, one can read this current book as 'Everything You Always Wanted to Know about Imaginative Dutch Post-war Films (But Were Afraid to Ask Psychoanalysis)'.

CINEPHILIA TIES THE BOOK TOGETHER

The careful reader may already have noted that most of the interesting Dutch titles mentioned so far draw influences from international cinema: DE DANS VAN DE REIGER and Resnais; HET GANGSTERMEISJE and Fellini; PING PONG E POI and Varda; EEN OCHTEND VAN ZES WEKEN and Lelouch; JOSZEF KATÚS and Godard; OBSESSIONS and Hitchcock; HELDEN IN EEN SCHOMMELSTOEL and Ray. In addition, JOÃO EN HET MES bears strong resemblances to the German film AGUIRRE, DER ZORN GOTTES [AGUIRRE, WRATH OF GOD] (Werner Herzog, 1971), also thanks to its setting in the Brazilian jungle (AGUIRRE was shot in the Peruvian jungle). In short, the more ambitious films gain their contours in relation to a huge variety of examples from international (art) cinema, and even Haanstra's FANFARE—popular in Holland but not abroad—was greatly indebted to the humour of the British Ealing Studios.[37] Favouring documentaries in the 1960s, Haanstra only returned to fiction features when the French director Jacques Tati, whom Haanstra greatly admired ever since he had seen LES VACANCES DE MR. HULOT [MR. HULOT'S HOLIDAY] (1953), suggested that they co-direct a movie. The collaboration did not really work out as expected, and Haanstra's contribution to Tati's TRAFIC [TRAFFIC] (1971) was reduced to a line in the credits—'with the participation of'. But my point here is that if even this director—considered 'more Dutch' than any other Dutch filmmaker—has such an international orientation, can we then properly speak of a 'Dutch cinema' at all in terms of characteristics and conventions? If there is not really a common denominator in Dutch film history, however—already illustrated by Koolhoven's claim that World War II films were the only significant genre in the Netherlands—then it is futile to attempt to determine a certain 'Dutchness' in cinema, implying that 'Dutchness' is an impure concept that is already tainted with an international flavour.[38]

This international orientation means that, in general, the context of national cinema will not be an overriding concern in this book and that, as already indicated in *Humour and Irony* (18-19), I will use elastic criteria for regarding a film as 'Dutch'. Thus this study can potentially include discussions of international films if they are directed by a Dutchman (such as Verhoeven's ROBOCOP and ELLE) and international co-productions (especially Dutch-Belgian collaborations, such as MIRA and DE VIJANDEN).[39] Apart from the cameo appearance by Rademakers, the only substantial 'Dutch' contribution to LES LÈVRES ROUGES was the cinematography by Eduard van der Enden. Following the example of the Nederlands Film Festival,[40] which applies flexible criteria to decide whether a film can be a contender for best 'Dutch' achievements—including several films by Welshman Peter Greenaway or Argentinean Alejandro Agresti—my criteria are at least as flexible.

Given the sheer diversity, I opt for the fairly loose structure of a database rather than trying to write a coherent narrative of developments. Each chapter revolves around a psychoanalytic concept—such as the mirror (stage), father figures, desire, paranoia, (historical) trauma, aphanisis, and perversion—and the selected films are categorized according to the relevance of one of these concepts. Why are DE DANS VAN DE REIGER (1966), KARAKTER (1997), and GLUCKAUF (2015)—apparently so unlike each other—analysed in chapter two? All three titles address the difficult relationship a son/man has to his father. This means that the order of the films is determined by association. On the one hand, this choice is born out of pragmatism, making explicit that it is hardly expedient to write a history of Dutch film, whether chronological or alternative. On the other hand, this method of association illustrates that this study is written by someone who likes to profile himself as a cinephile, even preferring this self-declared title over his professional identity as a scholar.

A cinephile can love big and critically acclaimed pictures, but his particular fondness also concerns those film titles that have been floating beneath the radar of canonical lists.[41] A cinephile will seriously defend underestimated movies, category B or C even against all odds, talking about them as unduly underrated gems. In a cinephile's eyes, such films can reveal privileged moments that are beyond scripting and explanation.[42] A film lover can find pleasure in obscure details or an uneven narrative structure and can hold a fascination for supporting actors rather than the stars (as a cinephile might say: 'When I talk about Brad, I mean Brad Dourif rather than Brad Pitt').[43]

Cinephilia is ruled by a certain atemporality: a gangster picture from the early 1960s—say, KERMIS IN DE REGEN [FAIR IN THE RAIN] (Kees Brusse, 1962)—can be compared to a B gangster film from the mid-1980s—for example, MOORD IN EXTASE (Hans Scheepmaker, 1984) or WILDSCHUT (Bobby Eerhart, 1985). The films are juxtaposed indiscriminately, as if their quality is a matter of fact, to ensure that the love for them will not extinguish. For the cinephile, cinema has an 'undead nature', as Thomas Elsaesser has suggested (197). The memory of a cinephile works analogous to Freud's notion of the unconscious, which consists of an endless and achronological reservoir of impressions. Psychoanalysis does not stick to a calendar-based temporality; on the contrary, the concept of *Nachträglichkeit* was introduced to indicate that an event is not experienced directly, but its impact can only be understood belatedly if it can be understood at all. Bearing the notion of retroactive temporality in mind, the unconscious is indifferent to historical logic and causality. The choice for 'deliberate anachronism' as a structuring principle for this study has to be understood against this background.

A cinephile usually does not appreciate a film for its realism. Whether something is historically accurate or could have possibly happened is not something a cinephile cares about. One of the reasons for a cinephile's fondness for genres is that they have their own conventions, regardless of the probability of situations. A cinephile tends to value a filmmaker's dedicated effort more than polished perfection: a film's flaws can also be part of its charm. And when we are watching a movie from some decades ago, the process of aging provides a 'necessary detachment', to quote Susan Sontag, from the outmoded film, but for the cinephile, it can also arouse 'a necessary sympathy' ('Notes', 285). What initially seemed a run-of-the-mill picture can, with the passage of time, become a special delight. On this condition, there is sufficient ground for a retroactive 'celebration' of Dutch fiction films, as I hope this study will illustrate. Cinephilia, then, functions as an antidote to the perspective of the scornful sceptics. Cinephilia enables us to 'look awry' at Dutch fiction features and invites us to consider their limitations as well as their sometimes charming failures from a benevolent attitude.

Some years ago, I started examining Dutch fiction features for the simple reason that these films are 'orphans' in an academic context. Apart from a study by Peter Cowie from the late 1970s, a volume edited by Ernest Mathijs in 2004 that included analyses of twelve Dutch films, and a few other books, mainly monographs on single filmmakers, there have been precious few studies exclusively focused on Dutch films. My research on Dutch cinema was meant to enter uncharted territory. This may read like I was sacrificing myself: if no one is doing it, I will do the job of sitting through these many hours of Dutch films. But the more I saw of them, the more they became an unexpected joy.

In my previous study, I already mentioned the tendency of Dutch film lovers to view a fine Dutch picture as an unexpected oddity. Their reaction goes like this: I am not generally a fan of Dutch cinema, but I would make an exception for this particular film. One of the aims in this book is to prove that a great number of exceptions add up to a norm. Needless to say, ALS TWEE DRUPPELS WATER is one of these early exceptions, and I became greatly enamoured by the 'art' films of the 1960s, which followed in the wake of Rademakers' war film that I earlier labelled as the repressed key film of Dutch cinema. The unfortunate fate of these films made me dedicate a book to them, and several directors have taken up the 1960s legacy to some degree—from Orlow Seunke to Alex van Warmerdam, from Marleen Gorris to Mijke de Jong, from Nanouk Leopold to David Verbeek, and from Jim Taihuttu to Michiel ten Horn.[44] I was not always immediately impressed by many of the titles I investigated, but in the process of taking a closer look which was required for writing of this book, several films started to grow on me. I was spellbound by overtly ambitious or idiosyncratic if not madcap enterprises such as the aforementioned BIG CITY BLUES, HET GANGSTERMEISJE, EEN OCHTEND VAN ZES WEKEN, DE DANS VAN DE REIGER, PARANOIA, and JOÃO EN HET MES but also ANGELA – LOVE COMES QUIETLY (Nikolai van der Heyde, 1973), MAX HAVELAAR (Fons Rademakers, 1976), SOLDAAT VAN ORANJE [SOLDIER OF ORANGE] (Paul Verhoeven, 1977), MYSTERIES (Paul de Lussanet, 1978), RIGOR MORTIS (Dick Maas, 1981),[45] VAN DE KOELE MEREN DES DOODS [HEDWIG: THE QUIET LAKES] (Nouchka van Brakel, 1982), DE SCHORPIOEN [THE SCORPION] (Ben Verbong, 1984), KRACHT [VIGOUR] (Frouke Fokkema, 1990), DE JOHNSONS (Rudolf van den Berg, 1992), DE VLIEGENDE HOLLANDER [THE FLYING DUTCHMAN] (Jos Stelling, 1995), VAN GOD LOS [GODFORSAKEN] (Pieter Kuijpers, 2003), the short WERELD VAN STILSTAND [STILL WORLD] (Elbert van Strien, 2005), GUERNSEY (Nanouk Leopold, 2005), LENA (Christophe Van Rompaey, 2011), GLUCKAUF [SON OF MINE] (Remy van Heugten, 2015), and BRIMSTONE (Martin Koolhoven, 2016).[46] If one of my concerns with Dutch cinema—in both this and the previous study—is to make unexpected and deliberately anachronistic cross-connections, here is one for you: this heterogeneous list of titles above can be taken as the offspring of Rademakers' attempts at cinema. Because of the sheer variety of his oeuvre, which comprises only 11 feature films—from 'art' to cult; from genre film to historical epics—every chapter will start with one of his titles[47] and introduce us to a key concept from psychoanalysis which will function as a leitmotif for the chapter.

NOTES

1 Rademakers had received an Academy Award nomination for Best Foreign Language Picture for his debut feature, the 'Ingmar Bergman Light' film DORP AAN DE RIVIER [VILLAGE BY THE RIVER] (1958). It was followed by the comic-tragic mosaic film MAKKERS, STAAKT UW WILD GERAAS [THAT JOYOUS EVE] (1960), while the coming-of-age drama HET MES consolidated his reputation as Holland's most promising director of fiction features.

2 Although Hermans was no longer involved, he showed his face on the set a few times, a fact that he himself, incidentally, later denied. On one of these occasions, he had dressed himself as a Nazi for fun, and the photograph was used for a brief moment in Rademakers' film.

3 Apparently, Hermans did not catch a second remark Ducker makes about his hairless chin. When his uncle, Frans, is angered that Ducker is in hiding while his mother and wife are arrested and then sees that his nephew has painted his hair black 'like an old lady', he calls Ducker a 'degenerate'. Ducker then replies: 'Is this because I have no beard?'

4 Hermans wrote in 'Blokker en Bommel': 'In het boek is voortdurend sprake van het feit dat Osewoudt geen baard heeft. In de film is dat allemaal geschrapt, op één enkele plaats na, waar hij zonder enige functionele reden gaat vertellen: ik heb geen baard. Tot overmaat van ramp zie je even later, in een grote close-up, dat de acteur die de rol speelt, wel degelijk een baard heeft.'

5 To mention three titles that were over an hour long: NIET TEVERGEEFS (Edmond T. Gréville, 1948), LO/LKP (Max de Haas, 1949), and DE DIJK IS DICHT (Anton Koolhaas, 1950).

6 In its 'unquestioned positivity in the portrayal of the resistance', DE OVERVAL did not set an example for future Dutch war pictures but instead was the 'last gasp of unrestrained patriotism' (Burke, 188)—that is, until the release of DE BANKIER VAN HET VERZET [THE RESISTANCE BANKER] (Joram Lürsen, 2018).

7 The film was broadcast on Dutch television only one time, in 1966, and, as Claudy Op den Kamp mentions, it was screened a few times on special occasions, but only after Heineken's express permission (55). One such screening was during De Nederlandse Filmdagen in Utrecht in 1987. The British critic Neil Roddick, in particular, was highly enthusiastic and considered ALS TWEE DRUPPELS WATER one of the best films he had seen that year (see Beerekamp). The English title Roddick used was THE SPITTING IMAGE.

8 'GROTE FONS! [...] Het grote pad bewandelt [...] een Nederlander.... eindelijk.......!' (qtd. in Bernink, 55).

9 'de misschien beste Nederlandse film van de vorige eeuw.'

10 To illustrate the scepticism towards Dutch cinema, let me cite a cartoon by Gummbah, one of my favourite absurdists. A man asks what present he should

give to a 'horrible asshole' ['vreselijke klootzak']. The salesman suggests a Dutch movie. The man replies: 'Is that not all too cruel?' {'Is dat niet wat erg wreed?'] (Published in *de Volkskrant*, 16-09-2019).

11 ALLEMAN, in particular, was a great success, with 1.6 million viewers. Haanstra had registered daily life in the Netherlands, almost half of the recordings shot with candid cameras: children learning to skate on ice, people chastely putting on their bathing suits near the beach, and the birth of the daughter of the director's assistant is filmed as well. The juxtaposition of scenes often created a humorous effect. DE STEM VAN HET WATER [THE VOICE OF THE WATER] (1966), with its widescreen images and longer takes, documented how the ever-present water influenced the Dutch.

12 'Het Hollandse landschap is een ondramatisch landschap [...] dat is niet een verschil waaruit grote spanning kan ontstaan. [De Hollandse mens] heet nuchter, tolerant, behoedzaam en zelfverzekerd – en dat zijn geen eigenschappen die snel conflicten uitlokken.'

13 'Hij [de Nederlander] is eerder geneigd tot observatie dan tot onderzoek [...]. Wij tonen geen mensen, maar wuivend graan.'

14 Een taal die 'scherp en leeg, eentonig' is. 'Luister naar het mannelijk Zweeds. [...] En Frans. Geweldig. [...] De rapheid en nuance in het Italiaans' [...] Het Amerikaans. 'Die taal is stoer [...]'.

15 The great majority of Flemish words are similar to their corresponding Dutch words, and the pronunciation is only slightly different.

16 The omnibus film was called GLI EROI DI IERI... OGGI... DOMANI [THE HEROES OF YESTERDAY ... TODAY ... TOMORROW]. Apart from Weisz, the other three directors were Enzo Dell'Aquila, Fernando Di Leo, and Sergio Tau.

17 More than 50 years later, Weisz eventually did make HET LEVEN IS VURRUKKULLUK (2018). Unfortunately, not everyone noted that the film is built on a historical tension: while it is set in present-day Amsterdam, its three protagonists display a 1960s carefree, 'love is in the air' mentality. This mixture of contemporary drama—the story of a cheating housewife, for example—and the frivolity of a Jacques Demy musical, including tap dances in the park, was appreciated too little.

18 See Verstraten, 'Theatrical Films and Cinematic Novels'.

19 Moreover, the actress Ellen Vogel, Rademakers' wife from 1953 to 1957, had also appeared in his second film, MAKKERS STAAKT UW WILD GERAAS. Only Mien Duymaer van Twist both acted in the play and repeated the same role as the protagonist's mother for the film.

20 Van Doude was born in Haarlem as Doude van Herwijnen. He had also played in Rademakers' previous film ALS TWEE DRUPPELS WATER.

21 Joszef Katús is a fictional character who participates in some public events taking place between 29 April and 5 May 1966, including a demonstration organized by so-called Provos, a pacifist countercultural movement.

22 BIG CITY BLUES is briefly discussed in chapter 6, note 3.

23 Verstappen's BLUE MOVIE, Verhoeven's WAT ZIEN IK!? and TURKS FRUIT, Van der Heyde's HELP! DE DOKTER VERZUIPT each had more than one million moviegoers, but none of them was selected for any important film festival, unlike marginal movies such as ZWARTZIEK (Jacob Bijl, 1973) and STRAF (Olga Madsen, 1973) (Hofstede, 123). MARIKEN VAN NIEUMEGHEN (Jos Stelling, 1974) had the honour of being selected for the main competition in Cannes.

24 Ditvoorst was the one exception who refused to compromise, unless one considers his gangster film FLANAGAN (1975) as an attempt to attain an audience. Yet FLANAGAN was too idiosyncratic a genre film to become successful. In the words of Ditvoorst himself, he was the only filmmaker who did not make bourgeois films but rather films about the bourgeois (qtd. in Van Scheers, 183).

25 In 2014, Tom Ook made the compilation 'Canon der godverdommes', consisting of fragments from Dutch films in which characters use the infamous curse word https://www.youtube.com/watch?v=hWR9HzDGIto [12 May 2020].

26 For a longer version of this argument, see Verstraten *Humour and Irony*, 179-182.

27 Scriptwriter Gerard Soeteman wanted a different ending for KEETJE TIPPEL. To hammer home the point that money turns people into bastards, he wanted a final scene in which Keetje goes outside in a beautiful dress and refuses to give money to a beggar. Keetje holds her hands to her ears in an attempt not to hear the screaming beggar, but she realizes all too well, to her shame, that she has forgotten her humble beginnings (qtd. in Van Scheers, 193).

28 See Verstraten *Humour and Irony*, 203-210 for a longer version of this hostile reception.

29 '[C]ocktail van leed en ellende' (Bovekerk).

30 The very best sex scenes, as Koolhoven explains in the first season of his *De kijk van Koolhoven* (episode six, broadcast 9 November 2018), are those scenes that indicate how the relationship between characters is about to develop. He gives the example of A HISTORY OF VIOLENCE (David Cronenberg, 2005) in which the first love scene illustrates their harmony and the second one reveals their growing tension.

31 Koolhoven argues this in the clip called 'Theatraal acteren', one of four brief interviews with Gerhard Busch, https://www.vpro.nl/cinema/nff/artikelen/Koolhoven-Busch.html [Accessed 13 April 2020].

32 Koolhoven, qtd. in Beekman 'Met Koolhoven', V5. Though less prominent than the World War II pictures, films that highlight the personal struggle with a strict religious upbringing can be called another genre (or perhaps mini genre) in Dutch cinema. Like the WWII movies, these films are 'realist' rather than 'cinematic'.

33 Similarly, the plane in NORTH BY NORTHWEST that is spraying pesticides over barren land looks like a 'steel bird' (Imaginary); Norman in PSYCHO has a collection of stuffed birds (Symbolic); and in THE BIRDS, we have actual seagulls mercilessly attacking people in Bodega Bay but as an 'instrument' of the rage of Midge's mother (the Real).

34 Mathijs writes that Kümel 'produced three different language versions (English, French and Dutch) and found himself in conflict over the final cut of the film, resulting in two different versions (one English-language version of 87 minutes, and a French-language version of 96 minutes)' (101). I have only seen the English-language version.

35 These four films are: DORP AAN DE RIVIER; MAKKERS, STAAKT UW WILD GERAAS; HET MES; and MIRA.

36 The working title of the film DE DRIE SOLDATEN [THE THREE SOLDIERS] was changed to DE VIJANDEN to emphasize their enmity.

37 Alexander Mackendrick, director of such Ealing productions as WHISKY GALORE! (1949) and THE LADYKILLERS (1955), had been an advisor to Haanstra's debut fiction feature.

38 Exemplary of this orientation beyond Holland itself is the British critic Peter Cowie who in his 1979 study on Dutch cinema frequently compares Dutch films to the work of international directors: a sequence from MIRA underlines Rademakers' 'admiration for Kurosawa' (78); the ingrown pattern of village life in Haanstra's DOKTER PULDER ZAAIT PAPAVERS 'is recorded with a gravity and precision worthy of Dreyer' (45); in MARIKEN VAN NIEUMEGHEN, Jos Stelling is 'obviously aspiring to the achievement of THE SEVENTH SEAL' (107); some moments in Ditvoorst's DE BLINDE FOTOGRAAF are 'worthy of Polanski at his best', whereas the guiding spirit in DE MANTEL DER LIEFDE is 'not Polanski, but Buñuel' (101).

39 Both DE VIJANDEN and MIRA were subsidized equally by Dutch and Belgian funds. For the Flemish, MIRA was primarily a Belgian production because of the setting, the scenario by Claus based upon a novel by the Flemish author Stijn Streuvels, and the role of the actor Jan Decleir. For the Dutch, MIRA was primarily a Dutch production because Rademakers had directed it and Willeke van Ammelrooy was the female lead actress. After MIRA, such co-productions had a majority share by either Belgium or the Netherlands (see Willems *Subsidie*, 93).

40 Het Nederlands Film Festival (NFF) is since 1993 the new name for De Nederlandse Filmdagen, established in 1981.

41 Preferably, the films are shown on 35mm, for most cinephiles are slightly suspicious of the 'cold' perfection of a digital projection.

42 Let me admit right away that I am a bit too idealistic here. I will reveal less 'privileged details' than I would have wished to. The lens of this study requires me to focus more on plot developments than a strict cinephilic project would have enabled me. 'When the cinephile selects a fragment', Paul Willemen argues, 'it has to be an aspect of cinema that is not strictly programmable in terms of aesthetic strategies'. Such a fragment 'reveals an aspect or dimension of a person, whether it's the actor or the director, which is not choreographed for you to see. It is produced *en plus*, in excess or in addition, almost involuntarily' (237).

43 I owe this pun on the name Brad to Jurgen Heinsman, who used to own the Dvd shop *All About Movies* in Nijmegen. The shop was specialized in old classics, art-house, and cult films.

44 I could also have mentioned the films by the Flemish Eric de Kuyper, but his work is very little noted, albeit highly recommended for cinephiles. De Kuyper worked as a film lecturer at the University of Nijmegen from 1977 to 1986. He made several art films with his colleagues and students, and they are littered with references to opera, theatre, and cinema. He also made genre movies such as the 'sad musical' NAUGHTY BOYS (1984) as well as silent films such as the short PIERROT LUNAIRE (1988), which was an homage to German Expressionist cinema and to Georges Méliès. With their aesthetic focus on the male body, his films clearly display a gay sensibility. PINK ULYSSES (1990), a retelling of Homer's novel in the German and Italian languages as well as English intertitles, has many naked torsos of 'Greek' heroes, and it has also excerpts from other films, such as Eisenstein's BATTLESHIP POTEMKIN (1925) with bare male bodies.

45 RIGOR MORTIS should have been part of my previous study, but I had not seen Maas's mid-length black comedy at the time. It is about a man, Karel Hemelrijk, who has buried himself alive in order to set a new world record by remaining under the ground for 248 days. Karel, whom we never actually see, receives food through a pipe in the garden. People can pay to visit him, but since there is hardly any publicity, his wife Truus makes very little money: only a German family with a dog named Adolf comes to see the 'attraction'. Truus, who used to have a sing-and-dance routine under the name of 'Annabella', runs a bar that has only one regular guest: a trigger-happy policeman who since the death of his colleague drinks double the amount of alcohol he used to. On Day 124, however, a television team arrives to shoot an item. The cameraman persuades Truus to leave Karel and to restart her singing career. Realizing that his wife has left him, Karel commits suicide, not knowing that Truus is about to return, an illusion poorer. In the final shot, two buses filled with tourists make a stop at the place.

46 Given the fact that Dutch cinema is not generally held in high esteem, it may seem that I am trying to compensate for this disregard by what the sceptics may consider an overestimation on my part. Well yes, maybe I happen to have a weak spot for cinematic wallflowers, but at the same time I can be unimpressed by some Dutch fiction features that receive too benevolent a reception or even win prestigious awards. Bear in mind that in the case of these latter films, I have decided not to include them in this study or have only mentioned them briefly in a footnote, for why spend energy on so-so pictures? The reader can take my scathing critique of KOMT EEN VROUW BIJ DE DOKTER in this introduction as an exception to this principle, but the analysis of this film served the purpose of making a specific argument regarding the use of sex in Dutch cinema.

47 Because of several comic scenes included in them, Rademakers' DORP AAN DE RIVIER and MAKKERS STAAKT UW WILD GERAAS were already discussed at length in my previous study.

BIBLIOGRAPHY

Baudry, Jean-Louis, 'Ideological Effects of the Basic Cinematographic Apparatus', 1970, *Film Quarterly* Vol. 28, No. 2, (Winter, 1974-1975): 39-47.

Beekman, Bor, 'Met Koolhoven de grens over', *de Volkskrant* (30 December 2015), V4-6.

Beerekamp, Hans, 'ALS TWEE DRUPPELS WATER', *NRC Handelsblad*, 21 August 1996.

Bellour, Raymond, 'Symbolic Blockage (on NORTH BY NORTHWEST)', *The Analysis of Film* (Bloomington and Indianapolis: Indiana University Press, 2000), 77-192.

Bernink, Mieke, *Fons Rademakers: Scènes uit leven en werk* (Abcoude: Uniepers, 2003).

Bordwell, David, and Noël Carroll, *Post-Theory: Reconstructing Film Studies* (Madison, Wisconsin: University of Wisconsin Press, 1996).

Bovekerk, Henk, 'Waarom kijken mensen naar films vol ellende?' Vice (11 December 2015), http://www.henkbovekerk.nl/waarom-kijken-mensen-naar-films-vol-ellende [Accessed 3 February 2020].

Burke, Wendy, *Images of Occupation in Dutch Film: Memory, Myth and the Cultural Legacy of War* (Amsterdam: Amsterdam University Press, 2017).

Cowie, Peter, *Dutch Cinema* (London: Tantivy Press, 1979).

Elsaesser, Thomas, 'Specularity and Engulfment: Francis Ford Coppola's and BRAM STOKER'S DRACULA', ed. by Steve Neale and Murray Smith, *Contemporary Hollywood Cinema* (London and New York: Routledge, 1998), 191-208.

Hermans, Willem Frederik, 'Blokker en Bommel', *Podium* 18, 1 (October 1963): 38-48.

Hermans, Willem Frederik, *De donkere kamer van Damokles*, 1958 (Amsterdam: G.A. van Oorschot, 1997, 34th ed.).

Hofstede, Bart, *Nederlandse cinema wereldwijd: De internationale positie van de Nederlandse film* (Amsterdam: Boekmanstudies, 2000).

Kovács, András Bálint, *Screening Modernism: European Art Cinema, 1950-1980* (Chicago: University of Chicago Press, 2007).

Mathijs, Ernest, 'LES LÈVRES ROUGES / DAUGHTERS OF DARKNESS', ed. by Mathijs, 97-106.

Mathijs, Ernest, ed. *The Cinema of the Low Countries* (London and New York: Wallflower Press, 2004).

Metz, Christian, *The Imaginary Signifier: Psychoanalysis and Cinema*, trans. by Celia Britton, Annwyl Williams, Ben Brewster, and Alfred Guzzetti (Bloomington and Indianapolis: Indiana University Press, 1982).

Mosley, Philip, 'DE MAN DIE ZIJN HAAR KORT LIET KNIPPEN / THE MAN WHO HAD HIS HAIR CUT SHORT', ed. by Mathijs, *The Cinema of the Low Countries*, 76-85.

Mulvey, Laura, 'Visual Pleasure and Narrative Cinema', *Screen* 16, no. 3 (1975): 6-18.
Op den Kamp, Claudy, *The Greatest Films Never Seen: The Film Archive and the Copyright Smokescreen* (Amsterdam: Amsterdam University Press, 2018).
Schoots, Hans, *Bert Haanstra: Filmer van Nederland* (Amsterdam: Mets en Schilt, 2009).
Schoots, Hans, *Van* FANFARE *tot* SPETTERS: *Een cultuurgeschiedenis van de jaren zestig en zeventig* (Amsterdam: Lubberhuizen, 2004).
Sontag, Susan, 'Notes on "Camp"', 1964, *Against Interpretation and Other Essays* (London and New York: Penguin Classics, 2009), 275-292.
Van Scheers, Rob, *Paul Verhoeven: Een filmersleven* (Amsterdam: Podium, 2017).
Verstraten, Peter, *Humour and Irony in Dutch Post-war Fiction Film* (Amsterdam: Amsterdam University Press, 2016).
Verstraten, Peter, '"My Very Own CITIZEN KANE", Inspired by Godard and Fellini: Frans Weisz's Adaptation of Remco Campert's *Het gangstermeisje*', *Journal of Dutch Literature* 8, 1 (2017): 60-74.

Verstraten, Peter, 'Theatrical Films and Cinematic Novels: DE DANS VAN DE REIGER and L'ANNÉE DERNIÈRE À MARIENBAD', *Image [&] Narrative* 17, 2 (2016): 61-73.
Willemen, Paul, 'Through the Glass Darkly: Cinephilia Reconsidered', *Looks and Frictions: Essyas in Cultural Studies and Film Theory*, London: BFI, 1994, 223-257.
Willems, Gertjan, 'Hugo Claus, de snelste en goedkoopste filmer van Europa: De totstandkoming van DE VIJANDEN', *Zacht Lawijd*, 17, 1 (2018): 68-85.
Willems, Gertjan, *Subsidie, Camera, Actie! Filmbeleid in Vlaanderen* (1964-2002) (Gent:Academia Press, 2017).
Zizek, Slavoj, ed. *Everything You Always Wanted to Know about Lacan (But Were Afraid to Ask Hitchcock)* (London: Verso, 1992).
Žižek, Slavoj, *Looking Awry: An Introduction to Jacques Lacan through Popular Culture* (Cambridge, Mass.: The MIT Press, 1991).
Žižek, Slavoj, *The Fright of Real Tears: Krzysztof Kieślowski Between Theory and Post-Theory* (London: BFI, 2001).
Žižek, Slavoj, *The Sublime Object of Ideology* (London: Verso, 1989).

CHAPTER 1

Spitting Images, Blind Spots, and Dark Mirrors

Verstraten, P., *Dutch Post-War Fiction Film Through a Lens of Psycho-analysis*. Taylor & Francis Group, 2021
DOI 10.5117/9789463725330_CH01

ABSTRACT

Chapter one is structured according to a gliding scale: mirror scenes are discussed in a variety of films, but each case confronts us with ever more horrifying encounters with the unfathomable strangers within us. ALS TWEE DRUPPELS WATER is pivoted around presumed resemblance, whereas mirrors are avoided in MILO (due to the boy's abundant hair growth) as well as in RIPHAGEN (due to the protagonist's amoral principles). Shots of shattered glass are seminal in both the war picture SÜSKIND and the feminist GEBROKEN SPIEGELS about a serial killer. After explaining how mirrors can help to 'traverse the fantasy', the chapter ends with an analysis of the psychological thriller ZWART WATER about a girl with a gift for seeing spectral apparitions.

KEYWORDS
Mirror scenes – presumed resemblance – confining symbolic identities – traversing the fantasy – spectral apparition

One evening, the timid cigar shop owner Hennie Ducker in Rademakers' ALS TWEE DRUPPELS WATER (1963) sees a parachutist descend from the sky. This secret agent named Dorbeck turns out to be his spitting image, except that Ducker is blond and Dorbeck has black hair. Their encounter comes after a remark by Ducker's friend Hubach stating that the war would already have been over if everyone had joined the Resistance. 'Not everyone is a hero', Ducker replies, but the meeting with Dorbeck offers him the opportunity to do his bit. The secret agent gives Ducker a couple of assignments, and the latter is happy to fulfil them. Since Ducker becomes a fugitive after his own wife betrayed him to the Germans, Dorbeck brings him to a new home for shelter. Dorbeck has to leave right away, but Ducker takes his Leica camera because he wants to record 'this historical moment'. The next shot is shown via a big mirror, so that the camera seems to have crossed the 180 degrees axis: it looks as if Dorbeck and Ducker have switched places. Dorbeck says it is too dark in the room to take a photograph, but Ducker, while requesting his look-alike to stand still, takes one anyway. Dorbeck then asks Ducker to open a suitcase, and the latter complies with this request, which is still shown via the mirror. Then there is a transition to a medium-shot of Ducker who is surprised upon hearing that the content is meant for him: 'Me, in this?' A reverse shot shows Dorbeck in medium close-up on the left side of the shot, whereas we see Ducker in the background on the right via the mirror. They are apparently facing each other, but this does not seem that way due to the shot composition. Dorbeck: 'Try it on. It will fit you perfectly.' It turns out to be the costume of a female nurse, including a cap, and reluctantly, Ducker gives in to Dorbeck's command. The latter concludes: 'You see, it fits', and then quickly leaves, taking Ducker's other clothes with him.

Taking this fragment in ALS TWEE DRUPPELS WATER as a starting point, in this chapter I will close-read a variety of film scenes featuring mirrors, propelled by Lacan's idea that the mirror stage is a key phase in the Imaginary, one of his three orders. The mirror stage signifies both recognition ('that's me') and misrecognition ('that's not me, that's an external image').[1] The narrative function of the mirror shots in this chapter is discussed in relation to a variety of topics, such as the 'narcissism of small differences'; the mimicry of friendship; the impossibility to deceive the gaze of the Other; the coding of women with to-be-looked-at-ness; symbolic deception; and over-identification with mirror images. Ultimately, this chapter is structured according to a gliding scale: the mirror scene in each case confronts us with ever more horrifying encounters with the unfathomable strangers within us.

FROM IDEAL EGO TO EGO-IDEAL: *ALS TWEE DRUPPELS WATER*

It takes little imagination to understand that Ducker has a problem with masculinity. If we take a seminal motif from W.F. Hermans' novel into consideration, the protagonist (named Osewoudt in the book instead of Ducker) has always remained smaller than average, having been delivered prematurely as a baby. Due to his short stature, he is not permitted to join the army and therefore is not given the chance to prove he is a 'real' man. Moreover, as an obvious sign of his lack of a manly appearance, it is emphasized time and again in the novel that Osewoudt has no beard growth at all. In the film, this motif of lack/ absence is only mentioned twice, the first time when Ducker tells Marianne, who must dye his hair black: 'Don't tell me how clean I shave. I have no beard.' Further, Ducker is married to Ria, a woman who nags at him permanently. She commits adultery with Turlings, who sympathizes with the Nazis. To make Ducker's humiliation worse, the lovers do not hide the affair from him so that he knows he is being cuckolded. In the beginning of the film, after Ducker has said that not everyone can be a hero, he and Hubach see Ria and Turlings kissing through the frosted glass of the door. Hubach watches Ducker, but the latter does not react to the embrace and seems to act as if he has not noticed it. It confirms his earlier statement that not everyone is a hero: Ducker apparently lacks the courage and bravado that might befit a man. He turns out to be very good at judo, but that, he complains, is no longer of any use these days, although this talent will be very helpful in one of the later scenes.

As a resolution to Ducker's crisis in masculinity, a man literally falls from the sky—a man whose name also starts with a 'd' and has a 'ck' in it. The status of this man will be a riddle throughout the film. Is he some agent working for the Resistance, as Ducker claims? Or is Dorbeck only a figment of Ducker's imagination? The old doctor will reach the diagnosis that Ducker, just like his mother, is suffering from delusions. To support this hypothesis, the arrival of Dorbeck is preceded by three brief jump cut shots of Ducker at a table, from a close-up of his face to an extreme close-up.[2] In the last part of ALS TWEE DRUPPELS WATER, when the war is already over, Ducker is accused of being a collaborator who has harmed the Dutch Resistance. Ducker defends himself by claiming that he was instructed by Dorbeck, but this claim is only legitimate if he can prove that Dorbeck does exist. He tries to contact people who might have set eyes on Dorbeck or preferably might have seen them together. These people are either dead or not sane enough to give witness reliably, such as his Uncle Frans who is traumatized after his return from a concentration camp. The lover of Ducker's wife is not qualified either, because he was a backstabber. Some objects that Ducker kept in custody, such as Dorbeck's camouflage overalls and goggles, are too corroded to provide a conclusive answer. And thus, Ducker places his hope on the return of the Leica camera but, alas for him, when he gets hold of the apparatus again, a potentially compromising photograph featuring Obersturmbannführer Ebernuss is visible on the film strip, but the adjacent image that is supposed to reveal Dorbeck is too obscure to detect anything.

For the sake of my argument in this chapter, I will consider Dorbeck a hallucination of Ducker to attribute to him the status of his ideal ego. When Freud introduced his ideas on narcissism in 1914, he mentions that in the first phase, a child only yearns for the fulfilment of its lust and totally disregards its environment. A subsequent phase is described by Freud as primary narcissism, when a child's exclusive self-love in the phase of auto-eroticism is supplemented by some affection for objects in the outside world, albeit no more than modestly. These objects, like a cuddly toy, mainly function to confirm the child in his narcissistic perfectionism. According to Lacan, this shift from auto-eroticism, with a total focus upon one's self, to primary narcissism, with some attention to the child's environment, is facilitated by the so-called mirror stage. The act of seeing itself is an estranging experience for the child. So far, it has seen its own belly, and it could move its own quite uncoordinated hands and fingers. Owing to its agility, it was able to grab its legs or even suck on its toes. But this perception of oneself as quite helpless and fragmentary is somehow belied by the image in the mirror which presents the child as in one piece. In the mirror, the child can watch itself as fairly coherent, and what is more, Lacan argues, at this point the child identifies with this mirror image as an improved version of the self. The child longs to possess one day the motorial capacity of the child-in-the-mirror. Apart from this identification, the mirror confronts the child with the illusion of a unity of the self but in the guise of an external image. The child recognizes itself—'That's me'—but this recognition is also a fundamental misrecognition—'That's not me'—for it is only an image out there. The experience of watching oneself in the mirror is alienating, since 'I' observe myself as an 'other', as an imaginary creation, which suggests a physical totality that 'I' apparently do not possess.

The mirror scene in ALS TWEE DRUPPELS WATER is a displacement of the mirror stage in the imaginary order. The child's version tells us that the kid may think he sees a better self, whereas the adult Ducker sees two men reflected of the same height: his blond self and a dark-haired Dorbeck who is his almost total look-alike—almost but not quite. This 'not quite' makes a great difference. According to Freud, once a child comes to realize it is not a perfect being, it will sacrifice its primary narcissism.[3] In giving up the belief in its own grandeur, the child creates its own ideal ego (or image of an ideal ego): 'Okay, I am not perfect, but this image-in-the-mirror is what I would like to become.'[4] Likewise, Ducker constructs Dorbeck as his ideal ego, as we can gather from an earlier mirror scene. After Dorbeck has left his overall and his goggles behind in the cigar shop, Ducker tries them on. The still blond tradesman climbs on a chair in order to see his face in a small mirror, wondering whether it will make him look like a hero. In a conversation with his then-girlfriend Marianne, Ducker discloses that his immediate thought upon seeing Dorbeck for the first time was: That should have been me. Ducker is a passive character with an expression of slight panic on his face, but it is only once his blond hair is dyed black that there seems to be a change in character. He states that his life can start anew, and he immediately makes a pass at Marianne. When she replies that he shouldn't move too fast, he answers that there is no time to waste. As soon as the one directly perceptible difference between Ducker and Dorbeck is neutralized, he acts much more assertively, as if his black hair justifies an identification with the self-declared secret agent rather than with his very own self. In bed with Marianne, he says: 'Perhaps you would have chosen Dorbeck, if you knew him. [...] Apart from the very first ten minutes, you've only known me with black hair, like his.' She reassures him by saying: 'You'll see I will love you just as much when it's blond again.'

But even though Ducker looks more like Dorbeck than like himself, the identification is not total. Just as the mirror image remains external to the child as its ideal ego, Ducker will never become equal to Dorbeck, despite the now perfect resemblance. He is convinced that Marianne would have chosen his double if she had met him, simply because Dorbeck is a daredevil thanks to his symbolic position as a 'secret agent', whereas he himself is no more than the owner of a cigar shop. In a clear reference to Hermans' novel once more, Dorbeck was accepted into military service because he had made himself taller by stretching himself during the medical examination. Insofar as this can be regarded as a form of deceit, it definitely serves as an example. Thanks to passing the test, Dorbeck has a mental advantage over Ducker which creates in the eyes of the latter an insurmountable difference between the two. In the words of Ducker: 'I could only justify my existence by doing what he said.' The hierarchy is irreversible: Dorbeck gives instructions, and he will not take no for an answer; Ducker obeys his commands no matter whether his hair is blond or dyed black.

On the one hand, Ducker has no problem with this hierarchy at all. The meeting with Dorbeck has given him the satisfactory opportunity to help the Resistance, or so he believes. He can exchange his nagging wife Ria for the much more attractive Marianne. His attempt to take a picture in the mirror of both him and Dorbeck is an expression of Ducker's gratitude for the secret agent's role in such turning points in his life. On the other hand, it is impossible for him to shake off the impression that, whatever he does or achieves, he will always be second-rate in comparison to Dorbeck, and thus anyone or any girl might prefer his double over him. In terms of the imaginary, a Ducker with black hair is the exact spitting image of Dorbeck, but on the level of the symbolic, there remains a gap nonetheless. The black hair is just cosmetic and will in the course of time become blond again. As Freud has hinted in introducing the notion of the 'narcissism of the small differences': if two persons are practically alike, the one minor detail that distinguishes them becomes highly significant. This kind of narcissism has an impact on Ducker, for he seems haunted by the idea that Dorbeck's black hair automatically asserts his heroism, whereas his dyed black hair is a mimicry, illustrating that he is no more than a wannabe hero.

This risk of an unmasking is enacted in another mirror scene in ALS TWEE DRUPPELS WATER. When Ducker is interrogated by two inspectors who doubt the existence of Dorbeck and suspect Ducker of war crimes, a military policeman brings a mirror. The mirror is held up to a blond-haired Ducker, whereupon one of the inspectors yells in contempt: 'The face of a guy who has helped in the Liberation. Bloody hell.' This scene recalls my earlier description of the adult who holds the child in his arms and points at the mirror: 'Look, that's you', the adult says, but the result is much more opprobrious in the case of Ducker. In the case of the child, the observation is self-alienating (as described above), but the accompanying words of the adult are an indication that one is always embedded within a larger community: one lives in an inevitable reference to the big Other. The child itself is engaged in an I-you relationship, but there is a third person who, by naming this relationship, subjects the child to the symbolic order. Let's assume this third person is the father, stating: 'Look, that's you', and adding: 'Daddy's big boy.'

The situation during the interrogation is far worse for Ducker. Dorbeck is his ideal ego, the character he dearly wants to be/become. Taking a photograph via the mirror of himself and his spitting image was his way of saying: 'Look how closely I resemble my ideal ego.' If Dorbeck were present or if Ducker were to produce a photographic image of his double, he could show his interrogators how he wants to be judged. With Dorbeck as his ideal ego, Ducker could present an ego-ideal in front of the interrogators, to be paraphrased as: you may think I am a short, ordinary guy, but look at the heroic and charismatic Dorbeck, and you will probably realize that you underestimate me. In other words, Ducker wants to be seen through the lens of Dorbeck. In the absence of Dorbeck, however, Ducker's imaginary identification with this 'perfect' figure is built upon a void and lacks any ground of comparison. Ducker will now be judged without the symbolic support of his ideal ego and is therefore left to his own devices. The judgement of the one inspector is harsh: no one will believe that you are a war hero, and probably when you see yourself in the mirror, you yourself probably won't believe it. In the eyes of the Other, Ducker is a phoney.

The three mirror scenes (out of a total of four) in ALS TWEE DRUPPELS WATER are based on a shift from imaginary to symbolic identification.[5] The very first one showed how Ducker imitated the parachutist by wearing his goggles and is based on an imaginary scene: can I convince myself to be like Dorbeck? The second scene concerns the transition from imaginary to symbolic: Ducker dearly wants to recognize himself as Dorbeck and therefore wants to record the historical moment by making a double portrait in the mirror. But as the narcissism of the small differences implies, if a look-alike is not a total look-alike, any deviation is seminal. This deviation is formally underscored in the shot we see after Ducker has opened the suitcase with the nurse's uniform. We see Dorbeck straight on, while Ducker is represented as a mirror-image in the background, as if to suggest that he may want to be like his dark-haired ideal ego but will not be acknowledged as such within the symbolic order. The encounters between Ducker and Dorbeck have an imaginary dimension throughout, because Dorbeck makes sure they are never seen together. Only Ducker's mother sets eyes on them simultaneously, but since she cannot fathom how she could see her son 'twice', the doctor explains that it is due to her nerves. The third mirror scene confirms that the imaginary relationship between the two men has remained outside the symbolic domain. In the eyes of the general public, represented by the two inspectors, Ducker's appearance immediately demonstrates that he cannot be a hero. This is so obvious that a mirror is held up to him, so that Ducker—without the back-up of Dorbeck—can see for himself with his very own eyes how far removed he is from any masculine ideal. The exquisite photography by Raoul Coutard gives credence to a scenario in which Ducker's imagination seems overexcited. The widescreen shots often present empty silent streets, and the contrast between black and white in many outdoor shots creates a certain depth of field that makes Ducker stand out as a loner, as was mentioned in a review in *Haagse Post* (qtd. in Bernink, 53).[6]

In the encounter with Dorbeck, whether he is a figment of Ducker's imagination or a 'real' agent, Ducker meets his ideal ego: this identification is imaginary, for Ducker wants to be like him. Hence, a subject puts immense pressure upon himself, for he practically knows in advance that he will never be that perfect. But the subject's desire (in this case, Ducker's longing to be like Dorbeck) is embedded in the desire of the Other, as Lacan has instructed us (*Écrits*, 201). There is a shift from Dorbeck as ideal ego to Dorbeck as his ego-ideal, and this latter entails Ducker's symbolic identification with him. Let's consider that Ducker's insistence on taking the photograph delights him because it shows how close he supposes he has come to embody his ideal ego. This almost total resemblance (i.e., Ducker's imaginary identification) is of little significance when he is not acknowledged as such by others. If desires are not our own but, as Lacan says, the desire of the Other, this means in this particular case that rather than regard himself as a mimicry of Dorbeck, Ducker wants his environment to see him as (a) 'Dorbeck', as an indispensable link in the fight for the liberation of the Netherlands. For the one inspector, however, Ducker is an immoral character who cowardly puts the blame for his corrupt actions onto a fictive figure. The other inspector, Wierdeman, wants to give Ducker the benefit of the doubt but nonetheless demands proof of Dorbeck's existence.

The viewer of Rademakers' film cannot decide which scenario is correct: the arguments that Dorbeck is a hallucination dreamed up by Ducker or the arguments that he does exist. The final shot of ALS TWEE DRUPPELS WATER brilliantly contributes to this ambiguity. After the photograph has failed, Ducker is distressed, and since his desperate run is taken for an attempt to escape, he is shot in the back. On the verge of dying, a priest holds Ducker in his arms. Barely able to speak, Ducker asks him to find Dorbeck, but in a frontally staged close-up, slightly high-angle, the priest says: 'You must stay alive. You have to find Dorbeck yourself. No one else will find him for you.' While the priest puts his hand on Ducker's body, which is covered in blood, there is a dissolve to a female hand on another man's body, only wearing swimming trunks and bathing in sunlight. We then see Marianne in close-up: 'I knew someone in the war who looked like you.' We then have a close-up of Dorbeck, eyes closed: 'He looked like me?' And while the camera zooms out to a bird's eye perspective, we see the two on a rock near the sea, while the woman repeats the film's title: 'Like two drops of water.'[7] This final shot gives as much proof of Dorbeck's existence as that it can be taken as Ducker's posthumous hallucination, answering the priest's call that Ducker has to find Dorbeck himself—and he thus discovers him where he had always been: in his imagination.

In terms of morality, ALS TWEE DRUPPELS WATER delves into shades of grey. I would like to suggest that another World War II picture—one of the very few types of film with some tradition in the Netherlands—shows the other side of the coin of moral considerations, as I will explain below. This is made evident via a brilliant mirror scene early on in SÜSKIND (Rudolf van den Berg, 2010), which is of a totally different nature than the mirror shots in ALS TWEE DRUPPELS WATER.

PUTTING ON A CHARADE: *SÜSKIND*

In the beginning of Van den Berg's film, set in 1942, the German-Dutch Walter Süskind of Jewish descent visits a theatre in Amsterdam with his wife Hanna in the company of five young children, for his daughter Yvonne is having her birthday party. Upon seeing a banner at the entrance of the theatre that reads 'Only for a Jewish audience', he scoffs: 'Back to the dark ages.' At the cash desk, Walter puts a star of David on his jacket, and then we have a medium close-up of him with a slightly forlorn look. In a subsequent shot, Walter's mirror image is multiplied in 15 vertical reflective columns: we see him from his head to his waist, but due to the minimal width of the mirrors, his arms are absent from the image. While he is still shown via the 15 high but narrow mirrors, Walter looks over his shoulder, with the effect that the star of David only remains visible in some outer mirrors but disappears from the middle ones. When we see in the mirrors that Walter turns back to look at himself again, the camera starts to scan some of the multiplied stars at a relatively close range and then tilts up so that we see two mirror reflections of his face. This is followed by a cut to a close-up of his still forlorn facial expression.

At this point, some five minutes into the film, the formal shooting of the scene is of no significance, but it can be seen as a prelude to the problematic situation Walter will soon be caught in. He has already become slightly aware of the atrocious fate awaiting Jewish people, but when visiting the Jewish Council where he is mistaken for a Mr. Polak, he secretly checks the list of names of Jews who are selected for transportation to Camp Westerbork. He has every reason to worry, for it includes the names of his own family. They can only be removed from the list when Walter proves his 'indispensability' by helping the Germans to organize the transportation of Jews on behalf of the Jewish Council. He has moral quibbles, but his wife persuades him to take this job as a 'Nazi stooge' (Walter's words), for 'if you don't, ten others will, twenty, a hundred'. Walter willy-nilly agrees to fulfil the task, for it means he will have to work in close collaboration with Hauptsturmführer Ferdinand aus der Fünten, who demands that everything proceed flawlessly without tears and emotions. A woman who jumps from the roof enrages the Nazis, for a suicide equals chaos.

Walter does everything to win the trust of Aus der Fünten: he refers to his own German upbringing, he presents himself as a realistic tradesman, and he openly acknowledges him as his superior. Thanks to his contacts with Felix Halverstad, who attempts to manipulate the bookkeeping of the Germans, his strategy will change after he witnesses the shooting on site of a Jew who was trying to run away. Walter no longer just uses his appointment to save his own skin; he decides he wants to help some Jewish children to escape. Piet Meerburg provides Walter with good cigars and expensive wine in order to conciliate Aus der Fünten who might be susceptible to such favours, for Walter believes the German is unscrupulous but also very lonely and in need of company. Nonetheless, they realize that their room for manoeuvre is limited. They will have to operate with the utmost care, since the Germans are meticulous about numbers and become angry when only 387 Jews are put on transport instead of the expected 400. They put pressure on Aus der Fünten, who in turn puts pressure on Walter. So Walter realizes that they have to deliver a great many to save a few, which is best summed up by a conversation between Piet and Walter halfway through the film. Piet notes that they rescued 338 humans, whereupon Walter replies that he is rather mindful of the 40,000 scared faces he had to put on trucks. Though Hanna objects that she wants a husband and not a hero, Walter continues to socialize with Aus der Fünten and pays a visit to the latter's birthday party.

Aus der Fünten thinks he does Walter a favour by arranging a prostitute for him, but this blonde-wigged Jewish woman who regards Walter as a 'horny Kraut' speaks with an Amsterdam dialect. When she realizes he is not a Nazi and not interested in sex, she reveals that the Jews are being exterminated systematically, which until then Walter had taken for British propaganda. Her entire family had already been gassed in showers. It is at this moment that the gruesome destiny of the Jews put on transport really dawns on him. Walter wants to quit because he does not want to act as an 'undertaker of the Nazis', but one man at the Jewish Council persuades him to continue. They are probably doomed anyway, but thanks to Walter's contacts with the Germans, a few might be rescued. From this moment onwards, Walter redoubles his efforts to help as many Jews as possible, but it also prompts him to go into hiding with his family. Once Walter, Hanna, and Yvonne are detected, they are first sent to Camp Westerbork and then to Germany (see chapter four for a lengthier analysis of this episode). None of them will survive the war.

This plot description will not meet much disagreement from the viewers of SÜSKIND. What I would like to suggest, however, is that the early mirror scene delivers the promise of a much darker scenario, which is repressed in the story itself. When Walter looks into the mirror behind the cash desk, he sees a man quite pleased with himself: he is happy with his wife and child, and he has a decent job as a company manager at the Hoogovens steel company. He is, however, deeply annoyed by the situation he has been caught in. He has fled from 'that stinking country' Germany to Holland because of that 'bastard', 'only to find that he follows me here', since the Netherlands is now occupied by the Nazis who have ordered Jews to wear a yellow star. If Walter's look into the series of mirrors is one of contempt, it indicates how much he does not want to be a man wearing such a star. The fact that he has given in to this ridiculous and humiliating rule decreed by the Germans results in a certain kind of self-loathing. While standing in front of the mirrors, he looks around, as if checking whether someone might be watching him. Being detected with such a star could be taken as proof of his apathetic acceptance of the current situation.

Strictly speaking, Walter then decides to do something that is far worse than that. He makes the immoral choice of taking charge of the transport of the Jews, but he legitimizes this by referring to a 'noble' goal: I hate to do this, but this is the only way to protect my family, and moreover, my wife has encouraged me not to be a plaster saint. As regards the historical figure of Walter Süskind, it is not my aim to denigrate the heroic part he has played, and though the film goes to great pains to honour his courage, there is something perverse about his play-acting.

Walter's explicit stance is clear. When Piet gives Walter another bottle of wine for 'our friend', Walter complains that the bastard (Aus der Fünten) makes him sick, to which Piet answers: 'Okay, our bastard then.' But on the surface, it takes relatively little effort on Walter's part to act as the deputy of Aus der Fünten and to comply with the German regulations about order and efficiency. Walter can only continue the strategy by play-acting a close friendship with Aus der Fünten. Consequently, he is a collaborator and a 'filthy Kraut' in the eyes of some of the Jews who have been brought together in the Hollandsche Schouwburg before they are transported. Walter is very much aware of the impression that he is a traitor. After he has stopped one of the Jews from singing and has taken the key of a furious woman, he says to Felix, in a sarcastic tone: 'We're getting quite Teutonic already.' Once he comes to realize at Aus der Fünten's birthday party that the 'lifeboat doesn't exist' and that the Jews are just a 'big heap of offal', he asks his wife while raising his voice: 'Look at me. Look at me! Look at me!! What do you see? What do you see?' Intimidated by his rude approach, Hanna answers: 'A Kraut, a fucking Kraut.'

Apparently, Walter is quite convincing in feigning camaraderie with Aus der Fünten, and as psychoanalysis would suggest, there is a thin line between feigning/mimicry and one's symbolic identity. Walter hates the job he has to fulfil, but he does it anyway because there is no other option left for him. He can only execute his job by putting on a mask, the mask of a collaborative Kraut. But as Žižek has argued, once we start wearing a mask, we risk losing the 'inner distance' from this mask in the process: 'first, we pretend to be something, we just act as if we are that, till, step by step, we actually become it …' (*Enjoy*, 34). At this point in SÜSKIND, even Walter's wife yells at him that he is a 'fucking Kraut', so it is no sign of naïvety on Aus der Fünten's part that Walter could really be a dear friend. This is not to say that Walter truly has become a Nazi, but he has become an excellent executioner of his job. On the one hand, his convincing performance is required to be able to save Jews. On the other hand, Walter is only able to become a reliable accomplice for the Germans—or, in psychoanalytic terms, a 'pure instrument-object of the Other's *jouissance*' (Žižek, *The Plague* 232)—on the condition that he derives a perverse enjoyment from the role allotted to him, which also includes his friendship with Aus der Fünten. To enjoy, as Lacan has posited, is not related to realizing one's appetites and pleasures; it is 'rather something we do as a kind of weird and twisted ethical duty' (Žižek, *How to Read* 79).[8] Enjoyment encompasses those acts that we do against our explicit wishes and our own self-interest but that we cannot help doing anyway. These acts result in discomfort rather than satisfactory feelings, but we simply cannot 'get rid of the stain of enjoyment' (*Enjoy*, 22). There is a limitless bliss that keeps on repeating itself, beyond the subject's control. On the one hand, Walter wants to stop the whole charade with Aus der Fünten, but on the other hand, he enjoys the feigning of the friendship because the German does not realize that he is being deceived. For the Nazi, it is a truthful camaraderie: 'Süskind will never betray me', Aus der Fünten tells his superior Willy Lages. For the sake of succeeding in his strategy, Walter therefore has to act as if it is a truthful bond. As a token of Aus der Fünten's deception, the German passes the very same series of mirrors in the Hollandsche Schouwburg, but he is in so much of a hurry that he blatantly ignores the reflections that the viewer sees.

At some point in the film, Walter becomes fully aware that he is part of a machinery that drives many Jews to their deaths, and the fact that he continues to do his horrific task can only be justified by a minor remark in the beginning. He says to Felix that the Jews who arrive at the Hollandsche Schouwburg behave so meekly and obediently. Here we can explain why the scene with the series of mirrors is so significant: Walter's very own meek gesture of putting on the Jewish star, which has marked him as a passive follower of German rules, is projected upon those Jews who are gathered in the Dutch theatre. The look at himself in the mirrors—a mixture of disbelief and self-contempt—mediates how he sees other Jews. If Walter looks over his shoulder, it is to register whether someone might loath him for his obedience as much as he loathes himself, but in fact, it is already too late, for the big Other has already registered his meekness. Once Walter is appointed the theatre manager of the Hollandsche Schouwburg, he becomes an observer of Jews who also commit the fallacy of obedience. The dislike of his own star-wearing image in the mirrors translates into a latent contempt for the Jews who remain idle. This may seem a far-fetched reading, but remember that Walter is most sympathetic to those people who display a form of resistance: the nurse Fanny has escaped the fate of deportation because of a last-minute rescue by Walter. He undertook this utterly daring attempt out of admiration for her courage in not betraying Walter after she had been arrested for concealing a baby under her coat. In another example, Mrs. Waterman regularly bursts out in anger in the Hollandsche Schouwburg, even calling Walter a 'filthy Kraut', but thanks to Walter's endeavours, her two children Roos and Simon—who are permitted to call him 'Uncle Walter'—will be reunited after the war, as the final melodramatic shots of SÜSKIND illustrate. Walter's painstaking share in their survival suggests that he is more appreciative of someone like their mother who expresses her relentless fury at him than the great majority who just tacitly accept the situation in the hope that things will not get worse. Walter is willing to take a risk for those who either display their despair (Mrs. Waterman) or defy German pressure at all costs (Fanny).

Walter's position and behaviour in SÜSKIND are inversely proportional to Ducker in ALS TWEE DRUPPELS WATER. Ducker presumed he was involved in actions aiding the Resistance, although he is accused of siding with the Nazis. His focus on Dorbeck at an imaginary level was to become/be like him, but symbolically he is not acknowledged as a hero at all. The inspectors make Ducker look into a mirror to show that he simply does not have the appearance of a courageous man, but he remains convinced until the bitter end that he has done some brave acts. By contrast, when Walter looks at his image multiplied in a series of mirrors, he can symbolically identify with the image because of his social success, but his imaginary identification falls short, signified by the fractured imagery. The mirror embarrassingly confronts him with his obedience. When he is appointed the theatre manager, he extrapolates his meekness: Yes, Mrs. Waterman, you are right in calling me a filthy Kraut, for I play along with the Nazis, indeed. Walter shows little affinity for the Jews who are as docile as he is; instead, he prefers those who confront him with the man in the mirror he has witnessed to his own dismay. To put it crudely, he so desperately wants to erase his own docility that, despite all the 'scared faces in the dark', it is easier for him to accept when the non-resisting Jews are transported to Germany than when the few insurgent ones are.

In the fractured mirror shots at the beginning of SÜSKIND, he observes his own submissive character that is a prelude to his role as a 'Nazi stooge', but the angry reproaches at his symbolic position as the theatre manager who cooperates with the Germans have an impact on him. His bonding with Aus der Fünten is no longer just a necessity, it develops into a strategy as a minor form of subversion. Walter perhaps does not take delight in his camaraderie with the Hauptsturmführer, but he does enjoy the feigning of it, no matter how thin the line is between the act and the actual. In performing his friendship with the Nazi, Walter has to exaggerate his meekness on the surface in order to rescue some human lives, for which he cannot openly take symbolic credit, only to a very small in-crowd (Felix, Piet, Henriette Pimentel, Fanny). Meanwhile, his wife Hanna complains that he takes too many risks to save other people. So, the trick here is that in order for Walter to get any symbolic recognition for his actual contribution, he must be categorized as a scapegoat and a dirty collaborator. Thus, Süskind only receives some posthumous acknowledgment. This is clearly what Van den Berg's film does: it applauds the courage of the real Süskind who, as the text mentions at the end, saved about a thousand lives.

Whereas Walter plays the evil part of a Nazi stooge in order to be able to rescue some human lives—if only a drop in the ocean—Andries Riphagen in Pieter Kuijpers's RIPHAGEN (2016) is his polar opposite. Like Süskind, Riphagen is a historical figure, but this titular character was known as one of the most cunning Dutch traitors during the Second World War. With his likeable appearance, Riphagen wins the trust of a great many Jews, among others by staging a fight with a blackmailer, but his aim is just to rob them of their belongings and to deliver them to the Germans. In the film, the only time we see this Riphagen in a mirror is when the camera is positioned to show his reflection. When he is having sex with Greetje for the first time, for example, one of the shots shows him with his back to the mirror. In other words, mirror shots merely reflect his body, but the man himself never scrutinizes his own image. The most remarkable of these reflections is when his re-entrance into his former house is shown via a mirror: it is the first shot of the title protagonist after his opponent Jan van Liempd has read an official paper that certifies that Riphagen has died. Riphagen's wife Greetje believes that her husband is benevolent—yes, she knows he works for the German SD, but she is convinced he does not serve the purpose of the Nazi machinery. Instead of shots in which characters look into mirrors, Riphagen tends to pose for photographs, together with his victims-to-be. We never see him look at these pictures; he only collects them in a box for his personal archive, and in contrast to the photograph made by Ducker in the mirror, these pictures are all in sharp focus. At no point in RIPHAGEN does the protagonist reconsider his own moral stance—for that would require mirror shots. He is only keen on preserving symbolic evidence: see me posing among Jewish people who regard me as their benefactor. These photographs, which he keeps as a mere memento if not a 'trophy', may very well deceive the big Other but in the end are used by Jan to convince Greetje that her husband is a war criminal.

RIPHAGEN is a film about a treacherous character, but the potential darkness of the scenario is neutralized by the invention of a fictive character, Jan, who is too unblemished to come across as credible. He infiltrates the SD on behalf of the resistance group led by Gerrit van der Veen, and he functions as the morally upright benchmark for the film's viewers. He is bent on killing Riphagen, but in the end he is not sufficiently ruthless and Riphagen immediately takes the opportunity to strangle Jan when the latter has a moment of inattention. In order to do justice to the historical fact that Riphagen escaped to Argentina and only died in 1973, the film scenario had to opt for this ending in which the bad guy gets away with his dirty business.

HAIR, HAIR, FLOW IT, (DO NOT) SHOW IT: *MILO*

In SÜSKIND, imaginary identification constituted via fractured images initially presides over symbolic identification. In MILO (Berend and Roel Boorsma, 2012), this emphasis is reversed from the start.[9] In the opening shot, the steam on a mirror is wiped away by the ten-year-old Milo Mulder, for the boy has to put cream all over his body on a regular basis. The next time we see Milo give himself this treatment, he also puts the cream on the mirror itself so that he cannot see his own image. We hear Milo tell Caitlin, the girl next door who is new to his class, that he has a skin condition and that he is not allowed to take a shower after gym. At school, the teacher instructs her pupils to define themselves as an individual in what is called the '*identity project*'. Milo is singled out by the teacher who says he must include baby pictures, but he says he has none, for his father lost them when they moved home. A boy in the classroom jokes that Milo can go to the zoo and take a photograph of a baby skunk instead. After Milo beats up the boy after class, his Romanian mother Nadia is called in to have a talk with the teacher. She is told that Milo will not be suspended, but the teacher advises the mother to encourage Milo to try to be more socially integrated and to make some friends. The upcoming school camping trip is an excellent occasion for this, but Milo's father Brand does not give his son permission to join his classmates. When the family visits Milo's grandfather, Lucas Mulder, Milo complains about his father's decision, and as always, his granddad is on his side. While Milo's parents are present, Lucas is very clear: '*He's going. No argument.*' He even hands him money for the trip and lends him his single-lens reflex camera, for Milo's own camera has been confiscated by his father. Later, Brand warns his son that his grandfather has no authority over him. Dismayed by this reprimand, Milo sneaks away the next day, but the school bus has already departed.

On his own, Milo is hit by a car in the dark, but he is uninjured. The driver, Star, takes him in her car. She and her boyfriend Mickey are an old hippie couple with a dog. In hiding from the police, they are squatting in an abandoned caravan at an old camp site near a cement factory where they dance to the song 'Back Home' by Golden Earring. Initially, Mickey is a bit grumpy towards the kid, but once he finds out the boy has quite a sum of money with him, he is no longer ill-disposed. Moreover, Mickey sees that Star is very attached to the boy, evoking motherly feelings in her. Despite the rough conditions, Milo feels quite comfortable with the couple. At the supermarket with Star, he gives her a bottle of perfume and buys himself many jars of cream, for he has lost his rucksack. One evening, he secretly sneaks out of the caravan through a window, and while covering his face with a hoodie, he phones his parents' home from a pub. His father picks up, and apart from wanting to know where Milo is, the only thing he says is: '*Don't let anyone see you, under no circumstances.*' When he repeats this command, Milo hangs up before he has revealed his location and before his mother can take over from his father.

In a subsequent scene, when Milo is back at the caravan, his skin condition becomes visible: the cream was meant to prevent hair from growing all over his face and body. Mickey and Star take it light-heartedly: there is no shame in our house, Mickey tells him. He adds that men with a lot of hair often have an '*enormous pecker*', but this joke is lost on the boy. It is clear to them that the boy dislikes his father, so Mickey tells him about the problems he had with his own tough dad, named Bulldog, who taught him to '*filch, to fight, and to f…*' Though Star hates to see the boy leave, it is also obvious to her that Milo—who has started to wear a balaclava—misses his mum. They decide to bring the boy home, but if he does not get a warm welcome, Mickey and Star promise to take him with them on a trip to Portugal. Mother Nadia is all too happy to take him back in, while father Brand gives his son a hug and hands the old hippies money for expenses. But the tension between Brand and Mickey is perceptible.

The two men are polar opposites. Mickey is unshaven and has a weatherworn face with unkempt hair; Brand is properly groomed and impeccably dressed. Mickey is a restless character, and in order to capture his movements, the camera is restless as well. At Brand's place, however, the camera is much more static. The house is designed according to the feng shui method to bring things in harmony with their surroundings ('*feng shui horseshit*', according to Milo's grandfather). Milo's parents always knew of their son's rare genetic condition, called hypertrichosis, which is an abnormal amount of hair growth on one's skin. While Milo was away, the father reminds his wife of their '*deliberate decision to keep him sheltered*'. Milo only knows that he has to use cream but not why, and Brand wants to disclose the details of his condition when his son has reached a more mature age. The father fears the kid will be bullied by his peers if they find out. When Milo is all wet with water while playing on a trampoline, Caitlin laughs. According to Milo, she was making fun of him, but Brand corrects him, for in the father's view, the girl next door was laughing at him because '*we are judged by others*' incessantly.

Brand is obsessed with appearances, and indeed, we see him suntanning in his solarium at the beginning of the film. He has built a business out of '*energizing your wealth area*', as he explains in his video using typical jargon; his ambition is to become an Irish version of Martha Stewart. He sells new bamboo fabric by Eco Skin, and in short web films, his wife and '*my wayward*' son are forced to confirm how fantastic the clothes are. Milo pulls them off as soon as the camera is off. The official reason the parents kept the hypertrichosis a secret is that they were doing so for the benefit of their son, but after Milo's return it becomes clear that it was only for the sake of Brand. Upon Nadia's suggestion, Milo decides to make a presentation on his condition for his school 'identity project', but when he starts rehearsing, Brand becomes angry. Maybe '*you want to be a laughingstock*', he yells at Milo, '*but I care*'. In turn, Nadia gets furious at her husband for his selfishness. He calls her a '*fucking gypsy*', whereupon she hits him in the face. He locks her up and drags Milo into the bathroom. He takes a razor and wants to shave his son's face, but when Brand looks into the mirror, he is suddenly paralyzed. Milo grabs the opportunity to run away and unlocks the room where his mother is. In the following scene, the father looks on passively from behind a glass door as mother and son put their luggage into the car. Cut to sunny Portugal, where Nadia and Milo show a photograph of Mickey and Star to the owner of a gas station. The man becomes furious, for this couple had left without paying for petrol, but in a final shot, Nadia and Milo drive away quickly to escape the man's anger.

Lacan postulates that when you look at yourself in the mirror, you see yourself as an external image. 'That's me' in the mirror is a primary response, but on second thought you realize that strange eyes are scrutinizing you: you become a visible object for this particular object. A mirror has no eyes, but it gazes at you nonetheless. Brand is convinced we can deceive this gaze: if you make a good impression in terms of how you look, your social identity is secured, for others will judge you as a decent guy. His belief in the feng shui method is an extension of this conviction: if architectural space is arranged properly and if furniture is placed 'correctly', one feels oneself in harmony with the environment. A hairy boy does not make a good impression, so in his perception, his son will be a social failure, a laughingstock. Milo's skin condition is all the more problematic for Brand since it is a genetic condition, inherited from his ancestors. Brand is probably so narrow-minded that he thinks it is due to the lineage from his Romanian wife, as his outburst '*fucking gypsy*' suggests, but as the father of this boy, he cannot be blameless himself. Since no one has seen the hair on the boy's body except for the hippies on the run, Brand can still introduce Milo into the social community as a 'normal' kid with a proper appearance. To prevent Milo from revealing his condition for his 'identity project' at school, Brand resorts to violence. His sudden glance at the mirror as he is about to aggressively cut the boy's facial hair with a sharp razor appears to be a moment of self-reflection. He interrupts his brutal action as if he realizes that this is no way to impose his authority—as a father, that is. The strange eyes in the mirror—and of the mirror—have caught him in the act. A man who always prides himself on being in harmony with his environment thanks to his Eco Skin clothes and his feng shui practice has exposed himself as irrational to his external image. The mirror reminds him of his own dictum that 'we are judged by others': now that he has been seen in the reflection, he feels exposed. Brand's look into the mirror seems to work like an eye-opener. Of course, you can deceive the gaze of the Other, for the mirror merely reflects appearances. Strike a pose for the mirror and that's how you are. But here he has been caught by his mirror-image, and the impression that he is a well-balanced father has been shattered now that his violent underside has been exposed. In MILO, mirror-images are practically banned to avoid further self-alienation, but what if you live in a world that is dominated by reflections in the mirror?

NO SHEIKS OF BAGHDAD: *GEBROKEN SPIEGELS*

GEBROKEN SPIEGELS [BROKEN MIRRORS] (Marleen Gorris, 1984) is Gorris's second feature after the international success of DE STILTE ROND CHRISTINE M. [A QUESTION OF SILENCE] (1982). Like JEANNE DIELMAN (Chantal Akerman, 1975), DIE BLEIERNE ZEIT [THE GERMAN SISTERS] (Margarethe von Trotta, 1981), and DUST (Marion Hänsel, 1985), her debut feature belongs to a series of movies about women who turn into angels of vengeance. Though there are no female killers in GEBROKEN SPIEGELS, Gorris's first two films owe their impact to the fact that they use the narrative codes of realism, Anneke Smelik argues, but the viewer is 'impelled to interpret their meanings metaphorically' (350). The seemingly gratuitous murder of a male boutique owner by three women in DE STILTE ROND CHRISTINE M. is a brutal and violent act, but if the viewer does not also take it as a 'female fantasy of revenge' upon men's 'hostile incomprehension' of the position of women in society, then one is 'excluded from the subversive laughter' of the female characters at the end (Smelik, 352-355).[10]

GEBROKEN SPIEGELS is split into two parts that alternate with one another. The film opens with a man carrying a body bag in a deserted area, but it is too dim to discern the contours of his face. When he puts the bag on the cold earth, we get a close-up of his gloves. He then takes a Polaroid camera from inside his coat and takes a picture. It is then revealed that the bag contains a dead woman. It will turn out that this first scene is part of a story, shot in desaturated colours, about a male serial killer who has the habit of chaining his female victims in a garage until they starve to death.[11] Pinned on the wall is a series of photographs that show three women in various stages of despair and fear, whereas each final picture of the series testifies to their passing away. The man abducts another woman, Bea, who keeps on asking what he wants from her, but the man remains silent. Then she suddenly decides to stop talking, and from that moment onwards, the man insists that she speak, promising her food and even her release if she utters another word, but Bea does not open her mouth again and will end up in a body bag. In a conventional narrative film, the viewer will come to understand 'what exactly gives the man pleasure or what makes the woman guilty' (Smelik, 359), but we never get a clear motivation in GEBROKEN SPIEGELS why the man holds the women in captivity and whether he has any criterion for selection except their sex: he does not touch them but only objectifies them in pictures. The perpetrator remains an enigma to us, for his face is consistently beyond the edges of the frame or he is shot from the back in long shots (and sometimes extreme long shots). We only know that, on the surface, the man is a 'decent' citizen who neatly arranges his pen and pencil at the office and is so helpful as to do some extra work for a colleague. When he comes home from work, his wife has prepared him a dinner as usual.

The second story, which is intertwined with the one about the serial killer, takes up a bigger part of the film and is about prostitutes working in a brothel called Happy House. In an early scene of about one minute, we see the women together, and the 'manually operated camera starts moving on its own in the cramped drawing room, in an almost dancelike choreography' (Smelik, 356). The harmonious mood is interrupted when the doorbell announces the arrival of the first customer: 'The music stops, the camera comes to a standstill and the women remain motionless for just a second before moving into action' (ibid.). This scene marks the transition from the women as subjects with their everyday joys and concerns into pin-ups as objects of the male look, surrounded by mirrors.

Dora, who is considering quitting, is particularly sarcastic of the profession and she hopes that men who refuse to use rubbers will soon 'piss razorblades' as a punishment for their stubbornness. To Irma, who is watching herself in a mirror, she says: 'You are a unique beauty, especially your thighs, the more they're seen, the better.' This quote succinctly explains why the brothel is almost a house of mirrors. Their function may seem imaginary, for the women have to see for themselves whether they look fabulous and, if necessary, they dress themselves up or put on some extra make-up. However, since they are doing so in order to attract the attention of male customers, the function of mirrors in the brothel is basically symbolic: an appealing appearance is required, for the women are constantly subjected to the eroticizing looks of men with money in their pockets. When Dora is explaining the rules and tricks of the business to newcomer Diane, she is clear that emotions should be withheld for the single purpose of money-making: one has to make the john feel as if he is the 'Sheik of Baghdad'. Due to this hierarchical situation in which the customer is king, the women tend to be humiliated. The men who visit Happy House are 'assholes', Dora informs Diane, and 'even the kind ones are not kind'. When the depressed Linda hangs herself in the brothel, Irma puts a towel over a mirror as a sign of mourning, a habit adopted from her grandmother. Francine, slightly annoyed by the homage to Linda, pulls the towel off, causing the mirror to fall from the wall and break.

Francine's annoyance was also triggered by the fact that Linda had 'stolen' her best client, for this man had always been polite and paid her well for a 'quick screw'. This 'polite' customer who visits the brothel regularly happens to be in Happy House when a dreadful accident takes place: Irma is severely cut with a knife by a psychotic john. While Irma is badly injured, the 'polite' man takes her to the hospital in the company of both Dora and Diane. Upon their return to the brothel, the women tell their colleagues that Irma is seriously disfigured and will probably remain blind in one eye. Hearing the news, Francine is not in the mood for work, and her customer gives in to her request to come back another time. It is part of the women's business to switch off their emotions, but they are clearly taken aback by the incident. One man, the 'polite' one who had been driving Irma to the hospital, does not leave, however. We see him in a medium-shot profile while some prostitutes are visible in a mirror on the wall. One of the women thanks him for his help, but the man does not make a move. It is a most remarkable shot composition, for at this very moment when the distressed women want to take a break from their job, their being framed in the mirror indicates that they are cornered. The shot indicates that the man demands their service anytime: a woman in a brothel has a strictly objectified status and is no more than a man's tool. We get a close-up of the man's gloves and he then takes his wallet from inside his coat to show how dearly he wants to pay the woman who will offer him sexual pleasure. Only at this point do we fully realize that this man, Francine's favourite customer, is the serial killer, for the way he pulls off his gloves and takes his wallet from inside his coat is an exact formal repetition of the shots in the opening scene when he took the Polaroid camera to photograph the dead woman.

The fact that the man does not make a sound is reminiscent of the way he treats the chained women: as long as they talked and begged, he remained silent. We now also get a few shots of his occiput, which we have also seen frequently in the 'other' story. Once it is revealed that the friendliest customer is the serial killer who is so keen on objectifying women, the shot of the women in the mirror on the wall a few moments ago gains significance, as if this particular framing should be equated with the visually recorded mistreatment in the garage. The representation of the women via the mirror on the wall underscores the function that in the man's mind, they have to serve him regardless of the circumstances. The difference, however, is that these women have a work ethos of making men believe they are the 'sheik of Baghdad', but they are not chained. As 'Fac me vere tecum flere' from Joseph Haydn's *Stabat Mater* sets in, Diane takes a gun from a desk and fires a bullet at him, deliberately only creating a flesh wound to scare him off. She then shoots three more times, breaking three mirrors. Asked whether she will come back to Happy House, Diane answers 'No, never!', whereupon Dora departs with her. Strictly speaking, the mirror is identified with the imaginary order and gives one the opportunity to judge one's own appearance: the mirror is a tool to articulate one's self-identity even though, as mentioned before, this always-already is a form of self-alienation: 'I see myself in the mirror, but that's not me (but my reflection).' But the shot that frames the women in the mirror is a powerful reminder that in the world of the brothel, appearances exclusively serve the purpose of man's desires and that no situation is exempted from the rule that men such as this presumedly friendly customer confine women to a symbolic cage. In bringing the two storylines together at the end, the viewer has to take the cracking of mirrors as a 'ritualistic act of resistance' against imprisonment (Smelik, 362): we are invited to note the resemblances between the working conditions in the brothel as a house of mirrors and the way the unfortunate housewife in the thriller story is chained and photographed.

Significantly, there is one really friendly man in GEBROKEN SPIEGELS. Every day on her way to work, Dora walks past a barrack with no windows. An old man named André often hears her pass by, or he correctly guesses it must be Dora. He starts talking to her, and she stops to listen to his stories. Though his words make little sense, Dora often has a smile on her face. A neighbour leans outside her window with a disapproving look on her face, but Dora waves at her to scare her off,. The neighbour pulls back, shy because Dora makes explicit eye contact. It articulates why Dora takes pleasure in the nonsensical conversations with André: there is no visual register, let alone a hall of mirrors. Here she escapes visualisation, and she is really disconcerted when she finds out one day that, as a consequence of complaints from the neighbour, André's shack has been torn down.

THE AMBIGUITY OF (AN) AVATAR: *R U THERE*

Whereas the shooting of the mirrors by Diane in GEBROKEN SPIEGELS is a form of resistance against symbolic confinement, the mirror scenes in R U THERE (David Verbeek, 2010) are characterized by a striking inarticulateness.

The twenty-year-old Jitze stays in a large hotel room in busy Taipei, for he is part of a computer game team that participates in tournaments all over the world. Despite the presence of his teammates, he is often isolated in shots. We see him doing physical exercises in the gym or listening to music, cutting himself off from his environment. We get many close-ups of his face focused on the computer screen, while a huge crowd can watch him play his first-person shooting game. A recurring device is that we either see Jitze in sharp focus and his environment quite shallow, or the other way around. In several long takes, the camera just follows Jitze from behind, and this also happens in the key scene of R U THERE. Jitze, dressed in black and in sharp focus, is about to go outside, on his way to a sushi bar. We can hardly discern the environment, but the noise of the streets is clearly audible. In a subsequent shot, the camera tracks forward, first predominantly showing the sky, then tilting down to show heavy traffic. Then there is a sudden cut and once again the camera tracks forward to a crossroads, but now it turns out, as a token of the viewer's disorientation, that Jitze is approaching from the other side of the street. The camera slowly zooms in while cars and buses pass by, obstructing our view of Jitze. Then we hear a sound of a crash and the camera follows a scooter slipping over the asphalt that has lost its driver. In a reverse shot, the camera then very slowly pans to the left, gradually centralizing a flabbergasted Jitze, whereas the noise in the street is about to die away. The pan continues until Jitze is central in the shot, and then the camera very slowly zooms in on his face. There is a cut to an over-the-shoulder shot: Jitze's occiput is in shallow focus, and the camera zooms in slowly onto a woman with a helmet on her head. She is lying on the asphalt, motionless, and her eyes stare right at Jitze, but he seems paralyzed. As soon as there is blood on her face, a reverse shot zooms in on Jitze again—very slowly once more—and he even seems to take a small step back instead of coming to the woman's assistance. Shown over Jitze's shoulder, there are people bending over the unfortunate woman. Only then does Jitze continue his walk and the street sounds become a cacophony again.

Jitze wants to give the impression that the incident has not affected him. In one of the subsequent shots, he watches himself in the huge mirror in his room after a shower, but we only see his usual blank facial expression. When a virtual soldier on his computer screen falls down in the exact same position as the woman in the street, however, his reaction is too slow and his avatar goes down, and one might presume that his loss is not unrelated to the incident. The fact that his right arm is in pain has the advantage that he asks the Taiwanese girl Min Min whom he fancies to give him a massage for money. He continues to socialize with her and also meets her in the virtual reality world of Second Life, which Min Min describes as the best place to relax: she is a fairy; his avatar is a soldier. When Min Min wants to pay her family a visit, he offers her money whereupon she permits him to accompany her to her small hometown. At the end of R U THERE, Jitze is back in Taipei and he and his teammates are congratulated on their success in the computer game. Jitze is a bit hesitant to share in the celebration of the victory. There is a cut to Second Life once more, where Jitze's avatar is totally naked amidst an empty, paradisiac landscape near the sea. Then there is a shot transition to the crossroads, practically deserted this time. Shown via a high-angle, Jitze walks towards the spot where the woman had been lying on the street. This time, he does kneel down and, with the camera close to him, we see him touch the street with his fingers. In a subsequent Second Life scene he is dressed in modern clothes, and when the fairy comes along, she compliments the avatar on his outfit and wishes Jitze a safe trip. In the airplane, Jitze gets up from his seat, walks through the aisle, opens the door, looks over his shoulder with a smile on his face, and then steps out into the open air.

There are quite a number of mirror scenes in R U THERE, but they are all in between the incident and Jitze's return to the very same spot. It would be tempting to suggest that being a witness to the immediate aftermath of the accident has made Jitze more self-reflexive and that his encounter with Min Min and the subsequent visit to the countryside, with its river, mountains, and woods, has made him re-appreciate the materiality of Mother Earth over virtual worlds. R U THERE, however, does not really support such a reading, if only because its protagonist does not give up gaming and keeps on returning to Second Life. As a gamer who has travelled the world, Jitze is so enwrapped in what director David Verbeek calls 'a-cultural non-places'[12] (qtd. in Graveland) like hotel lobbies, airports, and security sites that the accident is a derailment of his daily pattern and it is too difficult to process what impact it really has on him. Traditionally, the mirror is regarded as an object for self-reflection, but not here. R U THERE shows us the biggest mirrors in such 'non-places' as the hotel elevator, his room, and the public bathroom in which he only expresses his frustration after a poor gaming performance. With mirrors in such non-distinct spots, it is no wonder that Jitze remains quite self-alienated throughout the film until the very end. The mere fact that he returns to the spot and touches the asphalt gives us the idea that it has affected him somehow. But the viewer is given no more than that, and it remains ambiguous whether it causes any substantial change in him. Insofar as we might take the last shot as a dream-thought about a suicide attempt, we could also say that it refers to the moment that the fairy in Second Life encourages Jitze's avatar to use the fly button.

It is a staple in many fiction films that mirror shots articulate a character's increasing self-awareness, but in Verbeek's film, they seem to hint at Jitze's self-alienation, which would be more in line with Lacanian psychoanalysis. I use the modest term 'hint' here, for the elliptical storytelling and the lack of clear-cut causality due to the protagonist's blank expression throughout R U THERE prevent the viewer from drawing such definite conclusions. His interest in Second Life can be a form of what Sherry Turkle describes as 'acting out':[13] he could be so ashamed of his apathy that he wants to escape into a virtual world. Turkle distinguishes this escapist logic from 'working through', a trajectory advocated by psychoanalysis: by looking at himself in the mirror, Jitze realizes he has to address his issues. What is too unbearable for him in 'real life' is then projected onto one's avatar. This virtual double becomes the container for the subject's repressed content. The mask/identity assumed in Second Life is then closer to one's 'being' than the face he spots in the mirror in real life. The barrier between a virtual landscape and the ordinariness of existence has been shallow throughout: a shot of a computer game also contains the white ceiling of the actual space, as if these two worlds easily merge together. For that reason, the status and function of Second Life remains unclear: is it a means to help Jitze gain a grip on reality, or does he aim to refashion his identity, preferring a virtual world over the actual one?

When Jitze looks at himself in the mirror, it is a moment of imaginary deception: this is how I present myself, but this is not who I am. At the end of Verbeek's film, Jitze is a member of a successful gaming team, but we know he feels lost but cannot give vent to his particular emotions. In Second Life, the domain of symbolic deception, he can take on the guise of a hero (wishful thinking) or of a doubter (disclosing his actual despair), but it is indecipherable what option he chooses in the end.[14] Does Second Life offer him an escape route or is it a domain that helps him to articulate his despair?

Virtual reality can, Žižek postulates, bring to light underlying fantasies: it makes present what is evaded in 'real life'. This may seem like a beneficial effect, but as psychoanalysis teaches us, it can be most nauseating when one's innermost fantasies are exposed in full. Virtual reality can be so obscene because, to quote Žižek, the 'phantasmatic intimate kernel of our being is laid bare (...) as a depthless surface' (*Plague*, 163-164). There is an inevitable distance between the subject's public symbolic identity (one may present oneself as a decent citizen) and his fantasies (one may wish to violate women), but the assumption is that this gap will be closed in cyberspace, for in a virtual world of almost total availability, 'everything will be written' (Žižek *Plague*, 164).[15] In order to explain the downside of this exposure, the Lacanian Real as the third of the three Orders must be introduced.

TRAVERSING THE FANTASY

The Real is at the heart of the symbolic order, but there is no language to adequately address the Real. On the cover of the 1973 French edition as well as the 1981 English translation of Lacan's seminar *The Four Fundamental Concepts of Psychoanalysis*, there is a reproduction of Hans Holbein's painting *The Ambassadors* (1533). Two well-dressed dignitaries are proudly posing among a variety of cultural accoutrements representing scientific and artistic achievements of the day—a clock, a globe, musical instruments—and this painting confirms the symbolic recognition attributed to them. Staring at the painter, however, the two men overlook a strangely shaped object at their feet, which is clearly visible to the viewer. It is an anamorphically depicted death skull, and if we were to see this skull in its correct form—e.g. via a lens that corrects the anamorphic distortion—then the entire cultural order would disintegrate. Obviously, accessing the impossible order of the Real is far from recommendable, and the role of our fantasies is to function as a protective shield against the utterly gruesome scenario that would be unleashed by a hypothetical confrontation with the Real. So fantasy does not trigger our wildest imagination in a Lacanian framework but is meant to prevent the subject from falling into a psychotic derailment: fantasy is on the side of the symbolic order and works to guarantee a safe distance from the Real.[16]

The function of fantasies is to keep the social order running, and they obfuscate what is potentially subversive. Žižek gives the example of an English publicity spot from the 1990s for a brand of beer in which a girl finds a frog. When she kisses the amphibian, the frog transforms into a beautiful young man. Her dream has come true, but then he starts to kiss her—and she turns into a bottle of beer. Žižek uses the spot to underscore Lacan's dictum that there is no sexual relationship. In terms of our social order, we have the familiar fantasy of the happy 'boy and girl' couple, but as the publicity spot suggests, this fantasy is a false illusion: whereas the woman favours a handsome man, any man apparently prefers an object—one that he can preferably share with his mates. This asymmetry, Žižek claims, exposes that a fantasy is supported by an inconsistent underside, in this case the figure of *a frog embracing a bottle of beer* ('Cyberspace', 509-510). In the symbolic network, fantasies function as logical cover-ups for inherent contradictions: even though we know that many marriages end up in divorce, we still tend to believe that both bride and bridegroom regard their wedding as the best day in their lives. Even though soldiers may occasionally go overboard in their violent behaviour, we still think they are disciplined and determined. Even when we know from experience that the judge is a nasty person, we still pay him respect when he enters the court in his toga.

One of the stakes of psychoanalysis is what Lacan called *la traversée du fantasme*, traversing the fantasy.[17] Surrealist art has the tendency to reproduce fantasies in all their inconsistencies. The Belgian painter René Magritte highlights the treachery of images, and he does so with a good sense of humour. According to the artist, a face is by definition a 'false mirror': 'Everything we see hides another thing' is one of his famous quotes, meaning that there is always a gap between the surface and the 'identity' underneath. There is a photograph titled *Le barbare* [*The Barbarian*] (1938) of Magritte himself with a bowler hat, posing with a hand on his chin, and next to him there is a painting—which looks like a mirror—of a man against a brick wall who is striking the same pose but wearing an eye-mask and a high hat. A key impression is that the reproduction on the right reveals the true barbaric nature of the man on the left—Magritte—whose appearance is so civilized. Similar to this example of painting, surrealist poetry 'was no longer to be an expression of ideas or emotions but the creation of a series of images', according to Anna Balakian (143). The function of a surrealist poem is to give its reader sight, and the vocabulary should be 'concrete in shape and colo[u]r, in texture and intent' (144). This is all quite conventional, but what is unorthodox about it is the 'unexpected linking of words' (147) in order to convey extraordinary if not incompatible mental images. André Breton wrote a poem with the lines 'I love you on the surface of seas / Red like the egg when it is green' (qtd. in Balakian, 152). It is a grammatically correct sentence written in the present tense with simple verbs (love, is), but the visualization of this phrase is beyond logic, laying bare a disparity between a 'normal' perception and a 'vital' one. Surrealist poetry has the habit of creating strange encounters between the images—such as Breton's 'a silver plate on a cobweb' (qtd. in Balakian, 149)—in order to trigger the unconscious to see the world from a new vantage point. The poets contended that by observing objects afresh, worldly phenomena were revealed more fully, and thus, as Breton hoped, people would feel the need to 'transform the world, change life' (qtd. in Balakian, 49). For the poets, absurdity as such was not a goal, but they intended to suggest that there is more 'truth' in bizarre or hallucinatory imagery than in prevalent conventional visuality, which was their way of traversing the fantasy.

I would like to refer to Luigi Pirandello's modernist novel *Uno, nessuno e centomila* [*One, No One and One Hundred Thousand*] (1926) for an additional example of 'traversing the fantasy', since the mirror plays such a pivotal role in detecting maddening inconsistencies in the symbolic network. The novel starts with a 28-year-old man, Vitangelo Moscarda, who is scrutinizing his face in the mirror when his wife says that the right side of his nose is a little lower than the left side. Moscarda is astonished, even more so when his wife mentions some other slight physical defects—eyebrows, ears, a little finger—and she is right about them, too. All these years he has not known his own body, and from that moment onwards, he thinks that when people are watching him, they are staring at his shortcomings. They are so obvious that of course everyone has seen them already, and he concludes: 'I was not for others what up to then I had inwardly pictured myself as being.' He then points out to a friend that he has a dimple in his chin, and the friend is amazed at this fact. Moscarda imagines that he sets a chain in motion and that his fellow citizens will soon use the mirror reflections of shop windows to study the slightly weird details of their appearance that they had not been aware of until recently. Thereupon a man asks Moscarda whether he knew he had a peculiar bobtail at the back of his neck, invisible to him in a normal mirror, and this question confirms that the 'someone' Moscarda thought he was does not exist: 'If I was not for others what up to then I had believed myself to be to myself, what was I?' He has discovered 'a certain stranger (...) *inseparable from me*'. For Moscarda, he can never be one person, for when he looks into the mirror, 'I (...) did not see myself, but was seen; and the other person, similarly, did not see himself, but saw my face and saw himself being looked at by me.' He wants to discover the stranger in himself 'with my very own eyes, (...) as if I were another', but this will be an impossible endeavour, which results in total self-alienation. The harder he tries, the more he realizes that he is no more than a 'poor, mortified body, waiting for someone to take it'. He ends his experiences in front of the mirror in his 'first madman's smile'.

If he is someone for his wife, someone else for his best friend, and again someone else for a third, he in fact becomes one hundred thousand somebodies. The net result of this multiplication is not 'a *more* but a *less*': for himself, Moscarda can only be no one. In the final part of Pirandello's novel, titled 'No Conclusion', Moscarda has gone to live in the open country and no longer cares about his appearance. He has stopped glancing in mirrors. The name 'Moscarda' has become irrelevant to him, just an 'epigraph'. The final sentence reads: 'I am dying every instant, and being born anew and without memories: alive and whole, no longer in myself, but in everything outside.'

Moscarda in *Uno, nessuno e centomila* verges on the brink of madness due to an over-identification with his mirror image. He has become perceptible to any detail he had missed on previous glances in the mirror, and he can only prevent himself from going crazy by withdrawing from symbolic etiquettes: living like a recluse, he no longer cares about his appearance, and names have become insignificant to him. The reflections in the novel testify to the fact that he has detected the inherent inconsistencies in the social system. According to Moscarda, his identity is not made up of the sum total of his characteristics—from facial features to his mood swings—instead, he is nothing because he cannot see himself as anyone else sees him. He wants to study his movements and his facial expressions by taking himself by surprise—in a mirror or a shop window—but he is always already too conscious of himself, and thus his actions seem unnatural and feigned. Moscarda can only be seen for who he is with eyes that are not his own. His reflections upon the inconsistency of his self-image are the polar opposite of the illusions of the majority of current users on social media that they can master how the public sees them: since they themselves can decide what they post on the internet, they can present themselves as 'shiny, happy people'. They live according to the fantasy that, to paraphrase the Freddy Mercury character in BOHEMIAN RHAPSODY (Bryan Singer, 2018), 'I decide who I am' (in his case: a born performer, born 'to give the people what they want'). By contrast, Moscarda has become all too aware that this fantasy is impossible. Traversing the fantasy equals the acknowledgement that one can never truly 'know thyself', for there is always an unfathomable stranger within us.

A TALE OF TWO SISTERS: *ZWART WATER*

A genre that can be said to be on the verge of traversing the fantasy is horror, and for that reason, Žižek is always particularly fond of using horror movies as examples. This film genre usually explores the limits of representation, offering the suggestion of a look into the abyss of the Real. In horror films, characters risk peeping through a glass darkly, so to speak, and can have the uncanny experience of meeting a stranger as part of themselves. In Dutch cinema, horror has never been a versatile genre, despite some proverbial exceptions: in the 1980s, two films by Dick Maas—DE LIFT [THE LIFT] (1983) and AMSTERDAMNED (1988)—proved to be both well-crafted and popular horror-thrillers, whereas the most noteworthy '*nederhorror*' film in the 1990s is the occult DE JOHNSONS [THE JOHNSONS] (Rudolf van den Berg, 1992). Since 2006, there has been a modest revival of *nederhorror*, with a few films that have had a big screen release, such as DOOD EIND [DEAD END] (Erwin van den Eshof, 2006), SL8N8 [SLAUGHTER NIGHT] (Frank van Geloven and Edwin Visser, 2006), the zombie-comedy ZOMBIBI [KILL ZOMBIE!] (Erwin van den Eshof and Martijn Smits, 2011), and DE POEL [THE POOL] (Chris W. Mitchell, 2014). One may call BUMPERKLEEF (Lodewijk Crijns, 2019), the comic slasher SNEEKWEEK [SCREAM WEEK] (Martijn Heijne, 2016), and the Nazi-zombie flick FRANKENSTEIN'S ARMY (Richard Raaphorst, 2013) as 'the good, the bad and the ugly' of nederhorror.[18] Only one film by Maas far exceeded all these films in box-office numbers: SINT [SAINT] (2010) with 335,662 cinemagoers.[19] An underrated movie of that same year, ZWART WATER [TWO EYES STARING],[20] directed by Elbert van Strien, was a psychological thriller with clear influences from horror.

The protagonist in ZWART WATER is the nine-year-old Lisa whose parents Paul and Christine inherit an isolated villa in Belgium. The enormous residence belonged to Christine's mother, and although Christine did not have any contact with her for many years, she is entitled to the mansion because her name is mentioned in the will. They decide to move there because it will save them rent and Paul is anxious to renovate the dilapidated place. Lisa is the internal focalizer in the majority of scenes, and we understand that she used to have an imaginary figure called Domlook: a child's drawing above her bed identifies Domlook as a 'liefe vrient' (a misspelling of 'dear friend'). Lisa, who has no siblings, is made to feel at home in her new environment and is given a rabbit named Daisy. Meanwhile, Lisa sneaks around in the attic and in the cellar and comes across an old diary that mentions Christine's twin sister Karen and the fact that no one is able to tell the two apart. In huge letters, Christine writes in the diary that she wishes that Karen were dead.

In the encounters Lisa has with the ghostlike apparition of the young teenage girl Karen, she is informed that Christine is responsible for Karen's premature death. Karen tells Lisa: 'Every time she looks at you, she is reminded of me, and she realizes what she has done to me', a sentence that resonates in Lisa's mind. She tells her father about how Karen was murdered, but he is puzzled by the account and thinks that she has turned her imaginary friend Domlook into a more morbid version. When he asks Christine about it, she replies that she has never had a sister. In a conversation with Lisa, Karen insists that her twin sister is like the evil stepmother from fairytales, and under the spell of the deceased girl, Lisa commits all kinds of seemingly irrational acts—tearing apart her mother's fashion drawings, cutting off the hair of dolls, and killing her rabbit. But while Lisa has become suspicious of her mother, the misgivings are mutual: Christine tells her husband that she thinks that Lisa is keen on killing her. At this point, however, we can wonder to what extent Lisa is still Lisa. While Lisa is lying on the floor, we see how a superimposed Karen has entered her body. Intercut with shots from a dreamlike meeting between Karen and Lisa in a cornfield, the child poisons the tea that her mother thereupon drinks. At the funeral of her mother, Lisa sees a wreath with a ribbon that says 'sweet sister ... Karen', which confuses her. Then Christine's nephew Geert discloses to Paul that the twin sister is still alive, but the two had avoided each other due to 'bad memories'. Paul then searches for Karen and meets a total look-alike of his wife, except that her hair is slightly different and darker. They used to do everything together, Karen tells him, but at one point Christine believed that her sister had stolen her personality and from that moment onwards, they both wanted the other dead. Christine started by cutting Karen's hair; Karen took revenge by stabbing her sister with a fork. When Christine prepared poisoned liquorice water, it almost killed Karen, and they parted ways for good.

Given this plot summary, one can attempt to make sense of where the spooky prologue scene fits into the narrative. We see the back of Lisa's head as she sits on a swing, moving it only slightly; her mother is out of focus and is reading a book and smoking a cigarette on a bench. Over the squeaky sound of the swing, we hear Lisa's voice-over: 'I remember how she looked at me ...', and it is barely visible how the mother, still out of focus, looks up from her book. 'There was something', and then there is a cut to Lisa on the right side of the frame in a room. 'She had seen something', and as Lisa moves forward, the camera makes a quarter-circle around her so that we have an over-the-shoulder shot of Lisa facing herself in a mirror with two smaller side-mirrors. 'Maybe it was that I always wanted to be near her', we hear her say as the camera slowly zooms in on Lisa's face in the mirror. Then the camera cuts to Lisa opening a door. The reverse shot, with the door post out of focus on the right side of the frame, shows Christine in front of the very same mirror, removing her lipstick. 'She never said anything about it', and while the shots alternate between a zoom-in on Christine and a zoom-in on Lisa, standing on the threshold, the voice-over continues: 'she always acted as if everything was all right'. Christine, looking at Lisa via the mirror, winks at her daughter, whom we see smile at her mother in a reverse-shot. Then there is a sudden cut to Lisa, once again in front of the mirror. There is a lengthy but slow zoom-in onto Lisa's face, while keeping visible one part of a side-mirror that shows half of her face. In the meantime, we hear her say: 'Each time I watch myself in the mirror I knew, there is another who looks at me. Was I me, was I not her? Who was that girl that resembled me so much?' And while the suspenseful music increases in volume, the screen goes to black before the begin credits start. Does this prologue precede the first scene of the film (which suggests that there was already something wrong between mother and daughter), or does it take place after the meeting with the spectral apparition of Karen (which may be more plausible from the point of view of the plot but it would mean that the prologue deviates from the chronological order of the film)?

Lisa's voice-over opens with the intuition that her mother has observed her in a special manner. This seems hardly worrisome, initially, for Lisa says that their bond is close: children often long for their mother's proximity, and a mother is in many ways all too happy to give in to that longing. But apparently it is not quite all right, for her mother is only pretending, Lisa's voice-over continues, and though she smiles at the wink her mother gives her, she doubts the sincerity of their relationship. Then there is a change in tone when the camera zooms in on Lisa's face in the mirror: she wonders whether there is another person looking at her when she sees herself. In other words, her mirror image belongs to someone else; her face is only a cover-up. Strictly speaking, this can be taken as the ultimate consequence of Lacanian alienation: in the mirror I see a most ideal version of me, implying that I am an other. But here it is not a more perfect exemplar of one's self; we can say in retrospect that in ZWART WATER, Lisa presumes that she might be (or be like) Karen, that her resemblance to the ghostlike twin sister is uncannily close. However, there is no Karen—at least, no one but Lisa can observe her. Focalized by Lisa, Karen is hanging in the cellar, but mediated by her father's look, there is nothing but an empty wall. The young kid Peter does not mention Karen when he is walking in the attic, though she is plain to see for Lisa. So if Lisa recognizes Karen as her alter ego in the mirror, there is no symbolic acknowledgement of Christine's twin sister at all. At best, one can say that Lisa has a 'sixth sense' for Karen's existence,[21] which puts the girl in limbo between the imaginary and the Real. The mirror in the prologue scene cannot produce her image, so Karen is beyond symbolization: the world of the visible can only produce a 'blind spot' that looks back at Lisa, which is a proper description of the gaze that haunts us.

Ontologically, she is either a figment of Lisa's imagination or a ghost with whom Lisa has conversations, as if for real. Insofar as Lisa does not see herself in the mirror but sees herself as if she is Karen, she has a glimpse beyond the order of symbolization: she sees someone who might have taken 'possession' of her, as we effectively see happen in one of the scenes. The idea that a spectral Karen might have entered Lisa's body is confirmed by the fact that Karen whispers the very same phrases from Lisa's prologue—'Was I me, was I not her? Who was that girl that resembled me so much?'—while we see an overhead shot of the two climbing a spiral staircase. Since it is not possible to determine when the prologue scene took place, it cannot be determined who is aping whom. Could it be that Lisa is the originator of the vivid imagination from which Karen has materialized as a phantom lady?[22] Or is Lisa in fact a ventriloquist, speaking Karen's words in front of the mirror, just as she poisons her mother's tea under the influence of Karen, who had reassured Lisa by promising: 'If you let me in your dreams, everything will be all right.' In that case, Lisa was no more than a vehicle for Karen's yearning to take revenge upon her sister, and as a tool of a vengeful ghost, she 'cannot help what has happened', as her unwitting father says to console her after Christine's death.[23]

CONCLUSION: THROUGH A GLASS DARKLY

In this chapter I have related Lacan's three orders to particular mirror scenes in Dutch films. It started with the idea of the look-alike in the case of ALS TWEE DRUPPELS WATER, which implied a transition from the imaginary to the symbolic: Ducker sees a resemblance in appearance, so he wants to be like

Dorbeck. In SÜSKIND, the process was reversed: the protagonist sees himself with the Star of David pinned on his coat as a token of his symbolic identity, but the shattered mirror image indicates that he refuses to imagine himself as a submissive Jew. In both RIPHAGEN and MILO, images in which the title characters look into a mirror are avoided, but for different reasons. In the first film, the absence of reflections—mirror reflections or self-reflection—parallels the protagonist's lack of moral principles. In the second film, the father wants to protect his son from an inferiority complex, but in fact it is the father himself who has the complex. His son's skin problem clashes with his idea of himself as a successful man/entrepreneur/father. In an attempt to disavow responsibility for his son's disease, he projects it onto his wife and her Romanian ('gypsy') descent, which understandably upsets her.

In GEBROKEN SPIEGELS, the prostitutes work in a brothel that is full of mirrors to remind them that their appearances are much more important than their identities. The shattered glass is a sign of Diane's wish to no longer be judged by how they look but instead to be taken seriously. Triggered by the disrespectful whoremonger, they refuse to be pinned down as objects of male desire. In R U THERE, the successful gamer Jitze is so numbed after he has witnessed an accident that he takes a leap into the virtual world of Second Life, since the many mirrors are not enough for him to realize self-reflection. Whether he is detached because of the mirrors or despite them is a question that remains unanswered in Verbeek's film, just as we do not know whether Second Life is an escape route for him or whether the virtual world really does confront him with his apathy in daily life and thus function as a token of his despair.

ZWART WATER is positioned at the opposite end of the spectrum from ALS TWEE DRUPPELS WATER, though they nonetheless have much in common. In Rademakers' film, both Ducker and Dorbeck stand before a mirror in one and the same shot, with Ducker seeing his spitting image as his ego-ideal. In Van Strien's film, the tables are turned: beneath the benign and common appearance of the young girl Lisa lurks an avenging force that makes the girl commit evil deeds. Lisa has a hunch that someone might take advantage of her resemblance to that other girl, and she looks into the mirror to detect the parasite, or to refer to Holbein's *The Ambassadors*, to experience whether she can see the death skull in its non-anamorphic form. In both films, symbolic acknowledgement was an insurmountable obstacle. Nothing could prove Dorbeck's existence and thus, people took him to be no more than a product of Ducker's wish fulfilment. Likewise, nothing could prove that there was indeed a 'girl in the cellar', especially since Karen has not died at all, and thus it was presumed that Lisa had been 'possessed' by a dark spirit—from a realm beyond symbolization and therefore invisible in the mirror.

In the mother-daughter confrontation in ZWART WATER, Lisa's father is reduced to the role of a mediator who is slow to comprehend what is going on around him. When he hears things from Lisa, he tells them to his wife, but he does not realize that this might create an explosive situation. When he tells people at work that strange things are happening to his daughter, a bespectacled colleague tells him that people can enter into contact with the dead: 'Our mind is like a house: when a room becomes empty, who comes to occupy it?' Paul is too down-to-earth to understand that his daughter could be a victim of her sensitivity, but it is just such level-headedness that puts a man at a disadvantage within the genre of the psychological horror—just like the unfortunate John Baxter in DON'T LOOK NOW (Nicholas Roeg, 1973) who is punished for his lack of affinity with what he pejoratively calls 'mumbo jumbo'. He does not realize that he is a psychic who is capable of having previsions, and this leads him astray, with fatal consequences. In the next chapter I will illustrate that such a father, one who is oblivious to practically everything, is emblematic of the pitiful father figures in Dutch post-war cinema.

NOTES

1 The mirror stage as formative of the 'I' is discussed in Lacan *Écrits: A Selection*, 1-5, among others.
2 In his detailed analysis of ALS TWEE DRUPPELS WATER, René van Uffelen also considers the four consecutive close-ups as Ducker's entry into his fantasy world (30). Moreover, a much quicker succession of jump cuts is employed later in the film when Ducker first sets eyes on Marianne: the camera jumps forward in two shots from long shot to extreme close-up of her face.
3 A child is gradually confronted with many cultural do's and even more don'ts, and it learns to understand that it is not the centre of the universe but part of a family or community.
4 Of course, a subject will never develop into this ego-ideal, except when he suffers from narcissistic disorders. A psychosis can result in delusions of grandeur.
5 The fourth scene is the one in which Ducker meets Marianne for the first time because she is supposed to dye his hair black.
6 Burke notes that the credits in ALS TWEE DRUPPELS WATER appear 'erratically [...] on the screen in either white or black text, or both—a pointer to the Ducker/Dorbeck duality at the core of the film' (117).
7 This Dutch expression is the equivalent of the phrase 'Like two peas in a pod.'
8 I will also discuss this notion of enjoyment in chapter nine in relation to ELLE, FLESH + BLOOD, and BRIMSTONE.

9 MILO is the debut feature of the brothers Berend and Roel Boorsma. Until this film they had made primarily video clips (among others for the successful Dutch rock band Lois Lane), commercials, and the short BRAT (2008).

10 For a lengthy discussion of DE STILTE ROND CHRISTINE M. see Verstraten *Humour and Irony*, 38-40.

11 Smelik remarks: 'The bleak colour scheme indicates that the "black-and-white" story is metaphorical in its extremity' (358).

12 'cultuurloze non-plekken'.

13 '[I]t helps to distinguish between what psychologists call acting out and working through. In acting out, you take the conflicts you have in the physical real and express them again and again in the virtual. There is much repetition and little growth. In working through, you use the materials of online life to confront the conflict of the real and search for new resolutions' (Turkle, 214).

14 This point about imaginary and symbolic deception is mentioned by Žižek in *Plague* (139).

15 Back in the late 1990s, Žižek hypothesized that with cyberspace, the play of (symbolic) appearances gives way to an (imaginary) simulacrum because of the total availability on the internet ('Cyberspace', 485). Before the advent of the digital, a selected number of photographs was made of the important moments in one's life: one was still very careful about what to show and, especially, what not to show. Nowadays, however, an unlimited number of pictures are produced and posted: everything is made visible on the internet or in the cloud. But because the web has been turned into a container of an endless bricolage of images, every (addicted or professional) user of social media may think that he or she creates self-stylized images, but it is unpredictable how an anonymous crowd will appropriate and use them. Now that 'Oedipus' as the key representative of the analogue world has gone online, the 'pacifying' function of the paternal figure—the symbolic father—has evaporated and the primordial father has been able to return: internet has become the domain of the big-mouthed political leaders and sexual harassers (Žižek 'Cyberspace', 491).

16 The Imaginary's role is supplementary to this function of fantasy. Since the Imaginary is identified with a strong attachment to the mother figure, it offers the particular illusion of plenitude. McGowan uses a comparison to explain this: 'Imaginary plenitude functions precisely like the cold medicine aisle at the grocery store, [but] a plethora of choices confront us. We can purchase a wide variety of brands and different types of each brand. (...) An imaginary plenitude bombards the subject, and this plenitude creates the illusion that relief must really exist if we just make the correct choice. Imaginary plenitude is a haven for the subject who would otherwise confront real impossibility' (40).

17 Žižek mentions the 'empty gesture' as an example of explaining the idea of traversing the fantasy (*Plague*, 27). If I apply for a job promotion, and my best friend is

second in this competition, I can decide to offer him the promotion for the sake of our friendship. And if he in turn decides to decline the offer, then our camaraderie is assured for the upcoming years, and I can accept the job promotion with a good conscience. There has been a symbolic exchange in which I make a gesture, which my friend politely rejects. So there is no change to the original situation at all, but it has nonetheless made all the difference since after our 'pact of solidarity' (ibid., 28) has been sealed, my friend cannot reproach me for taking the opportunity. But what if my friend had said: 'How generous of you to give me the job promotion! You truly are my best friend and I will gladly accept the offer.' That would probably be the end of our friendship. Fantasy, according to Žižek, entails the creation of a situation in which we think we are free to choose but in which unwritten rules tell us exactly how we are supposed to choose (ibid., 29). If my friend takes the offer literally and does not recognize what the socially acceptable choice is—i.e., to reject it so our friendship can continue—he traverses the fantasy and ruins the system.

18 'Ugly' can have positive connotations among cult lovers of horror, for they derive their pleasure from good trash and gore. Moreover, the creature design in FRANKENSTEIN'S ARMY, shot as a first-person movie, is much appreciated by its fans.

19 Most curious is the case of PROOI [PREY] (Dick Maas, 2016). This film about a lion on the loose in the city of Amsterdam initially had about 30,000 viewers, but then, to everyone's surprise, it was released in March 2019 in about 4,000 Chinese cinemas. During the first weekend, some 1.1 million Chinese went to see the film.

20 Guido van Gennep was director of photography of ZWART WATER but also of SINT and SÜSKIND.

21 The nine-year-old Lisa of ZWART WATER is clearly analogous to the nine-year-old Cole Sear from THE SIXTH SENSE (M. Night Shyamalan, 1999) who can 'see dead people'. On each and every photograph of the clairvoyant boy in THE SIXTH SENSE, there is a flare of light near his head as if it is a 'spectral record' of the child's 'extraordinary vision' (Stewart, 93-94).

22 PHANTOM LADY is also the title of one of those fine film noirs that Robert Siodmak made in the 1940s.

23 Though ZWART WATER had arthouse potential, the film was screened in the more competitive market of commercial theatres. In the trailer, the film was advertised as 'horror', but for die-hard horror fans, ZWART WATER was not scary enough. When Van Strien was a guest lecturer at Leiden University (3 May 2017), he suggested that it would have been more strategic for the trailer to have highlighted the psychological elements.

BIBLIOGRAPHY

Balakian, Anna, *Surrealism: The Road to the Absolute*, 1959, revised and enlarged (London: Unwin Books, 1972).

Bernink, Mieke, *Fons Rademakers: Scènes uit leven en werk* (Abcoude: Uniepers, 2003).

Freud, Sigmund, 'On Narcissism: An Introduction', *The Standard Edition of the Complete Psychological Works of Sigmund Freud, Volume XIV (1914-1916): On the History of the Psycho-analytic Movement, Papers on Metapsychology and Other Works*, 24 vols. (London: Vintage, 2001), 67-102.

Graveland, Mariska, '"Er knaagt iets": David Verbeek over R U THERE', *De Filmkrant* 382 (December 2015): http://filmkrant.nl/interview/david-verbeek-over-r-u-there/ [Accessed 14 May 2020].

Hermans, Willem Frederik, *De donkere kamer van Damokles*, 1958 (Amsterdam: G.A. van Oorschot, 1997, 34e ed.).

Lacan, Jacques, *Écrits: A Selection*, trans. by Alan Sheridan, 1977 (London: Routledge, 2001).

Lacan, Jacques, *Four Fundamental Concepts of Psycho-analysis*, trans. by Alan Sheridan (New York: Penguin, 1994).

McGowan, Todd, *Psychoanalytic Film Theory and* THE RULES OF THE GAME (New York: Bloomsbury, 2015).

Pirandello, Luigi, *One, No One and a Hundred Thousand* http://gutenberg.net.au/ebooks16/1600681h.html [Accessed 14 May 2020].

Smelik, Anneke, 'And the Mirror Cracked: Metaphors of Violence in the Films of Marleen Gorris', *Women's Studies International Forum* 16, 4 (1993): 349-363.

Stewart, Garrett, *Framed Time: Toward a Postfilmic Cinema* (Chicago and London: University of Chicago Press, 2007).

Turkle, Sherry, *Alone Together: Why We Expect More From Technology and Less From Each Other* (New York: Basic Books, 2011).

Van Uffelen, René. 'Op de montagetafel: ALS TWEE DRUPPELS WATER', *Skrien* (April 2001): 28-30.

Verstraten, Peter, *Humour and Irony in Dutch Post-war Fiction Film* (Amsterdam: Amsterdam University Press, 2016).

Žižek, Slavoj, 'Cyberspace, or, How to Traverse the Fantasy in the Age of the Retreat of the Big Other', *Public Culture* 10, 3 (1998): 483-513.

—, *Enjoy Your Symptom! Jacques Lacan In and Out of Hollywood*, 1992 (Revised Edition. New York and London: Routledge, 2001).

—, *How to Read Lacan* (New York: W.W. Norton and Company, 2007).

—, *The Plague of Fantasies* (London and New York: Verso, 1997).

CHAPTER 2

In the Name of Fathers – Overbearing, Flying, or Otherwise

Verstraten, P., *Dutch Post-War Fiction Film Through a Lens of Psychoanalysis*. Taylor & Francis Group, 2021
DOI 10.5117/9789463725330_CH02

ABSTRACT

Chapter two is informed by the question 'Why are there always two fathers?' (and sometimes even three). Starting with Rademakers' clearest attempt at 'art cinema' (DE DANS VAN DE REIGER), the chapter addresses the unbridgeable gap between actual fathers and the symbolic bearers of the father's name. Examining a heterogeneous list of film titles, father figures take different guises: as a preacher teacher (DORP AAN DE RIVIER), a mouthpiece of his wife (MAKKERS, STAAKT UW WILD GERAAS), an irresponsible bon vivant (CISKE DE RAT); a memory-image (PERVOLA), a great pretender (LEK; BLOED, ZWEET EN TRANEN; KARAKTER), a pathetic character (ABEL; DE AVONDEN; GLUCKAUF), an unwitting gangster boss (DE BOSKAMPI'S), and also a legendary ghost (DE VLIEGENDE HOLLANDER).

KEYWORDS
Two fathers (and sometimes three) – Freud's fable from Totem and Taboo – Hypermasculine and symbolic fathers – Unforgiving fathers

In the opening scenes of Rademakers' black-and-white DE DANS VAN DE REIGER, shot in widescreen format, a bald man plays the part of a horny master to a woman dressed as a chambermaid. She acts as if she is running away from him, but when she jumps upon the bed, she lets her ankles be kissed by him. When she gets up again, he goes after her, taking a bottle of champagne with him. They then start kissing each other, but suddenly they both listen up, for they hear a boy's laughter, offscreen. The camera moves around objects inside the apartment to end up peeping in through the window from the outside, and we now see the couple behind the bars, framed by curtains. As we hear an offscreen 'Dad, mom', the man swiftly takes the chambermaid's cap from her head. He then opens the window and says 'Eddie, my boy', to which the woman adds: 'Weren't you going to the cinema?' Any view from the kid is kept from us, for this frontally staged two-shot of the man and woman in the open window dissolves into a landscape shot of the Adriatic Coast, over which the credits are projected. The picture-postcard quality of the scenery is emphasized when yellow letters mention 'Greetings from Dubrovnik'.

Later it will become clear that this prologue is an episode from the boyhood of the protagonist, the 40-year-old Edouard ('Eddie'). A civil servant by profession, Edouard is on holiday with his wife Elena, who has brought an accidental Dutch tourist to their resort. This Paul, with his large moustache, is wearing ridiculously short pants, and with his suntan and his fondness for diving, he is the opposite of Edouard, who is dressed in a dark suit and has a white face, almost Pierrot-like. Little does Paul know that Elena has only asked him to pay them a visit in order to annoy her husband, for it turns out that the couple is in the midst of a marital crisis. They have been married for eight years, Elena tells Paul, but there is no hint of a pregnancy yet. That's because we love each other so passionately, she says scornfully, 'like a burning volcano, scorching everything'. In reality, Edouard plays solitaire all day, and he has found himself a spot in the shade on the beautiful terrace of the villa, for as it turns out, he stubbornly refuses to sit in the sun. By inviting Paul, Elena intends to trigger her husband's jealous nature, for at the root of Edouard's lacklustre attitude is his suspicion that Elena had a brief affair with a sailor during a costume ball one evening. In the presence of Paul, she says that it was only a whim and that he had promised to forgive and forget her, but apparently he cannot. Ever since the costume ball, he has behaved coldly towards his wife.

It definitely contributes to the ambiguity of narration in Rademakers' film that Elena and the sailor are shown in suddenly inserted flashback scenes leaving a dining room together, witnessed by Edouard, but we do not know whether she has made love to the stranger. We see Elena with her sailor-lover on the floor in a tight embrace, but this could be Edouard's imagination. In flashback, when asked why she has cheated on him, she repeatedly answers 'I wanted to', but this is no confession whatsoever. Perhaps Elena is only giving the impression that she has committed adultery simply to defy her husband, whom she calls a 'stubborn mule ... made of stone'. In Dubrovnik, she tries once again to provoke a reaction from her husband with her licentious behaviour. She starts to perform 'the dance of the heron' with both Paul and some local men, and as Paul discloses to Edouard, not very tactically, this dance is the typical foreplay for herons before they mate. She kisses Paul on the mouth but only when she is certain that Edouard's old mother—who is also present at the resort—is peeping through the window. She interrupts the kiss as soon as she hears the mother tell her son that he should do something about it. Later, Elena goes off with Paul to the beach, and it is clear that she only does so in an attempt to break Edouard's deadlock. When she asks him whether this is what he wants, Edouard has nothing more to say than: 'If you go swimming, beware of sharks.'

In the second half of DE DANS VAN DE REIGER, when Elena and Paul have gone to the beach, Edouard's mother, who had been inside the villa most of the time, is on the terrace to keep her son company. Edouard does not feel like playing a game, whereupon his mother asks him to tell her a story: she always says that Edouard owes his talent for storytelling to his father. Actually, you owe everything to him, she says, 'your fortune, your education ... don't ever forget him, my son'. No, Edouard declares, I will never forget him. The irony that is lost on Edouard's mother is that the son's very problem is that he cannot forget him.

The one action in the entire film Edouard announces to undertake is to commit suicide. His mother, however, persuades him to only pretend to hang himself from a tree on the terrace of the villa as an act of revenge for Elena's deceit. It will deliver her 'the fright of her life', his mother assures him. Her son has to stay alive because 'dead eyes can't see': he has to be witness to how she will beg for his forgiveness. Edouard is hesitant, for playing games is not one of his habits, but his mother climbs on a chair to help him put his belt around his neck. She stays on the lookout for Elena's return while Edouard takes a rest. After a long wait, she warns her son to prepare himself. With the belt around his neck, he hallucinates that Elena is sunbathing amidst a group of sailors, with Paul present as well. In an interior monologue we hear him say: 'Come here, I command you. I'm your lawfully wedded husband.' But as soon as he puts on the mask he was wearing at the costume party, his late father shows up in front of him and says: 'Eddie ... my son', an exact repetition of the phrase in the prologue, some thirty years earlier. The ghostly apparition of his father kicks the chair from under Edouard's feet, and as we see him walk away with his back turned to his son, he suddenly evaporates into thin air. Edouard is now really about to choke, but he is rescued thanks to the timely return of Paul and Elena. Paul soon leaves because he feels like an unwanted guest now that Elena seems to have regained interest in Edouard, who starts walking towards the water. She exclaims happily: 'Edouard, you are out in the sun!' and presumes that her strategy has worked. She caresses him and says that he did all of this 'because of me'. He denies it and answers that he simply did not want to be cheated on again, which she erroneously thinks is the same thing. From a window high up, Edouard's mother looks down upon the scenery below with a frown on her face: Elena puts suntan lotion on Edouard's bare chest, which is the end of the film. Nothing, however, guarantees that the 'game-playing' will not repeat itself the next day or the day after. The ending is thus no more than a temporary and fragile solution to the crisis.

That Edouard is a pathetic man who has alienated himself from his wife is visually underscored by Sacha Vierny's cinematography. Important scenes are set on or near a terrace, demarcated by a stone balustrade. Because the film is shot in widescreen, the protagonists are often at a distance from each other; the mise-en-scène emphasizes the awkward communication among them. The most striking scenes in the film are those in which we see Elena prominent in the foreground and the two men in the background—the one at the left and the other at the other edge of the frame—or the scenes in which Paul is in the foreground with husband and wife on either side of him in a visual illustration of the marital crisis. In one of the flashback scenes at the costume ball, when Edouard is looking for Elena in 'this ridiculous crowd', as his voice-over says, the shots succeed each other so quickly that the viewer is disoriented and doesn't understand how Edouard is positioned among the guests. In one of these brief shots, Edouard is in sharp focus while the crowd is out of focus, thus adding to the impression that he is confused.

Edouard is scarred by an indelible resentment, and this is suggested by the suddenness with which the present is interrupted by images from the past. The series of brief and brusquely inserted flashback shots in Rademakers' film have the effect of blurring temporal zones almost to the extent that past and present practically exist in the same timespan. It seems as if no real trigger is required: one only has to mention the term 'childhood' and the images are there on demand, without delay. This is probably why Edouard is such a high-strung person unable to enjoy his holidays, for there is the constant risk that the past can cloud over the present.

Strictly speaking, Rademakers' film presents its spectator with a psychoanalytic scenario in which the man's current sterile behaviour is determined by his upbringing.[1] Due to his parents' fondness for role-playing, he has difficulties discerning 'authentic' from fake: for the stodgy Edouard, everything is serious business. His father has remained a jester throughout his life: in the guise of a master, he seduces a 'chambermaid'. Moreover, Edouard remembers one embarrassing incident that occurred the day Edouard turned eighteen: one of his father's 'best jokes was reading my love letters in front of the whole family' during his birthday party. Edouard's mother acts surprised 'that you still remember that joke', which indicates that she has no clue about the traumatic impact of her husband's pranks upon her son. Edouard's resentment against his father is fuelled by his practical jokes and games of seduction, and as soon as Elena playfully imitates one of these games, Edouard is derailed. On the one hand, he is still unable to make an educated guess about his wife's presumed adultery: Was Elena serious about the affair or was it an irrelevant flirt? On the other hand, what seems to pique him the most, quite hilariously, is that it still irks him that the sailor was at the ball dressed up in his everyday duds—for he really was a sailor!—whereas it was officially a costume party. At the root of the current marital crisis, then, is Edouard's annoyance at his father's non-serious behaviour. That is why it is so ironic that when for once the deadly serious Edouard wants to play a nasty joke on someone—encouraged by his scheming mother—his father suddenly pops up as a hallucinatory image to spoil the game. The one time he follows in his father's footsteps, it almost kills him, illustrating how poor Edouard is at playing pranks.

A 'normal' trajectory for a boy presumes that he has to be patient and that as he grows older, one day he will be bigger than Daddy. Edouard is a tragic character in De dans van de reiger because no matter what he tries to achieve, he will never be able to step out of the shadow of his father, not even after the latter's actual death. This unfortunate fate for Edouard is presented in such a fashion that we can consider the film a comically exaggerated version of a father-son relationship that overclouds the son's marriage. Edouard is pathetic because he has not been able to overcome his Oedipus complex, and therefore he is unfit as a husband. According to this famous, or notorious, 'basic wish fantasy', as Freud called it, the son commits parricide and marries his mother. Edouard's identity crisis seems to be the inverse of this Oedipal scenario. He is a passive character with suicidal tendencies, but the spectral apparition of his father gives him a reason to live after all: if he were to die by hanging himself from a tree, that would have meant that his father had played one more successful trick on him, and Edouard could not grant the master jester this 'pleasure'.

Rademakers' film received mixed reviews, and this is perhaps due to the fact that DE DANS VAN DE REIGER is difficult to describe in terms of tone or genre. Is it a textbook case of psychoanalytic father-son conflicts, or is it a parody of psychoanalysis? Despite the preposterous content, it does not seem like a comedy or a parody,[2] for it was shot in the solemn vein of a Resnais art film. The film is an intriguing case, however, because not only does the protagonist lack the antennae to distinguish the authentic from the fake, the viewer of DE DANS VAN DE REIGER also has difficulty deciding what the status of the film is. And because of this hesitation, I consider this film a special delight.

The title of chapter five in Žižek's *Enjoy Your Symptom!* is a question: 'Why Are There Always Two *Fathers*?' This question is fairly easy to respond in the case of the Oedipus myth. Oedipus's father Laius occupied a symbolically powerful position until he was murdered by a young hothead who did not know that the victim was his father. The son was then rewarded with the right to marry Queen Iocaste, resulting in a generational confusion: by marrying the widow, the son literally usurps the place of his father. But there are also two fathers in DE DANS VAN DE REIGER, for in addition to the father-as-master-jester, there is the father-as-symbolic-authority. A father must fulfil a paternal function, one that is best summed up by the idea of a 'preacher teacher', to coin a phrase from George Michael's song 'Father Figure'. He is supposed to be a balanced man who lives up to the expectations of 'fatherhood', but the problem is that most fathers neither point their offspring in the right direction nor teach their children valuable life lessons, at least not in Dutch post-war cinema. This chapter will address this unbridgeable gap between actual fathers and the presumed ideal of 'preacher teachers'—from fairly 'benevolent' and jovial ones to god-fearing patriarchs, and from helpless and needy ones to powerless brutes.

A PREACHER TEACHER, A MOUTHPIECE OF HIS WIFE, AND AN IRRESPONSIBLE BON VIVANT

In spite of his short stature, the Dutch actor Jan Teulings, who played the father in DE DANS VAN DE REIGER, had 'paternal' roles in two earlier films by Rademakers. In DORP AAN DE RIVIER, discussed in *Humour and Irony* as a 'Bergman light', he was the mayor who concocted a cunning plan to have the village doctor Tjerk van Taeke dismissed from his job. Initially, this doctor from a region up north was met with suspicion by the community because of his seemingly laconic attitude that made it seem as though reading his newspaper was as important to him as the delivery of a baby. Presuming that the doctor considers the mentality of the country people despicable, the mayor checks whether Van Taeke wants to back him up in taking 'drastic measures'. Interrupting the mayor, the doctor lets him know that he disagrees with this arrogant attitude. It gradually turns out that Van Taeke is cut from different cloth. The inhabitants of the village come to trust him because, when the tide is high, he puts his own life at risk for the well-being of his patients. Since the mayor realizes that he cannot pull the doctor into his sphere of influence, his growing popularity piques him. The local elite conspires to give the doctor a dishonourable discharge because of what they call 'excessively high invoices' based on the bill the mayor himself received upon the diagnosis of a mild catarrh. The mayor is to give him an envelope with a thousand guilders as a farewell present, but during the ceremony, as the camera pans in a semi-circle, Van Taeke humiliates the mayor by holding the envelope, without looking at its contents, above a burning candle.

In DORP AAN DE RIVIER, two kinds of paternal figures face each other. The first is the mayor as a respected 'father of the community', with good connections among the local elite. In the eyes of the civilians, he fulfils his role properly, but owing to the doctor's actions, it is revealed that beneath the mayor's decent appearance lurk arrogance and contempt for the common people. By contrast, the doctor seems like a bumpkin but proves to be forthright and fair: he adamantly refuses to favour the rich over the poor and has a keen eye for the needs of the common people. Though the doctor's role as a father of four young boys is given little emphasis in DORP AAN DE RIVIER, in the few scenes with his sons he gives the same impression of a strict and principled man who is nonetheless not without empathy. When his sons secretly go out at night to blow the old village pump to smithereens with a self-made bomb, he cannot tolerate their behaviour and condemns the 'scoundrels' to a fortnight of bread and water. He sends the boys back to their beds but asks the oldest, Hendrik, how they managed to make the bomb. He can only smile at the exact description, as if he understands that boys have to be naughty brats sometimes.

The best proof of his empathy is the scene in which he asks his oldest son in a stern voice why he never visits his mother's grave. We get an extreme close-up of the son's face and suspenseful music. The boy does not know what to say because in an earlier scene we see him witness his father taking the corpse of his wife out of her coffin and using another coffin to bury her in his own garden. So this particular son knows that the official burial, which took place in the presence of the mayor, was a charade. When the music becomes softer and the camera in a reverse shot slowly tracks backwards from the father's face in close-up, we see that it dawns on him. He tenderly touches the boy's neck and tells him: 'Do not forget how she was.'

Whereas Doctor Van Taeke as a father comes close to the notion of a 'preacher teacher'—perhaps closer than any other character in Dutch post-war cinema—Mr. Keizer in MAKKERS STAAKT UW WILD GERAAS [THAT JOYOUS

Eve] (Fons Rademakers, 1960) is reduced to an empty signifier of 'fatherhood'. He never speaks on his own behalf but is a spokesperson for his wife's demands. His son Henk is seventeen years old and wants to spend his days with 'lazy bums' (his mother's words). At one point, Mr. Keizer, played by Teulings, enters the café that his son frequents with his friends. Henk is embarrassed by his arrival but ultimately ends up sitting with his father at a table. It is clear that Mr. Keizer is sent by his wife: he explains that she is very upset that Henk does not want to celebrate Saint Nicholas at home but with his friends. 'It is a special night for mother ... You are her son ... You disappoint her.' And when Henk refuses to give in, Mr. Keizer almost feels relieved: 'Very well, there is nothing I can do anymore', as if he can just return home and tell Mrs. Keizer that he has tried to persuade Henk but to no avail. Mr. Keizer is the docile type who has no more ambition than to do his proper duty as a mere extension piece of his wife's concerns and desires. The division of tasks in the household is pretty clear: Mrs. Keizer is the one who is the boss, but her husband has to be the spokesperson of the decisions taken, as a father is supposed to do. He is allowed to act like a boss, as if he is the father authority, thereby concealing that his wife is the one actually pulling the reins.

Mr. Keizer's attempt to perform his role as symbolic authority depends upon the willingness of his immediate vicinity to acknowledge him as a 'father'. Strictly speaking, his acts can be seen as a fulfilment of the paternal function, but it is all too evident that he underperforms. Upon entering the café, Henk's peers already start to laugh, knowing in advance that the father's efforts to bring Henk home will be unsuccessful. Whereas normally his wife is able to ask Mr. Keizer to do this or that 'as a father', she is irritated at his passivity when immediate action is required. When Henk is brought home drunk and needs some assistance, Mrs. Keizer repeatedly asks him to 'give me a hand' and adds 'don't just stand there'. In a situation of slight panic, it is clear that her frenetic activity implies that she has a low opinion of her husband: better not leave any initiative to him. And last but not least, now that Henk has reached an age that his mother's wishes are no longer his commands, Mr. Keizer's role as mouthpiece of his wife becomes all the more pitiful. Mr. Keizer in Makkers staakt uw wild geraas wears the social mask of 'father', but at the end of the day, he cannot speak with a voice of authority since everybody considers him a father only in the biological sense and not in a social-symbolic sense.

The importance of the mechanism of acknowledgement is illustrated by Ciske de Rat (Guido Pieters, 1984), which is set in the 1930s and proved to be hugely popular with its 1.59 million viewers. In the immensely successful number-one hit song, the eleven-year-old boy Ciske Vrijmoeth sings about his vindictive mother Marie who treats him badly. 'No wonder my dad has gone to sea', the kid continues, thereby legitimizing the fact that his father Cor has left him to his own devices. Upon his return, the father tries to file for a divorce, and when the mother refuses, Cor points to Ciske's two younger brothers and explicitly doubts whether he is their biological father. After having suggested that Marie is sleeping around, Cor also asks Ciske to keep an eye on his mother and to check who stays over at night. Ciske takes this question literally, and when caught as a peeping Tom, he is severely mistreated once again. In the meantime, we have come to realize that Cor has selfish reasons for wanting a divorce: he has a new girlfriend who is pregnant, so he wants to marry her. This girlfriend, whom Ciske is supposed to call 'tante Jans' [Aunt Jans], is really kind to him, but after the young boy has served six months in prison for the accidental killing of his brutal mother, it turns out that his father and tante Jans are no longer a couple, in spite of the birth of twins. Tante Jans reassures Ciske that this had nothing to do with him nor with the crime he had committed: it is strictly between Cor and her. When Ciske is acting as a babysitter for the twins, he has his father come over to see the kids of his own flesh and blood, but when tante Jans returns prematurely, she is enraged. Since we share Ciske's perspective most of the time, we have no clue why the relationship came to an end, but we are made to understand that Cor must have done something terribly wrong given that the very reasonable tante Jans reacted so fiercely when he visits.

Despite all signs to the contrary, Ciske continues to have full confidence in his father. If things do not work out fine in the kid's life, this is due to the father's absence, but as the opening song indicates, according to Ciske, Cor is totally justified in leaving his 'bad' mother. He has an idealized picture of his Daddy, which can be sustained because his father is away for long stretches of time and hence cannot spoil the picture. And as soon as he is around, the kid appreciates his father for doing convivial things with him. Thus, the young Ciske is not conscious of the fact that his father never takes responsibility for him. In fact, some other men bear the burden of taking pity on Ciske: a police detective, a chaplain, the schoolteacher Bruis who has agreed to become his guardian. These men are replacements of the father who only shows up whenever it suits him, but precisely because of Cor's frequent absences, Ciske can continue to idolize him, thinking that life would be much better for him if his father were around all the time. Though it is obvious that the father is a loafer and a bon vivant, everyone is careful not to open Ciske's eyes to his father's opportunism—but he will probably realize this once he has reached Henk Keizer's age.

FATHER AS A MEMORY-IMAGE: *PERVOLA, SPOREN IN DE SNEEUW*

An inverse way to 'idolize' the father is shown in PERVOLA, SPOREN IN DE SNEEUW [PERVOLA, TRACKS IN THE SNOW] (Orlow Seunke, 1985), selected for the Venice Film Festival that year. At the beginning, we see Simon van Oyen give a performance in a sold-out theatre; his brother Hein is a latecomer who takes a seat near the back, hiding his face. Simon tells the story of how his father left the profitable family firm to his brother, for he himself—a sensitive gay actor—was disinherited some twenty years ago. In a matte shot we see Hein working as a stockbroker amidst a great number of telephones and a lot of noise. When a telegram arrives announcing the severe illness of the father who lives with his second wife in a snowbound area in Norway, Hein asks a colleague to inform Simon because the message explicitly mentions: 'Warn Simon'. The actor takes it as a sign that his father might want a last-minute reconciliation with him, even though Hein wants to talk Simon out of visiting the dying man.

Once they arrive at the father's house, Hein makes sure he enters the father's bedroom first and quickly hides a photo of Simon in the drawer of a bedside table. When the sick old man asks whether Simon has come as well, he gets a nasty cough. Hein bends over him, and when Simon comes to father's bed, Hein brings the disconcerting news that he does not hear him anymore. It turns out that father's last wish was to be buried in Pervola, only accessible by a horse-drawn covered sleigh through the snow that will take about six days of travel. Simon is determined to grant him this final wish, especially when he sees Hein throwing into the fireplace a letter Simon had sent his father. Hein suddenly decides to join him on the trip after Simon shows him a lighter with the inscription: 'To father. From Simon', a scene in which we hear Simon's off-voice telling his theatre audience that this decision surprised him.

Most of Seunke's film concerns this trek, which is magnificently shot. But the events are presented in 'minor key' (Hinson), turning PERVOLA into a road movie without an actual road, for the characters have to make their tracks themselves, as the subtitle implies. During the journey, Simon discovers a few more clues that he was much dearer to his father than he had assumed. Once the coffin is opened because some skiers wanted to check its content, Simon sees a photographic portrait of himself near the corpse—which, as we saw earlier, the widow had put into it. This confirms for him once more that his father did not consider him the black sheep of the family. As soon as he discovers this, Hein confesses that he had obstructed all contact between his father and his brother and that the main reason for joining Simon and the guide Aapo on this track was to conceal his deception. Father had wanted to undo the disinheritance but could not reach out to Simon. Hein is prepared to offer him financial compensation for his deceit—from an initial 50-50 in the firm's revenues to a 70-30 deal.

During a quarrel, two gunshots are fired, which happen to set both the coffin and the covered sleigh in flames. First, Simon extinguishes the fire on the coffin with the help of the snow as well as his own wig. Then he helps his brother, who is in a state of shock, out of the sleigh but the sleigh itself burns down. Simon and Aapo leave Hein behind for the final part of the trek. Presuming that Hein may have frozen to death, Simon feels guilty and returns to find him but to no avail. In the meantime, Hein had been rescued by a group of skiers and while he is recovering from the terrible cold, Simon and Aapo must cross a bridge for the final spot. Unfortunately, the bridge is too fragile and breaks, causing the coffin to fall down into a stream. Simon and Aapo save themselves in the nick of time. There is cross-cutting between Hein and Simon who, miles apart, yell a similar scream.

After Simon receives a warm applause for his performance from the theatre audience, he meets Hein in the wings just when a photographer says off-screen: 'Van Oyen?' The two brothers look in his direction, and the film ends with a freeze frame of their looks into the camera, after which the photograph can be included in the family photo album.

In PERVOLA, SPOREN IN DE SNEEUW, Simon was made an outcast due to his father's verdict. He had every reason to hate his father: for twenty years he had not heard a single word from his father, who had humiliated him by disapproving of his homosexuality. The more his father was at a distance from him—both in time and in space—the more he was inclined to revere him as a memory-image according to the adage that desire is aimed at things beyond one's grasp. For Simon, the father as a flesh-and-blood individual had developed into a spectre from his past. Precisely on account of their long-time separation, he was keen to pick up on every sign that could give evidence of some affection, like bits of information transmitted from a posthumous entity. The father as an abstract, spectral agent, however, is more impressive than any flesh-and-blood father. No actual father can live up to the expectations required of a 'supersize dad', except for the dad who is too dead to contradict them. For the 'good' son Hein who owed his capital to the father's decision and still had some contact with him, the father was a man with fallacies and caprices—and one of these flaws according to him was father's idea to rehabilitate Simon. So Hein feels little inclination to grant the man his final and outrageous whim of being buried at Pervola. In fact, the 'bad' son Simon comes out the morally better of the two. He has interpreted several clues as indications that the old man had wanted to lift the disinheritance. He did not receive these signs from his father directly because he arrived too late to see him alive, hence the 'positive' messages circulated in the symbolic order—and one of them ultimately arrives at its destination when Simon finds the photograph in the coffin. The father was more a function and a benchmark for Simon, and as such he has become bigger in his mind than the fragile figure he must have been in the last years of his life. The signs that the father was willing to clear Simon's name only aggrandizes his symbolic status for the son. Since the father was always-already dead for him, it is only a small step mentally to be totally committed to the dead father's will. This is the purest variant of the worship of the father in his abstract-symbolic guise: the paternal function is stronger than any concrete embodiment, as a fable by Freud teaches us.

GREAT PRETENDERS: *BLOED, ZWEET & TRANEN; LEK,* AND *KARAKTER*

Since the father is removed from his position, son Oedipus no longer encounters obstacles to an incestuous relationship with his mother. What is more, marriage to the queen is the official reward for solving the riddle of the Sphinx. Freud supplemented this Oedipus myth with the fable of the primordial father in his *Totem and Taboo* (1912), whose lesson can be regarded as the 'exact observe' of the Oedipus story (Žižek 'The Big Other', 1). This fable is meant to explain the origin of moral law and indicates how the transition from an animalistic, tribal order to Culture came about. A violent and jealous father has kept all the women for himself and moreover expelled his growing sons. The brothers plan to eliminate him, for he stands in the way of their 'sexual demands and their desire for power' (Freud 'Totem', 142). The problem, however, is that once the father has been killed, one of the brothers might want to take up the paternal position. Each of the brothers might want to have all the women just as the father did, but in laying claim to a hierarchically privileged position, he might become a murder victim himself. In order to minimize mutual rivalry, they all equally 'renounced the fruits of their deed by denying themselves the liberated women' (Freud 'Totem', 142). Both out of a sense of guilt about the murder and out of the realization that inter-male competition would backfire on them, the brothers 'construct the patriarch as an impossible and unreachable figure, one that no individual could embody' (DiPiero, 113).

This symbolic patriarch comes to 'embody' the memory of the primordial and narcissistic father who sowed such fear. In fact, the primordial father becomes an even more powerful figure after his death. Strictly speaking, the brothers are his successors, but due to their agreement with each other, they cannot fully identify with or imitate him, for they bar themselves enjoyment of all women. What the father's presence had formerly prevented they now prohibit themselves (Freud 'Totem', 143). While their extremely dominant father was alive, the brothers could still dream of all the privileges that might befall them one day, but the symbolic patriarch is an abstract instance who fills an empty spot that is impossible to conquer. In other words, the dead father fills a symbolic place that cannot be occupied by anyone who is living, since his position and function must by definition remain a void. To relate this to the sections above, all fatherly characters—the mayor, Doctor Van Taeke, Mr. Keizer, Cor Vrijmoeth—attempt to fulfil a paternal duty, for better or for worse. They all derive a certain authority from this symbolic place of the father: the mayor because of his ceremonial job; Cor because his son believes in him as kids tend to do because he is the father. To Simon in PERVOLA, his old man has become such a grandiose figure in his mind—having not seen him for so many years—that he turns him into a moral benchmark.

Let us take once more the example of Mr. Keizer, who incidentally has no first name in the film, as a token of authority. Though his wife has the tendency to belittle him time and again, the roles in the family are divided in such a manner that she expects him to take up so-called paternal responsibilities: as a father, Mr. Keizer has to do this and that. Regardless of whether he is the best person for the task—and we are quickly made to realize he is not—his symbolic position requires him to have a chat with his son in the café, for example. This illustrates a widespread cultural legacy: any father is indebted to the dead and empty place of symbolic authority. At the risk of repetition, the most important function of the father in his symbolic guise is to teach the son that rivalry with the father is senseless. The son may think he is removing an obstacle, but an even bigger obstacle is erected: the ineradicable memory of the killing will induce a guilt complex in the son that will prevent him from appropriating the privileges that used to be his father's prerogative. The son desires to kill the father (the Oedipus complex), but the fable from *Totem and Taboo* explains why a murderous competition between father and son is prohibited. This comes with a proviso, however. This prohibition is only effective on the condition that the primordial and extremely dominant father figure remains repressed. The best guarantee that the symbolic father will prevail over the hypermasculine and obscene father is that he is not only dead but also ignorant of his own death.[3] Indeed, it is crucial for the balance within the symbolic order that the truth of his death is hidden from the father (Lacan *Écrits*, 300). The place of this dead agent as bearer of the symbolic Law is sustained, but only when the father is engaged in a certain 'eye-closing' of his sorry situation (Gallop, 182). This place is constitutively empty, but as a compensation, his surroundings treat the father as if he really is an authority. Hence, patriarchy is a play-act in which mothers may hold the reins but make their husbands believe that the voices of men are decisive.

As soon as a paternal figure disregards this tacit understanding and pretends to occupy the place of the symbolic patriarch, things become complicated. There are three excellent examples in Dutch cinema: BLOED, ZWEET & TRANEN [BLOOD, SWEAT & TEARS] (Diederick Koopal, 2015), LEK [LEAK] (Jean van de Velde, 2000), and KARAKTER [CHARACTER] (Mike van Diem, 1997), which won the Academy Award for Best Foreign Language Film. BLOED, ZWEET & TRANEN focuses upon three seminal phases in the life of André Hazes, an incredibly popular singer of sentimental songs. In 1960, at the age of only eight, the young boy is already known for his golden voice. His father Joop, an incurable alcoholic, drags his son into the café and wants him to sing so he can collect some money to pay for a drink. André gets a glass of beer too, for as his father says, the young boy likes to sip the foam. While André is performing at a market, he is discovered by the successful artist Johnny Kraaykamp who invites the boy to sing a song on his television show. When father Joop hears about the invitation, he is not impressed: why did they not ask Joop junior, much more talented than André? The father commands André to practice until the boy is totally exhausted. Because the television broadcast is a success, Kraaykamp asks André's parents permission to record a duet with the boy. The father is not very gracious towards the artist, but the prospect of money appeals to him. Against all expectations, the single is a flop, and father Joop starts behaving like a despot towards his wife and children. The mother receives serious blows and André even more so when he twice tells his father: 'I wish you were dead.'

These events in the year 1960 are consistently alternated in BLOED, ZWEET & TRANEN with the other two phases: the early 1980s, which chronicles the rise of the singing bartender to national fame, and the year 2004, when André is stressed out because of two upcoming concerts in the football stadium ArenA. The transition from one phase to another is at times prompted by visual parallels. When the eight-year-old boy is mistreated by his father in the corner of a room, there is a cut to a 53-year-old André who feels like a wreck, sitting in the corner of a hotel room in Noordwijk: he is diabetic, his liver is in bad condition, his hearing has deteriorated, and his wife Rachel wants him to follow the doctor's advice to reduce his beer consumption, which has resulted in a quarrel. Although André is not nearly as vicious towards his family as his own father was, he has inherited the habit of heavy drinking from the old man. He is caught in a vicious cycle: when he is under pressure, alcohol functions to control André's nerves, as Rachel knows all too well, but excessive use triggers his fits of anger, which impact both his wife and two children (aged ten and eleven). He is still successful as an artist, but his lifestyle ruins his health, resulting in his premature death at the age of 53.

The middle phase (1980s) highlights the period when André transforms from an ordinary lad into a best-selling performer of torch songs. The EMI record company instructs its staff producer Tim Griek to contact the bartender and track down Hazes. Tim is quite reluctant to see him as an asset for the company since this Hazes is much too plebeian for his taste, but their mutual preference for blues is a common denominator that brings them together. They create a number of Dutch hits, and André's fame hits an early peak when he is asked to perform in the Concertgebouw, the famous concert hall in Amsterdam. This opportunity is not only an artistic recognition, for this is the temple of serious music, it reminds André of the time he had once been smuggled into this building as an eight-year-old to watch a blues concert by Muddy Waters and B.B. King, of whom he was in total awe. Moreover, his father had once told André that the Concertgebouw was beyond his reach. There is a key scene in Koopal's film when, just before André's show is to begin, Tim tells him that there is a man at the box-office without a ticket who swears he is André's father. Tim is puzzled, for André had told him earlier that his father was no longer alive, but André only replies: 'He is not coming in.' When he adds that his father is dead to him, Tim understands that the man really is the father, but André is determined to keep him out: 'He can piss off.' During the concert, however, André recognizes his father's face among the crowd just as he has finished a song. He whispers something in the conductor's ear, pulls off his jacket, and sings a hit with lyrics such as 'Say no more, I'll go away, if you want // you look down on me // I have never believed in you.' He looks repeatedly in the direction of his father, and his voice is raised when uttering particularly dismissive lines. Father Joop gets the message, and before the song is over he walks towards the exit. After the concert, Tim is ecstatic about André's performance, but André is crestfallen: 'Why did you let him in?' and tells Tim that his father was only trying to provoke him with his presence.

For Hazes' devoted fans, the greatest attraction of Bloed, Zweet & Tranen consisted of the many songs in the film. The main actor Martijn Fischer, who had also performed the role of André Hazes in the theatre, gave a life-like performance, both visually and aurally. But the plot of the film is centred around André's troublesome relationship with his father and the problems he encountered at a later age in combining his existence as an artist with his own role as a father of two kids. André's father was an extremely dominant patriarch who did not want to be bossed around by anyone. Those who could not accept his will as the law were given a severe beating. This is a father who takes up the impossible symbolic position of the (dead) father: the dominant father acts as if he is entitled to be the even more dominant symbolic patriarch. Joop assumes he would be allowed free entrance into the Concertgebouw simply because he is André's father. And yes, most fathers would be granted that privilege by their children except the father who has always pretended that he occupies the place of symbolic law, that is, the father who does not accept any opposition. This pretence is so utterly false and inappropriate that such an authoritarian figure has forfeited the right to be considered a father. Such a father may be alive but, as André says, 'he is dead to me'. But when Joop appears as a most unwelcome guest, son André does not answer his presence with the 'language' of physical violence but instead uses a symbolic language: the lyrics, the tone of his voice, and the way he directed his singing at him. In this way he removes his father from the symbolic throne he had occupied for so long, and as we see Joop walk towards the exit, it is clear the father has lost his aura and that he has been reduced to an ordinary man who will no longer play a part in André's life. In that sense, the symbolic order has been re-instated, for the (dead) father from Freud's fable is no longer a haunting presence who can show up unannounced. Instead, he has become what he is supposed to be: an unpleasant memory.

LEK opens with one of André Hazes' songs, 'Kleine jongen' [Little Boy], in a karaoke version performed by the tough criminal Ben Haveman in the presence of his gang members. Meanwhile a man is hanging with a rope around his neck, but his hands can still cling to an iron rod that is gradually being heated until it becomes unbearably hot.[4] There is an immediate transition to a close-up of a baby crying loudly. The 25-year-old rookie policeman Eddy Dolstra and his wife Ria are visiting a gynaecologist in the hospital because they fear one of them might be infertile. There is no physical defect, the gynaecologist assures them, but she asks the couple how often they screw a month—after she has asked them whether they are okay with the word 'screw'. When Eddy responds 'Ten or fifteen times', Ria laughs and embarrasses Eddy by saying not only that it is no more than three times a month but also that he comes prematurely. The set-up is clear from the beginning: there is the all-male environment of Haveman, recognized by everyone as their boss, and the average but ambitious agent Eddy who has a problem with masculinity. Ultimately, these two polar opposites meet each other in a final confrontation.

Every man that Eddy encounters is somehow superior to him, either in rank or in masculine charisma and bluff. The chief of police Berg, his boss, has little confidence in Eddy and gets angry after Eddy makes an untactful arrest of the well-known criminal Patrick van Veen, who leaves the police station with a clean sheet. He is all the more irritated since Eddy and his closest colleague Franco acted on the request of the Criminal Investigation Department (CID) whose head is Berg's rival, Ferdinand de Wit. In turn, De Wit puts Eddy under pressure because of an 'illegal encounter' after he was spotted talking to Jack Boon, who happens to be an old pal who used to live on the same street during Eddy's childhood. Jack—or 'Sjakie' for Eddy—was a bit of a laughingstock at the time, but to Eddy's shock and surprise, this sad boy from the past had surpassed him. Eddy runs into him at the men's toilet in the hospital after the meeting with the gynaecologist, and 'Sjakie' is overjoyed because he has just become the father of a baby girl: he has created 'new life, new life', whereas Eddy has failed to make Ria pregnant. Moreover, 'Sjakie' drives away in a Lamborghini Diablo, and he learns from De Wit that Jack has made a fortune by dealing hash and coke, gambling, and trafficking in women and weapons. De Wit encourages Eddy to contact Jack, for as one of Haveman's henchmen, he can be an informer for the CID.

In the company of all these men, Eddy is constantly belittled, and as such, the Hazes song 'Kleine jongen' is also about him. Willy-nilly, he gets involved in events he is not very capable of handling. Jack refuses to meet De Wit, but he agrees to give valuable information regarding Haveman on the condition that Eddy will be the one and only mediator: he does not want to have contact with anyone else. In his role as errand boy, Eddy is informed by Jack how to intercept a huge drugs transport, but when the boat turns around before reaching the harbour, Eddy is certain that one of the policemen is in cahoots with Haveman's gang. Eddy's suspicion that there is a snitch in the force angers his colleagues: they consider him a backstabber.

When an operation a few days later in the Chinese restaurant Lin Wah goes wrong, Eddy discovers that Franco is the rat, but De Wit thinks that Eddy himself is the saboteur. He is suspended from work for two weeks by Berg, who is displeased when Eddy refuses to disclose the name of his contact. Eddy feels wronged and asks Franco to introduce him to Haveman's gang. He secretly tapes the meeting so that he has auditory proof against the rat. But before Eddy can reach either Berg or De Wit, his wife, who is now pregnant, is paid a visit by two criminals who mistreat her so badly that she loses the unborn child and ends up in hospital. Meanwhile, Eddy knows that Franco has found a picture of a young Eddy (who happens to be in a leotard) together with Sjakie. Eddy warns his old comrade, who has his little girl on his chest in a baby carrier. Sjakie gives him a head butt and once Eddy wakes up, he has the keys to Sjakie's car in his pocket. Two hitmen track down Eddy, for their assignment is to kill the man in a yellow Lamborghini. In his hour of need, however, Eddy is rescued by Sjakie. He tells Eddy to ask him what the name of his girl is—Jacky—and then Sjakie hands him the baby and shoots himself in the head. Devastated about the news that Ria will not be able to have any more children, he takes revenge upon the gang: Patrick shoots Haveman in the throat; Eddy kills Patrick. Franco is fired after Berg hears the tape made by Eddy, and the ex-cop is taken into a car by three dodgy men, apparently hired by Haveman who has barely survived the attack. In the final scene, Eddy is released from prison and both Ria and a five-year old Jacky await him; the girl shouts 'daddy' when she sees him.

Van de Velde's LEK is an American-style police thriller set in the Low

Countries. At one point in the film, which is quite gritty by Dutch standards, the gangster Patrick asks what he should do with 'Serpico' (meaning Eddy), a reference to the protagonist from Sidney Lumet's 1973 drama about a cop who blows the whistle on police corruption.[5] Although Patrick is being ironic here, for he undoubtedly does not think that Eddy deserves the name of Serpico, LEK is most commendable for the way it depicts how Eddy adapts to circumstances. In the beginning of the film, he is on good terms with his wife, though she does not accept his rosy depiction of his performances in bed, which he himself blames on his frequent nightshifts. He fails as a would-be father, but in the course of the film, he is confronted with a series of 'father figures'. To start with, he is sandwiched in the conflict between his direct boss Berg and the CID chief De Wit. Further, he is used as a pawn by Sjakie who behaves more like a man than he does in every regard. In turn, Sjakie is exceeded by Haveman, the alpha male par excellence in the film who imposes his fondness for torch songs on his environment.

Frustrated by Franco's betrayal, angered by the ridicule of his colleagues, and shocked by the mistreatment of Ria, Eddy rises above himself—or perhaps we could say he becomes the man he always was. Before Jack gives him the head-butt, he tells Eddy: 'You dream of being a big boy, but you don't play by the rules of the game.' Sjakie recalls when they first saw a Lamborghini as young adolescents, but despite his big mouth, Eddy did not dare to drive the sports car—Jack did. Eddy dreamed of burning down the school, but it was Jack who actually did this, claiming he did it to protect that 'little boy' who was being bullied partly because he was a stutterer. Though Eddy denies this and says that Sjakie was the stutterer, Sjakie challenges him to mention anything that Eddy is capable of and Jack himself is not. 'I even have a child, Eddy.' After Eddy reawakens, he is like Jack: he drives his Lamborghini; he is tracked down like a criminal; and, most crucially, Jack gives him Jacky, turning him into a father. Transformed into a substitute for the paternal 'Sjakie', Eddy is able to eliminate Haveman's gang.

In addition to father Joop in BLOED, ZWEET & TRANEN and gangster boss Haveman in LEK, there is an extremely dominant figure who acts as if he embodies the law in KARAKTER. There is, however, a crucial difference, which makes Van Diem's film the more unconventional of the three: in KARAKTER, the father himself takes responsibility for his unmasking. In the 1920s, a young man, on the very day he has become a chartered lawyer, walks into a building in an agitated manner and plunges a knife into an older man's desk. This young man, Jacob Katadreuffe, takes a step back and then announces his farewell: 'You no longer exist for me.' The man at the desk, named Dreverhaven, turns his back on Katadreuffe, whereupon the latter quickly starts to take his leave. Before he is at the end of the corridor, however, he hears a 'congratulations'. Katadreuffe turns around: 'You congratulate me? I cannot take the hand of someone who has opposed me my entire life.' Katadreuffe immediately heads for the exit of the building again, but he halts his step upon hearing Dreverhaven say '...or cooperated', which the older man then repeats after a few seconds. Ultimately, Katadreuffe leaves the building, visibly exasperated, but then quickly decides to return after all. As soon as he faces Dreverhaven, the young man is shown running in slow motion. Cut to a low-angle from the desk, with the knife in sharp focus, Katadreuffe takes a giant leap forwards, but the camera goes to black and shows us the title of the film: KARAKTER.

After Katadreuffe is witnessed leaving the building at five in the afternoon with blood smeared on his face, he is arrested sometime later for either manslaughter or murder. Van Diem's film then takes the form of an interrogation, intercut with frequent flashbacks that concern the relationship between the bailiff Dreverhaven and Katadreuffe.[6] The first flashback shows us the bailiff as a representative of the 'law without compassion'. When a woman lies on her sickbed during an eviction, he drags the bed outside into the freezing cold. It illustrates how Dreverhaven can operate in a ruthless manner, but we can also surmise from this that he is capable of unmasking malingerers, for the woman gets up from her 'sickbed' and starts swearing at him. In subsequent flashbacks, Katadreuffe discloses that Dreverhaven is his biological father who forced himself upon his taciturn maid Joba. She leaves him as soon as she discovers she is pregnant and obstructs all contact with the bailiff: she returns all letters and donations to the sender. At primary school, the kid is named a 'bastard', but when he inquires after his father, his mother's usual reply is: 'We do not need anything from him.' When the boy is later arrested with a few peers for some mischief, he gives his name as 'Dreverhaven'. The bailiff, who knows this boy is his son, comes to see the kid. After we see a subjective shot of Dreverhaven walking through the corridors, embedded in Katadreuffe's flashback narration, the bailiff deliberately misrecognizes the kid: I have never seen this boy before.

A couple of years later, when Katadreuffe is eager to leave his mother's home, he tries to start a business, but he fails and cannot pay his debts to the bank. Later while working at a law firm, he realizes that Dreverhaven was at his mother's place in order to calculate the value of Katadreuffe's personal belongings, which is no more than fifteen guilders. Soon thereafter he receives a letter with another request for bankruptcy, but thanks to his monthly income the debt can be repaid gradually. He is horrified, however, when he learns that the bank is owned by Dreverhaven. Remembering the earlier incident in which he was humiliated by his father, he stubbornly prefers a financial ruin over a settlement, which means he will have to pay back the entire sum. His extraordinary discipline helps him to cut loose the attachment to Dreverhaven, but not for long. Katadreuffe wants to challenge the father and asks for another loan. He receives the sum of 2,000 guilders, but in addition to an interest of eight per cent, there is a tricky condition: Dreverhaven can ask for the entire sum to be returned whenever it suits him. Of course, the father does so at a most awkward moment, and since there is a fly in the ointment, Katadreuffe is even put on trial. With the help of his generous lawyer, the son withstands the adversity.

Another confrontation takes place a few years later, when father and son meet by accident in a dark alley. Dreverhaven yells at Katadreuffe: 'Do something to me!' Despite his repetitive and aggressive command, the son does not make a move. The father pushes him to the ground, but the son retreats towards the exit of the alley. The father throws a knife at him, but it misses him. In a conversation with Katadreuffe's mother, Dreverhaven discloses why he will not back off their son: 'I squeeze him dry for nine-tenth, and that one-tenth remaining will make him stronger.' When Joba, who has fallen ill by that time, thereupon makes clear that his final attempt to persuade her to marry him is in vain, Dreverhaven grudgingly replies: 'Maybe I will squeeze out that one-tenth as well.'

Instead of venting his rage on Katadreuffe, Dreverhaven gives his tenants only three days to evacuate, and he does so 'in the name of the law'. Though he leaves his son in peace, Dreverhaven still haunts Katadreuffe's mind, for the latter knows that his father can strike mercilessly at any time. And since Dreverhaven knows that the son knows, the bailiff can postpone any action. According to an analysis of a lawyer, the reason Dreverhaven is so dangerous is because he is tired of life, and world-weary people are indifferent. After Joba dies, Katadreuffe goes to see his father once more. This is a repetition of the opening scene but with two seminal differences. First, the camera sides with Dreverhaven consistently, so Katadreuffe is a figure in the background. Second, we now see what happens after Katadreuffe's giant leap. There is a serious fight, but the son is no match for his father—until the moment the latter is out of breath. As Katadreuffe takes the knife in his hand, Dreverhaven holds his son's hand and asks him: 'help me', encouraging him to kill him. The outcome is then interrupted for a scene in the interrogation room, where it is reported that the autopsy proves that Dreverhaven died six hours after Katadreuffe left. Having been cleared of the charge of manslaughter, Katadreuffe is asked to imagine what happened in the meantime. We see Dreverhaven take the knife, a hard cut to a close-up of Katadreuffe's face, and then Dreverhaven puts the knife into his own stomach; in close-up we see his hands covered in blood. In the final scene, Katadreuffe inherits Dreverhaven's possessions, and we see the old man in the hour preceding his death, writing his will. This scene of Dreverhaven writing is intercut with a scene in which Katadreuffe's best friend, Jan Maan, reads out the letter. Katadreuffe is not very enthusiastic and remarks that it is probably signed 'A. B. Dreverhaven, bailiff', whereupon his friend says no—then a cut to Dreverhaven signing the letter with 'vader' (father). Back to Katadreuffe, who looks over his shoulder. If we presume that the subsequent shot is an eyeline match, it means that he sees his father, who halts his step and looks back at him, whereupon the end credits set in.

Katadreuffe was born because his mother was overpowered by her employer. As an act of resistance, the stubborn Joba refused to acknowledge Dreverhaven as the boy's father. There is only one moment when the boy himself uses 'Dreverhaven' as his family name for strategic reasons, but then the father disavows him: the one time he could have gained symbolic recognition as a parent, he rejects the offer. In terms of his official function, he induces fear among people: the 'law without compassion' is an apt characterization of his work as bailiff. But his methods are so ruthless—if not obscene—that he is like an extremely dominant, even jealous figure rather than a reasonable and even-handed man. He displays his power in such an excessive manner—as when he commands his tenants to evacuate within three days—that he resembles Freud's primordial father. The fact that he attempts to obstruct his son (or so the latter thinks) in his ambition to build a career reinforces this similarity. The peculiar situation in KARAKTER is that Dreverhaven tends to speak 'in the name of the law' on numerous occasions but then acts like the hypermasculine father. He can be said to make a claim upon this symbolic position, but not on the basis of charisma. Instead, he does so by acting aggressively. In his moments of great brutality, he pretends to be synonymous with the law: I am permitted to do so because I represent the law and thus no one is justified to contradict me. We thus have a robust character who is a father, albeit a non-father for mother and son. Since he acts as though he is untouchable, his powerful appearance seems to equal an unquestionable authority. In terms of the Freudian fable, the extremely dominant father pretends to occupy the impossible place of the symbolic patriarch by committing horrible deeds while constantly referring to 'the law'.[7]

As said before, this place only functions insofar as it is unoccupied, that is, filled in by a dead father who is plagued by a certain blindness. The flashbacks, narrated by the suspect Katadreuffe, go to great pains to suggest that Dreverhaven suffers from failing sensory perception. In the visualization of the flashback—a mental reconstruction by Katadreuffe—we have several point-of-view shots from the object of narration, Dreverhaven, one of which was mentioned above. Just after the boy's arrest, he meets the young Katadreuffe and then says he does not know the boy (but he does). If this misrecognition is a result of the boy's punishment for his illegal use of the name 'Dreverhaven', other scenes illustrate that his senses are failing him (or perhaps he only imagines this). One day at the law firm, Katadreuffe is perplexed to encounter Dreverhaven, who is on his way to a meeting. He climbs a flight of stairs in order to be able to have a clear view of his father. When the latter finally looks up in the exact direction where Katadreuffe is standing, we get a subjective shot; in it, however, we only see the stairs and not Katadreuffe. Either he got out of the way or, more plausibly, his father is incapable of seeing him, certainly not when the son is standing above him. In the eyes of Katadreuffe, he himself is no more than a mere abstraction to his father. In the scene following this one, Katadreuffe discovers in the archives that Dreverhaven was the acting bailiff when his first business went bankrupt. 'He came to our house', he realizes. After a dissolve, we see Dreverhaven visiting his mother, or, more accurately, we see how Katadreuffe imagines the visit. As Dreverhaven walks through the house, we hear the subdued conversation between the mother and the lawyer accompanying Dreverhaven. When Dreverhaven turns to Joba, however, the music drowns out the words. Next, there is a perception shot of Dreverhaven watching Joba and the lawyer. We see their lips move, but we hear no words. The wordless part of the scene lasts until Dreverhaven turns his back on them and the camera positions itself next to Joba and the lawyer. The scene implies that the bailiff is too dazed to listen to what is being said.

The subjective shots of the now dead object of narration illustrate above all how the narrating Katadreuffe views his father: Dreverhaven is incapable of adequate sensory perception. In the eyes of the son, the father is missing a certain level of sensitivity. That is why his sight is failing, his hearing is worsening, and why, in a later scene, he screams without uttering a sound. The fact that Dreverhaven's perception is flawed places the first subjective shot in a different perspective. At the eviction with the woman on her sickbed, we get an internal focalization by Dreverhaven when he bends over her. With the woman still on the bed, he drags it outside into the freezing cold. Immediately, she gets up from her 'sickbed' and starts swearing. Since this is the first flashback scene, we might suspect that he is capable of distinguishing ill people from simulators, but no, the later subjective shots only reveal that he lacks the quality to correctly assess situations. The first subjective shot does not show his capacity to recognize frauds but only emphasizes his insensitive and heartless nature. Even if the woman had been sick, he would have acted in the same way.

A father figure like Dreverhaven is guilty of behaviour that befits only an authority who thinks that he is not liable to error. Any such pretentious identification of himself as authority—'I act in the name of law'—is, as a rule, an exaggeration. Dreverhaven presents himself as 'the subject presumed to know' how to separate right from wrong. But a figure of authority owes his privileged position to his ignorance, to the fact that he does not know that the father is dead. A madly stubborn father who identifies too much with the paternal position is on the verge of collapsing. His supposed infallibility is only a posture, and thus he has to pay for this excessive display. There is no need for the son to kill this bluffing father, he just has to realize that he is a buffoon who is over the hill. His challenge to his son to stab the knife into him is a last, poor attempt to illustrate his extreme dominance, but the son avoids the trap. He had already declared him dead: 'You no longer exist for me.' From the perspective of Dreverhaven, it sounds like a death sentence when Katadreuffe contradicts him when he says he has been cooperative. It implies that he really was the obscene father who has to die first before he can speak on behalf of the law. His suicide with the knife that his son has returned to him is then a most logical consequence.[8]

FIRST REFORMED FATHERS: THE SUB-GENRE OF RELIGIOUS FERVOUR

In his seminar 'The Quilting Point' from *The Psychoses*, Lacan referred to the fear of God to explain the logic of the master signifier on the basis of Jean Racine's 1691 tragedy *Athaliah*, but, as Žižek suggests, instead of God, one could also refer to the fear of the Nazis on the part of the Jews or the fear of the shark in Spielberg's JAWS (*The Parallax View*, 37). The fear of God is presented in Racine's play as so ominous that any other fear pales in comparison to it. All fears, Lacan observes, 'are exchanged for what is called the fear of God, which, however, constraining it may be, is the opposite of a fear' (*The Psychoses*, 267). This fear is a mere master signifier that does not add any positive content: it is a strictly symbolic gesture, introduced in order to make a situation readable. All our everyday worries and anxieties become nothing as soon as we imagine ourselves a fear so encompassing that all fears can be made subservient to it. Once I start to tremble for an otherworldly fear that has no ground in reality, I can become 'fearless in all worldly matters' (Žižek, *The Parallax View*, 37).

Lacan's reading of this fear of God in Racine can be extended to a specific Dutch sub-genre in both literature and film, of the 'suffocating belief in doom and gloom'. In quite a number of cases, a film will present without much emphasis an environment pervaded by the Dutch Reformed Church, that is, as a story embedded in a more prominent story, as in SPETTERS (Paul Verhoeven, 1980). Eef, one of the three male adolescent protagonists in this film, tries to confess to his pious father that he is a queer, a sissy, a faggot, but these terms do not mean anything to his father. It is only when Eef cites Leviticus 20, verse 13—'If a man also lie with mankind, as he lieth with a woman, both of them have committed an abomination'—that it dawns on the father what his son is saying, and he becomes furious. It is such a disgrace to him and his family that he refers to the Bible to predict that blood shall be upon his son.

But the Reformed faith can also be used for a sub-plot that impacts the narrative as such. At first sight, the main story of DE STORM [THE STORM] (Ben Sombogaart, 2009) is about the young woman Julia who is frantically searching for her lost infant boy during the devastating flood disaster of 1953, but to add melodrama to this tragedy, there is the minor story about Julia's father who had denied the existence of his grandson because his daughter is unmarried. From an ideological angle, it is crucial that DE STORM is structured in such a manner that the reason for the flood is to challenge the father in his faith. It would have made sense to him if his wife and his 'good' daughter—Julia's sister—had survived, but what irrational turn of fate allows Julia of all people to still be alive? This father not only has to accept the death of his wife and his 'good' daughter as 'God's will' but, stricken as he is by misery, he has no other option but to reconcile with his one remaining, 'sinful' daughter.

Whereas this story about the father's mental struggle is a minor, albeit seminal narrative thread, in films such as EEN VLUCHT REGENWULPEN [A FLIGHT OF RAINBIRDS] (Ate de Jong, 1981), TERUG NAAR OEGSTGEEST [RETURN TO OEGSTGEEST] (Theo van Gogh, 1986), the dry comedy MATTERHORN (Diederik Ebbinge, 2013), DORSVLOER VOL CONFETTI [CONFETTI HARVEST] (Tallulah Hazekamp Schwab, 2014), and KNIELEN OP EEN BED VIOLEN [IN MY FATHER'S GARDEN] (Ben Sombogaart, 2016), the focus is on the religious fervour itself, often highlighting a circle of men and their brethren. Even though the influence of Calvinism and the Dutch Reformed Church has decreased in the last couple of decades, there are still some areas in the Netherlands—often rural—in which people are still well-read in the Scriptures.[9] This heritage in Dutch culture requires us to refer to another logic of 'the father' which is derived from a late study by Freud entitled *Moses and Monotheism*. In a variation on the fable from *Totem and Taboo*, the old Egyptian Moses, an epitome of rationality, was killed by his rebellious followers, who then out of regret substituted him for the Semitic Moses, or Jahweh, an extremely jealous God. So here, a symbolic father is replaced by a 'vengeful and unforgiving [...] God full of murderous rage' (Žižek 'The Big Other', 2).[10] This unforgiving God-the-father may resemble the obscene-primordial father from *Totem and Taboo*, except that the latter enjoyed many sexual privileges, whereas the 'uncompromising God' speaks to his followers and simply 'says "No!" to *jouissance*' (ibid., 2). The old Egyptian Moses was reasonable, but the new one is an 'irrational' and prohibitive father whose 'voice is inherently meaningless, nonsensical even'.

The authority of the father in TERUG NAAR OEGSTGEEST is grounded in his recitations from the Bible, which in turn are grounded in the 'inexorable orders' from a malicious God: 'It is like this BECAUSE I SAY IT IS LIKE THIS!' (Žižek, 2). When protagonist Jan Wolkers visits his father at his sickbed, even before we see him we hear the father reminding the son that he always kept to the text 'Serving the Lord, Romans 12:11', a line that Jan had used in a derogatory manner in one of his books. While the camera remains focussed on the protagonist, we hear the father still off-screen, reduced to a feeble voice. He says that to his embarrassment, Jan's book was mentioned during a sermon the previous Sunday to illustrate the narrowness of education in the past. The father felt guilty ('this is about me, your old father'), although he knows he has taught his offspring 'respect for the Almighty'. It is only after the son says 'It's only a book' and switches on a lamp that we see the father's face, who then recites from the Bible as if to redeem the son's sexually impertinent and blasphemous writings.

During the many flashbacks to the 1930s and the war years, the voice of the father is dominant throughout. When the family has gone to the beach on a sunny day, the father says his prayers, asking the Lord 'to bless us poor sinners', whereas the camera shows the young Jan in close-up. As soon as his father has fallen asleep, he asks his mother whether he can catch lizards in a tin can. After the lizards have died due to the father's carelessness, Jan becomes angry. The reply by the father is shown via a high-angle shot, as if he can act as a true representative of the Father: 'You dare raise your voice against your parents? Your hands will grow out of the grave and be trampled by stallions.' When in a later scene the father calls Jan a 'wayward boy', the son will continue to behave like that and hides the dead lizards in a cream pie. At the same time, the words of the father resonate in Jan's head when a slide show is accompanied by the telling of the fairy tale about Tom Thumb: 'Shall we send these gluttons in the woods too?' The apocalyptical messages often sent by the father via a voice-over create a culture of sexual repression: as the young boy Jan thinks about kissing the prettiest girl at school, the next shot shows us an image of a frog. At the same time, the recitations about a world of damnation unleash a morbid fascination on Jan's part: he is greatly interested in the stories by Uncle Louis—the 'black sheep' of the family—about the bones of the dead dug up after ten years in the grave, and we then see Jan's mental image of a barge with skeletons. And later, after Louis dies, Jan imagines his coffin leaving the soil like a 'V1' as Louis says out loud that he doesn't want to be buried. Jan also listens carefully to Louis's story about the horrible death of Jan's grandmother, who was 'encased in vermin'. This is followed by a scene in which we see the camera straight above the family while we hear the father say that one shall not eat creeping animals, for they are an 'abomination'. At other times, the father is shown reading from the Bible in low-angle so that his head seems to grow out of the book itself, or we see him recite with his mouth in extreme close-up.

While sitting at his father's deathbed and being overwhelmed by his many recollections and mental images, Jan himself quotes from the Bible at times, such as the verse in Corinthians about 'a house not made with hands, eternal in the heavens'. On the one hand, the verbatim quotes illustrate to what extent Jan has been indoctrinated by his religious upbringing. So many years have passed since he has stopped believing in God—since his late teens—and yet he can still recite passages. On the other hand, the biblical phrases are quoted with ironic gusto. For his father, every word is a sacred and serious business, but the son's imitation of texts from the Scripture is characterized by a sarcastic distance, underscored by Jan's remark to his father: 'When you die, what will become of God?' For him, the voice of the prohibitive God-the-father, in whose name his father tends to speak, is meaningless. Many flashback scenes, recalled by the astute non-believing Jan, give evidence of the seeds of doubt that are sown in his mind: despite the solemn tone of the father, the verses sound hollow and nonsensical. The descriptions of sexually frank passages in the novels of the real-life Jan Wolkers were attempts to resist the '"No" to

jouissance': for the father, sex is strictly functional, meant to procreate, but for the son, it becomes a source of great pleasure. While depicting the religious culture, Van Gogh's film ultimately sides with the son's perspective: it exerts a fascination with those objects that are the result of this religious repression (dead lizards in a cream pie; skeleton bones; a flying coffin).

In TERUG NAAR OEGSTGEEST, Jan visits his old father during the last days of the latter's life. In EEN VLUCHT REGENWULPEN, also from the 1980s and also based on a book about dispelling one's Reformist heritage, the situation is similar except that the protagonist, the 33-year-old biologist Maarten van Leerdam, is not at the bedside of a dying father but instead is taking good care of his old bedridden mother whom he used to worship as a child, as we see in a series of flashbacks.[11] Maarten has stopped going to church, which he used to frequent when his strict father was still alive. This does not mean that his morals have become loose—on the contrary, he is still very much under the influence of the Protestant culture, which implies that he lead a pious life; if not, God's vengeance will strike upon sinners. When two elders come to see Maarten's old mother and to pray for her, she says that it is of no use, for her sins are too scarlet to be pardoned. Maarten then chases the elders away and even throws one of them in a nearby water. This is the one violent eruption on Maarten's part in EEN VLUCHT REGENWULPEN and a clear example of how these films from the 1980s portrayed elders and preachers as hypocritical and insensitive creatures who talk hellfire and damnation while wagging their finger (Hoogendoorn).

Though this unexpected aggressive impulse may suggest otherwise, Maarten's main problem is that he is too balanced a character. He has never violated any rules, and his career is promising. He is doing research on cloning, which in the context of the film could be interpreted as the possibility of procreation without the necessity of sex. The regularity of his life is disrupted, however, when he hears at the beginning of the film the voice of God during a nightmare, asking him why he has drifted from the 'path of the fathers'. The voice commands him to lose his virginity within seven days, and if not, he will be cast into the outer darkness where the fire is not quenched and the worm does not die. Instead of the usual prohibitions, he has to cope, quite unexpectedly, with an order of enjoyment: Maarten has to taste the 'sin' of the flesh to prepare him for a life in which he will 'be fruitful and multiply'. Since he is a very self-disciplined character, prohibitions were never a problem for him, but he now has to act in a much more forthcoming manner than he is used to. In his adolescent years, he fancied Martha, but since this girl neglected him, he had no interest in seducing any other woman. In what could be his final week before being sent by God to the outer darkness, Maarten is accompanied by an imaginary alter ego, his womanizing look-alike (without glasses but with a moustache) who, as an extension of God's voice, bombards him with advice. Maarten, however, continues to behave like a coward in his contacts with women. Ultimately, he does have sex in the nick of time, just before the deadline, and it is no coincidence that he is only able to do so after the incident with the elders—in which he calls Christianity 'all deceit'—as well as after his mother's death. He sleeps with Zus, Martha's sister, and he only gets the courage to kiss her when he sees her combing her hair in a similar fashion as his own mother did in one of the flashbacks. At the end of De Jong's film, Zus asks after coitus what it felt like and he answers: 'I thought I was on the verge of dying.' If we grant belief in God's voice during the nightmare, this line is correct, for having sex was the sole way to escape God's death sentence. The line can at the same time also refer to the sexual experience as such, once we take into account that an orgasm is often called the 'little death'.

PATHETIC FATHERS AS ADDRESSEE: *DE AVONDEN* AND *ABEL*

Hollywood films such as the BACK TO THE FUTURE trilogy (Robert Zemeckis, 1985, 1989, 1990) and WAR OF THE WORLDS (Steven Spielberg, 2005) have employed a smart strategy to reinstall the paternal duty via a detour. In Spielberg's sci-fi adaptation of a novel by H.G. Wells, the father is represented as a 'loser': he is a divorced man in a mid-life crisis who is scorned by his ex-wife and is not taken seriously by his kids. Then there is a terrible 'crisis' on a much grander scale, for planet earth is threatened by an alien invasion of tripod fighting machines. Since it is the father and not the mother who takes up the grateful task of protecting the children, the teenage kids are ultimately prepared to see him as their 'daddy'. The moral of the story: when it comes to domestic trifles, mother may help you out, but when the need is highest, count on father.

In addition to this scenario of WAR OF THE WORLDS, there is the restored oedipal trajectory in BACK TO THE FUTURE (Robert Zemeckis, 1985). Marty's father has been bullied ever since childhood, but when the son travels back thirty years in time, before his own conception, the time-travelling son teaches his father-to-be how to become assertive. Thanks to the successful intervention of Marty, he changes the future of his own family. The father is able to stick up for himself, but when Marty returns to the present, everyone acts as if it has always been like this. Marty has gone back in time to 1955 to improve his father's character but—and this is important—there are no traces of his recovery operation.

Whereas the fathers in these films are remade to live up to the expectations of conventional paternity, it is much more common in Dutch cinema—and perhaps in European cinema in general[12]—to display an ambivalent attitude towards the father as bearer of symbolic authority. Any discussion regarding such an ambivalence must mention Gerard Reve's classic novel *De avonden* [*The Evenings*] (1947), which gives the impression that father-son relationships in post-war Holland are refractory, to say the least. Because *De avonden* is known as a literary milestone, it took several decades before a filmmaker dared to adapt it. Rudolf van den Berg's adaptation from 1989 opens with a nightmare by the twenty-something protagonist, Frits van Egters, who is in a slight panic on New Year's Eve: 'I have to tell it. I have to tell it, but how?' He hears the voice of a friend, Wim, outside. He then runs into the living room, where his father is smoking a pipe and reading a newspaper, but he is unable to express himself. He walks towards the window; Wim is still standing under the lantern light. He turns to his father, but the only thing he is able to say is 'father'. He then wakes up and sees that it is only Sunday 22 December: he still has nine more days to say 'it'. Unlike the novel, which is strictly chronological, the film viewers know that Frits must disclose something important before the year is over, and they will be wondering whether or not he will say what he has to say. Whereas the novel registers both daily events and dreams in plain but slightly archaic sentences, the film articulates some scenes, such as the dream sequences, in a slightly different style than scenes at the dinner table or at the office, which, alas, does not work for the better.

One of the scenes, shot in a divergent style, shows Frits when he hears about the suicide of the pretty boy Wim, for it uses out-of-focus shots to underscore that it shocks him. Given that Wim is rumoured to be homosexual, the shock Frits experiences suggests that the 'it' concerns Frits's repressed sexual desires. In the meantime, the viewers watch a series of uneventful events: Frits visiting the birthday party of a baby; Frits attending the reunion of his school, Frits at the swimming pool, Frits working at an office, Frits having dinner with his parents. At each event, he is bored to death. Frits shares an obsession with torture fantasies with his one-eyed friend Maurits, and he has a tremendous fascination for physical decay. He considers himself fortunate for still having all his hair and likes to make pestering remarks about friends getting bald. Most important for the sake of my argument is that Frits, while acting politely most of the time, is irritated by the habits of his father. The old man is hard of hearing, grinds his food, champs while eating, farts during dinner frequently, and uses his dirty porridge spoon in the sugar bowl. When Frits asks his father to tell stories from the past, the old man has no clue that Frits is not interested in the stories themselves; in fact, the son takes delight in the fact that, as we can gather from his body language, he knows exactly what the father will say, apparently because he has told these stories many times before. At one point, the father remarks 'Did I not already tell you this?', indicating that he is quite forgetful.

Insofar as Frits can be said to have an aim, it seems that he wants to annoy his parents, and his father in particular. When he is about to turn off the radio at the very moment his father complains about the terrible music, he turns up the volume instead and says that he likes the 'sharp violins'. When a friend asks him why he does not leave his parental home, he has no prompt reply but then shouts at him that someone has to keep an eye on his father and mother. He himself lacks the stability to be a beacon for them, but he speaks his most crucial lines when in a state of drunkenness: 'But God sees us all. He is Almighty. If you think I do not see you, remember that God watches over you. He is witness to your righteousness.' Rather than regarding this confessional statement as a straightforward reliance on a Supreme Being, this quote has to be taken with a grain of salt. Frits is possibly so confused about his own presence in the world that he tends to give ironic retorts all the time. But of course, it cannot be ruled out that a jester will use ironic phrases in an ironic manner to make truthful claims after all. In a later scene, when the bottle of wine his mother thinks she has bought turns out to be a sour fruit drink consisting of apples and berries, he talks to God: 'Eternal God, see the immeasurable goodness of my mother', and asks him: 'Protect them' (meaning his parents). The scene precedes the supposed climax of the film, for Frits had set his mind on telling 'it', but in one more dream scene, shot with a wide-angle lens to emphasize its surreal quality, he is ultimately only able to utter: 'People can sing', to which his father dryly replies: 'But birds can sing, too'. After he has woken up and the clock has struck twelve, he initially thinks that all is lost but then recuperates by repetitively saying to himself: 'I breathe, I move, I live.'

On the one hand, it is not only important what Frits has to say, it is above all crucial that his father is the addressee of his message. If one has no respect for the addressee, it would not be difficult to tell what is on one's mind. So the fact that Frits fails to confess 'it' is an implicit acknowledgement of his father as a symbolic authority. On the other hand, he treats his father as if he were a child, and he is annoyed by his behaviour. Moreover, his father is so absent-minded that it is easy to make fun of him. The two times Frits calls out to God, one gets the impression that he considers his own father such a failure that he is desperately searching for an alternative in order to keep the memory of a once powerful father intact. If need be, God is this alternative, though Frits is never serious about religion. At the same time, one cannot help thinking that Frits is belittling his father throughout so as to make the obstacle of telling him about 'it' an easier hurdle.

Whether Frits treats his father too harshly or not, burnt out and pathetic father figures have become recurring characters in Dutch cinema, perhaps propelled by the reputation of Reve's novel. Alex van Warmerdam's drily humorous debut feature ABEL [VOYEUR] (1986) is made in the spirit of the suffocating atmosphere in Reve's *De avonden*. Here we have a 31-year-old son who has not been outside for some years. In this hilarious 'caricature of a psychological drama' (Verstraten *Humour and Irony*, 278) in a domestic setting, the son's every action, or lack thereof, seems motivated by his attempts to annoy his father and to receive support from his overprotective mother after the father is driven mad by the son's attitude. Since Abel derives pleasure from the fact that his father is ashamed of him, he gives him all the more reason to be embarrassed by him, e.g. by deliberately acting like a retard in the presence of a psychiatrist. Since the father cannot control himself, he turns himself into a bigger fool than the son feigns to be. These fathers from ABEL and DE AVONDEN are yardsticks for fathers in Dutch cinematic culture: they become objects of ridicule, but at the same time they still radiate some symbolic power which is evident by the fact that they are still deemed worthy of provocations by sons.

A (BROKEN) CHAIN OF DEAD FATHERS: *GLUCKAUF*

This dialectic of slight derision and an unremitting belief in the father, despite everything, has been extended to a film like GLUCKAUF [SON OF MINE] (Remy van Heugten, 2015). Whereas the father in DE AVONDEN is a bit pitiful because he is hard of hearing and lacks table manners, Jeffrey's father Lei Frissen has a hot-tempered nature. In the beginning of the film, we see the gun-carrying Lei take his young boy from his mother before we arrive in the present, more than ten years later, when the two of them are hunting. It is clear that Lei is the experienced shooter teaching his son to become a 'real man'. It also becomes obvious to the adolescent Jeffrey, however, that his father is a wretched character. 'No father loves his son as much as Lei does', Jeffrey's girlfriend Nicole says at one point, but their interaction is one of constant attracting and repelling. The son has no problem with the fact that his father, who frequents the local café often, uses small-scale crime to keep his head above water. But Jeffrey soon discovers that his father has some debts with the charismatic crook Vester who complains to the son: 'In your father's world, money has no memory.'

It is the undeniable strength of GLUCKAUF, which won four Golden Calf awards, that the camera remains close to the characters in a hand-held style that is reminiscent of the cinema of the brothers Jean-Pierre and Luc Dardenne.[13] There are many tracking shots with the camera showing the characters from behind or with the camera in the rear seat of a car. The camerawork prompts the viewer to focus more on the facial expressions of the characters than on the object of their attention. This is a type of cinema that takes little notice of causality. We never get clear-cut psychological motivations, signified by the fact that flashbacks are absent, though we know that Lei has a troubled history. We can only gather bits and pieces of information in passing. Vester's contempt for Lei becomes most apparent when he tells Jeffrey how much he admires the latter's grandfather, 'big fellow, tough, with hands of stone', implying that it is unbelievable that Lei is his offspring. Jeffrey becomes aware that his father is unable to pay off his debts and starts doing some sleazy jobs for Vester without informing his dad, of course. The father gets furious when he discovers that son Jeffrey is involved with Vester on his behalf. He wants to seek redress, but one of Vester's henchmen prevents him from attacking the local crook, who by the way is usually represented in a friendly and polite manner: speaking in a soft voice; doing the dishes; feeding the pigeons.

Though Vester feels contempt for Lei—'you have burdened your son with guilt'—Lei nonetheless has a positive self-image. He wants Jeffrey to be like him and teaches him the things he himself is good at, such as hunting rabbits. But the son seems to outdo the father: he seems wiser, more restrained, less self-destructive. When the two of them carry out a drugs transport, the atmosphere becomes aggressive until Jeffrey intervenes with a good command of the French language. The fact that Jeffrey knows that Lei has debts with Vester frustrates the father, for his weakness is exposed. But the topic of money also discloses a key difference between father and son, and this time not to the disadvantage of Lei. Unlike the son, who in the beginning works as a small-time drugs dealer, the father is not interested in making money at all costs. When he and his son do another job for Vester, it turns out that they have to ride a group of women to some brothel. Halfway there Lei stops the van, for he has moral objections, and after having a fierce debate with his son, Lei walks away and Jeffrey takes over the wheel. Vester allows the son to keep a great amount of money—'we'll settle this later'—which puts Jeffrey under his influence, at least until the matter is settled.

Tragically, the possession of money will indirectly become fatal to the son. Jeffrey is celebrating his twentieth birthday in the café, and thanks to Nicole's insistence, Lei has come as well. He is drinking beer at the bar and is in a bad mood. To cheer him up, Jeffrey takes him outside to show him the car he bought the father as a present, thanks to the huge sum of money he received from Vester. Jeffrey wants to give his father a ride right away, and in a wave of nostalgia, fuelled by his state of near-drunkenness, Lei tells Jeffrey that he should never forget where he comes from. Lei then reminisces how his own father took him, a young boy then, into the mines. We do not see this visualized as a flashback, but we see the tears in his eyes as he remembers how he was left to his own devices when he lost his father's hand. Jeffrey then interrupts the story by saying: 'Vester was right. You sound like a bitch.' Whereas Lei has tried to be a caring and empathetic father despite his character flaws, Jeffrey's rude remark mimics the carelessness of his grandfather, Lei's own father. Keeping up with the soundtrack, the speed of the car accelerates, but the screen has gone black for a while. There is a transition to the funeral service for Jeffrey, and as the priest starts his sermon we see the father moving around in a wheelchair, with bruises on his face. Taking vengeance on Vester who is indirectly responsible for his misery, Lei robs money from Vester's henchmen. He is wounded in the skirmish but refuses to be treated. He delivers the money to a pregnant Nicole, but she only accepts the pictures of Jeffrey as a kid. After she says that it is going to be a boy, Lei leaves but hangs the money bag on the doorknob. Slowly walking on the road, he is picked up by Vester. The final shot is of a car on fire.

Since the very first shots of GLUCKAUF seem to show a burning car, beginning and end are connected, implying that Lei was in fact dead from the start. Van Heugten's film encourages us to distinguish between two kinds of dead fathers: one who is buried and remembered favourably (Lei's father) and one, though still alive, is the 'walking dead' because he gets little respect from others (Lei). Lei visits the tombstone of his old man during a very brief scene. We can read that his father died in 1975 at the age of only 33, and though this is not mentioned in the film, this was immediately after the closure of the last coal mines in South Limburg, in December 1974. We know very little of Lei's father, but a few remarks in passing give far from unanimous clues to what he was like. He is briefly mentioned by Lei's uncle Broos, who says that if he were alive, he would have ended up as an angry man and an alcoholic. To Jeffrey, Vester sketches a positive portrait of a 'proud' grandfather: he only did a job for Vester once, but when the victim ended up dead instead of frightened, he refused to accept any money. Lei associates his father with a traumatic youth memory, however, and he wants to spare his own son the feeling of being abandoned. After taking Jeffrey away from his mother, Lei keeps his son close, for better or for worse, educating him to become his mirror-image. Lei wants to be a caring father as a reaction to the carelessness of his own dad. Now that Jeffrey has reached an age of maturity, he is about to outgrow his father. The episode with Vester confirms that the son has become bigger than daddy, to Lei's frustration, for he is about to lose his original function as caregiver. It results in excessive drinking on Lei's part, but despite his drunkenness, he is able to intervene successfully when Jeffrey is attacked by a few men, one of whom Vester had ordered the son to beat up. Afterwards, Lei embraces Jeffrey so tightly that the latter almost chokes—a clear example of smothering love, as if he is very happy to fulfil his paternal duty of protecting his son.

The father-son relationship in GLUCKAUF is a complex one in the sense that it is too easy to discredit Lei. It is implied that the grandfather, as a former coal miner, was the victim of economic misfortune: the closure of the mines was a serious blow to him, but his son Lei remembers him as a ruthless fellow. This harshness can also be deduced from Vester's stories to grandson Jeffrey. Lei is represented as a much more empathetic father, someone who refuses to do the dirty job of delivering the prostitutes and who protects his son. He is, however, considered a marked man given that he is despised by Vester, and in a key scene, Jeffrey reiterates a contemptuous remark: 'You sound like a bitch.' Since this is followed by the fatal accident, Lei becomes a no-good father in the eyes of the community. In the chain of men in the family, he is branded the weakest link, not worthy of the name of father or even grandfather. When Lei visits his ex-wife, she initially does not want to see him, but after some deliberation she listens to what he has to say, keeping the door ajar. He tells her about Nicole's pregnancy but ignores the words 'grandmother' or 'grandfather'. And the fact that Nicole refuses to accept the money he has grabbed violently from Vester's men implies that he does not deserve the label of 'grandfather'. As a father, Lei is the outcast in the family heritage: he will be remembered less dearly than his own father, despite the latter's carelessness, and not as favourably as his son, despite the latter's craving for money eclipsing his moral principles.

GLUCKAUF seems emblematic of a state of affairs regarding father figures. There used to be a generation of authoritative men, to which Lei's father as well as Vester belong, but the chain has been broken with Lei. If Vester is at one point generous to Jeffrey, this is because he regards him not as a descendant of Lei but of his grandfather. Vester, almost acting as his surrogate daddy, thus believes Jeffrey has a promising future ahead of him, but this future is cut off due to the accident, which was caused by Lei. In an era of the decline of traditional power structures due to the contempt for authority exhibited by the generation of 1968, as Paul Verhaeghe keeps stressing in his work such as his best-selling study *Identiteit*, the void is filled by the liberal-capitalist doctrine of 'individual responsibility'. In Freud's time, if the father said 'no', the answer was 'no', so one could blame daddy for missed opportunities. In today's world, people are responsible for their own success given the assumption that everyone is given opportunities and that the point is just to grab them. This also means that one is responsible for one's own failures. If young/adolescent characters in films seem adrift in many movies, struggling to find a mode of living, this cannot but be related to the fact that fathers have been unable to adjust to a situation in which the idea of 'Ask daddy, he knows' is no longer applicable.

RESTORING THE IMAGE OF THE FATHER

Many films, not only Dutch films, represent fathers who are trying to cope with circumstances in which their authority is no longer self-evident. In DE PASSIEVRUCHT [FATHER'S AFFAIR] (Maarten Treurniet, 2003), Armin discovers after his wife's death that his son Bo cannot be his son because he finds out that he himself is infertile. The father regards himself as the weakest link in a generational chain, for when his very own father Huib is about to die, he hears that the old man had a one-time affair with his wife, so that his son is his half-brother. In a flatly spoken but nonetheless sentimental voice-over, Armin concludes that his anger has been replaced by gratitude, for without his father there would have been no Bo. CLOACA (Willem van de Sande Bakhuyzen, 2004) portrays four male friends in their forties, each of whom has manoeuvred himself into a most awkward situation: an upcoming divorce; an acute manic episode; sex with the daughter of his best friend; a charge of swindling. The one who is a father has the political influence to help his friend Pieter who is accused of fraud (unjustly, or so it appears), but of all people, he is too much of a coward to support him. Pieter's suicide in the final shot is shown via a dolly-in on the shower drain, in which blood is mixed with water, a clear reference to a similar shot in Hitchcock's PSYCHO (1960). This comparison suggests that modern-day fatherhood is morally bankrupt, as if it is as monstrous as Norman Bates' psychotic attachment to his mother. DE LIEFHEBBERS (Anna van der Heide, 2019) is a more light-hearted continuation of the mental struggles in CLOACA. Four 40-something siblings—one of them a depressed homosexual, another an autistic architect—reflect upon the impact of their once dominant father who is now suffering from Alzheimer's.

At best, fathers are likeable or become likeable again. They can be good companions, but that is also the death knell for their authority. After many years of neglecting his daughter, the father in MEET ME IN VENICE (Eddy Terstall, 2015) makes an enjoyable trip with her by train across southern Europe, disclosing at the end that his reason for inviting her is the fact that he is terminally ill.[14] The handicapped father in NENA (Saskia Diesing, 2015) wants to commit suicide so desperately that his sixteen-year-old daughter—the one remaining reason on his list of cons—accepts his death wish and accompanies him to the rail tracks. The father in WATERBOYS (Robert-Jan Westdijk, 2016) is a self-interested wiseacre who does not know that his son has been cohabiting with a girlfriend for three months. When both he himself and his son are requested by their partners to leave home, he takes along his only twenty-something child on a trip to Edinburgh for the promotion of his latest book. He is invited as a special guest, since his novel, which happens to be set in Edinburgh, has been translated into Scottish. The trip with his sensitive and cello-playing son teaches the father to behave less arrogantly, with the result that, instead of father and son, they become buddies who celebrate, in the words of the father, their 'regained freedom'.[15]

The dwindling influence of fathers means that they either have to accept such an egalitarian relationship as the best alternative[16] or they become frustrated for losing their grip on their offspring. The boxing trainer in LANGER LICHT [NORTHERN LIGHT] (David Lammers, 2006) is annoyed that his adolescent son is wearing a ballerina tutu, but when he tries to hang on to his position of authority, they become alienated from each other.[17] LANGER LICHT is an arthouse drama, but in popular films, there is usually a utopian solution to this kind of alienation. In DE ZEVENDE HEMEL [THE SEVENTH HEAVEN] (Job Gosschalk, 2016), a father has torn his family apart, all because this 'pig-headed' know-it-all wanted his oldest son to take over his Italian restaurant. We know that the film will end in a reconciliation because the characters address all crisis situations by singing well-known Dutch pop songs. These unrealistic musical scenes that constantly interrupt the story prepare the viewer for a happy ending: even Paul who has been insulted time and again comes to visit his parents in Italy, since this was the dearest wish of his terminally ill mother; father must drop his overly strict attitude and can only stutter his apologies.

If the image of the father as a father is to be rescued, then the hilarious approach of DE BOSKAMPI'S [LITTLE GANGSTER] (Arne Toonen, 2015), basically aimed at a youth audience, seems key. Rik Boskamp's father Paul is the prototypical nerdy bookkeeper who is made fun of at the office, though he is so oblivious to anything that he hardly notices the small harassments: practically daily, Rik has to remove post-it's from his clothes. And Paul is 'Mr. Nice Guy' who is 'incredibly gullible' and never says no. When Rik moves to a new town, he makes his environment as well as his classmates believe that he is of Italian descent ('Ricki Boskampi') and that his father is a Mafia boss. The father himself has no pretentions at all: he remains the very same absent-minded man as ever, unaware that his son has renamed him 'Paulo'. If people are nonetheless impressed by the man, it is thanks to the kid's convincing play-act. The charade seems about to collapse when Roderick, one of Rik's former classmates who used to bully him, moves to the same town and threatens to expose them as the Boskamp family. But Rik/Ricki puts some heavy laxatives in Roderick's drink so that the new kid in town instantly has serious stomach problems. The schoolkids, however, presume that he shits in his pants out of fear for Ricki, the son of a Mafia father. As in the case of BACK TO THE FUTURE, the 'modern' father can only be considered a true father on the condition that the son bestows him a mask of authority, even if it requires quite some smart and foul tricks to uphold the illusion. Finally, the truth comes out that the father is not a Mafia boss at all, but when Paul realizes that his son only invented all of this because he does not want a clumsy and forgetful father but rather a 'cool' one, he starts to behave accordingly, or at least to some extent. As a bonus, he marries Gina from the local pizzeria and he dares to say 'no' when a talkative salesman wants to sell him 'stainless steel knives'.

IN SEARCH OF THE IMAGINARY FATHER: *DE VLIEGENDE HOLLANDER*

Whereas Rik Boskamp transforms his father through make-belief, the status of the father in DE VLIEGENDE HOLLANDER [THE FLYING DUTCHMAN] (Jos Stelling, 1995) is in limbo. There could be a clear lineage, for the son is the spitting image of his deceased biological father, but it could also be the case that the father is the product of a fanciful narrator. To start with the first option: Stelling's film is set at the close of the sixteenth century when the reigning Spanish Catholics were at war with Dutch heretics. In this '*turbulent age*', as the opening text reads, '*thousands of statues, symbols of the hated power, were decapitated and pillaged*'. In the beginning, we see a sign of life from underneath a monstrously large image of a head, part of an apparently demolished gigantic statue. The image is straight from a Fellini movie such as CASANOVA (1976) and the toppled head is regularly shown in close-up to underscore its massive impact. A farmer's wife starts to dig the sand after she has detected a hand. A man emerges and the two immediately have sex up the hill next to the statue's head. Thanks to the intervention of the Italian storyteller Campanelli who witnesses the lovemaking, the farmer Netelneck and his men are so distracted that they arrive too late to catch Netelneck's wife in the act. The man crawls back in time under the head, but the farmer and his men drag him out of his hiding place. They keep the man tied up in the dirt of a cesspool. Campanelli liberates him from his unfortunate position, but only because he thinks the man knows where 'the gold' is hidden. During his escape, the man is hit by a bullet and Campanelli holds him in his arms in the man's dying seconds. The Italian only discovers that the man is originally a Dutchman, and when he asks him whether the gold is hidden in the cesspool, he takes the Dutchman's silence for confirmation. But the latter simply draws his last breath, and the Italian buries him. The lengthy prologue ends when the farmer's wife waits for the man's return beside the image of the large head. Seasons pass, and in wintertime, next to the head, the farmer's wife dies in childbirth, but the baby is alive and kicking. As long as this boy lives, Netelneck will hold a grudge against him, and this only becomes worse when at the age of 21, the physical resemblance with the Dutchman is unmistakeable—the same actor, René Groothof, plays both the Dutch father and son.

Campanelli, however, claims to be the boy's originator as well, his spiritual father. Apart from the fact that Campanelli sets the story in motion because of his search for gold,[18] the Italian, who calls himself a 'marvellous artist and comedian', acts as a storyteller, addressing the viewers.[19] In the beginning, he chases a crow away, for this symbol of death is a nuisance to a story that is about to start. Nonetheless, the crow announces its proximity time and again, for Campanelli's narratives always take a turn for the worse: 'This love story ends in shit', or later, 'I could invent a happy ending, but people have to pay for that'. He uses his rich imagination to manipulate the Dutchman's son who is eager to hear about his father. In exchange for food and for access to the cesspool on Netelneck's farmyard, Campanelli tells the then seven-year-old kid about the father's background.

Campanelli makes up the tale that the boy's 'real' father is a captain on a big ship with red sails and black masts. On the bow of the ship, there is a one-eyed lion's head. 'He can fly, above the waves. He is a wizard, just like me.' Campanelli requests the child to close his eyes, and then silently sneaks away to prove to the kid that he can fly. Fourteen years later, there is a renewed encounter, and Campanelli gives the now 21-year-old Dutchman a jerkin that belonged to his father. Wearing this heirloom will make the son invulnerable: he has to trust the wind and he will learn how to fly. He adds to this: 'You are the fruit of my imagination. In fact, I am your father. When I let you go, I will fly away, too.'

Campanelli dies about one-third of the way into Stelling's film, stabbed to death by Netelneck's real son. From that moment onwards, everything that happens seems instigated by Campanelli's imagination: on his way to the sea, the Dutchman finds a ship by accident in a swamp, and many voices resonate in his mind, among others the quote about the one-eyed lion's head. Just as his father had sex with his mother once, he has sex with Netelneck's daughter-in-law Lotte once and then loses track of her in the chaos at the beach. Some seven years later, Lotte recognizes the jerkin while visiting a prison with her husband and her own son. She insists there be a search for the Dutchman, and her son meets him first when the Dutchman performs a magical trick. To the astonishment of Netelneck's son, his wife Lotte reveals that the Dutchman is the father of their son and she wants father and son to spend some time together. The encounter is reminiscent of the encounter between Campanelli and the seven-year-old Dutchman. After the father has asked the boy, 'Can you hear the wind?' they sit together until daybreak. He then asks him: 'Do you believe I can fly?' He climbs up a wall and requests his son to close his eyes with his hands, for if not, he might fall. When the Dutchman is really high, the camera is at a low angle. The boy yells for his mother, but Netelneck's son walks into the courtyard. He looks up together with the boy, but the Dutchman is gone.

In 2003, IMAGO—the organisation of European directors of photography—published *Making Pictures* in which the most visually stunning European films from the twentieth century were collected. DE VLIEGENDE HOLLANDER is the only Dutch picture in the volume, and this honourable mention contrasts with the rather cold to lukewarm reviews the film received from the majority of the Dutch press. For Jos van der Burg, the film consisted of an admirable 'chain of tableaux vivants', a series of painterly shots that recalled the imaginative work of the Italian brothers Vittorio and Paolo Taviani, but the story is so drawn out and extended that it does not arouse any emotion at all. Peter van Bueren's review exposes how critics are in two minds about Stelling's film. It is an original and sensitive variant of the *commedia dell'arte*, in the vein of KAOS (1984) by the Taviani brothers, and its slow pace is idiosyncratic, but the historically incorrect film is so absurd that it borders on irrationality. For Van Bueren, the imaginative DE VLIEGENDE HOLLANDER becomes too imaginative, and whether or not Stelling's films are excessive becomes a moot question throughout. Since excess and an all-too-vivid imagination can have their benefits, I am inclined to support Stelling's own position that Dutch culture is too deeply rooted in Calvinism to really appreciate his cinema. Calvinists have the tendency to put their faith in verbal expressions and to distrust visuality. They prefer word over image, because they presume that unlike pictures, texts can be crystal clear. According to John Calvin, the sect's founder, the New Testament excels in clarity of expression, enabling an 'immediate experience of truth' for believers (McGrath, 159). It is the task of clergymen associated with a rigorous doctrine like Calvinism to boil down the words in the Bible to a single, unambiguous message. In contrast to the presumed unequivocalness of texts, images are not restricted to just one meaning. Because of their essential indeterminacy, images open up a space for ambiguity and leave room for interpretation by the viewer. An image always represents more than meets the eye, inviting the viewer to add meaning to it.

Out of dismay with the Calvinist tradition that incessantly insists on the virtue of thrift, Stelling creates an antidote in the form of spectacular cinema with a sparse use of words. And the one character who talks a lot, Campanelli, only produces endless babble, once more affirming that language in his films is a source of miscommunication, as in DUSKA (2007), with the uninvited visitor who only speaks Russian, and DE WISSELWACHTER [THE POINTSMAN] (1986) about a taciturn man who never has a conversation with the French woman who steps out at the small railroad station by mistake. He thinks she is named 'dégoutant', not realizing that she had described the black coffee he had offered her as 'disgusting'. Stelling's films are meant to transgress the Calvinist tradition that privileges word over image by radically conveying a visual imagination.

CONCLUSION: THREE FATHERS

Stelling's film DE VLIEGENDE HOLLANDER covers the three types of father that have been examined in this chapter. The son is in pursuit of a father who has no name but only a legendary and fanciful nickname, The Flying Dutchman. We know that he is dead, but the son does not know this, and for that reason, his father is imaginary rather than symbolic. This father is not an anchor for him in his social circuit but functions at the level of his imagination. One day, the son hopes, the nickname will be embodied, and then the father will definitely live up to the reputation the tales have made of him. The figure who comes closest to the symbolic position of the father—which is unoccupied by definition, for no man coincides with the Law—is the Italian storyteller Campanelli. He verbally depicts the biological but posthumous father as a product of his wondrous narratives. His eloquence persuades the son to believe in the character with miraculous qualities. In this triad, Netelneck is the unforgiving father, the one who says 'No!' to *jouissance*. He resembles the obscene-primordial father from *Totem and Taboo* except that he lacks the sexual privileges. Indeed, his own wife commits adultery with that rascal, named The Flying Dutchman by Campanelli. Netelneck develops into a repressive father and tries to prevent any bond between the Dutchman's son and Lotte, Netelneck's daughter-in-law. But saying 'no' also triggers sexual desires. History repeats itself. Though Lotte becomes the wife of Netelneck's son, and though her boy-child has the surname of her husband, the Dutchman's son is the boy's 'real' father but not officially—he is only tied to the boy by blood.

Theoretically, the Name-of-the-Father, this supreme signifier, is meant as a cover-up for a lack in the social system: any father is endowed with authority on account of this Name. But many of these father figures in this chapter do not live up to expectations: they are either great pretenders who exceed the 'norm' and misuse their position or they are pathetic characters who underperform in their function. Because of their disappearance, the fathers in De vliegende Hollander—both the 'original' Flying Dutchman and his son as father of Lotte's son—are of a different kind: they are imaginary rather than symbolic. But the manifestation of fathers as spectral apparitions, as Lacan explained in his seminar on *Hamlet* and the ghost of the father, always hint at a glitch in the symbolic order. The scenario for the son is then to either feign madness, as Hamlet does, or to persist in (un-Calvinist) fantasies.

NOTES

1 This scenario is reminiscent of Freud's case study of the 'Wolfman' who, according to his analysis of one of the patient's dreams, had as a toddler witnessed his parents having sexual intercourse. Though he was no longer consciously aware of this event, this early incident had so deeply ingrained itself in the child's unconscious, Freud claimed, that it had caused the man's current psychic problems. The patient himself considered Freud's diagnosis to be far-fetched, but his case nonetheless became a 'showpiece of psychoanalysis' (Sergei Pankejev, qtd. in Hughes, 102).

2 Claus had called his own play, on which the film was based, a 'nare komedie' [a grim comedy].

3 One of Freud's patients had the following dream about his father: '*His father was alive once more and was talking to him in his usual way, but* (the remarkable thing was that) *he had really died, only he did not know it*' ('The Interpretation of Dreams', 430).

4 The scene is clearly inspired by the moment in Reservoir Dogs (Quentin Tarantino, 1992) when Mr. Blonde cuts off the ear of a policeman while singing and dancing to the 1970s pop song 'Stuck in the Middle With You' by Stealers Wheel. The scene also recalls the hanging scene in Once Upon a Time in the West (Sergio Leone, 1968) in which a man with a rope around his neck stands on the shoulders of his younger brother until the latter collapses from fatigue.

5 Whereas Eddy in Lek is cynically called 'Serpico', in Baantjer: Het begin [Amsterdam Vice] (Arne Toonen, 2019), the protagonist Jurre de Cock is mockingly compared to Lieutenant Columbo, the homicide detective from the hugely popular 1970s American television series *Columbo*. Toonen's Baantjer film is set in April 1980, during the days preceding the coronation of Princess Beatrix. Jurre is new to the police force in Amsterdam and he thinks he has to work according to the rules. When he discovers a corpse in the canals with the word 'rat' carved in red

letters on the dead man's chest, Jurre is determined to file a report, to the irritation of his more experienced partner Tonnie Montijn. On the tumultuous day of the coronation, he discovers that this Tonnie is collaborating with an old schoolmate who trades in drugs. The next day, while witness to a shoot-out, he learns that Tonnie was also responsible for the dead 'rat' in the canals.

6 Van Diem decided to choose a flashback structure for KARAKTER upon watching AMADEUS (Milos Forman, 1984).

7 THE FAMILY (Lodewijk de Boer, 1973), the film adaptation of De Boer's own play, is the apt title for a degenerate band of two brothers (Doc and Kil) and one sister (Gina) who live in a run-down building. The film is wilfully weird, and the response has been divided, because viewers find it difficult to relate to the brutal and madcap characters. (I myself, however, appreciated the film, precisely because there is no ready-made guide as to how to read it.) THE FAMILY excels in an anarchistic disorderliness, which seems to be the result of the particular family situation. Their mother has died a long time ago, and they have only vague memories of their dominant father who used to gallivant with a great many women. They think he has been dead for about twenty years. Raised by a father who never taught them any rules of decency, the three—who are now adults—behave rudely towards any guest. Kil spills beer over the man from the insurance company, jokes about the man's baldness, and shows off his dirty feet. When the father unexpectedly returns, they do not believe his lies. Whereas the father has stories about his role in the resistance during World War II, Doc informs him that they were told he was a traitor who had even denounced his own Jewish wife to the Germans. They kick out the old man and continue to live according to their animalistic impulses. Kil has an incestuous relationship with his mute sister, and after she has slit the throat of a guest, a police force intervenes. This time, Gina screams out loud just before all three are killed.

8 The disturbed relationship between a 'not-so-tough' Jermaine Slagter and his rich father Stephen in CATACOMBE (Victor D. Ponten, 2018) is best expressed in the latter's line: 'Don't be afraid to be the best.' Jermaine is a 32-year-old right wingback in an average Dutch professional soccer team, about to go one division down. Since 'J' and the Belgian goalkeeper Kevin have money problems, he makes a business proposal to Stephen. J's father declines the offer by telling an anecdote: at the age of ten, Jermaine participated in a game of keeping the ball up without having it touch the ground. The stadium was packed, and the counter had reached close to 500 when Jermaine's only remaining rival made a mistake. As soon as he knew he had won, Jermaine stopped. He said to this father: 'I didn't want to frustrate the other boys by showing that I am so much better than they are.' At that moment, his father knew that Jermaine would not be competitive enough to make it to the top. It was then that he taught him: 'Don't be afraid to be the best.' His son did not have the merciless mentality to become an excellent soccer player. The point of

the father's story is that if Jermaine were a 'real' man, he would not have made this business proposal but would have asked his father upfront: 'Dad, I have debts and I need money.'

9 DUISTER LICHT [DARK LIGHT] (Martin Koolhoven, 1997), a mid-length television drama, is inspired by Job's sorry fate from the Bible. A peasant woman has to endure much grief: her husband has left her and her son has died at the age of 21. Moreover, she is suffering from terrible skin abscesses. Despite her misfortune, she has remained pious. At the beginning of the film, she knocks down a young burglar and chains him to the wall of the pigsty. Under threat of a gun, the thief has to do farmer's tasks: milk the cows, clean up the animal's feces, slaughter a pig. She wants him to say his prayers and read from the Bible. She informs the burglar that she is convinced that he has arrived to be the witness to her cure and that he will then become a believer himself. The thief, however, tells her that he is here so she can re-marry after she is cured, just like Job. When she puts on her wedding dress, the young burglar grabs the gun. Before he leaves, he tears a page from Job's story and makes her chew on it.

10 The concept of the Messiah is introduced as compensation for the guilt of the killers: the foretold arrival of the Messiah is the hope that the old Moses may return.

11 In the flashbacks, all characters speak with the voices of the adult actors so that it is immediately clear 'who is who'. This idea was prompted by practical considerations. First, it was always clear who the Maarten in the scene was. Second, the young actors were not very experienced, and thus the lines were spoken by professional actors. Third, the film had to be post-synchronised anyway, and in this way it was more efficient.

12 Think of the incestuous father in FESTEN [CELEBRATION] (Thomas Vinterberg, 1998) or the father who pretends for the sake of his son that the situation in the concentration camps is but a game with a great prize for the winner, as in LA VITA È BELLA [LIFE IS BEAUTIFUL] (Roberto Benigni, 1997).

13 The similarity between GLUCKAUF and the cinema of the Dardenne brothers also pertains to their choices for their films' setting: Van Heugten's film was set in the former mining area of South Limburg, and the Dardennes tend to shoot their pictures in the vicinity of Liège, which is only some 30 miles away.

14 In ONDER HET HART [IN THE HEART] (Nicole van Kilsdonk, 2014], Masha falls in love with Luuk, a divorced father of two children. Everything is fine, but then Masha's new boyfriend becomes incurably ill.

15 In JONGENS [BOYS] (Mischa Kamp, 2014), the fifteen-year-old Sieger has relative freedom to explore his sexuality. His father is a recent widower and he already has his hands full with Sieger's older brother who has become rebellious after his mother's death. Kamp's television film became such a 'tender and touching coming out' picture—the general consensus among critics—because there was no meddlesome father to interfere with Sieger's growing affection for his relay race teammate Marc.

16 In contrast to Olga's mother who vehemently objects to the fact that her daughter is dating the visual artist Erik in TURKS FRUIT, Olga's father has no quibbles with his son-in-law to be. It turns out that he can appreciate a good practical joke as much as Erik does. In other words, he is a jester rather than a figure of authority.

17 In NIEMAND IN DE STAD [OPEN SEAS] (Michiel van Erp, 2018), three of the main male characters who are members of the same student fraternity are alienated from their fathers. Jacob acts as if he is fulfilling his father's expectations but he has secretly quit studying medicine, secretly has a boyfriend, and ultimately commits suicide. Matthias's father lives in Spain with a young woman and has built up a huge company at the neglect of his son. In a final confrontation with his terminally ill father, Matthias yells at him that he is his only true legacy. In the last scene, we see that Matthias has inherited his father's business after all. A few times in NIEMAND IN DE STAD, protagonist Philip is about to call his father, but he never does, so we never find out what is bothering him. This film about life in a dorm was Van Erp's debut fiction feature after he had made a television series and a great number of excellent documentaries. I did not like NIEMAND IN DE STAD as much as the critics did, partly because the character Jacob was made to recite the themes of the film too explicitly. He tells the slightly immature Philip: 'You were never at open sea. You're still on the inland waterways. But when the fresh water around you has turned into salt water, we'll know what kind of sailor you are.' Or he remarks that there are no windows at the fraternity 'to save us from looking out so that we can escape the choking inevitability' (of adult life).

18 Campanelli's narrative role is considerable: When he tells Netelneck that a treasure is hidden in the cesspool, the farmer goes into the dirt, a rope around his belly. Campanelli cuts the rope, drowning the old Netelneck.

19 Campanelli is played by Nino Manfredi, famous for numerous roles, such as two films directed by Ettore Scola. He features in Scola's masterpiece C'ERAVAMO TANTO AMATI [WE LOVED EACH OTHER SO MUCH] (1974) and in BRUTTI, SPORCHI E CATTIVI [UGLY, DIRTY AND BAD] (1976). But an absolute must-see is the Spanish dark comedy EL VERDUGO [THE EXECUTIONER] (Luis García Berlanga, 1963).

BIBLIOGRAPHY

Claus, Hugo, *De dans van de reiger: Een nare komedie in twee delen*, 1962 (Amsterdam: De Bezige Bij, 1965).

DiPiero, Thomas, 'The Patriarch Is Not (Just) a Man', *Camera Obscura* 25–26 (1991), 101–24.

Freud, Sigmund, 'The Interpretation of Dreams', *The Standard Edition of the Complete Psychological Works of Sigmund Freud, Volume V (1900-1901): The Interpretation of Dreams (Second Part) and On Dreams*, 24 vols. (London: Vintage, 2001), 339-622.

—, 'Moses and Monotheism', *The Standard Edition of the Complete Psychological Works of Sigmund Freud, Volume XXIII (1937-1939): Moses and Monotheism, An Outline of Psycho-analysis and Other Works*, 24 vols. (London: Vintage, 2001), 3-137.
—, 'Totem and Taboo', *The Standard Edition of the Complete Psychological Works of Sigmund Freud. Vol. XIII (1913-1914): Totem and Taboo and Other Works*, 24 vols. (London: Vintage, 2001), 1-161.
Gallop, Jane, *Reading Lacan* (Ithaca: Cornell University Press, 1985).
Hinson, Hal, 'Tracks in the Snow', *Washington Post* (August 24, 1987).
Hoogendoorn, Maurice, 'Religie in films is nu exotische folklore', *Nederlands Dagblad* (19 February 2016).
Hughes, Judith M., *From Freud's Consulting Room: The Unconscious in a Scientific Age* (Cambridge, Mass.: Harvard University Press, 1994).
IMAGO, ed., *Making Pictures: A Century of European Cinematography* (New York: Harry N. Abrams, Inc., 2003).

Lacan, Jacques, 'Desire and the Interpretation of Desire in *Hamlet*', *Yale French Studies* 55/56 (1977): 11-52.
—, *Écrits: A Selection*, trans. by Alan Sheridan, 1977 (London: Routledge, 2001).
—, *The Psychoses: Book III, 1955-1956*, trans. by Russell Grigg (London: Routledge, 1993).
McGrath, Alistair E., *A Life of John Calvin: A Study in the Shaping of Western Culture* (Oxford: Basil Blackwell, 1990).
Van Bueren, Peter, 'Absurd en kluchtig spektakel van een gevoelig fantast', *de Volkskrant* (11 May 1995), https://www.volkskrant.nl/nieuws-achtergrond/absurd-en-kluchtig-spektakel-van-een-gevoelig-fantast~b6c1bb1b/ [Accessed 12 May 2020].
Van der Burg, Jos, 'De stront wordt duur betaald: De vliegende Hollander', *De Filmkrant* 156 (May 1995), https://filmkrant.nl/recensies/de-vliegende-hollander/ [Accessed 12 May, 2020].
Verhaeghe, Paul, *Identiteit* (Amsterdam: De Bezige Bij, 2012).
Verstraten, Peter, *Humour and Irony in Dutch Post-war Fiction Film* (Amsterdam: Amsterdam University Press, 2016).
Žižek, Slavoj, *Enjoy Your Symptom! Jacques Lacan In and Out of Hollywood*, 1992 (Revised Edition. New York and London: Routledge, 2001).
—, 'The Big Other Doesn't Exist', *Journal of European Psychoanalysis*, Spring – Fall (1997), http://www.lacan.com/zizekother.htm [Accessed 7 May 2020].
—, *The Parallax View* (Cambridge, Mass.: MIT Press, 2006).

CHAPTER 3

That Obscure Object of Desire

Verstraten, P., *Dutch Post-War Fiction Film Through a Lens of Psychoanalysis.* Taylor & Francis Group, 2021
DOI 10.5117/9789463725330_CH03

ABSTRACT

Chapter three puts into practice Žižek's claim that cinema teaches us how to desire. Starting with Rademakers' HET MES, it is argued that desire is incessantly frustrated: the satisfying object cannot be appropriated. The film analyses are inspired by the question of what conditions are needed to trigger desire. Films like LIEFDESBEKENTENISSEN and EEN OCHTEND VAN ZES WEKEN demonstrate that love blossoms by virtue of obstacles. Both HAVINCK and DE GROT are centred around a posthumous infatuation with a love object. In DE POOLSE BRUID, desire is mediated by violent acts, whereas the girl in HEMEL imitates the behaviour of her Casanova-like father. In INSTINCT as well as LOOS, sexual desire is used as a trap for a male character.

KEYWORDS
Obscure objects of desire – Courtly love – The virtue of obstacles – A fantasy staged for the sake of the Other

It is pretty clear what piques the thirteen-year-old Thomas in Rademakers' third feature film, the black-and-white coming-of-age drama HET MES [THE KNIFE] (1961). Since his father passed away eight years ago, his mother is now living with Oscar, who fought in the East Indies, just as Thomas's father had. They both used to have the rank of lieutenant. Thomas hardly knew his father, so he and the girl Toni, with whom he is on close terms, can only talk about him on the basis of rumours and hearsay. When Toni says that his father died of a 'simple cold', for he had a 'weak constitution, like you', Thomas immediately contradicts her diagnosis and claims that a serious pneumonia proved fatal to him. According to Toni, her mother once said his father was the most beautiful man she had ever seen. But he was also a daredevil who always drove too fast, even at night, Toni asserts, to which Thomas proudly adds that the yokels in the village were 'scared stiff' of him.

In the eyes of Thomas, Oscar is an intruder who has disrupted the bond with his mother. Not only does Oscar occupy the empty place left by Thomas's father—that might have been fair enough—he is also far removed from the idealized picture Thomas has of his father. This is shown in a quite surreal dream sequence, which is brightly lit and is practically without shadows. Thomas is riding on horseback, but then a sports car catches up with him, his father behind the wheel in a lieutenant's outfit. The car makes the horse fall down, whereupon the father takes a gun and aims at his son: 'No, it's me! Thomas!' In a subsequent shot, it turns out that the father has been replaced by Oscar in the very same uniform, but then the shot freezes and is cut in two halves.[1]

Oscar does not care at all about what Thomas's mother wants, often frequenting the pub and showing up at Thomas's place whenever he feels like it. Thomas realizes that Oscar's behaviour makes his mother very unhappy, and he cannot stand the fact that she remains hooked to him. As a son, he is unable to offer any comfort, since his mother locks herself up in her room during Oscar's absence. One night when he hears a noise, he peeps into their bedroom when the door is ajar and witnesses how his mother is on her knees for Oscar and 'crying like a stable maid', the son says in a voice-over. Thomas is so disgusted by this sight that he runs away from home.

After having slept in a barn, he meets a soldier named Ratte who teaches him many things, including how to approach the enemy with a bayonet. As soon as he is brought back home to his worried mother, he keeps thinking of Ratte's words: 'I had to be a man. Act in cold blood.' Thomas sighs deeply, and in a reverse shot we then see his mother in the distance with Oscar. The upcoming scene is shown in slow motion, accompanied by Thomas's voice-over: 'She had not changed. She came up to me to hurt me. But no one is supposed to hurt me again.' We then get a medium close-up of Thomas walking towards his mother: 'I'm a soldier. In cold blood.' We then hear his imitation of the rallying cry he learned from Ratte—drowned out because of the slow motion—as well as the jazzy score performed by Pim Jacobs that functions as the theme music. But before Thomas encounters his mother, he falls onto the grass, a knife in his hand – the very knife that is so precious to him, as we learned in previous scenes. The punishment for this attempt to stab his mother is that Thomas is sent to boarding school. His mother admits that the situation has become impossible because she cannot live alone in the house, or anywhere else, without Oscar.

So far, it seems this is just another run-of-the-mill story about growing pains and about a boy who has problems accepting his stepfather-to-be. If a mother is a boy's first object of love, there is reason to presume that the bond between Thomas and his mother was particularly close. We can presume his father was on a military mission abroad when Thomas was very young—the battle in the East Indies lasted until the end of 1949. Moreover, at some point Toni implies that the father's room is still forbidden territory for Thomas, emphasizing the fact that the daddy was an aloof character. Due to the father's detachment and his subsequent premature death, the relationship between mother and son was probably more intimate than average. This is affirmed when Thomas visits a gypsy fortune teller at the fair, who sees in her crystal ball that 'your mother loves you a lot. Remember, a mother is the most precious gift in your life.' It is at least significant that Thomas talks—in voice-over—about the knife episode of last summer 'as if it had happened to somebody else', suggesting that this kind of aggressiveness towards his mother was totally alien to him.

In the case of an imaginary mutual relationship between mother and son, there are two different scenarios. The child thinks that he alone can fulfil the mother's needs, and according to the opposite scenario, the child demands that the mother fulfil his needs and only his (Verhaeghe *Love in a Time*, 64). The child scribbles a drawing for his mummy and exclaims 'Look, a sun!' The mother will confirm it by saying 'That is the most beautiful sun I have ever seen'. And the child may continue to please his mother by drawing a picture of a horse or a house, and the mother will greet each drawing with invariable enthusiasm. This example explains in a nutshell that the logic of Lacan's dictum 'love is giving what you do not have' is based upon a 'pretence' (Verhaeghe *Love in a Time*, 70). By drawing, the child has found a means to satisfy his mother. Perhaps the kid does not really feel like making pictures, but he does so anyway out of love for his mother. Whereas the child may be convinced that his mother is on cloud nine because of the 'really beautiful' pictures, the mother's praise is motivated by encouraging her child in his activity, though the actual scribblings may end up in the dustbin. So, both mother and child pretend as if the pictures are fabulous, but they are only made as an expression of mutual love. The mother's stance can be summed up as: You do not draw beautifully but nonetheless I act as if you do, since I love you. The child's stance: Actually, I wanted to do something else, but because of your spontaneous reaction I continue to draw, since I love you.

This harmonious relationship is broken due to the intervention of a stranger. Oscar takes on the position of substitute father, and though he had served with Thomas's father, in the eyes of the son he is not really entitled to this position because he makes his mother miserable. In order to illustrate his disagreement with Oscar's claim, he shows him the knife, but Oscar is quick to get the better of the boy. When Thomas later takes out the knife to try and stab his mother, it is to express his annoyance with the fact that she remains docile and has decided to side with Oscar. Thomas's action is fairly ambivalent, though. On the one hand, he wants his mother to choose him over Oscar. On the other hand, he is at the age where he can cut himself loose from his mother. This ambivalence has its parallel in a scene at the beginning when Toni's mother brings her face close to Thomas and says: 'You're looking more and more like your late father.' And while laughing: 'You will drive women nuts. You've the same eyes as your father. The eyes of a cheat.' On the one hand, Thomas is pleased with the remark because of the noted resemblance with the man his mother was married to—as if he would be a better substitute than Oscar. On the other hand, it also means that he has to have an eye for other girls/women, provided it is not his mother. Afterwards, Toni tells Thomas that she was very embarrassed that her mother treated him as if he were an adult, but for Thomas it means that he is no longer seen as a (mama's) boy. That's why the words of Ratte keep resonating within him: 'I'm a man, I'm a soldier.'

In this ambivalent but inevitable process of separation, the boy has to choose another girl/woman over his mother. He has to divert his love for his mother towards an eroticized object of desire that is not his mother (or sister), but he will choose a love object that can be traced back to his first love.[2] The problem, however, as noted by Freud, is that the reciprocity of love (for/with the mother) can transform into an autoerotic sexual drive (chasing women like a Don Juan, without commitment), which brings to memory the all too familiar split between the Madonna and the lowlife whore. With this distinction in mind, I will examine the role of Toni as well as other possible objects of desire.

Rademakers' HET MES is structured as a series of flashback scenes in which Thomas reminiscences why his mother decided to send him to boarding school. In the first scenes, we see Thomas being taken by car from his home to the station, shown in extreme long shots. In subsequent scenes, Oscar is behind the wheel, the mother is in the passenger's seat, and Thomas is in the rear seat of the convertible, but since the camera is at the back of the car, we only see his head from behind. When a funeral procession passes by, the car has to halt next to the driveway of a convent garden. Suddenly we hear Thomas's voice-over (but we still have not seen his face) about this garden as a 'blasted place'. As soon as the car continues its journey, the camera goes another direction, tracking forward into the driveway. There is then a dissolve to the garden, while we hear Thomas say that the events seem as though they occurred more than a year ago but that they happened this summer. Thomas walks into the shot and continues: 'It is as if it has happened to somebody else. As if I was somebody else. An ignoramus. An ignorant fool.'

Both the voice-over and the camera movement indicate that there are two Thomases; the one before and after the incident with the knife. In the recent past, Toni is his closest pal; they take a great liking to each other, but they are not in the phase of kissing, at least not yet. When he steals the knife from the exhibition, he shows it to her first. She is impressed, as he expected, but also urges him to return the object. He refuses and calls her a 'scared pussycat'. In a later scene, halfway through the movie, Thomas boasts in her company that he is going to visit the place of the so-called Falcons, a type of boy-scout group for late teenagers. Thomas behaves very boldly but is chased off their territory. He is determined to return, and when he does so, late in the evening, he and Toni, while hiding in the bushes, see two boys and a girl coming their way. We can hardly see what is happening, for the camera is mainly focused on Thomas's face. It is clear that he cannot help watching, and Toni condemns his lustful observation, calling it a 'mortal sin'.

In voice-over, Thomas mentions that he had never felt so strange and that everything was buzzing. After Toni says: 'I know I am a boring girl. Say it.', he takes out his knife and half-seriously threatens to cut open her belly in one slash. Toni is not really impressed, taking it as boyish bluff, but the moment is nonetheless decisive. It expresses his yearning for initiation into a more mature world, a world of sexual mores. Toni, as his closest friend with whom he has teamed up for life, refuses to take this route, however, and thus Thomas remains stuck. Toni could function as the ideal companion with whom he can cut himself loose from his mother, but renounces the possibility that she could be his object of desire by saying: 'I know I am a boring girl.' After witnessing his mother in the bedroom with Oscar, which Thomas takes as a scene of depravity, he goes to Toni's place but does not find her at home.

Since she cannot offer him the comfort to break the bond with his mother, he ultimately takes up the knife, though he proves too weak to really approach her. In the final scene of the film, in the train together with his mother on his way to boarding school, Thomas has one flashback: in the company of Toni, he buries the knife in the woods. 'Do you swear you will never dig it up?' Toni asks him. Before he gives her a reply, we hear his voice-over: 'I felt ridiculous, but Toni still believed in those games.' Then we hear him say to Toni: 'I can't play with you anymore, Toni.' If he wants to develop into a man (like his father) and not remain a mama's boy, Thomas will have to get rid of someone like Toni who keeps him from maturing. His mother will continue to live with Oscar, but he himself, he has no clue. Once he discovers that his childhood friend is too shy and cowardly, he provokes her by taking out a knife—and he later repeats this act with his mother in a failed attempt to pretend he has become a man. HET MES may seem like a simple title for any film, but it is an appropriate one for this movie. He uses the knife to separate himself from his mother, but due to the immaturity of Toni, who still believes 'in those games', she is no alternative, and thus the adolescent Thomas remains in search of a proper object of desire, as the great majority of the protagonists I examine in this chapter do.

AMOUR FOU: LOVE ROMANCES IN DIALOGUE WITH FRENCH CINEMA

The 1923 silent film COEUR FIDÈLE by French filmmaker Jean Epstein was a deliberately simple love story because, as the director explained, the superficiality of the narrative enabled him to focus all his attention on the formal aspects of the film. Epstein's aim was to explore the properties that are unique to the medium: frontally staged close-ups, changes in focus, and dazzling camera movements, for example when the protagonists are in a carousel. The love romance served as a starting point for young aspiring directors in the mid-1960s in the Netherlands which did not yet have a fiction film tradition. Owing to the success of his debut feature DE MINDER GELUKKIGE TERUGKEER VAN JOSZEF KATÚS NAAR HET LAND VAN REMBRANDT (1966), Wim Verstappen grabbed the opportunity to shoot another picture without a second thought. LIEFDESBEKENTENISSEN [CONFESSIONS OF LOVING COUPLES] (Wim Verstappen, 1967) was too low-budget (only 60,000 guilders) to have any true artistic aspirations, but the mode of working was unorthodox, for there was even less of a script than in the case of JOSZEF KATÚS. There was no more than an outline of a narrative and the sense of an ending. Indeed, the loose structure of these two Scorpio productions ensured that they were included in a DVD release by the Filmmuseum as Dutch exemplars of the *nouvelle vague*, the French new wave. Thus, the main question was, as actress Shireen Strooker memorized, how to arrive at the beginning of the film. Dialogues had to be improvised on the spot, whereas the budget limited the possibility of a second take. While improvisation had worked greatly in JOSZEF KATÚS, a quasi-documentary filmed on the streets amidst a bunch of long-haired hippies who were called Provos in Amsterdam, Verstappen had underestimated just how much preparation a funny rendition of a romantic rendezvous requires for it to work (Den Drijver, 106).

In LIEFDESBEKENTENISSEN, the protagonist-writer Frank Jansen has just published a novel that is quite a success. When a woman he sleeps with asks him: 'Do I end up in your next book?' he replies, 'Yes, as a peculiar nun', which is more or less the same answer another mistress receives upon the same question in a later scene. In voice-over, we hear the letters he and his former lover Mascha, a translator by profession, write to each other. Frank explains to her that he appreciates their correspondence and that she is her mental pal, but Mascha answers that she herself feels very feminine, both in spirit and body. While Frank is making love to yet another flirt, we hear in voice-over that Mascha's message had a counterproductive effect, and that infidelity is a consequence of every good love letter. In the meantime, Frank starts to fancy Marina, though he knows he will never have high-level conversations with her. Keeping in touch with Mascha is therefore essential because playing games is indispensable for Frank: he wants to create situations that he cannot predict the outcome of. Since he himself cannot visit London due to tax debts, he makes sure that both Marina and Mascha go to the city in each other's company. Upon her return, Marina becomes angry at Frank because he had kept it a secret that her friend Peter had come over from London to pay her a visit in Amsterdam. She only happened to find out thanks to her premature return, since the trip to London had bored her to death.

Because of Marina's dismay, Frank is too reluctant to face her, and as a ten-minute intermezzo in the film exposes, he starts writing a harem story inspired by Denis Diderot's first novel *The Indiscreet Jewels* (1748). Frank himself plays a sheik who can point a magic ring at all women in his harem which makes them disclose their intimacies. When Frank hears Mascha confess that only his happiness counts, he says in voice-over that she is smart enough to guess that her part will be omitted. This is followed by Frank's confession that he never dares to point the ring at Marina. 'I am scared of her. She is the worst we can imagine: she is plain. She can do practical things that we are not capable of. We are the misfits; I will remain the silly clown.'

After Mascha has spent quite some time with Peter in Amsterdam, Marina is annoyed with her and also presumes that Mascha actually wants Frank. Mascha is amazed that Marina does not realize that Frank is infatuated with her. And thus in the next shot, Marina ends up in bed with Frank denying that he is a silly clown. Instead of the habitual question Frank got from his lovers about whether she will have a part in his next book, Marina asks: 'What kind of book are you writing anyway?'

Made on a shoestring budget and to a great extent via improvisation on the spot, it should not surprise us that LIEFDESBEKENTENISSEN merely illustrates some proverbial notions regarding love. First, Frank loves Marina, or thinks he loves her, according to the commonplace that 'opposites attract': he is the narcissistic intellectual—or in his own words, 'the silly clown'—but he envies her because she is so very common and uncomplicated. This is proven by the fact that she does not even know what kind of a writer he is, as if his status is entirely indifferent to her. All the other flirts seemed to hope they would end up as a muse in one of his novels. Second, in the embedded harem story, Frank wants to know about the hidden desires of all women, but he doesn't want to know Marina's because she has to remain a mystery. This chimes with the idea that love falls flat as soon as one knows too much of a partner. Once Frank is able to read Mascha's thought via the magic ring, she is removed from the story, which in this case means that she is no longer a possible love interest for him.

Whether LIEFDESBEKENTENISSEN was a great film or not was irrelevant to producer De la Parra and director Verstappen, aka Pim and Wim.[3] Since the number of movies in the Netherlands was so limited at the time, their adage was to make movies regardless of production values. Quantity was of primary importance (shoot as many pictures as you can); quality only came second as a criterion.[4] Most critics considered LIEFDESBEKENTENISSEN a disappointment after the refreshing JOSZEF KATÚS, although François Truffaut, who took the effort to scribble down critical notes, was apparently delighted by Verstappen's second feature.[5] In comparison, there was near unanimous praise for Nikolai van der Heyde's debut feature with the bilingual title UN PRINTEMPS EN HOLLANDE – EEN OCHTEND VAN ZES WEKEN (1966). Like Verstappen and De la Parra, Van der Heyde had attended the Film Academy in Amsterdam, and the three of them founded the film journal *Skoop* in 1963, together with Gied Jaspars, as a Dutch equivalent of *Cahiers du cinéma*. The budget for EEN OCHTEND VAN ZES WEKEN was limited (130,000 guilders), but it was more than twice the budget for LIEFDESBEKENTENISSEN. Van der Heyde's film also used a love romance as a backbone which seemed to give him some liberty to experiment, predominantly with chronology. Since the title gives a clear indication of how long the affair between the Dutch racing driver Jimmy and the French model Annette lasts, Van der Heyde could permit himself to present scenes in a relatively random order; some scenes are cut back-and-forth, as when Annette's telephone conversation with a man is interrupted a few times by brief dancing sequences. The film has no specific mention of dates, except that a voice-over tells that they meet on 24 May and that Annette's modelling assignment in the Netherlands ends on 18 June, but then she decides to stay on a few more weeks.

Whereas LIEFDESBEKENTENISSEN showed the conditions for a romance to blossom, EEN OCHTEND VAN ZES WEKEN focusses upon a romance doomed to come to an end. However, what is most striking if not stunning are the strong analogies to a certain French film that was much more famous released some three months after Van der Heyde's picture. Like EEN OCHTEND VAN ZES WEKEN, UN HOMME ET UNE FEMME [A MAN AND A WOMAN] (Claude Lelouch, 1966), which won both a Golden Palm and an Academy Award (for Best Foreign Language Film), is about the love between a French woman from Paris and a racing driver. Each film has lengthy scenes of cars speeding around race circuits. Both films have shots of silent, pensive characters alternated with elaborate, reflective voice-overs (spoken by male protagonist Jean-Louis Duroc in Lelouch's film and on behalf of male protagonist Jimmy in Van der Heyde's). Both men have a scene with an unnamed woman in a hotel bed, only to make it clear that she is no match for the female protagonist: Jean-Louis reads aloud from a racing magazine the fake news item that he is spending all his time with another woman; Jimmy is too distracted to hear the words of the stewardess in his bed because his mind is set on his past affair with a French model, who is the mother of a son. Van der Heyde's film starts after the affair is over and Jimmy is left with his recollections.

The tremendous efforts by Jean-Louis as well as Jimmy to convince Anne / Annette of their love border on despair. When Jean-Louis receives a telegram from Anne after participating in the Monte Carlo rally, he immediately drives to Paris and then to Deauville to prove to her that he appreciates the gesture, but as in Van der Heyde's film, the affair will not endure. Although Jean-Louis and Anne embrace at a train platform with a camera circling around them in the final shot, this tender moment seems only a frail basis for a relationship. Anne has made clear to Jean-Louis that her memory of her deceased spouse, the stuntman Pierre, shown in colourful flashback scenes, is stronger than her affection for him. Jean-Louis muses in a voice-over: 'It's crazy to refuse happiness ... Maybe if he had lived, he'd have become an old fool, but as it is, he'll always be quite a guy', and thus Pierre remains an unbeatable rival for Jean-Louis. In EEN OCHTEND AAN ZES WEKEN, Jimmy goes to Schiphol Airport to keep Annette from going back to France, but later she decides to leave for Paris anyway. As in UN HOMME ET UNE FEMME, the obstacle to an enduring relationship between Jimmy and Annette is of a mental nature. She tells him: 'Do not try to impress me. I want you to be your very own self.' He replies: 'I can be anything you want me to be.'

This brief dialogue illustrates an unbridgeable discrepancy: whereas she points out that he should not change, he expresses his readiness to change, although we can doubt his sincerity. Later in the film, when Jimmy is in training on the race circuit, she is reading a French book. In a shot that lasts about half a minute, the viewer is made to understand that every man is unhappy with his wife because he cannot understand her, while he himself cannot be understood by her. The 'sensation of forward motion' was the one and only guideline for him as a single man, but when in love, he is no longer sure of the direction of movements. This is underscored in EEN OCHTEND VAN ZES WEKEN by both the jazz-tinged score and the cinematography, which captures Jimmy's mood of insecurity and disarray. When they spend their time in a modern villa while their relationship is at a dead end, some static wide shots seem to capture the alienating atmosphere of an Antonioni film. In several other scenes, Van der Heyde's film copies the dynamic cinematography of an early Godard: e.g., seven overlapping takes show how Jimmy—who has the air of a

young Jean-Paul Belmondo, especially when wearing his sunglasses—arrives at a hotel by car. A restless camera depicts how Jimmy—'as long as he was driving [fast in his car], he felt alive and kicking', a voice-over says at one point—is too restless for a lasting relationship with the equally restless Annette ('as long as she worked, she felt alive and kicking', a voice-over claims). At times, the camera makes semi-circles, moves behind objects, shifts in focus, goes from long shot to close-up and back—in short, it goes to and fro. The voice-over says twice: 'Instead of loving her, he tried to conquer her, but he did not know how.' We then have a scene in which the camera shows his face in close-up, slightly in low-angle and constantly switching positions (left, right, left, right ...). We hear his inner monologue, but because of the editing it seems as if he is split. Hence, his indecision regarding how to cope with a woman he truly loves makes it impossible for him to be his 'own self', which was Annette's one and only request.[6]

POSTHUMOUS INFATUATION: *HAVINCK*

In the introduction to this book, I mentioned that the year 1966 was a most remarkable year in Dutch cinema (and 1967 the second best) because of the ambitious attempts by some directors to create 'art' films: DE DANS VAN DE REIGER; EEN OCHTEND VAN ZES WEKEN; JOSZEF KATÚS. HET GANGSTERMEISJE by Frans Weisz was another bold film. In the article 'My Very Own CITIZEN KANE', I went to great lengths to elaborate upon its alienating devices, its references to Fellini and Godard, and the idiosyncratic adaptation process, for the film was the result of conversations between Weisz and novelist Remco Campert, whose book *Het gangstermeisje* had yet to be written. The film is about a writer named Wessel Franken who has published a successful novel, *Het gangstermeisje*, which features an image of his own wife Leonie on the cover. He is asked by an Italian director to make his book into a film script, but much to his wife's chagrin, a woman named Kitty is chosen to act as the gangster girl. Wessel has no experience in writing a screenplay and therefore accepts an offer to go to Menton, in the south of France, for inspiration. It is also a form of escape because he is uncertain whether to continue his marriage, and while in France, the enthralling image of Kitty keeps coming to his mind. HET GANGSTERMEISJE is a challenging debut feature by Weisz because of the ambiguousness of many shots. When a scene with Kitty is brusquely inserted, we are not sure whether we are seeing the actress in her everyday life or whether it is a scene imagined by Wessel or a shooting of the actual film. To complicate matters further, Wessel is distracted from his screenplay time and again because he actually wants to write a story about a psychotic bass player living in a hotel room near the seaside. The scenes of this story-to-be-written are seemingly quite randomly inserted in the film. When Wessel sets off for Rome in the final part of the film, the Italians praise him for the script but nonetheless demand considerable changes. They want to have the detective, the gangster girl's adversary, to be less of an introvert, but Wessel disagrees. In the concluding scene, he walks onto the set during shooting, takes control of the sound equipment and tells the crew—including the baffled director Jascha—that he wanted to tell the story of a man pursuing his own happiness who becomes a prisoner of his own fantasy.

> I fell in love with a woman I had created myself. A word, an image, the gangster girl. I got caught up in a shadow play that only seemed a play to you, indeed, but for me it was a serious matter. I do not want to become a victim, so finish playing the game, but without me.

Wessel then walks away from the set in the direction of the Colosseum while shooting continues with the scene in which the gangster girl Kitty kisses the detective just before killing him. I refer to HET GANGSTERMEISJE here because Wessel's disappointment is related to his awareness that Kitty as his presumed object of desire was only a mirage. In that regard, it is most fitting that in most scenes Kitty is probably represented as a woman he fantasized about—or a woman he had to fantasize about in his role as screenwriter because she was supposed to be the main protagonist in the film that still had to be shot.[7]

The discrepancy between an actual woman and her sublime image is a prelude to a film Weisz was to make more than twenty years later, HAVINCK (1987), an adaptation of a 1984 novel by Marja Brouwers. In the opening scene, we see Lydia sitting at a table in a static long shot, writing a letter; it is quite dark, only some light peeps through the window. This seems to set the tone for a morose picture, and indeed, throughout HAVINCK, white, grey and blue will predominate. In a subsequent shot, Lydia is behind the wheel of a car, close to the motorway. We see her face in the rear mirror. While she is smoking a cigarette, she readjusts the mirror so she can look at herself. When she starts driving again, the camera remains static and shows us the one direction sign, with the text 'go back' underneath it. We then hear Cole Porter's 'True Love', and a two-shot shows the lawyer Robert Havinck and his teenage daughter Eva attending the funeral service, but soon they are presented in separate shots. The father is displeased with the selection of this particular song: 'How original', he says ironically, but Eva claims her mother always had to cry upon hearing Porter.

HAVINCK has a number of flashback scenes, but they are never articulated as such in order to suggest the impact of the past upon the present. There is

a shot of Eva after the cremation of her mother, but when she turns her head, the background comes into sharp focus. We hear a quarrel between her parents, and when her father walks away, Eva and her mother hug each other. This makes it clear to the viewer that Eva blames her father, who is having an affair with a singer-actress, for Lydia's unhappiness. Robert is represented as a particularly cold character, lacking any emotion. After the service, Eva's art teacher even tells him he is an accessory to murder due to neglect of his wife. Lydia's father reproaches him that he did not bury Lydia but instead cremated her. For him, it is a sign that Robert really wanted to banish Lydia from his life. Robert takes little time to mourn and goes back to the office much earlier than expected.

Meanwhile, Robert has flashbacks as well, but time and again, they are represented via camera pans, not via a cut. He sits in his car, heavy rain outside. A pan to the left, and Lydia starts singing 'Baby Love', whereupon he joins in. In another apparently very early flashback, she wonders whether she will be able to commit himself, but he wants to persuade her by calling himself a 'sensualist'. The good memories are replaced by more sour ones, once he has read her suicide note ('Why did I not get what had been promised to me?'), originally discovered by his daughter, who in turn is angry because she is not mentioned in the brief farewell letter. In one of the key flashbacks, once again shown via a pan, Lydia asks Robert what he thinks of the painting she has made. When he says it is 'nice', she gets furious, because he does not recognize its quality nor the fact that she has made a portrait of her daughter with her own blood for the red parts. 'You are my fatal mistake!' she yells at him. He tries to make up with her by saying it is really good, but then the camera pans to the right and shows Robert in the present, on his own, at the kitchen table.

In retrospect, Robert realizes he has not given her due attention—he did not appreciate Lydia for the woman she was but, as befits a lawyer who is accustomed to technicalities, as his wife. Lydia is reduced to a symbolic role within the family. While all flashbacks are introduced via pans, there is one exception in which Robert is presented as an attentive observer of a scene. Lydia has demolished several objects, and as she pulls him by the hair, she cries desperately: 'Here I am. I exist.' There is a close-up of Robert, as if he is still looking at the scenery, implying that it finally dawns on him. He has failed to live up to his self-declared label of a 'sensualist'; in practice, he was a calculating lout.

Lydia only comes to exist for Robert in his remembrances of her, which are cued as extensions of the present. She had to die first before he could gain an interest in her particular motives. Lydia wanted to be an object of his 'true love', but Robert could only desire her once he no longer 'possesses' her: she was 'his' wife, but he has lost her. In the physical absence of Lydia, he develops a belated fascination for her. As a consequence, his mistress ends their affair because she is fed up with his 'posthumous infatuation'. Robert's self-reflections have a direct impact upon his work as lawyer. Robert has to defend a client who has fired some shots through a door that killed his girlfriend, but he claims he only shot 'out of love'. In his defence in court, Robert tries to put the severity of the crime into perspective by arguing that his client is charged because he did something drastic, while many people are considered free of guilt, though they commit thousands of minor offences, such as contempt and disinterest, that also lead to death and murder. His boss considers Robert's defence 'unprofessional mumbo-jumbo', but by this time he considers it much more important to reconcile with his daughter Eva and to prove himself a worthy father.

LOVE REGAINED AT THE POINT OF DYING: *DE GROT*

Aforementioned films like HET MES, OCHTEND VAN ZES WEKEN and HET GANGSTERMEISJE end with the suggestion that the lovers will not meet again. HAVINCK is based upon the proposition that one can only truly appreciate what has been lost: there is no second chance for Robert as a husband, but perhaps the tragedy will make him a better father. But what if there is a second chance? DE GROT [THE CAVE] (Martin Koolhoven, 2001), based upon Tim Krabbé's novel from 1997, offers a possible follow-up. The opening scenes only start to make sense once they are revisited later in the movie. Via a high-angle, we see an extreme long shot of a market in an Asian country. A man with a photo camera is near a blood-stained spot, though this spot does not get any emphasis. In a subsequent scene, we see a bespectacled Dutch man arrive at the airport, check in at a hotel, have a drink at an outside cafe, take a shower, drive by rented car, have a rendezvous with a woman at an empty market square at night, and put a suitcase in the trunk of her car while their hands touch each other. Though DE GROT is constructed as a non-linear film in which we are going back and forth in time, the narrative ordering of scenes becomes clear in retrospect. The man in the Asian country is the 43-year-old geologist Egon Wagter. He is anything but an adventurous character, as we will learn, but he has one specific professional ambition. He wants to do fieldwork in South America to examine a unique rock formation, but he needs money to participate in an expedition. Because his job as a geography teacher at a secondary school does not pay him enough, he rings his old friend Axel van de Graaf, whom he has known since he was fourteen (and Axel fifteen). The phone call to Axel is a most remarkable step for Egon for, until this moment, Axel has always been the one to take the initiative, and this reversal of roles is, of course, a dark foreboding.

Throughout DE GROT, Egon has shown himself to be a pliant character who has the perseverance to obtain a PhD but when fate obstructs his academic career, he is satisfied with his job as a schoolteacher. In short, Egon is a model citizen, whereas Axel defies all rules of good behaviour. Axel is able to realize his plan, announced at the age of fifteen, to throw his life away: he will eventually turn into an international drugs criminal. He is a daredevil who survives three bullets in his body, but he also becomes rich and influential. The seeds for this division of roles are already laid at a young age, when Axel simply does whatever he wants. During a camp in the Ardennes, he sneaks out of his tent to fuck young girls, and when Egon and Marjoke wonder about the content of some big silos, which they describe as 'upside-down salt-shakers', Axel steps between the two and suggests that Egon have a look. Egon is hesitant, so Axel himself immediately climbs up the endlessly long stairs and gives the answer: 'There is nothing'. Axel is always on the move, and thus Egon is pushed in all kinds of directions by his 'youth friend', most of the time willy-nilly. From their mutual glances, it is clear that Egon and Marjoke are in love, but time and again, Axel prevents them from getting together. When Egon sees Marjoke in the train, Axel pinches him in the back to make him move forward; when they are playing in the water, he calls out to them to come with him to the cave (not that Axel is at all interested in the cave); when the youngsters have to pick berries in pairs, Axel arranges that Egon is paired with Vera.

DE GROT concludes with a scene in which the youngsters go sightseeing in a stalactite cave, and since it is the only time that Egon and Marjoke are not interrupted by Axel, it is deliberately lit to create a paradisiacal sphere. They exchange glances, their hands make contact, and they even kiss—the very final shot of the film. Hence, DE GROT ends with a romantic encounter—indeed, a highly romantic encounter if one believes the camp leader Kees, who tells the youngsters during a campfire about 'the secret of true love': a simple, affective gesture can be more satisfying than sexual intercourse. Despite this finale with the promise of pure happiness, we also remember from an earlier scene why the feelings Egon and Marjoke have for each other ultimately do not crystallize into an everlasting affair. Egon is one of four youngsters who are expelled from the camp by Kees after he has caught them having sex in a tent at night. This was, of course, a plan concocted by Axel, who had managed to drag Egon into it as well as the girls Vera and Florrie—even though none of them really wanted it, as Egon later tells Axel. 'No, you were only interested in that dud Marjoke', the latter replies. And since this Marjoke woke up that very night, alarmed by the noise, Egon knows that she knows. To make him feel embarrassed, she passes in front of him the next morning without a word, only deeming him worthy of a reproachful look. Due to Axel's persuasion, Egon has done something he did not want to do in the first place, and which—even worse—will cost him the love of his life.

The entire film by Koolhoven is geared towards bringing the love couple together—again. Unlike the comedy of remarriage from the thirties and forties —such as THE AWFUL TRUTH (Leo McCarey, 1937), THE PHILADELPHIA STORY (George Cukor, 1940), HIS GIRL FRIDAY (Howard Hawks, 1941)—the repetition is not an improved version of their original teenage love. Almost one hour into Koolhoven's DE GROT, there is a sudden intermezzo about a woman in Canada who owns a shop called 'Marcie's Gems'. When she is with her adolescent son David near a small lake, she shows her talent for throwing stones over the water surface. The attentive viewer may soon realize that this Marcie is the adult version of Marjoke, for it was a fourteen-year-old Egon who taught her how to throw stones like that at the camp. Another important clue is that Marjoke/Marcie is usually in focus, more than any of the other females in the film. When Egon accidently ends up with Margriet in bed, there is a two-shot, and when Egon bends forward to the camera, she is no longer sharp. Similarly, Adriënne, Egon's wife, is out of focus when she tells Egon in passing that she has slept with Axel once. It foretells that, despite their marriage, she is not the true love of his life.

It will be clear to any viewer that Marcie equals Marjoke when, after arriving at Schiphol Airport, she insists on meeting Axel. She says that she has second thoughts about the assignment. Axel's response is rhetorically sharp: 'You contact me all of a sudden after 25 years, asking if I can help you out financially. And now you say, I am too scared. Don't you want to know what is in this salt shaker? What did a life without risks offer you?' The answer to both these questions is 'nothing', and this makes the transition to the journalist, Michiel Polak, with the photo camera in the opening shot of DE GROT logical. It is the journalist who is acquainted with Egon and who is covering the career of Axel

('Axel v.d. G.') for his newspaper. Michiel interviews a market salesman who testifies that he found the two lovers in each other's arms. Michiel doubts the term 'lover', but the salesman is convinced that it was an amorous encounter. There is a cut to Egon and Marcie/Marjoke on the night-time market square, shown from behind a balustrade. Cut to Axel who asks Michiel whether it was true that they were found 'in each other's arms'. After an affirmative answer, Axel says: 'I went too far with Egon, but I was right.' An immediate cut to the market where Egon and Marcie are violently attacked by street hoodlums. Lethally wounded in a pool of blood, they stare at one another. The key question of the film is whether they instantly fall in love or whether they recognize each other. The salesman's words reverberate: they held each other so tightly that they had to be pulled apart—which means that they crawled towards one another despite their serious injuries. After a close-up of Marcie/Marjoke first and then Egon's face, there is a dissolve to the cave scene, which suggests that they recognize the other character. A close-up to the face of a badly wounded Marcie, and another dissolve to the very same flashback scene: they share this memory. In the cave they had their first romance, which ended so brusquely; on the market square, they come together again, just before dying.

First, it is significant that Axel has functioned as an obstacle to the adolescent love between Egon and Marjoke throughout the film. Time and again, he interrupts their exchange (except in the cave itself) and fixes Egon up with other girls. At the same time, Axel is an arch matchmaker, and ironically, he is the only one who knows that he is arranging a renewed meeting between Egon and Marjoke/Marcie, 29 years later. Second, DE GROT leaves it up to guesswork why Axel is so intrigued by Egon. As we can gather, Axel was already dealing drugs by the time he met Egon, and he may have been struck by his peer's naïve innocence, by the fact that he was not yet corrupted by the evil in the world. By moving Egon in any direction he wants, Axel turns Egon into an object of his homosocial desire: Egon is his friend insofar as Axel can prove himself the superior one in an implicit mutual rivalry. And because he is an adventurer, he bets that the meek Egon will admire him. For that very reason, Axel asks him as a running gag at each and every encounter over the years what was inside the 'salt-shakers'. In front of Marjoke, Axel showed he had the chutzpah to take a look inside the big silo, something Egon didn't have the courage to do. By repetitively confronting Egon with this question, Axel confirms his own superiority and thereby Egon's mediocrity. Since the hierarchy between them is time and again fixed in favour of Axel, the latter can keep on referring to Egon as his 'friend'.

Third, it is worth noting that because of the film's non-linearity, the two lovers can only enjoy moments of intimacy posthumously. By the end of the film, the romantic scene is immediately framed with dark overtones: we know that the love between Egon and Marjoke will not materialize. Looking into each other's eyes at the point of dying, the scene in the cave is a dreamlike memory from the past that contrasts with the gruesome present. DE GROT owes this effective contrast to its functional non-chronological order of events. The scene can be presented as an idyll because we know it will never become reality. Since it is restricted to this one moment, it is a short-lived idyll that lacks the inevitable ups and downs of a relationship. Even 29 years after the event, they can still continue to dream how great it might have been.

Strictly speaking, the scene of tenderness at the end of DE GROT has a gooey feeling, but we accept it since it is mediated by our knowledge of its tragic aftermath. In other words, its aesthetic effect comes at a price: it is not just love but an already doomed love.[8] It is congruent with Lacan's lesson about courtly love (*The Ethics*, 150-154). As soon as one captures one's object of desire, a feeling of disappointment comes to replace its preconceived expectations of ecstasy. The presumed sublime object disintegrates into 'just' an ordinary object. Hence, as Lacan hypothesized, desire requires a necessary distance and will never be possessed by the subject. The courtly lady may be close, but any physical encounter with her is postponed, and with each postponement, the desire for her may increase. Egon and Marjoke may have kissed each other at a young age in DE GROT, but the forte of Koolhoven's film is that its non-linear structure indicates that the consummation of love is represented as 'too late'. The idea of love in DE GROT is propelled by the presence of a structural hindrance, which takes the shape of the character Axel, who radiates a certain authority over the lovers. This obstacle is absent in the scene in the cave (for Axel is not around then), but Egon and Marjoke had no idea then that this moment of intimacy would never be repeated. They can only properly appreciate it some decades later as a shared posthumous memory—a fitting final shot of the movie.

THE PROS AND CONS OF GOOD ETIQUETTE: *HET MEISJE EN DE DOOD* AND *WILDSCHUT*

Though DE GROT is smartly executed, its theme of male homosocial desire and missed romances as such is not new. Film noirs in particular can be regarded as an apt variation of this theme because of the way this genre stages the structure of a triangular relationship: a relatively young man falls in love with the femme fatale, but she is already tied to a wealthy and influential paternal figure, as in GILDA (Charles Vidor, 1946), THE KILLERS (Robert Siodmak, 1946), or THE LADY FROM SHANGHAI (Orson Welles, 1949). In film noir, this older man is the constitutive obstacle, for he will often refuse to give her up. And when the younger man believes that the woman chooses him because of his virility, he can never be sure whether she is playing a deceitful game out of self-interest. This clash is reiterated in HET MEISJE EN DE DOOD [THE GIRL AND DEATH] (Jos Stelling, 2012), and the title already suggests that this story is as classical as a tale by Pushkin, whose poetry the main protagonist Nicolai likes to cite.[9] In this film by Stelling, which won a Golden Calf for best film as well as for its cinematography, the aged Russian physician Nicolai revisits a derelict hotel near Leipzig as well as a grave marked 'Elise'. He reminisces about the time he was on his way to Paris as a young student of medicine and decided to spend a night in the hotel. As soon as he is about to leave after breakfast, his eyes catch sight of the young Elise, and he decides to postpone his departure for one more night, and another, and another. He is unable to consummate his love for her, since she is the property of a rich and 'dirty, old' Count. The courtesan begs him to forget her, since this is 'our destiny'.

Upon his return a few years later, the young Russian is severely beaten by one of the Count's henchmen. Elise thereupon defies the Count's commands and comes to the aid of the bleeding Nicolai. From that moment, the Count makes sure that she is being watched by his servants so that the two lovers cannot run off together. She then goes back to the Count again, or so it seems in the eyes of Nicolai, for he considers this an act of betrayal. After a brief absence, he comes back—this time with a moustache—and wins huge amounts of money at the expense of his old adversary. The Count dies of a heart attack after his immense loss, but Nicolai nonetheless leaves in a bitter mood, for he yells at Elise: 'Once a whore, always a whore.' The hotel where Elise has hidden herself closes down after the Count's death, so she is left locked up in it. Back in the deserted hotel many years later, the old Nicolai can only love her belatedly, as a phantom. Wrapped up in his reveries about her, he dies on the hotel bed, surrounded by cobwebs and insects. Thus, HET MEISJE EN DE DOOD fully conforms to the Lacanian scenario that a permanently unfulfilled desire is what can keep alive the idea of love as a sublime idea.[10]

Though at first glance the polar opposite of HET MEISJE EN DE DOOD, the gritty WILDSCHUT [STRONGHOLD] (Bobby Eerhart, 1985), advertised at its release as the 'best Dutch B-film ever' (Van den Tempel), offers grounds for comparison in the way a woman is sandwiched between male interests. WILDSCHUT was a box-office failure, since exploitation pictures were simply not done at the time (Van den Tempel). But in an era that post-dates Tarantino's *nouvelle violence*, Eerhart's film has been re-appreciated as a fantastic cult movie, with sharp-witted lines and Hidde Maas as the 'Dutch Robert Mitchum' (producer Henk Bos, qtd. in Van den Tempel). Two tough gangsters are on the run after robbing a bank, but the black guy Charlie gets a bullet wound in his leg after they steal gasoline in the night without paying. Jim and

Charlie take shelter in the farmhouse of the poacher Deleye who lives in the woods and near a military firing range. The family consists of mother Sibyl, stepfather Deleye, son Hugo, daughter Lisa and her baby Ruben, and the five of them are kept hostage to give Charlie the chance to recover from his bad wound before the two gangsters travel to a 'faraway place'. Since there is the constant threat that the gangsters will harm the little Ruben, the family members keep their lips sealed when the local bulky policeman—whose presence offers some comic relief—or the near-by soldiers arrive for inspection.

The official reason for the visit of the soldiers in their jeep is to take water from a pump at the farm, but it is obvious that they fancy the blonde Lisa, for she plays, as gangster Jim guesses, the 'camp follower', with Deleye as her pimp. At one point, Jim pushes Lisa in front of the window and clearly acts as if he is her lover, causing the soldiers to leave. Throughout WILDSCHUT, Lisa is trapped in a situation in which men vie for her. Her brother comes to her bedroom, proposing that he run away with her provided that he finds the money the gangsters have stolen. Jim considers the blonde woman 'gaga', as he says repetitively, but Charlie, who occupies her bedroom, has an ear for her problems. Quite casually, Lisa discloses to him that Deleye —her stepfather— is Ruben's father. It is no wonder that Lisa also has her own fantasy country, which she has drawn on her bedroom door, and that she even speaks a non-existent tongue: in her language, Ruben is named 'Wanjamo'.

Though Charlie tells her that her country is a safer place than his world of hideouts and escape routes, Lisa sees in the arrival of the gangsters an opportunity to get away from her family, knowing that her mother and stepfather do not mind: 'They tell me each day, you can go, we can take care of the baby.' That Lisa is attracted to Charlie becomes evident when the policeman comes to scrutinize the place. Upon seeing Lisa with Ruben in her bed, the agent tells her that in fairy tales, the big bad wolf is sleeping in the bed, but here he could be hidden underneath the bed. He does not see that Charlie is indeed in bed next to Lisa under the sheets, and in a later scene they are caught in the act of lovemaking by Jim who comes to tell his partner that Hugo was killed in a fight. Before they continue their flight, the two gangsters carry Hugo's corpse into the woods, but when it is discovered by the soldiers nearby, things move on apace. Jim shoots a soldier in the forehead, whereupon the military jeep leaves as quickly as possible; the policeman has shown up in the meantime and is about to shoot Jim, but his moments of hesitation are fatal to him. While Charlie is waiting in the car with Ruben—using him as a sort of protection shield—Jim surrenders to Deleye, who ruthlessly shoots the gangster in his chest. This is the moment for Lisa to grab the baby from Charlie's arms and to give it to her mother. She takes the wheel of the car and drives away. The couple on the run is chased by tanks and a helicopter, but after some time the manhunt is put to a stop. Lisa makes eyes at Charlie, but suddenly she opens the door of the car and, in a reference to the chicken run in REBEL WITHOUT A CAUSE (Nicholas Ray, 1955), she jumps out of the vehicle, whereupon the car, with Charlie still in it, drives off the cliff, followed by an explosion.[11]

This surprise ending contrasts with the predictable closure of HET MEISJE EN DE DOOD—predictable, for tragedies all too often end with dead women. Elise in Stelling's film had a faint hope of 'liberation', but her potential rescuer Nicolai misjudged her strategy. His misinterpretation is to a great extent related to the aristocrat environment in which one is supposed to keep up appearances. One's intentions can then easily be mistaken, and thus Nicolai leaves the hotel in frustration, not seeing that Elise's choice to return to the Count was just a cover-up. Such not-seeing is the root of tragedy. Unlike HET MEISJE EN DE DOOD, the characters in the B-gangster film WILDSCHUT are not restrained by the conventions of good etiquette. On the contrary, they are quite degenerate, with a scent of incest, and hence Lisa's audacious escape seems as logical as it is justified. By choosing to run with Charlie, she grabs the opportunity for another life. She apparently prefers a ride with a handsome tough guy over a domestic life in which her stepfather exploits her as a camp follower. She can even believe that her departure is in the interest of her baby Ruben. Her anguished remark that she is such a terrible mother that any gangster would be better equipped to raise her kid reinforces the idea that her absence would benefit Ruben's future life, as if this sacrifice is the best she has to offer as a young mother. Moreover, Charlie offers her the alluring prospect that they will be a new 'Bonnie and Clyde', and when Lisa says she does not know the couple, he explains that they are the 'Romeo and Juliet of crime'. In fact, because it is shot in a relatively restless style, one can regard WILDSCHUT as an homage to BONNIE & CLYDE (Arthur Penn, 1967) or to its B-predecessor GUN CRAZY (Joseph H. Lewis, 1950). Penn's film starts with some disorienting close-ups of Bonnie, who is much too energetic for the small bedroom and is all too happy to join Clyde, which feels like 'liberation' for her. But just as we begin to think that her choice for an adventurous love life, outside the 'blessings of civilization',[12] makes sense, it turns out to be the ultimate trap for Charlie. Lisa makes him believe that she loves him, but while she comes across as a pretty naïve and straightforward woman, she suddenly proves herself to be as treacherous as a femme fatale from a film noir.

Another Dutch film in which a farm is used as a hideout is DE POOLSE BRUID [THE POLISH BRIDE] (Karim Traïdia, 1998): the fugitive is not a gangster but a Polish woman on the run; the farm is not inhabited by a large family but by a lonely bachelor. Whereas WILDSCHUT was an underrated B-movie that was only appreciated in retrospect, predominantly by cinephiles, DE POOLSE BRUID was an instant arthouse success which had the honour of winning the

Audience Award at the International Film Festival Rotterdam, a rare achievement for a Dutch picture.[13]

LOVE AFTER AN ACT OF VIOLENCE: *DE POOLSE BRUID*

It is highly significant that in the opening shot of DE POOLSE BRUID, the woman running barefoot in the city streets of Groningen has a blood-smeared face. After the beginning title she is still running, this time in the countryside, before she arrives exhausted at the farmhouse of the reclusive Henk Woldring. He takes her in his arms and gives her a shower. She will have a blood-smeared face again in a much later scene, but this blood is of an entirely different origin. Because Henk does not ask questions about her past, we can only reconstruct from bits and pieces what the nature of this 'first blood' is. Flashes of a nightmare reveal to us that she has been sexually abused in a brothel; a blond man arrives at the farm, inquiring after a Polish runaway woman named Anna; later he arrives once more in the company of Anna's 'employer' who is her pimp; and a child's drawing is a sign that she has a daughter. Since the woman only speaks some broken Dutch and Henk is taciturn by nature, the two only exchange the absolute minimum of words. There is only a slow mutual advance—he teaches her how to feed the chickens and how to ride a bike; they go to the market and she chooses his blouses; they play checkers and she cheats at it when he has his back turned to the game. Anna's presence offers him distraction from his worries about late payments, and in addition to that, her help in the household is most welcome, although it annoys him that she wants him to pray before dinner. The swift and aggressive manner in which Henk recites the Lord's Prayer implies that he must have prayed a lot in the past but has since abandoned religion.

Anna is already around for a couple of days when he tells her that the photograph on the wall is a picture of his mother who passed away twenty years ago. From the shyness with which he hands her his underwear—for she is about to wash his clothes—we can already surmise that Henk is inexperienced with women. When he buys her a dress, he chooses the one she had been admiring in a shop window the other day. She is delighted with the present and asks him to wait while she tries it on. A sexual advance is to be expected, but at that very moment a car arrives with Anna's employer and his assistant, who demand financial compensation for her lack of services. Upon their return the next day, they instantly kill Henk's dog and he himself gets away with only a flesh wound. Henk is prepared for their subsequent visit and shoots the employer dead. After a suspenseful scene, the assistant is killed as well—not by Henk but by Anna, who hits him so vehemently that her face is smeared with the man's blood. After Henk cleans her face, once again, they make love in the shed with the camera at a considerable distance. Not another word is said in the remainder of the film. While Henk buries the bodies, Anna takes her suitcase and leaves, but it is only a temporary departure: in the final scene, Henk hears a child's joyful laughter and from afar we see Anna with her daughter.

What gives DE POOLSE BRUID its poignancy are the many landscape shots, frequently used as intermezzo, in-between scenes: the barren acres, a yellow cornfield, the painterly clouds, or rather, the 'unfinished sky', to quote the title of the Australian remake (Peter Duncan, 2007).[14] Such shots suggest that the farmer is determined by his environment: he is as unchanging as the landscape. And just as this nature can only be taken by force, such as a typhoon or an earthquake, the actual lovemaking only takes place after they both have murdered a man. The second time she has blood on her face signifies that her act of killing has been a transformative event. Contrary to his character, Henk has undergone a change, and he opens himself up to a woman other than his late mother. He can love Anna once she has proved that she is as resilient as the landscape.

PERHAPS LOVE: *BOVEN IS HET STIL*

Closest in spirit to DE POOLSE BRUID is, perhaps, BOVEN IS HET STIL [IT'S ALL SO QUIET] (Nanouk Leopold, 2013), even though there is hardly a female character involved in this film, let alone a bride. Like DE POOLSE BRUID (and WILDSCHUT), BOVEN IS HET STIL is set on a farm and also features many shots of the agrarian environment, but they are quite idyllic: we see morning dew, sunlight through the reed, lens flare, a child with a donkey or sheep passing by accompanied by piano sounds. The atmosphere indoors, however, is less serene. Helmer is a middle-aged farmer who takes care of his ill and old father, but only reluctantly. At the beginning of Leopold's film, Helmer has to go to great pains to lift his father, who can no longer walk, up the stairs. It is unclear whether Helmer is annoyed by his father or whether he is surly and taciturn by nature, but the entire film has hardly any dialogue. When his father wants him to get a doctor, Helmer refuses to call one. When his father asks him what he sees outside, he says 'nothing', while there is a hooded crow on the top of the tree. The one time the old man comes out of his bed, he looks for the crow—obviously taken by him as a sign of his impending death.

Apart from the daily work with sheep, cows, and donkeys, not much happens in BOVEN IS HET STIL, but as a result, tiny details become all the more significant. Helmer decides to paint the room of his late brother Geert so that a new farmhand can stay there. It is unclear why he hires the teenager Henk, for there is not very much work to do. Helmer takes Henk upstairs to meet the old man, who only asks him: 'Show me your hands ... No, the inside', but does not seem very impressed. The dairy driver who visits Helmer's farm daily remarks that this new farmhand does not work very hard but then adds: 'Sturdy lad, though.' A clue to why Helmer hired Henk is given in one of the very brief conversations between Helmer and his father. The old man says out of the blue: 'When Geert died, it was as if I died.' After a few moments of silence, Helmer calmly replies: 'And you were left with the wrong son', but the father cannot remember whether he thought so. Geert was the brother who was supposed to become the father's successor as a farmer, but Helmer took over willy-nilly. Hiring a farmhand who lives with them gives Helmer good reason to remove Geert's stuff from the room, which seems to have remained untouched ever since the brother's death. At one point, Henk creeps into Helmer's bed, and though Helmer calmly asks his farmhand not to do this, they end up holding each other tightly while Henk weeps. Soon thereafter Henk departs.

The point for Helmer is not that Henk is a young man instead of a woman but that he seems to have a problem with intimacy and physical contact as such. When the corpulent dairy driver is in his yard, he spies on him but avoids being seen. The other day the dairy driver had said: 'I missed you. I didn't see you the last few times.' 'I was upstairs, perhaps', Helmer lies, 'Father's ill'. The exchange of words is usually brief, and especially Helmer strikes uncomfortable poses. In a long shot, early in Leopold's film, we see the farmer naked, studying his body at length before a mirror. Retroactively, one might say that he is wondering how someone might admire that body or would like to be intimate with its bearer. Probably insecure about his own physique, Helmer seems too shy to have contact with others, let alone make any advances. While he is sitting next to his sleeping father, he says in a soft voice, talking about the dairy driver: 'He has beautiful hands. Very strong hands. Sometimes I look at those hands. You wouldn't understand that. Your hands were only used for beating.' This is the one clue in BOVEN IS HET STIL that suggests that touch is identified with aggressiveness (being hit by the father) rather than caressing. When the dairy driver says that he is quitting his job and going back to Mechelen, Belgium to live with his sister, Helmer is able to keep his demeanour: 'Okay, good luck, goodbye.' As soon as the dairy driver has left, however, Helmer has to regain his composure against the wall, which indicates that he is a restrained character in the company of others. If in his dying moments the father says that his son is a strange bird, we are supposed to think that the father has produced this strange bird, who has come to believe due to the father's behaviour that Geert was always preferred over him. At the end of the film, when the burial of the father takes place, the dairy driver unexpectedly shows up as one of the attendants.[15] We see him out of focus until Helmer turns around and sees that he has bruises on his face. After the funeral, they walk on the farm's yard, and Helmer has only two questions: 'So you're back again?' and 'Does it hurt?' The final shot shows Helmer lying amidst the reed, staring at the sky. We understand that there is little chance that he will get intimate with the dairy driver.

Given that this is a movie by Nanouk Leopold, who in all her previous films (discussed in chapter eight) had used static shots, it is remarkable that the camera is never static in BOVEN IS HET STIL; even in the long shots we see the camera move slightly. The restless camera in combination with the editing, which is jerky by Leopold's standards (including jump cuts, transgression of 180 degrees axis), can be seen as an expression of the Freudian wisdom that repressed desires always return in other forms. The fact that the camera is never static, no matter how minimal some of its movements, can be taken as a manifestation of Helmer's reluctance to submit to intimacy, despite his yearning to make contact.

THE FREQUENCY OF LOVE: *170 HZ* AND *OUT OF LOVE*

Helmer was never his father's favourite son. It is perhaps due to this lack of affection and the resulting lack of self-confidence that he has never developed his emotional range. In small gestures, we see the longing between him and the dairy driver, but it is basically restricted to furtive glances. Animosity towards one's father can not only obstruct a love affair, it can also unite a couple, as is the case with the teenagers in 170 HZ (Joost van Ginkel, 2009), who spoil no opportunities to express their bond, in opposition to their fathers. Van Ginkel's film stands out for the consistent use of gestural language, for both the sixteen-year-old Evy and her nineteen-year-old boyfriend Nick are deaf. Hence, the confrontations between Evy and her father take place in silence, but as the subtitles make clear, they are no less vehement. They live in a beautiful but coldly decorated home filled with glass walls, and Evy's father clearly does not want her to be intimate with that long-haired motorcycle boy in the leather jacket. In the beginning of 170 HZ, Evy is sitting in a bathtub with her knees bent up. The scene is intercut with happy moments with Nick, who lives in an abandoned bus. At the end of the film, she is in the very same position in the bathtub, and it is obvious that everything we see seems squeezed in as she reminisces her turbulent relationship with Nick.

The one time that Nick comes over for dinner at Evy's place to meet her parents, his answers are arrogant. 'Why don't you have a hearing implant, like the one Evy will get?' Evy's father asks. Whereas the daughter protests that she does not want one, Nick replies: 'Apart from Evy, no one has ever said anything of interest.' It is not clear what annoys Nick, perhaps an overall ennui with the bourgeois world in general. His mother points out his father's new car, but he is clearly not interested, even though he earns his money as a car mechanic. Meanwhile, Evy becomes so angry with her own dad that she agrees to the plan Nick has mentioned before: the two of them will run away together. She suggests that they return only when she is five months pregnant. To her surprise, Nick comes to pick her up one night, earlier than expected.

It only becomes clear later that Nick has deliberately run over his father with his motorcycle, and this accident is the reason he wants to leave prematurely. The father appears at uneven intervals as a memory image. On their way to their new hiding place, an empty submarine, Evy caresses Nick's fingers, but a reverse shot reveals Nick's father in the passenger's seat, complimenting the son on his beautiful hands. Slightly irritated, Nick responds: 'You've told me before.' When the father requests a kiss, they kiss each other tenderly, until Nick draws back, which results into a puzzled look by Evy: 'You've such a strange expression sometimes.' At one point, the two adolescents are swimming under water towards each other and their facial expressions are cheerful, until out of nowhere Nick sees the stiff body of his father, impeccably dressed, in the water. Nick gets out of the water, visibly in shock. Initially, his father was a primary source of annoyance to him, also triggering his competitive nature. The rivalry with his father seemed to energize Nick. But once the son kills him, his dead father shows up as a posthumous phantom, as a manifestation of Nick's guilt complex.

Van Ginkel's 170 Hz loses its momentum, however, when the two lovers are entirely on their own, away from the outside world that irritates them. Without a hostile environment, they soon resort to quibbles. Evy is writing her diary on a typewriter, and Nick rewrites it with lines such as 'I hate my mother'. When she asks him why he did so, he has no more to say than 'Would you love your child more than me?' 170 Hz is never explicit about motivations, but Nick seems so fearful of being left to his own devices—'Would you miss me if you were not here with me?' 'Will you stay with me forever?'—that his actions are counterproductive. When Evy sends a text message to her mother, he gets a fit. He becomes angry again after she denies that she is scared of him: 'This is the first time you've lied to me.' He suspects her of wanting to leave him, but she says she is only going for a swim. He wants her to prove this, and so Evy jumps into the cold water, but eventually she swims away from him. There is an insert of Evy in the bathtub, apparently reflecting upon her bygone period with her lover, then a cutback to Nick who puts his foot in a rope with an anchor attached to it. In the end, Evy is a single mother, with a small baby whom she baptises in water.

The problem with 170 Hz is pinpointed precisely in a review by Kieron

Casey. Van Ginkel's film is a 'formal triumph' and astonishes the viewer with its 'technical bravura'. Its brilliance is displayed in the alternation of shots with sound and those without—during the silent shots we 'listen' with either Nick or Evy; the slow motion scenes in which the lovers throw paint at each other; and the unexpected camera angles, of which the top-down shots of Evy in a bathtub—an homage to REQUIEM FOR A DREAM (Darren Aronofsky, 2000)—are particularly eye-catching. But Casey found himself 'underwhelmed by the plot', for when Nick and Evy run away, the film 'sadly finds itself in a storytelling cul-de-sac'. More critics have mentioned that the story of 170 HZ was too meagre, and Van Ginkel admitted so himself, after he had made his more impressive successor, THE PARADISE SUITE (2015).[16] The problem, however, is not so much the meagreness as such but rather, paraphrasing Casey, that the story about the 'burning intensity of first love' clashes with the rather cold 'technical brilliance' of the film's formal devices. In that sense, OUT OF LOVE (Paloma Aguilera Valdebenito, 2016) can be taken as its counterpart. From their first encounter onwards, it is a game of attract and repel between the Greek Varya and the Russian cook Nikolai. She is happy to taste his delicious chili, but it burns her stomach. When she thinks his food makes her fat, she turns the kitchen into a mess. At one point, she turns the apartment into a romantic place by decorating it with many heart-shaped balloons. To her anger, Nikolai does not return from the bar—which is just one illustration of his 'biggest fear': that his behaviour gets out of hand when he drinks too much.

There is quite a number of scenes in which the two make love passionately, but their affinity for each other can easily turn into a quarrel or even a physical fight. Nikolai is disturbed that Varya puts parmesan on her pizza with prawns; Varya hates the smell of his badly washed clothes, and she ridicules the name 'Nevaeh' that Nikolai's best friend has given to his daughter. He first sleeps at another guy's place, and later she confesses that she has been kissing someone else, simply because their chemistry is too much for her to bear: 'Everything is you', she says. During a fight, he fractures her eye socket, which results in their definitive break-up.

In order to emphasize the suffocating impact of an affair that is too passionate, the camera is very close to them most of the time, as if there are no other people around, just the two of them. If Nikolai and Varya move a lot, the camera does so as well, and it does not really distinguish between lovemaking or a quarrel. Hence, the way in which OUT OF LOVE is shot implies a close but apparently paradoxical congruence between love and hate, which Lacan explained with the neologism *hainamoration*.[17] If you love someone for the person they are—and not because of that person's cooking skills, bank account, beautiful blue eyes, or their habit of buying you presents—you love the other because of something in him/her more than him/herself. There is something indefinable that your partner does not share with anyone else. It may seem disappointing to hear that someone only loves you because you are a millionaire, but it is also more comforting, Žižek points out: you will continue to attract your partner as long as you remain rich and allow the partner to share in your wealth; if you lose your millions, your partner will abandon you, 'no deep traumas involved' (*Interrogating*, 291). But how do you make sure that you keep that 'indefinable X' if this is only in the eye of the beholder? Moreover, and more problematically, this indefinable X can also be a cause for disturbance. The particular idiosyncrasy that makes me love you is also the main reason for me to hate you. That there is hectic camerawork throughout OUT OF LOVE is an affirmation that a burning love can slip into deep hatred and vice versa: what moves you can also start to irritate you—just as the camerawork can both energize and fatigue the viewer. If 170 HZ was rooted in a deliberate clash between content and form due to its 'technical bravura', OUT OF LOVE displays a perfect match between story and cinematography thanks to its raw energy.

ONLY THE BASTARDS: *HEMEL* AND *INSTINCT*

The slippage between desire and love at the heart of this chapter is emblematically tackled in HEMEL (Sacha Polak, 2012). Hemel, meaning 'heaven', is the peculiar name of the 23-year-old protagonist, a city girl who behaves very much like an adolescent. She has not taken on any responsibilities, but though she lives on her own, she is still attached to her old room at her father's place. Polak's HEMEL has eight intertitles, referring to one-night stands ('genital phase' and 'Mohammed'), to a specific dance ('Sevillana'), or to a kitschy slogan ('You make me human'). Perhaps the most crucial one is the third 'chapter' called 'Father and daughter', for Hemel's behaviour seems to mirror that of her father Gijs. He has always lived on his own, with many open-ended relationships. Hemel's birth was a 'great gift after a tiny accident', but ever since the mother passed away, father and daughter have regular contact. When Hemel is introduced to her father's latest conquest—Sophie, who is much younger in years than he is—she speaks bluntly as usual, irritated by the fact that she had to wait a while for the two to show up: 'Are you late because you had sex first?' The father is both slightly embarrassed and slightly amused, and calmly responds: 'Yes'. Hemel then addresses Sophie: 'He kicked out his last girlfriend because of the bad sex.' Her father quasi-strangles her and says: 'You're like me, aren't you?'

In an imitation of her Casanova-like father, Hemel has sex three times in the first half of Polak's 80-minute film, none of which is very satisfactory. The third time in 'chapter' five (called 'Where God lives') was particularly tiring. The viewer is witness to the choke sex she had with an 'SM guy', and she recounts the experience at a party to Annabelle, of all people, who has decided to remain a virgin until marriage. With her fourth lover, in chapter six, she only has a post-coital conversation, but she ultimately becomes 'infatuated' with an older man, closer in age to his father than to hers. This Douwe is the faithful type, and upon his question 'How many conquests do you remember?' she answers: 'Only the bastards.' She clearly enjoys Douwe's company, but during a walk on the beach he tells her, to her disappointment, that the relationship cannot last. When her father announces in the next chapter that he intends to start living together with Sophie—something that up to then had never happened—Hemel is confused at first. She visits Brechtje, one of her father's colleagues, who recalls how her father always took care of her, and as Hemel listens, her nose starts to bleed. Brechtje embraces her tightly, and the film ends on this moment of intimacy. This closure suggests that it might mark a farewell to her period of relentless pursuit of desire, of hedonistic pleasures. Whereas Thomas in HET MES used a knife in an attempt to cut the umbilical cord with his mother and was sent to boarding school by her instead, Hemel's nose-bleeding marks her separation from her father and symbolizes that she is ready for her state of independence.

If Hemel's relationship to her father complicates her sexual life, in Halina Reijn's debut feature INSTINCT (2019), which premiered with a Variety Piazza Grande Award at Locarno International Film Festival, we get only minor but unmistakable hints that protagonist Nicoline has sex-related mental scars. To start with some telling scenes, her mother comes over to watch television with her and decides to stay over, though there is no urgent reason. We then have an overhead shot and see the two spooning, the mother only wearing a slip. In a later scene, Nicoline is dancing with her sister's daughter and the mother starts crying: 'It's so great to see you all so happy.' And towards the end of the film, mother sends a text message: 'Never forget that you are a very strong woman', a clear indication that her daughter has had to endure things in the past. Given the fact that the mother is trying to be so comforting throughout, one can only guess that she is trying to make up for the things Nicoline's dad did to her, who is absent and not mentioned once throughout the film.

Meanwhile, her sister tells her not to be too self-critical when Nicoline discloses that she has slept with a male colleague. This advice is also a reminder that her biological clock is ticking. Shown in brief fragments, the sex scene between Nicoline and co-worker Alex stands out because he is surprised by her impatience and by the fact that she evades eye contact. Nicoline is not after anything romantic but starts lying on the floor, inviting him to take her from behind; in the eyes of Alex, she looks like a 'rabbit'. Later Alex tells her that he senses—'intuitively', he says—that she has issues and that he will be there to help her. She gets angry at his suggestion that she needs a protective man, and Alex then drives away in his car, angered by this 'evasive non-conversation', which signals the end of their brief affair.

At the beginning of INSTINCT, psychotherapist Nicoline starts a new job at a penal institution as a successor to a man who has a burnout. Despite her professional experience, she does not want a tenure position at the detention centre. The challenge that viewers of Reijn's film have is to decide how to consider the encounters between Nicoline and her client, the sex offender Idris. Since the viewers have only bits and pieces of information about Nicoline's background, we do not really know what she has up her sleeve. Whereas her colleagues are in favour of granting Idris unaccompanied leave to reward his positive attitude, Nicoline is sceptical, suggesting they should also regard the crimes he did not commit. We know hardly anything about Idris except what is on his record—the aggressive treatment of young women—and he refuses to describe his misdemeanours in his own words when Nicoline asks him to. She thinks this sex offender knows too well how to give socially appropriate answers instead of honest ones. To test him, she casually mentions the loaded term 'long stay', but he does not even blink. Idris's behaviour is volatile: he can act nice and friendly but also be hot-tempered and intimidating. Though Nicoline tries to resist his charm, she becomes more and more intrigued by him. But cause and effect could also be the other way around: her fascination could be the result of her resistance. Her growing obsession with him is best indicated by her visit to Kentucky Fried Chicken after Idris tells her that he has a son named Milan who works in this fast-food franchise. It is clearly a first-time visit for Nicoline, for she has no clue what it means to order two buckets of chicken. But it is another sign of Idris's unreliability that the intern Marieke claims that the son has a job at McDonald's.

During his first unaccompanied leave, which lasts no longer than four hours, Idris says he wants to see the sea. Nicoline follows him at a distance, but in the dunes he is aware of her proximity. With no witnesses around, they approach each other, which challenges the viewer to consider the nature of this cat-and-mouse game. As several film reviews have mentioned: who is the hunter here, and who is the prey? Are they both like animals following their 'instinct'? To support this idea of the bestial nature in us all, in an early scene at Nicoline's home, we hear in the background the narrator of a nature documentary about predators and vultures on a television set. And in another scene, Nicoline hallucinates that there is a black dog sitting on her bed. The idea that she lacks control and is led by her impulses is emphasized by the many mirrored reflections that duplicate her image—in the bathwater, in the windows of the tram or train, or in the glass protecting a painting—by the frequent use of soft-focus (either Nicoline sharp and the background blurry or vice versa); and by a soundtrack with much static noise.

Her fascination with Idris can only go in one direction: to even closer encounters with him. When they are in an isolated space in the clinic and Idris starts to French kiss her, he suddenly pushes the red button that warns security.[18] Nicoline feels pressed to excuse herself to the two guards and tells them there was nothing wrong. But during a subsequent unaccompanied leave, Idris is suddenly at the door of Nicoline's apartment. She tells him he has to go away, but the fact that she does not close the door on him abruptly is taken as an invitation by Idris. He acts smooth and casual, but the visit ends predictably: she is raped on the couch from behind. Nicoline is too stunned to resist during the act and is in tears after he has left. Back at the institution, she walks into Idris's room and takes off her underwear. In his eyes, her action is a confirmation of his earlier statement that women have rape fantasies, even more frequently than men. As he is about to penetrate her, she pushes the red button, and to the guards who come running in, it looks as if she is being raped. He yells at her 'You love me', but it is in vain. While the camera remains focused upon Nicoline until the credits, we know Idris will end up in the isolation cell because in the opening scene of the film this is what happens to Nicoline in a roleplay with the guards when she pretends to be a furious client.

Reijn's INSTINCT is a psychological arthouse thriller, but at the end there is a shift in genre to a slasher film. I discuss the conventions used in slasher films and Carol Clover's idea of the Final Girl in this sub-category of sleazy horror in the last pages of chapter five in an analysis of one of my favourite Dutch cult movies, DE JOHNSONS, but here, in Reijn's film, the combination of slasher and thriller does not quite work. In several slashers, a rape victim concocts a strategy to take her revenge and when she succeeds in her payback, she deserves Clover's title of Final Girl. The strength of INSTINCT was that the two protagonists were playing a dangerous game in which the roles of cat and mouse were indeterminable. As a psychotherapist, however, Nicoline uses the power of the institution to bring her client down: she is the catwoman who has trapped the mouse. Moreover, Nicoline is also 'victorious' in the debate with her colleagues, because her minority opinion that Idris is not ready for a return in society is confirmed. In the light of the #MeToo movement, it may seem justified that a woman settles a score with a charming psychopath, but Nicoline's payback overshadows the intricate reflection on the darkness of desire that took place throughout much of the film. In addition, the viewers are left wondering at the end whether this is not the only time that Nicoline has trapped convicted sex offenders. Is this something she did before at other institutions? Is that the reason why she refused a tenure contract in the first place?[19] In other words, one may wonder whether Nicoline is a Final Girl re-offender.

THE DEVIL'S ADVOCATE: *LOOS*

When Erwin Olaf designed the controversial poster for LOOS (Theo van Gogh, 1989)— fully nude female buttocks and legs in high heels and black stockings and suspenders, wrapped in chains—it was a clear hint of the dark desires addressed in the movie. The poster was grist to the mill of Van Gogh, who always liked to play the role of an *enfant terrible*. I have already written extensively about this 'agent provocateur' and his three best-known films—06, BLIND DATE, and INTERVIEW—in *Humour and Irony* (192-195). After his tragic and abrupt death in November 2004, all three films were remade in the US. Nonetheless, I think that LOOS is his finest achievement, despite Van Gogh's overt eagerness to insert sleazy scenes. And though his treatment of dark desires is a bit too tongue-in-cheek, LOOS has become a curious delight with the passing of time, all the more so because it has always remained under the radar.[20]

LOOS starts with a shot of a scantily dressed woman who is offering her services to a man in a point-of-view shot from the perspective of the man: 'Shall I kneel for you?' She then goes down the stairs into the depot. After we have seen an insert of a woman entering the store, the tone changes. We hear the invisible man's voice with a heavy Surinamese accent: 'Shut up, you filthy white whore.' We then read the news headline that the 26-year-old Marlies B. has been killed in a shoe store. The prime suspect is the nightclub owner Harry Wery. The criminal barrister Willem Loos is asked to defend him, not for the first time. Loos is not sure whether to take the assignment, but Wery puts pressure on him by threatening to hurt his daughter if he doesn't defend him. During his investigations, Loos attends the kinky nightclub Showtime (where a leather-clad man hits a nail through his foreskin) where he is introduced to videos of bondage and torture. Loos is not attracted to these scenes, but he comes under the spell of a mysterious woman named Anna. When he is drinking at a bar, she takes his glass, calls him 'Tommy', and offers him champagne. She takes him to room 77 of Hotel Atlanta, and the next morning, his keys are missing, which are returned by one of Wery's henchmen. All that Anna does, whose family name is Montijn, is unpredictable: she disappears regularly and shows up suddenly, usually in room 77. The meetings are arranged by Wery, who tells Loos to consider her visits a 'business gift'. Anna's sexual wishes are of an uncommon kind, too uncommon for Loos, but he gives in to her demands. In a fancy restaurant, he has to tell her the story about when she was mistreated as an object at a market for slaves, which excites her. In another scene, Anna wants him to take her to a subway tunnel and chain her to a wall. She tells him to leave her there for a couple of hours, but when he returns, she has vanished.

With the day of the court hearing approaching, Wery's case is not very favourable, but Loos does not seem to mind. He tells his client that if Anna does not return, he hopes Wery will be convicted for murder in the first degree. But there is a sudden twist that brightens Wery's chances in court. Apparently, there was a female witness in the shoe store, and Loos places an ad in a newspaper asking this woman to contact him. He meets a blonde woman who only wants to testify in exchange for a substantial amount of money. She tells him she heard a man with a Surinamese accent say 'Shut up, you filthy white whore' and points her finger at the victim's black husband. Wery is thus saved, and to celebrate his release, Loos visits the man's loft where he happens to see a wedding picture of the nightclub owner, with Anna as the bride and the blonde woman standing on the other side of Wery. Reminiscent of the plot of WITNESS FOR THE PROSECUTION (Billy Wilder, 1957), Loos realizes that he has been fooled by his client, and to aggravate the embarrassment, Wery gives a perfect rendition of 'Shut up, you filthy white whore' in a Surinamese accent. The bad news does not end there, for it is reported that Anna's body has been found. Apparently, she jumped from a balcony, but police inspector Dorrius gives Loos a warning: you are apparently the last one who saw her alive, so we have to keep an eye on you.

In distress, Loos goes back to the bar, and this time he is seduced by the blonde witness, Maria, with the very same phrases that Anna had used. Almost hypnotized by the repetition of this seduction technique, he follows her, quite flabbergasted. Maria takes out handcuffs and says 'this is love'. He does not resist when he is tied to a bed, but then Wery walks down a staircase, whom Loos had threatened in a previous scene. Before Wery can act, however, he is shot in the back by Maria. With a 'I loved her, too' to Loos, and the announcement that the charwoman will arrive in two weeks, she bids farewell to the solicitor.

Notwithstanding some shortcomings—including the script and some of the acting performances—one of the attractions of LOOS is that its femme fatales have a neo-noir sensibility. Though Anna ends up dead, Maria gets away with revenge at the expense of the two men who think they are involved in a rivalry with each other. Both Wery and Loos share a perspective in which women are objects of exchange among men, and thus they pay dearly for their blindness to lesbian desire, which is at the root of Maria's intervention. Moreover, Loos, an experienced solicitor, was barking up the wrong tree. Anna as well as Maria made it clear that they were playing games, confirmed by their use of the same seduction technique, including the verbal repetitions. As Žižek has postulated, while the classic femme fatale tries to conceal her manipulative tactics, the neo-noir femme fatale is completely transparent: she is so outspoken about her cunning ways that the man presumes, out of conceit, that her explicit stance is a false move. It is because Anna and Maria are so obviously acting the role of dangerous women that Loos cannot believe that they are really dangerous. In the words of Žižek, this strategy—which he relates to the neo-noir femme fatales in BASIC INSTINCT (Paul Verhoeven, 1992) and THE LAST SEDUCTION (John Dahl, 1994)—can be paraphrased as follows: 'Why do you act as if you are just a cold, manipulative bitch when you really are just a cold, manipulative bitch?' (*The Art*, 16). By means of Maria's revenge, Wery is punished for his false pretension that he is a master manipulator while Loos is chastised for his naivety.

In addition to several kinky intermezzos that have been included, Van Gogh's feature film also has a few characters sing children's songs. One of these is called 'Papegaaitje, leef je nog?' (Tiny parrot, are you still alive?'), where the word 'advocaatje' (small advocate) is substituted for 'papegaaitje' (tiny parrot). Having barely survived the adventures, Loos is given ample time to reflect on why he was duped by attractive women not once but twice.

CONCLUSION: DESIRE OF THE OTHER

Desire is a forward movement. A character misses something essential in his/her life and wants to obtain it, but as psychoanalysis teaches, desire is incessantly frustrated: the satisfying object cannot be appropriated. The male subjects in this chapter, however, do not want to give up their pursuit of this object, and against their better judgement, they persevere. The men try to conquer yet another woman, just like Casanova, but once they have made love to that woman she becomes part of a chain of flirts (as in LIEFDESBEKENTENISSEN). The man and the woman in EEN OCHTEND VAN ZES WEKEN are only 'alive and kicking' once they are both free to do their favourite activities (driving, modelling), but Jimmy makes the error of trying to conquer Annette, which goes against the rule that love blossoms by virtue of obstacles. Havinck learns that true love is essentially a fascination that one experiences 'too late'. The most intimate moment in the lives of Egon and Marjoke in DE GROT can only be experienced as a posthumous memory. The gangster girl is an unattainable fantasy, part of the fiction created by the scriptwriter. The love between the farmer and his Polish bride is mediated by violent acts, and this is likely to create an obstacle: for an average man and woman, such murders usually come with a sense of guilt that will loom over their relationship.

But, as one of Lacan's most famous phrases runs, 'desire is the desire of the Other' (*Écrits*, 201). At the imaginary level, desire accords with the structure of envy: perhaps the scriptwriter loves the gangster girl because director Jascha is so enthralled by her image. But desire can also be determined by the symbolic network: guilt-ridden, Havinck learns to loves his late wife after all because his environment expects him to mourn her death and it can bring him closer to his daughter. Perhaps the Polish bride loves the farmer all the more now that he has killed a man for her, and vice versa. The young couple in 170 HZ love each other because their fathers disapprove of the affair, but once they are on their own, the love soon evaporates without the opposition of their parents. Desire is not just a matter of choosing a favourite object; it is a fantasy staged for the sake of the Other. And for that very reason, desire is all the more impenetrable to the subject itself (Žižek *Interrogating*, 74-75), resulting in morally diffuse pictures such as HEMEL and INSTINCT, which respectively portray the slippage from desire to love and the slippage from desire to revenge. LOOS is another, and more interesting, variant on this latter slippage: the neo-noir femme fatales openly put their cards on the table, but the solicitor nonetheless falls into the trap of his desires.

NOTES

1 The dream sequence in HET MES gives expression to Rademakers' preference for an 'anti-naturalistic realism' ['anti-naturalistisch realisme'] (Bernink, 42).

2 As Verhaeghe mentions, the 'shadow of the past' will fall over the present relationship 'like a lead weight' (*Love in a Time*, 60).

3 Another Pim and Wim production, RUBIA'S JUNGLE (1970), De la Parra's second feature as director, was also a low-budget film and also about unrequited love. Despite its lack of success, it is quite interesting, especially thanks to the beautiful black-and-white cinematography. Rubia used to live with the writer Lukas, but she has gone to live at her godfather's place on an island near Amsterdam. She fancies the black man Albert, but he is not prepared to leave his wife Helen. Lukas follows Rubia like a detective and then informs Helen about the frequent contacts between her husband and Rubia. But Albert had already told her everything. One day, Albert gives in to Rubia's frequent requests and decides to spend an entire day with her. Rubia still has a key to Lukas's house, and one day when the writer comes home, he hears some people making love and therefore leaves again. The next day, Albert tells Rubia that while he doesn't regret what happened, he nonetheless chooses to continue his marriage: it is impossible for him to pay attention to two women. She goes to Lukas's place to get a gun and then visits Albert. In the

presence of Helen, she fires two shots at the black man and then shoots herself in the head. Lukas's voice-over mentions that it took her six hours to die. Her last words were addressed to Lukas: *Leave me alone*.

4 As a follow-up to the idea that quantity is at least as important as quality, De la Parra took the initiative for so-called 'minimal movies' in the late 1980s, in financially difficult times in the Dutch film industry: people had to make films on a shoestring budget in a brief time-span. Between 1988 and 1993, fifteen minimal movies were initiated, but six of them remained unfinished. Paul Ruven was also actively involved in the most noteworthy of these minimal movies: he co-scripted LOST IN AMSTERDAM (Pim de la Parra, 1989) and DE NACHT VAN DE WILDE EZELS [THE NIGHT OF THE WILD DONKEYS] (Pim de la Parra, 1990); he co-wrote and co-directed, together with Sabine van den Eynden, MAX & LAURA & HENK & WILLIE (1989); and he wrote and directed HOW TO SURVIVE A BROKEN HEART (1991).

5 The Belgian director Harry Kümel invited Truffaut to see Verstappen's second feature, translating all the dialogue on the spot into French.

6 Despite a selection for the Berlin Film Festival, Van der Heyde's second feature, TO GRAB THE RING (1968), about a gangster on the run for the mob, was not very successful. The gangster was played by Ben Carruthers who had acted in SHADOWS (John Cassavetes, 1959) and THE DIRTY DOZEN (Robert Aldrich, 1967). For his third feature, the highly idiosyncratic ANGELA – LOVE COMES QUIETLY (1973), Van der Heyde went to great lengths to contact Barbara Hershey for the main role. He had seen her in 1969 in Frank Perry's LAST SUMMER, after which he started writing her many letters, all of which were returned unopened. When she paid a visit to the Netherlands, he was finally able to get her consent, but just before shooting she insisted she be credited as 'Barbara Seagull' because she was convinced that a dead seagull was living inside her. Hershey played the title heroine, Angela, stepdaughter of a rich American—played by another star actor on Van der Heyde's wish list, Ralph Meeker—who returns in the 1930s to his native soil, a village in the province of Friesland. He wants to see Louise, an old flame from his former days. The village is quite conservative, and therefore disapproves when Louise's adolescent son Harm-Wouter, who failed his studies, runs away with Angela. Van der Heyde's film turns into a kind of hippy fantasy, with Angela walking barefoot and milking cows on the way. A farmer catches them in the act and makes them one of his hands. When the farmer tries to rape Angela, Harm-Wouter comes to her rescue and they escape. While swimming naked in a small lake, Harm-Wouter discovers that Angela is pregnant, and at the doctor's office, he introduces them as 'Mr. and Mrs. Dijkstra'. The last five minutes, however, are simply enigmatic. As they are sitting near a tree in the grass, they are suddenly surrounded and beaten by a company of men headed by the farmer. The beatings are intercut with shots that suggest the marriage of the youngsters, with Harm-Wouter's parents in a happy mood and Angela with a baby on her lap. Is this a posthumous fantasy? The

camera goes back and forth between the violent beatings and the cheerful dancing at the wedding. Suddenly there is a shot of a little girl in an impeccably white dress on the railway tracks. She seems to turn around because she hears Angela's scream (or does she?), but then everything is quiet. While the girl continues to play on the railway in slow motion, the film ends. Van der Heyde's four subsequent features were far removed from his artistic ambitions. HELP! DE DOKTER VERZUIPT (1974) was a tremendously popular comedy, but the three films that followed were not only artistic failures, they also bombed at the box office.

7 Unlike the film, Campert's novel ends with Wessel returning home, though he has no clue whether he and Leonie will continue their marriage or not.

8 A great example of doomed love in Dutch cinema is VOOR EEN VERLOREN SOLDAAT [FOR A LOST SOLDIER] (Roeland Kerbosch, 1992), based upon the memoirs of Rudi van Dantzig, a well-known choreographer (1933-2012). The film is set in the present, with Jeroen rehearsing with young dancers. The choreography is meant to be a 'memory of memories', which recalls for him the celebration in 1980 of the soldiers who liberated the Netherlands in 1945. Jeroen has received note that his foster father during the war, 'Hait', has passed away. The envelope also contained a pair of sunglasses and a picture of him with his foster family. When he attends Hait's funeral, he sees the church door. A boy comes out, an eleven-year-old Jeroen who leaves the service temporarily to pee against a tree. The brief conversation with his younger self brings the older Jeroen back to 1944 when he was transported with other children from Amsterdam to the Frisian countryside where food was not that scarce. He lives with a Christian family that reads from the Bible daily. When Canadian soldiers arrive, he has a good time with one of them named Walt. At one point, Hait tells Jeroen that he caught him in the act, and while we expect him to say he has found out about the sexual nature of Jeroen's friendship with the soldier, Hait says it is not decent to keep all the sweets he receives to himself. When the entire country is liberated, Jeroen has mixed feelings since it means that Walt will depart. Before his farewell, Walt made some photos, and when Mem, Hait's wife, does the laundry, Jeroen thinks the pictures are ruined. On the boat back to Amsterdam after the funeral service, the old Jeroen once again meets his younger self (also heading back home to Amsterdam with his mother) and tells him that there was a photograph after all. When working on the ballet performance with his dancers at the end of VOOR EEN VERLOREN SOLDAAT, he receives another envelope. It contains not only an enlargement of the photo but a second item as well: it is the soldier's dog tag with Walt's family name on it ('Cook'). Jeroen can now search for his lost soldier if he desires, but Kerbosch's film wisely ends here, for those happy days are not likely to be relived again.

9 The title of Stelling's film also recalls the famous German poem *Der Tod und das Mädchen* (1774) by Matthias Claudius.

10 Gordel van smaragd [Tropic of Emerald] (Orlow Seunke, 1997) is built around the idea that love can be interrupted by historical events. This can fuel desire or obstruct it, depending on the gravity of the situation. Theo Staats goes to the Dutch East Indies and falls in love with Ems Pons, an Indo-European singer from the poor kampong who is married to a much older nightclub owner. The husband tolerates their affair on the condition that it is kept a secret, but people begin to gossip. Seunke's film is regularly intercut with archival footage, accompanied by voice-over commentary by either Theo or Ems. Footage from the Japanese invasion in the East Indies is a prelude to another obstacle to their relationship, for once Ems's husband is shot by Japanese soldiers, Theo ends up in a camp. Ems continues to sing and also plays the 'Jap whore'. In return for her sexual favours, Theo is transferred to the kitchen, which considerably increases his chances of survival. And indeed, Theo is able to leave the camp after the war, albeit with a serious eye infection, but instead of thanking her for her sacrifices, he is angry at Ems's collaboration. Another problem arises when Theo's uncle is murdered by Indonesian rebels in their fight for independence. Theo takes over the plantation, but due to his work he has little time for Ems, who now has to amuse herself for the first time in her life, as she says. Theo and Ems get married after all, but as Theo says in voice-over, he wonders whether they can ever love each other again. The military campaign by the Dutch against the Indonesian Nationalists presents another obstacle for the couple. Theo no longer feels safe and wants to go back to Holland. Though Ems agrees to join him, in the end she steps off of the train and remains in the country where she was born, which is the end of their relationship.

11 In an interview with Bor Beekman, Jack Monkau who played Charlie explains that his character got away with the girl, but the American studio Cannon Film insisted that the black man had to die. Monkau had to return from his holidays to reshoot the ending.

12 When the escaped convict cowboy Ringo and the prostitute Dallas are permitted to ride away into the great wide open in Stagecoach (John Ford, 1939), Doc Booth remarks that they are 'saved from the blessings of civilization'.

13 It took some fifteen years for another Dutch film to win the Audience Award at IFFR, Matterhorn (Diederik Ebbinge, 2013).

14 Chris Keulemans mentions that for Traïdia, De Poolse bruid is reminiscent of his childhood in Besbes, Algeria. In the magnificent countryside of Algeria, farmers regularly take the law into their own hands, and thus beauty can change into violence instantly (264-265).

15 Later a neighbour asks the dairy driver at the reception after a funeral service: 'Have you never been inside at Helmer's place? Did Helmer never offer you a cup of coffee?' Helmer dryly responds: 'He's having coffee now.'

16 See Van Ginkel in an interview with Berend Jan Bockting.

17 Lacan introduces this term in Seminar IX on 20 March 1973; see *Encore*.

18 It is clear that Idris has triggered Nicoline's desire: she does nothing to resist his charms. This is reminiscent of the notorious scene in WILD AT HEART (David Lynch, 1990) when Bobby Peru begs Lula to say 'Fuck me!' When she finally gives in and utters a barely audible 'Fuck me', he answers that he is sorry that he has no time today. According to Žižek, this unexpected rejection is particularly traumatic. Peru 'has attained what he really wanted: not the act itself, just her consent to it, her symbolic humiliation, [a] rape in fantasy which refuses its realization in reality' (*Plague*, 185).

19 These questions were suggested to me by Hans Beerekamp.

20 Another reason I am sympathetic to LOOS has to do with a most remarkable series of rare cameo appearance: by the writers Maarten Biesheuvel, Karel van het Reve, and Edgar Cairo. The writer and columnist Max Pam has a more substantial role as the suspect, whereas producer Matthijs van Heijningen plays the part of a prison guard who tells dirty jokes.

BIBLIOGRAPHY

Bernink, Mieke, *Fons Rademakers: Scènes uit leven en werk* (Abcoude: Uniepers, 2003).

Beekman, Bor, 'We hébben al een neger', kreeg Jack Monkau te horen. De acteur kan er nog om lachen', *de Volkskrant* (4 March 2020), https://www.volkskrant.nl/cultuur-media/we-hebben-al-een-neger-kreeg-jack-monkau-te-horen-de-acteur-kan-er-nog-om-lachen~b09d0427/ [Accessed 16 May 2020].

Casey, Kieron, 'BIFF Film Review: 170Hz', *The Totality*, http://www.wondrouskennel.com/2013/04/film-review-170hz.html [Accessed 17 May 2020]

Clover, Carol J., 'Her Body, Himself: Gender in the Slasher Film', 1993, ed. by Mark Jancovich, *Horror: The Film Reader* (London and New York: Routledge, 2002): 77-89.

Den Drijver, Ruud, *Circus Bloteman: Biografie van Wim Verstappen, Filmpionier uit de West* (Amsterdam: Stichting Wim Verstappen Scorpio Films, 2015).

Keulemans, Chris, 'Karim Traïdia: een Algerijnse dromer die meer wil weten dan er te weten valt', ed. by Wim Willems, *Cultuur en migratie in Nederland: De kunst van het overleven* (The Hague: Sdu Uitgevers, 2004), 247-275.

Lacan, Jacques, *Encore: Book XX, 1972-1973*, trans. by Cormac Gallagher (Eastbourne, Antony Rowe Ltd., 2004).

—, *Écrits: A Selection*, trans. by Alan Sheridan, 1977 (London: Routledge, 2001).

—, *The Ethics of Psychoanalysis: Book VII, 1959-1960*, trans. by Dennis Porter (London: Routledge, 1991).

Van den Tempel, Mark, 'Dutch Treat: De opkomst en ondergang van Cannon', *De Filmkrant* 379 (September 2015), https://filmkrant.nl/artikel/filmslot-de-opkomst-en-ondergang-van-cannon/ [Accessed 12 May 2020].

Verhaeghe, Paul, *Love in a Time of Loneliness: Three Essays on Drive and Desire* (London: Karnac Books, 2011).

Verstraten, Peter, '"My Very Own CITIZEN KANE", Inspired by Godard and Fellini: Frans Weisz's Adaptation of Remco Campert's *Het gangstermeisje*', *Journal of Dutch Literature* 8, 1 (2017): 60-74.

Žižek, Slavoj, *Interrogating the Real*, ed. by Rex Butler and Scott Stephens (London: Bloomsbury, 2013).

—, *The Art of the Ridiculous Sublime*: LOST HIGHWAY (Seattle: Walter Chapin Simpson Center for the Humanities, University of Washington Press, 2000).

—, *The Plague of Fantasies* (London and New York: Verso, 1997).

CHAPTER 4

From Ordinary Men and Rabbles to Heroes

Verstraten, P., *Dutch Post-War Fiction Film Through a Lens of Psychoanalysis*. Taylor & Francis Group, 2021
DOI 10.5117/9789463725330_CH04

ABSTRACT

The fourth chapter takes the ethical distinction Jacques Lacan makes between a hero, an ordinary man, and a rabble as a lead, and it detects hitherto unexplored affinities between ALS TWEE DRUPPELS WATER and SOLDAAT VAN ORANJE. As the chapter progresses, the definition of heroism becomes increasingly complicated, discussing 'authentic' partisans versus characters who walk a thin line between treason and heroism, such as the female teacher in PASTORALE 1943. The final four films focus on male characters who dedicate themselves to a self-declared mission and are determined to persevere, no matter what. This reaches its climax in the nail-biting film SPOORLOOS, which tries to explain why a hero should be seen as someone 'capable of excess'.

KEYWORDS
Heroes and rabbles – martyrdom – excluded from a symbolic network – capable of excess

Is Ducker, the blond-haired protagonist in ALS TWEE DRUPPELS WATER, a hero, a rabble, or perhaps an ordinary man? This question seems fairly easy to answer at first sight. In the eyes of the resistance, he is a rabble: they do not believe there is a Dorbeck, so Ducker has to take full responsibility for all his outrageous activities. Ducker himself believes he is an ordinary man-turned-hero, for he did his courageous deeds merely on the request of secret agent Dorbeck. In the eyes of the priest who stands by him in the last moments of his life, Ducker is an unfortunate ordinary man. The priest might have presumed that Dorbeck was only a figment of Ducker's imagination, but he fully supported him in his quest of proving the existence of Dorbeck. Hero or rabble are irrelevant categories to the priest; in his perception, Ducker was just a woeful guy trapped in an awkward situation. Ducker was in need of spiritual help, and the priest was ready to give it to him according to the commandment 'Love thy neighbour'.

Following the reading above, the distinctions between hero, rabble, and ordinary man are basically a matter of perspective in ALS TWEE DRUPPELS WATER. The qualification depends on whether one believes Ducker's story to be true or not. The differences between an ordinary man and a hero are, as Lacan states in his *The Ethics of Psychoanalysis*, 'more mysterious than one might think' (321), and his brief reference to the rabble in *Television* contributes to the confusion. It is only a thin line between the rabble and the ordinary man. The rabble does not suffer from his superego, for he ignores the moral voice that commands him not to do 'bad' things. He can do them without feeling bad, and because he has no regrets, Lacan claims, 'analysis should be withheld from the rabble' (*Television*, 43): therapy will be ineffectual for those who are not prepared to atone for a sinful life. The ordinary man, by contrast, feels guilty even when he has done nothing wrong. When a police officer calls out 'Hey, you!', the ordinary man is the one who immediately presumes that the agent is addressing him. He thinks: I am not aware that I made an offence, but it is highly probable that I am to blame for something. The problem of the ordinary man is that he gives credence to the superego, bombarding him with unjustified 'recriminations'. He is lured by the superego, the equivalent of a bully's whisper, which makes him believe that he is an unscrupulous man who pursues solipsistic pleasures (Schokker and Schokker, 152). Analysis is supposed to teach him to turn a deaf ear to this 'moral' interior voice of the superego. So the ordinary man who might erroneously think he is a rabble has to learn to ignore the superego if it tries to talk him into a guilt complex. In Lacanian terms, this ordinary man can become a hero on the condition that he does not compromise his desire, regardless of circumstances or consequences. One does not become a hero by 'accomplishing' an admirable act, but one can be called a hero when one is radically transformed by 'undergoing' an act and one is fully prepared to accept the consequences of what one's words or actions have set in motion. In the words of Žižek, a hero

> does not step aside when the arrow that he shot makes its full circle and flies back at him—unlike the rest of us who endeavour to realize our desire without paying the price for it: revolutionaries who want Revolution without revolution (its bloody reverse). (*Enjoy*, 14)[1]

Saying 'no' out of principle is the exemplary case of such an act, as when Antigone insists that her brother receive a decent burial, even though this demand means that she is consciously excluding herself from the community. A heroic and ethical act implies taking a position that goes against one's self-interest: Antigone chooses the status of *objet petit* '*a*', the object-cause of desire, which is beyond the confines of the symbolic order. The pursuit of an object of desire results in frustration as soon as one captures it and sets a chain of events in motion: one's 'I' is never satisfied (see chapter three). By contrast, *objet petit* '*a*' cannot be symbolically articulated and relates to a desire one does not rationally pursue because it does not serve one's personal concerns at all. Antigone acquires the status of *a* because there is no reasonable justification for her choice except that she states 'this has to be done, no matter what'. She sticks to a position even though she has everything to lose, and thus she puts her 'I' at stake. This chapter will show a gliding scale from a relatively common-sense idea of the distinction between the ordinary man and the hero to a different one, one that is informed by a Lacanian notion. This gliding scale will correspond to a change in emphasis from 'I' to '*a*'.

ACCIDENTAL 'HERO': *SOLDAAT VAN ORANJE*

Ducker suffers from a minority complex, and Dorbeck is required as a mediating Ego Ideal. By giving in to Dorbeck's precise instructions, he hopes to become an 'I' himself, fully integrated in the symbolic order. His desire for acknowledgement obviously serves his self-interest and is therefore at odds with Lacan's ethical axiom: do not give up your desire. A case slightly more complex, which I have already discussed in chapter one, is SÜSKIND. It seems that history speaks favourably of this historical figure, also thanks to Van den Berg's 2012 film, but despite his actions, he does not meet the criterion of a Lacanian hero. Walter Süskind is led too much by opportunistic behaviour. He takes the job first and foremost because he feels the responsibility of fatherhood. Having seen his name on the list, he realizes that this is the only way to save his family. It makes sense that he favours his symbolic mandate over his desire: he would never have wanted to take up the job or to enter into a collaborative relationship with the Nazis if it were not for the survival of his own family. At the same time, Walter is not a rabble, for he clearly feels guilty about his sly strategy. Out of pity for the young victims as well as to soothe his moral conscience, he goes to quite some lengths to rescue a number of children. After he is arrested with wife and daughter, some children are locked up to keep them out of sight of the Germans. Suddenly, Walter is given permission to go back to Amsterdam for one day. The official reason for the journey is to get some precious stones to hand them over to the Nazis, but the tacit reason is to save the Jewish children in hiding. Separated by barbed wire, his wife tells him 'not to ask anything', but he can guess that he owes his temporary leave to her willingness to sleep with Obersturmführer Gemmeker (Walter had seen that this commander had selected her from the crowd). He returns in time to the camp, but Gemmeker did not keep his 'promise' that his wife will be his again 'and only his'. Much worse, Hanna and daughter are put on the train to Germany. It turns out that Aus der Fünten who felt betrayed by Walter, had overruled the commander, and Walter is left with the choice to go back to the camp or to join his wife and daughter in wagon number fourteen. He chooses the latter, which means that he sticks to the symbolic mandate: the family is together again, but at a terrible price, for all three will be dead before the war ends.

The final scene of Van den Berg's film SÜSKIND suggests that the protagonist has not died in vain. Thanks to his efforts to protect young children, we see that the reunion of the siblings Roosje and Simon, shown in slow motion and accompanied by violin sounds, is watched over by Fanny, one of Walter's assistants. If historians were a bit ambivalent as to how to judge Süskind's role in the war, the film not only emphasizes that his sacrifice saved the lives of others, he is also symbolically acknowledged as a heroic martyr: Fanny knows, as we know now, that the emotional embrace between the siblings was enabled by Walter's intervention. One might say that Van den Berg retroactively honours the historical Süskind by giving the film the man's name. Such martyrdom is a Biblical notion of heroism rather than a Lacanian one: he dies so that others can live.[2]

It is but a small step from the sacrificial Süskind to the war hero par excellence in Dutch film history: Erik Lanshof, based upon Erik Hazelhoff Roelfzema whose memoirs were source material for the scenario of SOLDAAT VAN ORANJE (Paul Verhoeven, 1977), number twelve on the all-time list of Dutch box-office successes.[3] Insofar as Erik is a hero, however, he is an accidental one. Some thirteen minutes into SOLDAAT VAN ORANJE, there is a photographic picture, made with a delayed action shutter, portraying six friends on the eve of World War II. The actual result is shown in freeze-frame so that the audience has the time to linger over this picture. In each and every case, a minor detail will determine the life course of the friends. Alex is partly of German descent, and due to this family tie, he comes to side with the Nazis; Erik wants to help Jan to escape to England, and thus he offers him his place on a plane, but on his way there Jan is captured and later executed; Nico is known as a real stickler but he is hit in a hail of bullets while Erik is miraculously saved; Guus gets beheaded at the end of the film after he has taken revenge upon Robbie; this Robbie who is not present on the photograph, had become a traitor, because, if he did not, the Germans would arrest his Jewish fiancée Esther.[4]

The particular strength of SOLDAAT VAN ORANJE is to suggest that each path could have been Erik's, a suggestion that gains in emphasis when he watches the photograph once more at the end of the war in the company of Jacques, the only other person in the photo to survive the war. If Erik had been as reckless as Guus, he would have been dead; if Erik had had German ancestors, he might have sympathized with the Nazis like Alex who is blown to pieces as a soldier on the Eastern Front;[5] if Erik had not given Jan the chance to escape to England, he would have died prematurely; if Erik had preferred to pursue his studies, like Jacques, he would have remained anonymous. And one can add to this: if Erik had started an affair with Robbie's fiancée who frequented his apartment, he might have become the traitor.

These 'what if ...' scenarios can be supplemented with a most intriguing one if one considers SOLDAAT VAN ORANJE alongside ALS TWEE DRUPPELS WATER. While Jan is still held in prison, the Germans arrest Erik for investigation. During the last night before his execution, Jan is able to send a coded message to Erik, who is released the next day: a man named 'Van der Zanden' is a spy, working for the Germans. When in London, Erik meets this Van der Zanden, who turns out to be a personal advisor to the Dutch Queen. Erik intends to kill this traitor on his own initiative, but his attempt fails, since Van der Zanden outsmarts him. Soon thereafter he understands his utter naivety: the Germans kept Jan alive in the hope that he would send a coded message to Erik that would blemish Van der Zanden's reputation. The question then becomes: 'What if Erik had acted effectively and had killed this important figure?' In that case, Erik would have been like Ducker from Rademakers' film and would probably have met the latter's sorry fate. In other words, Erik could only become a hero, a soldier of Orange who at the end of the war was a trustee of the Dutch Queen, because he failed to see his planned assault through, in contrast to Ducker who dies as a doomed anti-hero and a despicable outcast because he was successful in executing all the assignments given to him. SOLDAAT VAN ORANJE illustrates that Erik is everything but a natural-born man of courage but rather fell into the position by complete accident and was subsequently celebrated as a hero upon homecoming.

SOLDAAT VAN ORANJE is one of the very best films made in the Netherlands, and it ended as number two in a public poll for best Dutch film of the twentieth century (after Verhoeven's TURKS FRUIT from 1973). The film has narrative pace, is tailored to American cinema, has a fantastic musical score by Rogier van Otterloo, great acting—including a performance by prolific British actor Edward Fox—and has black-and-white newsreel footage strategically interwoven into the adventure story. In addition, SOLDAAT VAN ORANJE is no exception to the rule that a Verhoeven film ends irresolutely. As J.P. Telotte mentions in his analysis, the film is 'prone to resist neat conclusions' (14). For example, Verhoeven's film asks its viewers what has been accomplished by the end of the war. Who did the right thing? In answer to the question why the ending is so curiously 'non-judgemental', Verhoeven said he did not know whether Erik's lifestyle was better than Jacques'. 'Should you be a war hero and have all your friends killed because of your audacity? Or should you be this student who didn't do anything and who prepared himself to be a good member of society?' (qtd. in Bouineau, 70). Another example is the opening and concluding airport scenes with Erik as a dutiful 'soldier' of the Dutch queen, which Telotte considers inconclusive because plot-wise they illustrate the victory over fascism, but its imagery uncannily recalls the military establishment they have just defeated. As the Queen's adjutant, Erik seems ready to submit to '*blind* obedience' of her majesty (Telotte, 15). Moreover, early in the film, we are introduced to the bizarre rules and regulations of student associations when Erik is forced to sing with a bleeding head wound while soup is being poured over his skull. The brutality of their habits is a bit like the aggressive methods of torture employed by the Nazis.

Above, I argue that SOLDAAT VAN ORANJE and ALS TWEE DRUPPELS WATER were closely affiliated on account of the reversed mirroring of the protagonist's fate (Erik would have been like Ducker if ...), but the ambiguous ending of each film underscores the idea that there is no clear-cut manifestation of old-school heroism in Dutch cinema, except for Paul Rotha's well-attended but completely forgotten DE OVERVAL (1962)[6] as well as the recent BANKIER VAN HET VERZET [THE RESISTANCE BANKER] (Joram Lürsen, 2018).[7] This conventional notion of heroism within the Dutch resistance during World War II is downplayed even further in PASTORALE 1943 (Wim Verstappen, 1978), released one year after SOLDAAT VAN ORANJE. A voice-over introduces the

Dutch as a 'kind people, because they have hardly any heroes'. More relevant for this chapter, however, is that Verstappen's film also suggests in passing an instance of what Lacan coined 'an ethical act'.

FEMALE DAREDEVILS: *PASTORALE 1943* AND *HET MEISJE MET HET RODE HAAR*

The story of PASTORALE 1943 consists of a chain of miscalculations as well as poor attempts at deception. In the very first scene, a man at an outside cafe, Van Dale, is deceived by a blonde woman, Mies Evertse, who asks him if he can help her find a hiding place for anti-Nazis: he doesn't realize that she is collaborating with the Germans and is soon thereafter arrested. Later, protagonist Johan Schultz, who has renamed himself Johan Schults to make his German name sound more Dutch, invites a woman whom he suspects to have been the traitor. They meet in a café, but Van Dale fails to recognize Mies due to his terrible eyesight. Meanwhile, the masquerades of four Dutch men who raid a distribution office are so amateurish that one of them, Piet Mertens, is immediately recognized. Unfortunately, the collaborator Henri Poerstamper, the local pharmacist, has also witnessed him. Mertens has to take shelter at a nearby farm, but at one point the persons in hiding are captured by the Germans. The resistance immediately assumes that Poerstamper has betrayed them. Since the naïve farmer's daughter Marie is dating the pharmacist's son Kees, one might think that Marie informed Poerstamper out of anger at the persons in hiding, who delivered her a dead crow as a representation of her boyfriend. Poerstamper, however, had kept silent, because he assumed that everyone would suspect him. The actual traitor, as only we know, is Marie's former boyfriend Jan, but because Marie yelled at the Germans that Poerstamper had promised her they would be left in peace, the conclusion is inevitable for Mertens' friends: Poerstamper deserves to die.

The friends dress themselves up as German soldiers, and Johan, who teaches German at school, persuades Poerstamper to ride with them. But the plan is clumsily executed, for one of the moustaches hangs loose. Poerstamper starts calling for help and they have to use force to take him into the woods. Originally, the resistance wanted to read him fragments from the Bible out of decency, but they have to shoot him on the spot because the Germans are on their way to rescue the pharmacist. And as if to emphasize their inexperience even more, their victim—Poerstamper—survives.[8] To their abhorrence, they realize that they had mentioned each other's names in front of Poerstamper, so they are forced to undertake another mission to shoot him in the hospital. It is difficult for the viewer to judge whether their masquerades as his NSB friends is convincing, for we see them from the perspective of Poerstamper's blurred vision. After Schults promptly executes the patient, they quickly run away. Immediately thereafter, the Germans arrest Schults, but this fate only befell him because he had been too indiscreet in his contacts with Mies. In the end, Schults is liberated thanks to his Nazi brother August Schultz—played by Rutger Hauer who starred in SOLDAAT VAN ORANJE.[9]

More than any other error, the mistake that humiliates Schults the most is his misjudgement of his colleague Miep Algera, who teaches English language. The entire staff suspects her of having an affair with a Nazi officer, and they decide to use the 'weapon of the mind': they refuse to speak to her anymore. She is indeed seen with a German, frequenting a café. Then she is suddenly taken from the school by the German secret service. Her colleagues are sceptical, believing that the arrest must have been an oversight or that her lover had dumped her. Schults is annoyed by these reactions, for it dawns on him that she was using her affair to obtain information for the resistance. Just before her arrest there is a scene in which we have a brief glimpse of Miep secretly meeting a Dutch man at an early hour in the woods. She tells him 'I love you', which confirms Schults's hypothesis.

What is most interesting about Miep's case is that she is only able to do her 'illegal work' in total secrecy. The price she pays for this is the contempt of everyone in her direct environment, which means she is effectively excluded from the community she belongs to. Walter Süskind was at least surrounded by a number of people who knew that his strategy showed that he had some kindness in his heart, but Miep was an isolated figure in three separate domains: she had to keep her secret to herself in her daily life: she play-acted a romance with a German Luftwaffe officer; and she gave information to her Dutch lover in the resistance. Or rather, she could only be effective by strictly keeping these domains separate. In retrospect, Schults considers her brave, for he thinks she suffered from the suspicious looks she often received, even though she never expressed any complaints. Though played by star actress Sylvia Kristel, Miep's role is too marginal to know whether she is disheartened by the negativity she meets from her colleagues. Since her expression is basically blank, it may be that she actually enjoys acting out an illicit love and suffering the contempt of others in order to be able to transfer secrets. The fact that she tells her Dutch lover that she loves him is then a consequence of her dedication to the cause. From this perspective, she is not as radical a hero as Antigone because she is fighting for the greater good of a community (those fighting for a liberated Holland), but she can only do so by accepting that the great majority of this community expels her. And the one man who can testify to her moral conscience is her Dutch lover, but a German fire squad has already executed him.

In order to underscore my argument, let me contrast Miep with another, even more famous female war hero, Hannie Schaft, whose life story was chronicled in HET MEISJE MET HET RODE HAAR [THE GIRL WITH THE RED HAIR] (Ben Verbong, 1981). This film has been criticized for taking many liberties with the facts surrounding this historical resistance fighter. Unlike the somewhat enigmatic Miep from PASTORALE 1943, Hannie is a fully subjectivized character, but as critic Egbert Barten laments, Verbong downplays her political motives and too often suggests that she acts quite irrationally, driven by fear and feelings of revenge (235).[10] Verbong's film is structured as a flashback memory recounted by fellow resistance member An at the end of the war. After a zoom-in on a freeze frame dated October 1942, the picture begins. Hannie is determined to quit her law studies, for she prefers direct action to talk. She wants to join a small resistance group, of which An is a member. She is asked by the leader of the group to shoot a blindfolded man through the head, but she cannot pull the trigger. She soon realizes it was only a test, for there were no bullets in the gun. She loses all hesitance, however, when she reads a letter from her Jewish friend Judith, and the superimposition of a shot of a train makes it clear that Judith has been sent away. After witnessing the brutal murder of two strikers, she is ready for her first assignment. She shoots an informer, and though she claims it felt pretty normal, she also sheds tears out of stress. Later she postpones the execution of a female traitor, Mrs. De Ruyter, because the supposed victim is in the presence of a child. When Hannie later shoots this woman after all, she starts fidgeting her hair afterwards. Her lover and fellow resistance fighter, Hugo, says that it makes her look like a little girl. She responds that she does this when she feels uncomfortable, and indeed, the attempted assassination has failed. The survivor tells the Germans that the shooter was a red-haired girl. The next assignment goes terribly wrong: the target is hit successfully, but Hugo is also shot and begins bleeding to death. Hugo's last words are spoken to the doctor: make sure the Germans do not find the photograph in my coat. The addressee turns out to be a German officer masquerading as a doctor, and he now knows what the red-haired girl looks like. After An dyes Hannie's hair black, she becomes more unsparing than ever, ruthlessly killing both the dog and its owner out of revenge for Hugo's death. When she is captured some time later, Mrs. De Ruyter does not recognize her, but the Germans decide to wash her hair so that the original red returns. Hannie is executed a few weeks before the war ends.

Verbong's HET MEISJE MET HET RODE HAAR conforms to the classical build-up of a character. She is convinced of her good cause, but initially she is too compassionate to kill. Each and every event gives her reason to become more ruthless. Hence the film meticulously traces her development into the role of a vengeful woman according to conventional psychological motivation. We as viewers can perfectly identify with Hannie: she has become a full-fledged 'I' with 'human' emotions (including tears and the wish to spare a child the memory of a killing). In her analysis of Verbong's film, Wendy Burke notes that the barren countryside with its muddy fields (128), 'bitter weather and plaintive cries of seagulls (...) mirror [Hannie's] increasingly desolate frame of mind until finally she is executed' (131). The 'unusual muted colour film stock (...) deliberately draining out most of the film's colour tones in post-production' adds to this effect of desolation (ibid.). Hannie stands out as a character among the crowd because her hair has a red glow, whereas the entire film appears almost monochrome. There is no question that Hannie has been brave, but she is also represented as a common-sense hero, unproblematically embedded in a symbolic network, for all her steps are comprehensible. But not giving in to one's desire—which means choosing '*a*' over '*I*'—means pursuing objectives that are beyond comprehension because they violate one's self-interest. The option of choosing '*a*' is never hinted at in the case of Hannie, but it is in the case of Miep from PASTORALE 1943. It could be that she loves the Dutch man from the resistance because this affair requires her to play-act a liaison with a German officer. Perhaps she detests this play-acting as much as she enjoys it, in which case she derives satisfaction from fulfilling a 'dirty duty'. She has an affair with the German, probably for the sake of her Dutch lover and only secondly for the sake of the resistance, even though the secrecy of her mission means that her colleagues feel contempt for her.[11]

THE PARTISAN AND THE SCHEMER: *IN DE SCHADUW VAN DE OVERWINNING*

When does a play-act make a hero and how is a hero to be distinguished from a rabble? These are the key questions in a dialogue between two inmates who share the same cell in IN DE SCHADUW VAN DE OVERWINNING [SHADOW OF VICTORY] (Ate de Jong, 1986). The first hour of the film consistently juxtaposes their two storylines: one is about the resistance group led by Peter van Dijk who has his wife in a hiding place and a pregnant mistress within the resistance in addition to having fallen in love with a third woman. In the beginning of the film, the group dresses up as Germans and with their masquerade succeed in bombing the population register. The other narrative is about the Jewish David Blumberg, who is interrogated by the German officer Kohler early on in the film. This Blumberg claims to have made a cunning deal with Eugen von Spiegel, a German general in Berlin who is granting permission to rich Jews to escape to Switzerland. Blumberg has persuaded him that for every rich Jew, Blumberg may write down the name of a poor Jew on a list, and that the Jews on this list will not be put on the train to Poland. Kohler initially respects the 'Von Spiegel list', but he exerts pressure on Blumberg as soon as it turns out that there is no General Von Spiegel.

It is immediately made clear to us that Blumberg himself is impersonating Von Spiegel. While he is telling Kohler about the deal, we see him write a letter on a typewriter and sign the document. Kohler, however, presumes that someone else is taking the guise of Von Spiegel, and he wants to use Blumberg as a decoy. The Jew must bring either 'Von Spiegel' or his assistant Baron Van Tuyl to the Nazis or the entire list will be abolished. In the meantime, Peter van Dijk has been requested to liquidate Blumberg because 'London' suspects him of collaborating with the Germans. Van Dijk, however, wants to make sure that Blumberg truly is a traitor. This is where the two stories start to interact. Thanks to a greedy mediator, Peter van Dijk is introduced to Blumberg under the name of 'Jan-Paul'. Van Dijk performs a kind of 'audition' for the role of Van Tuyl but only agrees to present himself publicly as the baron after some deliberation. Unbeknownst to Blumberg, Van Dijk does so as part of a plan to liberate two of his female peers from the resistance. In the meantime, another German officer, Schwarz, has put Blumberg under pressure as well: he has to pay him 100,000 guilders or deliver Peter van Dijk to him, and if not, the 600 Jews on the Von Spiegel list will be put on the train to Poland. Blumberg has no choice but to collect some precious jewels, for as he tells Schwarz: 'I do not know Peter van Dijk' (and, as we might recall, Blumberg only knew Van Dijk as 'Jan-Paul'). After they take possession of the money, the Germans arrest Blumberg for trading on the black market.

When Blumberg and Van Dijk are put together in prison, Van Dijk is 'Jan-Paul' for Blumberg, but he is arrested for identifying himself as 'Baron Van Tuyl' to the Germans. It then turns out during their conversation that Blumberg already knew that Jan-Paul is Peter van Dijk, and he begs him to turn himself in. Van Dijk considers this an outrageous request coming from a man who might be working together with the Germans. Blumberg's reply goes something like this: That is easy for you to say—you can choose to join the resistance because you long for a great adventure, but I do not have any other option than to collaborate, for if not, I will be sent away together with my entire family. So collaboration is the only mode of survival for us Jews. Moreover, do not underestimate my contact, for this general Von Spiegel actually is a German resistance agent. So, how dare you say that you are a hero and I am not? If you live by the standard of human dignity, then you would turn yourself in, for that would save the lives of the 600 Jews on the list.

Van Dijk does not do as Blumberg says but instead is involved in an adventurous rescue operation. The rescue is successful, except that he himself gets wounded. When Schwarz is close to killing him, Van Dijk plays a final trick on him by handing Schwarz a grenade which then explodes and kills them both. Hence, Van Dijk is a passionate 'resistance "martyr," placing his calling to carry out resistance tasks above his duties to his wife, children, friends, and lovers' (Burke, 204). Whereas Van Dijk sacrifices himself, the fate of Blumberg is undetermined.[12] He confesses to Kohler that he had invented both Von Spiegel and Van Tuyl, to the embarrassment of the German officer. Kohler cannot report the non-existence of these figures, because that would mean he had made a total miscalculation and that his career would be over. He tells Blumberg to make something up since he is apparent so skilled at lying. While Blumberg confirms he has told the truth this time, the Jew is made to witness—from a low-angle that tracks backwards—a train leaving for the East, with his loved ones and many 'Von Spiegel Jews' on board. Kohler tells him his family will be spared the concentration camps if Blumberg collaborates with the Germans.

The merit of De Jong's IN DE SCHADUW VAN DE OVERWINNING is to consistently juxtapose the two narratives via crosscutting. The viewer is inclined to sympathize with the daredevil Peter van Dijk, a brave partisan who sacrifices

his life. The pregnancy of his mistress ensures his legacy: in the final images, she holds their baby. He is contrasted with the Jewish double-crosser Blumberg, who is introduced in a scene in which Blok, another Jew, begs him for help, whereupon the camera tilts up to show Blumberg via the mirror as the listener. The film is structured so as to culminate in the dialogue between Blumberg and Van Dijk about forced choice versus choice. Blumberg in fact admits that he may be a liar and a cheater but that the art of deception may perhaps require more courage than Van Dijk's adventurous mentality. Van Dijk plays a game of hide-and-seek with the Germans, and as long as the Nazis do not identify him, he can quit his partisan activities any time he likes. In De Jong's film, Van Dijk's reputation has been built already: his name is on everyone's lips, for the Germans are intent on capturing him. By contrast, Blumberg's strategy can only be successful on the condition that he maintains his reputation of cooperating with the Germans. He is the ordinary man who in the eyes of the resistance has turned into a rabble. It is only by performing the act of feigning by granting belief in the existence of both General Von Spiegel and Baron Van Tuyl—that is to say, until Kohler knows he has been deceived and Blumberg is forced to assist in administering the camp—that he can effectively save the Jews on the list.

The character of Blumberg begs comparison with Süskind from Van den Berg's 2012 film. Walter took up the role of theatre director, and he did his secret work while he was embedded in an already existing symbolic network. He succeeded in fooling Aus der Fünten by acting as a good friend, or rather by acting as a substitute sibling, since the Nazi is downhearted by the death of his brother. Once Aus der Fünten knows Walter has led him astray, he gives him the choice to join his family on the train. In other words, Walter is offered the option to sacrifice himself in the company of his beloved ones. Blumberg, by contrast, is a humble schemer who has created a figure, Von Spiegel—an artificial 'father' so to speak—who is superior in rank to Kohler. Blumberg has deliberately constructed an empty position with the aim of fooling the ruling Nazi order. His creation provides him with authority himself, for he is the ordinary man who maintains close contacts with a German general. Hence, Blumberg has constructed a surplus adjacent to the symbolic order, and he has to believe in his own universe to make it effective. In other words, Blumberg has to perform his role perfectly or perish. He can derive a certain perverse enjoyment from setting up his intricate scenario—shown to us in brief flashback scenes when we see him at his typewriter signing a document.

Whereas IN DE SCHADUW VAN DE OVERWINNING implies that Peter van Dijk's partisan actions have a romantic whiff about them, both Walter Süskind and Blumberg act out of strict necessity. Walter is a man who makes as much use as possible of his difficult and limited circumstances. From the German perspective, his deceit is regretful because the Nazis are keen on maintaining the correct numbers, but the escape of a few Jewish children does not really damage the organization as such. In that sense, Aus der Fünten can 'pardon' Walter and at least grant him the option to embrace his family. Unlike Walter, Blumberg has invented a scenario out of nothing. Provided that the Germans think the Von Spiegel list is authentic, his plan works. As soon as he tells the truth ('there is no father figure'), however, it has dire consequences not only for Blumberg and the people on his list but also for Kohler. The Nazi machinery as such is short-circuited: if there were an impostor, that would be alright, but Kohler cannot file a report stating that there is no Von Spiegel at all, for that would be too much of a disgrace. Blumberg's punishment is that he is made to witness the transportation of the Jews on his list: now he is as lonely as hell. Although my analysis here may suggest that Blumberg is the most heroic of these characters since the effect of his approach proved to be particularly subversive up to a certain point, bear in mind that he can just as easily be suspected of collaboration: in his paranoid universe, he is the one who likes to pull the strings, but if it comes to saving his own skin and the lives of his family members, he may be less altruistic than the others.

THE JOKE OF BEING A HERO: *DE IJSSALON*

'*Was its der Witz ... um ein Held zu sein?*' These German words, which can be translated as 'What is the joke (or fun)... of being a hero?', are the final ones spoken by the most unlikely of heroes, the German Otto Schneeweiss in DE IJSSALON [THE ICE CREAM PARLOUR] (Dimitri Frenkel Frank, 1985). He has fled Berlin where he had a renowned sweet shop, but now, February 1941, he is the owner of an ice cream parlour in Amsterdam. The atmosphere is unpleasant from the start. There are two teams of thugs in front of his shop: one affiliated with those collaborating with the Germans, and the other is anti-fascist. There is an impending threat that violence will ensue, but as a good host to his clients, Otto tries to act as if it is business as usual. Then an old friend comes along, Gustav Reinecke—played by Bruno Ganz, some twenty years before his role as Hitler in DER UNTERGANG [DOWNFALL] (Oliver Hirschbiegel, 2004). Reinecke has become a major in the German army, and as he was on a visit to Amsterdam he wants to taste whether Otto still has that terrific plum cake he used to have in Berlin. On leave for two weeks, Gustav comes over to the ice cream parlour quite often, always wearing his uniform. He happens to fall in love with the blonde Trudi, with whom Otto himself has been infatuated for a while.

At one point, Otto joins his friend Gustav and the latter's latest conquest Trudi to a dinner party at the German *Sicherheitsdienst* [security service]. Otto is introduced as a professor of history from Berlin, and the Obersturmbannführer Müller considers him a most amusing fellow. Müller laughs out loud at 'the professor's' dirty joke, which runs like this: The Nazi Göring visits a performance by Josephine Baker at the Folies Bergère in Paris. Someone asks him: *Quelle age a t'elle*? [What is her age?] to which Göring responds: 'Probably brown, too', since he hears the French term âge (age) as the German word Arsch (ass).

When the fake news goes around that one of the collaborator thugs died during a fight, the Nazis swear to take revenge by way of a raid on the ice cream parlour, since the anti-fascist strong-arm boys like to defend this particular spot. Otto is informed about this upcoming disaster, but he prefers to listen to Mahler's fourth symphony on his record player at his home above the parlour. Two of the anti-fascist boys, Luuk and Louis, are hiding behind the counter and use ammonia on the intruding NSB group. Luuk and Louis run away without being seen, but Otto—who in the meantime has become quite drunk—is arrested and awaits execution. Trudi wants Gustav to use his influence with Müller to have Otto released, but he does not dare to do so, so Trudi takes this into her own hands and seduces Müller quite easily, for the Oberstürmbannführer has been flirting with her throughout the film. While he is about to undress, she takes his gun and orders him to call the office to annul the execution. There is crosscutting now: the camera zooms in on a frontally staged Otto to a medium close-up. A few seconds before the actual firing, we hear him say to no one in particular: '*Was ist der Witz ... um ein Held zu sein?*' There is an immediate transition to Müller with a telephone in his hand, but we already hear the shot of the firing squad on the soundtrack. Müller tells Trudi that he has intervened in time, but she does not believe him and shoots him. Later,

Gustav is among the small crowd that watches how the body of Müller is taken from the ice cream parlour. As soon as Trudi sees the German major, she grabs a black-and-white photograph of the three of them (with Trudi in the middle) and tears off Gustav from the picture, making sure that he sees her doing it.

DE IJSSALON is not a particularly great film,[13] but Otto's final words are highly inventive, especially because they are in striking contrast to an earlier embarrassing scene in which he had used the very same expression. When the leaders of the thugs were facing off in his parlour, the anti-fascist Luuk put a scoop of ice cream on the black suit of the collaborator Hans. Fearing an escalation, Otto got on his knees and started polishing the stain from Hans's pair of trousers. After Hans and his men departed and Trudi entered, Otto started apologizing: 'I am not a hero and I do not want to be one, Trudi, please, *Was ist der Witz um ein Held zu sein?*' Otto, who had been called a chicken before by both Luuk and Trudi, has only one objective. He wants to keep the peace at all costs, even at the expense of humiliating himself. But once Obersturmbannführer Müller whispers in his ears what the Germans will do to the Jews, Otto instantly becomes sick to his stomach. We see him nostalgically remember some moments from his childhood on the basis of family pictures. During the raid upon his parlour, he wants Trudi and Gustav to leave him alone with his Mahler music and his booze. When he is interrogated after his arrest, he keeps confessing that he alone was responsible for everything, even though he knows of Luuk's act of sabotage. At the end of the film, Trudi mentions to Luuk, her brother, that Otto has apparently kept his mouth shut about his resistance activity since the Nazis are not after Luuk. Hence, Otto is symbolically acknowledged as a brave man and not the coward the brother and sister had called him, though he himself is not aware of the change in Trudi's perception. His very own '*Was ist der Witz um ein Held zu sein?*' addressed to the camera / firing squad becomes a painfully ironic question: it is anything but funny. It is ironic, however, that the man who made every effort to prevent the use of violence is facing the firing squad. What makes this ordinary man a bit of a hero is that he has ultimately accepted his death as the consequence of his attempts at peacemaking.

'DU KANNST, DENN DU SOLLST': *BEYOND SLEEP* VERSUS *DOKTER PULDER ZAAIT PAPAVERS*

So far, the reflections on heroism in Dutch films have had to do predominantly with subversive action rather than desire. As mentioned earlier, a Lacanian hero does not compromise his desire, even though common sense might tell him to choose other options. In order to clarify this notion of desire, I would like to discuss Beyond Sleep (Boudewijn Koole, 2015) alongside Dokter Pulder zaait papavers [Doctor Pulder Sows Poppies] (Bert Haanstra, 1975). Koole's adaptation of W.F. Hermans' novel *Nooit meer slapen* (1966) was widely considered a bold enterprise, for the novel was thought to be one of those 'unfilmable' classics. The main difficulty is that the book consists of many mental observations of the young geologist Alfred Issendorf, so that we can never tell what is actually happening and what is the protagonist's projection. The almost unanimous reception of the film was that the adaptation was well done, for Koole made clever use of out-of-focus shots, the alternation of close-ups and wide shots, a flashforward in the prologue of the film, a sound design that emphasizes such things as the unrelenting presence of mosquitos, and jump cuts to further mark Alfred's dissociation. The best indication that we are in the 'quicksand of Alfred's brain' (Broeren) is the scene in which he is so mad at one of his companions that he kicks him repeatedly, but a few moments later Mikkelsen has no wounds at all. Moreover, several other films in which characters are 'beyond sleep' and suffer from insomnia—Taxi Driver (Martin Scorsese, 1976), Cría Cuervos [Raise Ravens] (Carlos Saura, 1976), Insomnia (Erik Skjoldbaerg, 1997 / Christopher Nolan, 2002), and Fight Club (David Fincher, 1999)—also make it difficult to draw the line between 'reality' and sleep-deprived hallucinations.

In Beyond Sleep, Alfred is on an expedition to Finnmark, the north-eastern part of Norway, to see whether or not the hypothesis that the holes in the landscape there are meteor craters is true. He is accompanied by two light-haired, bearded Norwegians and Arne, who looks quite like him. He quickly falls behind his travel companions, as he is ill at ease in the environment. Alfred is presented as every inch a geek: he falls a couple of times, has to wade through a swamp, and arrives in the midst of a fog. His mother (whom we never see in the film) has given him a compass so he doesn't get lost, but the compass falls into a rock crevice. But, perhaps worst of all, his peers do not take him seriously. The Norwegians claim that humans inhabit a sadistic universe in which God conspires against them. When Alfred wonders why the mosquitos sting him all the time, Arne says that perhaps his sole purpose on earth is to feed the insects.

Each time Alfred mentions he is a geologist, he makes it sound as if he has to convince himself he is one. In the eyes of the old Norwegian professor Nummedal, he is certainly not a true geologist, given that he comes from a 'swampland without hills'. This professor is never seen in Beyond Sleep but his words keep resonating in the protagonist's head. The scorn for Alfred's research is made most tangible when he sees that Mikkelsen has the aerials of the area that Nummedal refused to give him. In fact, it should not surprise us that in this hostile environment, Alfred's self-confidence is damaged to such a degree that he is more prone to misperception than to reliable observation, no matter how obsessively he counts steps out loud to have some kind of data to hang on to. At one point, a backward tracking shot reduces him to a mere dot in the landscape, accentuating that Finnmark is everything but a natural habitat to him. Significantly, however, once he is entirely on his own, released from any social pressure, he starts to travel more effortlessly. But it is only a matter of irony that he looks the other way at the very moment a meteorite flies through the air behind him. His mission not accomplished, he goes back to the civilized world after having reported Arne's death to the police. In the bus, he reads a newspaper with an item about the meteorite.

The main protagonist in BEYOND SLEEP has a clearly defined aim and ambition: he wants to be acknowledged as a great geologist by finding proof of the impact of meteorites in Finnmark. He perseveres in his mission, even though the film only includes clues of scepticism and animosity. It becomes clear, however, that Alfred's mission was originally his father's project but that the man had died during a research expedition in Switzerland when Alfred was only seven years old. Alfred was trying to achieve what his father was no longer capable of achieving due to his premature death. Even if we were to assume that no one has even the slightest interest in Alfred's project, and even though he has had to withstand overall contempt, the mission still has value for him. Alfred's motivation is not so much geared towards serving science; instead, his desire seems to be first and foremost to redeem a symbolic debt. Alfred took up the project either to honour his late father and/or to surpass him. But no-one, it seems, is prepared to support his project. In pursuing this ambition, he is trying to establish a link with his dead father, but he does so at the risk of expelling himself from a social community, which is expressed in a twofold manner. First, his Norwegian companions are highly uncooperative, apparently sabotaging his research. Second, the only one who does not take an adverse attitude is Arne, but the viewer slowly comes to realize that he may be an imaginary figure, a figment derived from his insomnia.

BEYOND SLEEP suggests that the son feels morally obliged to continue his father's project. He does not have a specific talent for this kind of research; he is not very passionate about it; it was simply the duty that awaited him. This obligation is what Žižek describes as the 'standard motto of ethical rigour': 'There is no excuse for not accomplishing one's duty!' (*The Plague*, 222). This is based upon Immanuel Kant's quote '*Du kannst, denn du sollst!*' ('*You can because you must!*'), but, as Žižek argues, this motto must be complemented with its 'much more uncanny inversion' (ibid.), as I will explain below in my analysis of Haanstra's DOKTER PULDER ZAAIT PAPAVERS.

As an antithesis to the typical undertaking of a son in BEYOND SLEEP, Haanstra's film can be seen as an acerbic portrayal of a father's wilful neglect of his duties. In his younger years, Haanstra was a man who excelled in what Schoots calls existential optimism (*Bert Haanstra*, 256): people may quarrel with one another, but in the end a sense of community will prevail, as illustrated in his box-office success FANFARE (1958). In this comedy full of visual jokes, members of a brass band have a conflict, but the solution is one of perfect harmony. Since the 1970s, however, scenarios of increasing doom and gloom came to replace Haanstra's positivism (Schoots, 256). In general, critics were delighted by this turn towards a certain bleakness, but the audience clearly missed the cheerfulness of his films from the 1950s and 1960s (Schoots, 266).

The first half of DOKTER PULDER ZAAIT PAPAVERS is a remake-with-revisions of DE EEKHOORN [THE SQUIRREL] (1972), a film made by second-year students from the Film Academy under supervision of Harry Kümel based upon Anton Koolhaas's novella *De nagel achter het behang* [*The Nail behind the Wallpaper*] (1971). When the country doctor Kees Pulder is about to leave for Amsterdam with his wife to celebrate their son's discharge from military service, he gets a phone call from a former fellow student, the now famous neurosurgeon Hans van Inge-Liedaerd. He is so pleased to meet this respectable man after so many years that he decides to say nothing when his wife calls her husband an 'asshole'. While Pulder always regarded himself as an average and dull student with no sense of humour, to his surprise, Van Inge-Liedaerd is very complimentary during the copious dinner the two 'friends' share: he claims that he and their fellow students considered Pulder a connoisseur and appreciated him for his wit and wisdom.

Haanstra uses crosscutting, one of his tested devices from previous films, in order to clarify the obsession Pulder has developed for Van Inge-Liedaerd. Overwhelmed by the appreciative words of his guest, Pulder is in his bed, tipsy because of the alcohol, and looks at the photograph of his wife and teenage son. He has only scorn for them, but with each counter-shot of the picture on the bedside table, the smile on their faces transforms from barely imperceptible to an ever-larger grin. Whereas Pulder is about to hallucinate, we see Van Inge-Liedaerd lying on the guest bed as the medicinal drugs he took from Pulder's well-stocked supply cabinet take effect: he is having fantasies as well, which are shot in an overexposed fashion. We go back to Pulder, who thinks he hears the sound of a little mouse behind the wall and throws a shoe to make it silent. It is alternated with the scene in which Van Inge-Liedaerd's happy fantasy is interrupted by the equally delusional sight and sound of rats. He throws a shoe at the wall as well.

The pattern of crosscutting functions as the formal means to indicate that Pulder has had an 'awakening': the realization that he has more affinity with his old pal than with anyone else. The next day, Pulder realizes that Van Inge-Liedaerd had only been play-acting camaraderie in order to steal the doctor's entire supply of very precious medicines. With Pulder's wife and son back home, Van Inge-Liedaerd even throws a brick through a window at night to express his contempt for the country doctor. These incidents, however, do not diminish the impact the deceitful colleague has had upon Pulder.

Instead of being angered by the humiliation, Pulder gains a fascination for the neurosurgeon and attends the man's funeral service a little later. Except for Van Inge-Liedaerd's daughter Kitty and his mistress, Mrs. Mies, accompanied by the local poultryman, no one else is present. Though everyone he meets is scornful of the deceased because he had cheated on many people, Pulder says that his deceit was insignificant compared to the wake-up call he had received from their reunion. He has become a provincial drudge, lost in worrying about his patients who keep complaining about minor ailments and who always expect him to see them immediately. After this insight, he starts to neglect his professional duties to the dismay of his wife and son.

DOKTER PULDER ZAAIT PAPAVERS could have become a movie about a suburban father's mid-life crisis, like the celebrated AMERICAN BEAUTY (Sam Mendes, 1999).[14] In the latter film, Lester Burnham is so fed up with his domestic responsibilities that he chooses a lifestyle that befits an adolescent: he buys a flamboyant car, listens to music he liked when he was eighteen years old, and lusts after one of his daughter's girlfriends. The merit of Mendes' film is that these options are not as appealing as they seem to be, and by the end, Lester has annoyed practically everyone around him. Haanstra's picture takes a slightly different direction. In ignoring his responsibilities, Pulder gets on everyone's nerves, very much like Lester Burnham, but the difference is that he chooses options that are not very attractive. He starts to pay visits to Mrs. Mies, who is an alcoholic and an addict and generally regarded as a weirdo, even by the poulterer who keeps an eye on her now and then. Even though this woman can have angry outbursts about trifling details—e.g. when Pulder wants to nibble some crackers—Pulder's identification with Van Inge-Liedaerd is so total that he keeps coming back to visit Mrs. Mies. She may tell him that the neurosurgeon was 'pure evil', that he left a 'trail of ruins', and that he in fact hated Pulder, but this does not decrease Pulder's fascination in the least. Since he continues to see her, she at one point mentions what was supposed to be her lover's 'last heroic stand': after sowing poppies with her, Van Inge-Liedaerd wanted to drift into unconsciousness from the milk-like liquid that could be derived from the poppies. And now, as the film title implies, the doctor will sow those very poppies together with Mrs. Mies, as he keeps on calling her. He seems ecstatic, and late in the evening, he drives home, but while drunk, he causes an accident. After a jail sentence, his wife and son are waiting for him at the train station, but he does not show up, for he has taken the bus to Mrs. Mies. No one answers the door, however, and he then hears from the poultryman that it is rumoured she has poisoned herself. Amidst the poppies, he finds a note: 'Throw this brick through a window, empty the half bottle of vodka, go home, and forget about me and Hans. Well, not quite about me.' There is a relatively quick alternation between shots of Pulder and of his mirror image in the reflecting glass. After some hesitation, he throws the brick, shattering his image.

DOKTER PULDER ZAAIT PAPAVERS is deceptively simple, shot without striking formal devices. Perhaps the opening scene with the camera on a boat through the harbour is the closest the film comes to a bravura shot. The light is generally bright, as in a cheerful film by Haanstra, and the burst of red from the field full of poppies looks stunning. Thus the style of DOKTER PULDER ZAAIT PAPAVERS does not prepare its spectators for the sour tone of the movie and its dark ending. When Pulder throws the brick through the window of Mrs. Mies's house, he repeats what Van Inge-Liedaerd had done to him. Although the differences in context are considerable—in the case of Van Inge-Liedaerd, it was a vile act; in the case of Pulder, it was an act to commemorate Mrs. Mies—the repetition as such is more striking here. For Mrs. Mies is in effect telling him that if he wants to identify himself with the ignoble Van Inge-Liedaerd, then Pulder will do what Van Inge-Liedaerd did. It is Pulder's desire to become like Van Inge-Liedaerd, and that means that he would rather die than be recognized as a reliable country doctor—or in his words, he would rather die than 'keep up this crap'. By throwing the brick, he affirms his wishful identification with the degenerate neurosurgeon, and like him, Pulder is on a trajectory of becoming so despised by everyone that, just as with Van Inge-Liedaerd, only a handful will attend his funeral. The brick punctuates that he is on the brink of being excluded from the symbolic order, underscored by the sound of breaking glass. In the case of BEYOND SLEEP, the son at least wanted to pay a symbolic debt to his late father, but Doctor Pulder only seems intent on completely marginalizing himself, identifying himself with deplorable outcasts.

According to Žižek, Kant's motto that there is no excuse for not accomplishing one's duty—which was the motivation for the son in BEYOND SLEEP—should be 'rejected as hypocritical' (*The Plague*, 222). The motto can easily be misused, for example by a teacher who gives his pupils loads of homework and then claims he is not to blame since he is simply doing his duty. The problem is that one can be acquitted by saying that one is not responsible for one's acts, by claiming that one was supposed to do this (because it is in one's labour agreement or because one was given the order to do so, etc.). For that reason, Žižek claims that a careful reading of Kant's *Du kannst, denn du sollst!* reveals the 'uncanny inversion' that one should not do something simply on the grounds that one considers it one's duty: 'There is no excuse for accomplishing one's duty!' (ibid.).

Doctor Pulder can be said to act according to this inverted scenario. He is not distancing himself from his social duties because he wants to pursue the pleasures of his pre-adult years, as Lester in AMERICAN BEAUTY, but he makes the uncommon choice to identify with a most unfortunate impostor. Such an attachment seems devoid of any self-interest, especially since the doctor puts all his hard-won securities at stake: he positions himself at the margins of society. It is a bold step, for sure, but in the eyes of many, such as his wife and son, he is a good-for-nothing who takes the easy way out. We are inclined to say that the doctor has given evidence of his empathy, but no one, including himself, will consider him a hero for that. Is it possible to reconcile the ethical demand not to compromise one's desire with a heroic stand? To answer this question, I will venture into a discussion of two films that are adaptations of Tim Krabbé novels, the baroque gangster film FLANAGAN (Adriaan Ditvoorst, 1975) and SPOORLOOS (George Sluizer, 1988), a suspense thriller that Stanley Kubrick reportedly watched three times and then rang the director to congratulate him on this eerie movie. The first film represents the rabble version of desire; the second one the heroic variant.

THE FURY OF A PATIENT MAN: *FLANAGAN*

FLANAGAN opens with a father trying to take a picture of his two young sons, Peter and Paul,[15] but it takes some time before they each place an arm over the other's shoulder. In a subsequent extreme long shot, it seems as if the father is encouraging them to romp around. And in another brief scene from the prologue, Paul crosses a body of water on a thin board, and Peter only dares to do so after some hesitation. Then we are suddenly in the present, in Brussels. A cab takes Paul to Kitty's place. She is surprised to see him but wants to make love to him right away. He says he wants to talk, but in the next scene they are in bed together. Kitty tells him she feels as though he had never been away. Paul's main reason for his visit is to ask for his share of a heist, but she replies that only Peter knows where the money is and that he had told her he burnt it because it was too dangerous to spend the marked notes. Paul does not believe this excuse and throws a random object to shatter the mirror in Kitty's bedroom.

From here onwards, Paul starts to behave unpredictably. He can be very polite and charming. When no one opens the door at Peter's affluent residence in Amsterdam—according to the nametag near the door, he is Peter Babel, architect—he contacts the nanny Lily. Initially, she seems pleased by Paul's seduction of her, but she soon realizes that Paul can be violent and brutal as well. In her company, he points a gun at a salesman just for a pack of cigarettes. Lily has no option but to take him inside the house. When Peter's wife Dorna comes home, Lily nonetheless introduces the dominant intruder as an acquaintance.

To Paul's shock and amazement, the name 'Paul Flanagan' does not ring a bell to Dorna, but he promises to reveal Peter's past 'bit by bit, for it is no fun when you know everything at once'. We eventually find out—though we only gather this from conversations in the present, never from flashback scenes—that Paul stole 600,000 guilders at the Dutch-Belgian border as Peter and Kitty served as the lookout. Peter panicked because Paul fired a shot (or so Peter says), and by the time Paul arrived at the car he had already vanished, whereupon Paul was arrested.

The full title of Krabbé's novel from 1970 is *Flanagan, of de dood van het beest* [*Flanagan, or the Death of the Beast*]. Even before he is shot dead at the end, this wild beast acts as if he is symbolically dead. He has been treated as a total nobody, completely left to his own devices. He served eight years in prison, but not one of his family or friends ever paid him a visit. His family name is Flanagan, but no one else bears that name (except perhaps for his mother who is rumoured to have gone back to Ireland). Paul goes to see his bed-ridden father Augustus Babel in an enormous castle, in a mise-en-scène reminiscent of Orson Welles' patriarchal Cassavius in MALPERTUIS (Harry Kümel, 1971). Father's room has a huge sculpture of snakes and birds of prey, whereas the wall is decorated with wallpapered paintings from a forest. Meanwhile the old man likes to listen to a pre-recorded track of the singing of birds. This ambient surrounding is characteristic of the style of the film. Since the director cast predominantly theatre actors and often used (extreme) long shots, FLANAGAN has an effect of theatricality. The most crucial sets have a sense of grandeur and are meticulously designed. The neatly dressed Paul easily adapts to all these fancy surroundings, but while the camera shows him within a larger space, he comes to figure in many a scene as the detail that sticks out due to his erratic behaviour. When he finally meets Peter after having left the castle and being yelled at by his father's second wife, Peter's mother, that he is a good-for-nothing, the encounter begins on a calm note. His half-brother Peter shows him his collection of bird's eggs and, acting clumsily, Paul breaks one of them. After a fake apology, he ruins them all. Paul's demands are capricious: he wants one-third of the loot, then he wants the full sum, but his volatility is only a cover-up for his one and only aim. He is absolutely determined for Peter to turn himself in. Explaining that he has nothing to lose at all and that, in fact, he no longer exists, Paul wants Peter to undergo the same fate as he. He wants Peter, this mama's boy and coward, to experience the utter humiliation of breaking his mother's heart.

Paul finally obtains the hidden money in exchange for the release of

Peter's child he had kidnapped. Since Peter feels too sick to ride with him, Paul brings the boy back to his mother and proceeds to have sex with her. Then he rings Kitty and wants to share the money with her. He buys her an expensive ring and frequents a café with her. He asks her to watch the bag, goes to a café across the street and rings the police. A car quickly arrives to arrest her, since she is in possession of the marked notes. He goes back to the castle and tells Peter that he better call the police himself. Peter's mother screams that Paul has to go, for he only brings disgrace to the house. A few moments later, she takes a hunting rifle and shoots Paul in the chest. We then get a shot of the bed-ridden Augustus amidst the twittering of birds who chuckles: 'Typical Paulie', but it is unclear whether he thinks Paul fired the shot or whether he knows that Paul was the target.

THE FURY OF A PATIENT MAN could have been an appropriate title for FLANAGAN: driven entirely by revenge, everything else is secondary, at best a strategic means to this one end.[16] Paul has cut all ties to society, and perhaps the only one who may slightly understand him is his father ('You are an artist, you are free.') whose name he does not bear. They have all given Paul the idea that he no longer exist, so he believes nothing can prevent him from giving those cowards who deserve it their due. At the end, he pushes a mother over the edge, and she then protects her dearly beloved son by shooting Paul. His death is hardly a sacrifice, for Paul was so keen on revenge that the forced assassination by the mother becomes part of his mission—a victory rather than a defeat. For it is now not only mama's boy who will be under investigation from the police but his overanxious mother as well.

IN THERE, NO ONE CAN HEAR YOU SCREAM: *SPOORLOOS*

When nothing else matters for a man like Paul Flanagan but chaos and destruction, he becomes a loose cannon and, in the words of Dorna, Peter's wife, a downright 'rabble'. In *Het gouden ei* [*The Golden Egg*] (1984), a favourite novella on the reading list of secondary school pupils, Krabbé introduces two related man-types: an ordinary suburban father who after a 'heroic' act turns deliberately into a rabble, and an ordinary man who takes a heroic risk.

SPOORLOOS, the neo-Hitchcockian adaptation of Krabbé's novella, is an example of superb scriptwriting and an intelligent temporal structure. In the words of Scott Foundas upon the inclusion of the DVD in the prestigious *Criterion Collection*, Sluizer's 'elegant, sleight-of-hand filmmaking (...) splinters the narrative into a series of nonlinear fragments and shrewdly misdirects our attention throughout'. A first strand focuses on Saskia Wagter and her boyfriend Rex Hofman driving in a car to their holidays in the French countryside.

There is some bickering on the way. The most notable argument occurs after their car runs out of gas in the middle of a dark tunnel. Rex is angry that Saskia reacts in a 'hysterical' way and leaves her behind to get some petrol, ignoring that she is scared.[17] When they later make a stop at a heavily trafficked roadside gas station, she goes to buy some refreshments but never returns. Rex starts a desperate search for her, but to no avail. After the screen goes black for a brief moment, the second strand starts with the camera positioned in an uncultivated garden, and from a low-angle it shoots the arrival of a car. A man steps out, and we recognize him from the first part of the film where he was briefly shown in his car putting a fake cast on his left arm and waiting at the shop of the gas station. Raymond Lemorne, in his early forties, is the father of two teenage daughters and works as a chemistry teacher. He owns a remote villa thirteen kilometres from his home in Nîmes. When he is eating with his wife and daughters in the garden of the villa, one of the girls sees spiders in the drawer of a dinner table and starts screaming.[18] The family turns it into a fun game: each tries to scream as hard as possible. The next day, Raymond asks a neighbour whether he had heard any loud noise, but the answer was no.

We see Raymond doing some experiments and rehearsals, '... well like an actor preparing a role' (Foundas). How long does it take to regain consciousness after one is intoxicated with chloroform? How does one ask women to step into his car? What is his heartbeat once he has actually approached them to ask for the way to the supermarket?[19] Both his youngest daughter and his wife suspect him of adultery because of his frequent trips, but after he denies this, there is a sudden jump to a scene in which Raymond is adjusting the fake cast in his car. Then we see him waiting at the gas station, while Rex and Saskia arrive in their car, a scene we have seen near the beginning of the film. The image of Saskia is mirrored in both of his spectacle lenses.

In the third strand, posters with Saskia's portrait are hung in public places in France, with the accompanying text: 'This woman disappeared three years ago'. Raymond passes by a poster and tells a colleague that he admires the guy's obsessive 'perseverance'. He invites Rex to come over to France, for the fifth time by an anonymous postcard, this time to a terrace on a square in Nîmes. Rex tells his new girlfriend Lieneke, who has joined him on his trip to Nîmes, that the perpetrator is probably summoning up the courage to address him: 'He's watching me. I can feel it. I'm afraid he will stop sending me postcards, or that he is dead, for then I will never know.' When the camera makes a 180-degree turn, we see Raymond standing on a balcony in the background, looking in Rex's direction. Some time later, Raymond takes a seat at the terrace as well, all the time out of focus, even when Rex is looking in his direction. The lack of focus is an indication to the viewer that Rex does not recognize him—and Raymond is at this moment assured of that fact as well, as he later tells

Rex. When Rex is interviewed on French television, he says that he believes the perpetrator is a very intelligent man and a perfectionist as well. At one point he turns towards the camera and talks directly to the television viewers, addressing the felon: 'I do not hate you, but I want to meet you, for I want to know.'

In the fourth strand, this message is repeated when Rex watches a videotape of the broadcast back home. Lieneke is about to end their eight-month-old relationship, which is predictable given his ongoing obsession with Saskia. As she leaves the apartment, Raymond is outside the building, waiting to speak to Rex. He has come to propose a deal: if you go with me in my car to France, I will disclose what happened to Saskia. By proposing this deal, Raymond is clearly taking a risk, but he thinks that Rex has no proof against him, and above all he gambles on Rex's curiosity. Moreover, it is likely that, after all these years, Raymond wants 'to make someone privy to the genius of his perfect crime' (Foundas).

During their trip, Raymond recounts three key moments in his life. At the age of sixteen, he was standing on the ledge of the balcony at his home. No one in his sane mind would jump, he reasoned, so if he wanted to go against what was predestined, he had to jump. It is a 'slight abnormality, but unnoticed by the people around me', he tells Rex. 'You can find it in an encyclopaedia under "sociopath"'. The second moment was some 26 years later, when he saved a girl from drowning. His youngest daughter was bursting with admiration for her father the hero, but he warned her: 'Watch out for heroes. They are capable of excess.' After his much-appreciated good deed, Raymond realized that his daughter's admiration was not worth anything unless he could prove that he was perfectly capable of committing evil deeds. Since there is no hero without a villain, no white without black, he obviously had to conceive the worst thing he could think of. His victim should not be a prostitute, because no one would mourn them. And so when Saskia's image was reflected in his spectacle lenses, he knew he had the perfect victim, as she and Rex came across as a fine couple, especially since he had witnessed them kissing each other.

The third key moment was when he received birthday presents from his family. He was given a key ring with the letter R as well as a photo album covering his life. As soon as he saw the picture of himself as a sixteen-year-old boy in a sling after his fall, he understood that women will start to trust him if he comes across as a weakling. That he finally abducted Saskia was a matter of coincidence: she started talking to him at the gas station shop because she wanted to practice her French, and then she became intrigued by his key ring and wanted to have the same one with an 'R'. He told her that he had many more in his car, and when he invited her to step inside his car, she hesitated initially until she saw the family picture of Raymond with his wife and two daughters.

In the film's famous dénouement, Raymond brings Rex to the gas station and tells him that if he wants to know what happened to Saskia he will have to undergo the same thing Saskia did. He will have to drink a cup of coffee in which a sleeping pill is dissolved. It is a maddening choice, for if the same fate awaits Rex, it is not likely that he will survive. But the uncertainty, the not-knowing is perhaps the worst thing, as Raymond tells him slyly. The camera is filming from inside the car as we see Rex running frenetically to and fro in the thunder and rain. Even though the camera goes left and right to keep Rex in the frame, the thermos flask with the drugged coffee remains in the middle, telling us that it is inevitable that Rex will decide to drink the drugged coffee. In an almost verbatim repetition of a phrase used by Raymond, Rex says: 'To go against what is predestined, one must drink' (drink instead of jump). Rex drinks the cup, after which the screen goes black. In the next scene we see a coffin being covered by sand on more or less the same spot where the second episode started, in the uncultivated garden. The next shot is from inside the coffin, which is lit up when Rex uses his lighter to see where he is. He cries for help, but in a coffin, no one can hear you scream. In a final shot, the camera pans just above the grass and moves from Raymond's wife watering the garden to Raymond sitting quietly on a bench. The camera then goes back over the ground, tilting up to the rear window of a car, revealing a newspaper article about the vanished lovers.[20]

For author and co-screenwriter Krabbé, the recurrent motif of 'the golden egg' was most significant in both novella and film. In the beginning of SPOORLOOS, Saskia is telling Rex about a dream she had the night before, one she regularly has. As always, she is drifting in space, locked in a golden egg,[21] and to her it is a haunting image of unbearable loneliness. This time, however, there is a second egg far away, but she knows that once they collide in space, everything will vanish. It is unclear whether this is to be taken as a nightmarish scenario of chaos and disaster or that the collision will result in liberation and eternal affinity. It is soon thereafter that they are stuck in the middle of a tunnel because their car has run out of gas. A truck comes their way and its lights scare Saskia because, she says, they are like golden eggs. They have a quarrel, and Rex walks away by himself to get a jerrycan with petrol. He has a strange, perhaps even malicious, smile on his face—the first crack in his psyche, according to Steven Jay Schneider ('SPOORLOOS', 182). Upon his return, Saskia has vanished, but when his car arrives at the end of the tunnel, it has the form of the brightly lit egg from her dream, with a faint silhouette inside. The next shot shows that Saskia was that silhouette, waiting for Rex's return. She accepts his excuse that it was because he was in a slight panic that he had acted silly by leaving her behind to fetch some petrol.

Just before her vanishing, Saskia sits on Rex's stomach as he lies down on the grass. She makes him swear that he will never ever abandon the 'exquisite and always sweet' Saskia again; he swears to it, but the pledge is not very serious, since both of them are laughing. Once Saskia is gone, he desperately searches for her, but his playful vow is never taken as a cast-iron promise in Sluizer's movie. On the French television, Rex explains why his search has become so frenetic. It was because he has had the very same dream about golden eggs as Saskia had the night before her disappearance. He regards this recurrence as a 'sign' that he has to bring this 'homage' to his vanished loved one. For Rex's second major decision—whether or not to drink the cup of coffee—the golden egg motif is pivotal as well. He starts digging the earth near a tree and finds the two coins Saskia has buried there to seal their relationship. The two coins glisten in the dark like the eggs from Saskia's dream. Rex apparently interprets this as an omen, and the discovery of the coins prompts him to drink the coffee. We have two more egg references near the end: Rex's lighter, which he uses in the coffin, resembles an egg as it starts to die out. Finally, the newspaper item has an oval-shaped portrait of both Saskia and Rex.

When interviewed on French television, Rex claimed that his search is an 'homage', paying a symbolic tribute to Saskia. In that sense, it is appropriate that his disappearance makes headline news: he is remembered as the man who remained faithful to his vanished girlfriend, which is also a kind of homage. One may conclude from this that Rex is fully immersed in a universe of symbolic gestures, as if his aim is to show himself off to the community as a dedicated lover. I will claim the exact opposite, however. Remember that Raymond told Rex that he defined a hero as someone 'capable of excess'. Rex is such a hero in relentless pursuit of an impossible fantasy scenario: desire is privileged over knowledge.

Strictly speaking, Rex wants to know what has happened to Saskia. That is what he says while looking into the French television camera: I want to know. At one point, he had even told Lieneke that if he had to choose between his not-knowing of her happy existence somewhere else and knowledge of her death, he would opt for the latter. Raymond's guarantee that he will know about Saskia's fate does not make him drink the drugged coffee, however. He only decides to intoxicate himself upon seeing the coins buried in the ground near the tree, which resemble two golden eggs. The image from the dream of eggs colliding in space spurs him to go against the logic of predestination, just as Raymond did when he was a child. This utopian collision of the eggs is the object-cause of his desire, and the coins are the confirmation that this is his one and only goal: he has no other option but to stick to it, at whatever cost.

In discussions of *Antigone*, it is made clear that this hero, with her excessive demand to give her brother a decent burial, positions herself outside the symbolic community. If I were to draw an analogy between Antigone and Rex in the sense that both do not compromise their desire, it is emblematic that Rex is a protagonist about whom we never see even a tiny slice of his social life. While we get to know a lot about the other male protagonist Raymond, we know absolutely nothing about Rex regarding family, work, and friends, except that he has a relationship with Saskia, and later that Lieneke breaks up with him because he is so consumed by his obsession to find information about Saskia. When he switches on his computer, the screen briefly sums up a number of female names, apparently former lovers, but they immediately vanish in favour of the name of 'Saskia', which appears in several sizes as if his only symbolic connection is with someone who has left him and is no longer around. Perhaps Rex suffers from a fear of abandonment, and this has resulted in his obsession with his former beloved and his giving up on all social connections.

Very much like Raymond who meticulously prepares his most evil deed,[22] Rex displays an uncompromising perseverance. Hence, Rex is represented as someone who has already excluded himself from the symbolic community, and he shares this exclusion with Raymond who himself has become preoccupied with Rex because of the latter's stubborn search. Originally, Raymond is a father who is admired by his wife and kids, but he puts this admiration at stake by committing a crime that might turn him into a social outcast. Whereas Raymond shows himself capable of excess, without the option to confess this to anyone but Rex, the latter is excessive in his pursuit at the expense of his social ties. Thus, an imaginary dream-like collision with Saskia is the one and only pivot around which his desire is structured. When buried alive at the end of SPOORLOOS, he is in a panic, shouting 'I am Rex Hofman', a symbolic gesture *par excellence*. But he also starts to laugh, saying this is 'weird', for it is a hollow scream: he was already lost to the social circuit, some time ago. The fact that the flame of his lighter starts to resemble a golden egg in total darkness seems reassuring, as if this image will bring him closer to the fulfilment of his desire.

CONCLUSION: CAPABLE OF EXCESS

Ducker fulfils the assignments given to him by 'secret agent' Dorbeck for the purpose of gaining social recognition. And in his private world, this ordinary man definitely becomes a hero, but in the symbolic network he is named a rabble, since there is photographic evidence that he is on close terms with Ebernuss but there is no trace of Dorbeck. Ducker's ambition to be included in a symbolic circuit as a courageous resistance fighter turns into its opposite: he is expelled from the community as a dirty traitor. Insofar as Erik Lanshof is celebrated at the end of the war as a soldier of Orange, he owes this honour to his failure to fulfill a naïve assignment he had imposed upon himself. After this 'failure', he develops into the 'typical' war hero: a man who puts his life at risk for the benefit of the common good (the liberation of the Netherlands). Just like Erik, the red-haired Hannie Schaft as well as Peter van Dijk (from IN DE SCHADUW VAN DE OVERWINNING) are authentic partisans: if they die during their missions, they will be memorialized as martyrs for the cause. What I have tried to point out is that a character such as Miep Algera from PASTORALE 1943 goes beyond this 'common-sense heroism', for she really jeopardized everything: her work for the resistance was so secretive that she had to accept humiliation in the form of the condescending glances of her colleagues. Her espionage could only be successful if she wilfully excluded herself from a social network. Similarly, the characters Blumberg (IN DE SCHADUW VAN DE OVERWINNING) and Otto Schneeweiss (DE IJSSALON) had to walk a thin line between treason and heroism, without betting on receiving any recognition for what they did. In the case of Blumberg, it is not clear whether he can be judged a rabble or a hero. At the end of Frenkel Frank's movie, however, Trudi remarks that Otto apparently kept his mouth shut during his interrogation by the Nazis, and thus Otto's martyrdom is acknowledged after all.

The final four films are specific cases of male characters isolating themselves from their environment. Alfred Issendorf thinks he does the world a favour by following in his late father's footsteps, but he lacks support in his efforts. As befits a 'hero', he perseveres but increasingly withdraws into a private world, also due to his insomnia. In turn, Doctor Pulder identifies with two sad outcasts to such an extent that he deliberately ruins his solid reputation as a reliable rock within the community. Finally, FLANAGAN and SPOORLOOS have been read as two sides of the same coin: Paul Flanagan chooses the path of the 'rabble', and retribution for his years of imprisonment can only be paid for by making his family miserable: the cold satisfaction of revenge rather than any financial compensation is his sole gain. Rex Hofman in Sluizer's thriller proves himself to be capable of excess. He isolates himself from the symbolic network and dedicates himself heroically to the pursuit of Saskia's dream: he more or less knows that a bad fate awaits him, but he bets on an imaginary collision of two golden eggs.

NOTES

1 In Hitchcock's ROPE (1948), as Žižek mentions, a professor proposes a theory about Supermen, but when two of his students put this theory into practice by strangling a friend, the professor is shocked that his lecture has caused a murder and 'shrinks back from the consequence of his words, unprepared to recognize in them his own truth' (*Enjoy*, 13). A hero would unconditionally accept the consequences.

2 This fantasy of a 'heroic martyr sacrificing his own life to redeem a corrupt, stagnant world from the brink of destruction' has been popular in Hollywood disaster movies, from THE POSEIDON ADVENTURE (Ronald Neame, 1972) to ARMAGEDDON (Michael Bay, 1998), as Dan Hassler-Forest asserts (210).

3 Reportedly, Steven Spielberg was very much impressed by SOLDAAT VAN ORANJE, even considering Paul Verhoeven as a director for one of the STAR WARS episodes. The film also proved to be a calling card for its two main actors, Rutger Hauer and Jeroen Krabbé, for an international career. In the early 1980s, Hauer starred in NIGHTHAWKS (Bruce Malmuth, 1981) with Sylvester Stallone, EUREKA (Nicolas Roeg, 1983) with Gene Hackman, THE OSTERMAN WEEKEND (Sam Peckinpah, 1983) with John Hurt, and, of course, BLADE RUNNER (Ridley Scott, 1982) with Harrison Ford. Jeroen Krabbé had substantial roles in NO MERCY (Richard Pearce, 1986) with Richard Gere, and THE FUGITIVE (Andrew Davis, 1993) with Harrison Ford, and was also a Bond villain in THE LIVING DAYLIGHTS (John Glen, 1987).

4 With hindsight, Verhoeven remarked that Robbie, a youth friend of Erik, should have been depicted on the photograph as well, for dramatic purposes (Juttmann, 87).

5 Before going to the toilet, Alex had thrown a tiny crust of bread to a begging Soviet kid. The kid then throws a hand grenade into the WC, presumably in anger at being given only crumbs. In retrospect, Verhoeven regretted this scene: Alex should have given the kid a sandwich, for then the bombing could be taken as a sign of the boy's indoctrination (Van Scheers, 519).

6 The public appeal of DE OVERVAL in 1962 is understandable: with memories of war still relatively fresh, the viewers were treated to a patriotic picture in which Dutch resistance fighters are depicted in a most courageous fashion. Good and brave men rescue companions from a prison guarded by the 'bad' Nazis. Moreover, the film was advertised as based on true events and the famous historian Lou de Jong had been one of the scriptwriters, which further assured the film's authenticity.

7 In BANKIER VAN HET VERZET—which won five Golden Calves including Best Feature Film—the brothers Gijs and Walraven van Hall run an 'underground bank' to finance the resistance with fake credits. Moreover, they successfully plan a heist to steal millions of guilders from de Nederlandsche Bank to the frustration of the Nazis. Because the actual protagonist Walraven is represented as an idealistic and righteous hero, BANKIER VAN HET VERZET has more in common with DE OVER-

VAL than with other Dutch war pictures depicting a moral grey area. In September 2010, a fallen tree in bronze was unveiled in Amsterdam to commemorate Walraven van Hall as a 'fallen giant'.

8 Though Poerstamper is fully committed to the NSB cause, he is nonetheless portrayed as a 'jolly character, a family man who cares very much for his wife and two sons' in order to underscore the greyer incarnations of the enemy (Burke, 161).

9 This August has a particularly perverse motivation for his affiliation with the Nazis: he has taken the side of the Germans because he thinks they are about to lose the war and he likes joining lost causes.

10 The novel (1956) by Theun de Vries about Hannie Schaft is explicit about her communist sympathies, and upon her arrest she had copies of the Communist newspaper *De waarheid*, but this is not addressed in Verbong's film (Barten, 235).

11 In her study *Images of Occupation in Dutch Film*, Wendy Burke is particularly attentive to the 'greyer incarnations' of the German soldiers in Dutch war films from the mid-1970s onwards: the enemy is no longer represented in a one-sided manner, highlighting grotesque and pompous assets; instead we see German soldiers relaxing on the Scheveningen beach with Dutch families in SOLDAAT VAN ORANJE; Miep's German lover in PASTORALE 1943 is depicted as 'kind and courteous' (99); the SD man in this film is very interested in Johan Schults's poster of the Quinten Massijs painting *The Old Duchess*; and the kindest of them all is the German desk sergeant Schulz who looks after Anton Steenwijk in DE AANSLAG after his traumatic night and offers him nutritious food (104).

12 The role of Blumberg in De Jong's film is inspired by the so-called 'Weinreb affair'. Friedrich Weinreb was a Jew in his thirties who promised other Jews an escape route during the war. His profitable plan fell apart in 1944, and he was imprisoned after the war for fraud and collaboration for more than three years. It remains debatable whether he was a cunning parasite or a merciful man.

13 Barten mentions that most World War II films in the 1980s tended to interpret historical facts too loosely. Significantly, he observes, the more accurate pictures, such as Weisz's CHARLOTTE and Rademakers' DE AANSLAG, have been more successful than the inaccurate ones. According to Barten, DE IJSSALON belongs to the latter category: the German attack of the Koco ice cream parlour in Amsterdam in February 1941 is only used as a backdrop to the film's narrative (236).

14 AMERICAN BEAUTY won five Academy Awards, including Best Picture.

15 Paul Flanagan was brilliantly played by Guido de Moor, who acted in just a handful of films but excelled in theatrical plays. He won the Louis d'Or for best theatre actor no less than four times, the last time just preceding his death at age 52. One of his rare performances was his fantastic role as the small-time crook Freddy Freeze in one of my favourite little gems of Dutch cinema, KERMIS IN DE REGEN (Kees Brusse, 1962). Freddy steals cars for his boss Wadman. One evening, he is about to drive away when the drunken owner of the car shows up. Freddy hits the

man and drives off, and the next day he reads in the paper that the drunk was taken to the hospital due to an unfortunate fall. He is worried about the man's health but is happy to hear from his friend Willy that the patient died before he regained consciousness. When he hears that a woman has witnessed the beating, he thinks it best to disappear to Spain. He hopes to get the required money for his departure by robbing a bank. With Willy and Bertje, he does the job while the fair is in town. The bank director has a gun in his drawer, however, and they run away. Willy and Bertje are chased by the police by car until they have a fatal accident with a truck. Freddy himself will not survive: after a bullet was fired at him, he is slowly bleeding to death. In the meantime, Annie, the female witness who hardly ever participates in social events, has been asked to the fair. Another of Freddy's mates, Hugo, kills her in the dark of night, but he is arrested the next day.

16 TARDE PARA LA IRA [THE FURY OF A PATIENT MAN] (Raúl Arévalo, 2016) is a Spanish thriller about a taciturn and apparently gentle man who takes revenge for the eight years he has spent in prison after a robbery.

17 For Steven Jay Schneider, Rex's temporary abandonment of Saskia reveals 'an unacknowledged (and ultimately unsatisfiable) desire to run away from his relationship' with his girlfriend (SPOORLOOS, 182). Still sore about his departure, Saskia makes him solemnly declare at the gas station ('repeat after me') that he will never ever abandon her. This promise, as Schneider argues, is at the root of Rex's obsessive search for Saskia rather than 'genuine' love for her. Schneider even claims that Rex has 'repressed homoerotic impulses', and thus he 'ends up trapped not so much in a coffin as in the closet' (185).

18 A few minutes earlier, Raymond had put a corkscrew in this drawer, so he knew about the spiders. When he then asks his daughter to give him the corkscrew, he knew she would spot the spiders and betted on her screaming.

19 Foundas hits the nail on the head when he claims that 'it is Raymond's calm, scientific composure—the way he toys with human lives as a child with a magnifying glass does with ants—that makes the blood run cold'.

20 Sluizer himself remade SPOORLOOS as THE VANISHING (1993) in America, and because of a last-minute rescue ending, the US version was met with much scorn, as Steven Jay Schneider explains in his article 'Repackaging Rage': a brilliant thriller was turned into a spineless run-of-the-mill product. Critic Roger Ebert called THE VANISHING 'a textbook exercise in the trashing of a nearly perfect film' and other reviewers backed this verdict up by calling the remake an affront to the American public. Sluizer's response, quoted in Schneider, was pretty laid back: 'The No. 1 fascination for me was to be able to recreate characters in a different culture, in a different movie with different actors, but based on the same story.'

21 As Foundas mentions, this image of Saskia in a golden egg floating through space resembles the Star Child of 2001: A SPACE ODYSSEY (Stanley Kubrick, 1968).

22 Killing someone is not the worst, Raymond says to Rex, which makes us wonder what deed exceeds this. Then we have this minor and seemingly irrelevant scene in which a policeman on a motorbike stops Raymond for driving without a seat belt. Raymond replies that a doctor's certificate dispenses him from the obligation to wear one because of his 'claustrophobia': in retrospect, we realize that being buried alive is the worst that can happen to him.

BIBLIOGRAPHY

Barten, Egbert, 'Toenemende vrijheid: De verwerking van de Tweede Wereldoorlog in de Nederlandse speelfilm', ed. by D.H. Schram and C. Geljon, *Overal sporen: De verwerking van de Tweede Wereldoorlog in literatuur en kunst* (Amsterdam: VU Uitgeverij, 1990), 213-251.

Bouineau, Jean-Marc, *Paul Verhoeven: Beyond Flesh and Blood* (Paris: Cinephage, 2001).

Burke, Wendy, *Images of Occupation in Dutch Film: Memory, Myth and the Cultural Legacy of War* (Amsterdam: Amsterdam University Press, 2017).

Foundas, Scott, 'THE VANISHING: The End of the Road', *The Criterion Collection* (29 October 2014), https://www.criterion.com/current/posts/3340-the-vanishing-the-end-of-the-road [Accessed 12 May 2020].

Hassler-Forest, Dan, *Capitalist Superheroes: Caped Crusaders in the Neoliberal Age* (Alresford: Zero Books, 2012).

Juttmann, Bart, *Op zoek naar* SOLDAAT VAN ORANJE*: De geschiedenis van de Nederlandse filmklassieker* (Amsterdam: International Theatre & Film Books, 2020).

Lacan, Jacques, *The Ethics of Psychoanalysis: Book VII, 1959-1960*, trans. by Dennis Porter (London: Routledge, 1991).

—, *Television: A Challenge to the Psychoanalytic Establishment*, trans. by Denis Hollier, Rosalind Krauss, and Annette Michelson (New York: W.W.Norton and Company, 1990).

Schneider, Steven Jay, 'Repackaging Rage: THE VANISHING and NIGHTWATCH', *Kinema: A Journal for Film and Audiovisual Media* 17 (1 April 2002): 47-66.

Schneider, Steven Jay, 'SPOORLOOS / THE VANISHING', ed. by Mathijs, *The Cinema of the Low Countries*, 177-185.

Schokker, Johan and Tim Schokker, *Extimiteit: Jacques Lacans terugkeer naar Freud* (Amsterdam: Boom, 2000).

Schoots, Hans, *Bert Haanstra: Filmer van Nederland* (Amsterdam: Mets en Schilt, 2009).

Telotte, J.P., 'Narratives of Resistance: Verhoeven's SOLDIER OF ORANGE', *Film Criticism* 30, 3 (2006): 3-16.

Van Scheers, Rob, *Paul Verhoeven: Een filmersleven* (Amsterdam: Podium, 2017).

Žižek, Slavoj, *Enjoy Your Symptom! Jacques Lacan In and Out of Hollywood*, 1992 (Revised Edition. New York and London: Routledge, 2001).

—, *The Plague of Fantasies* (London and New York: Verso, 1997).

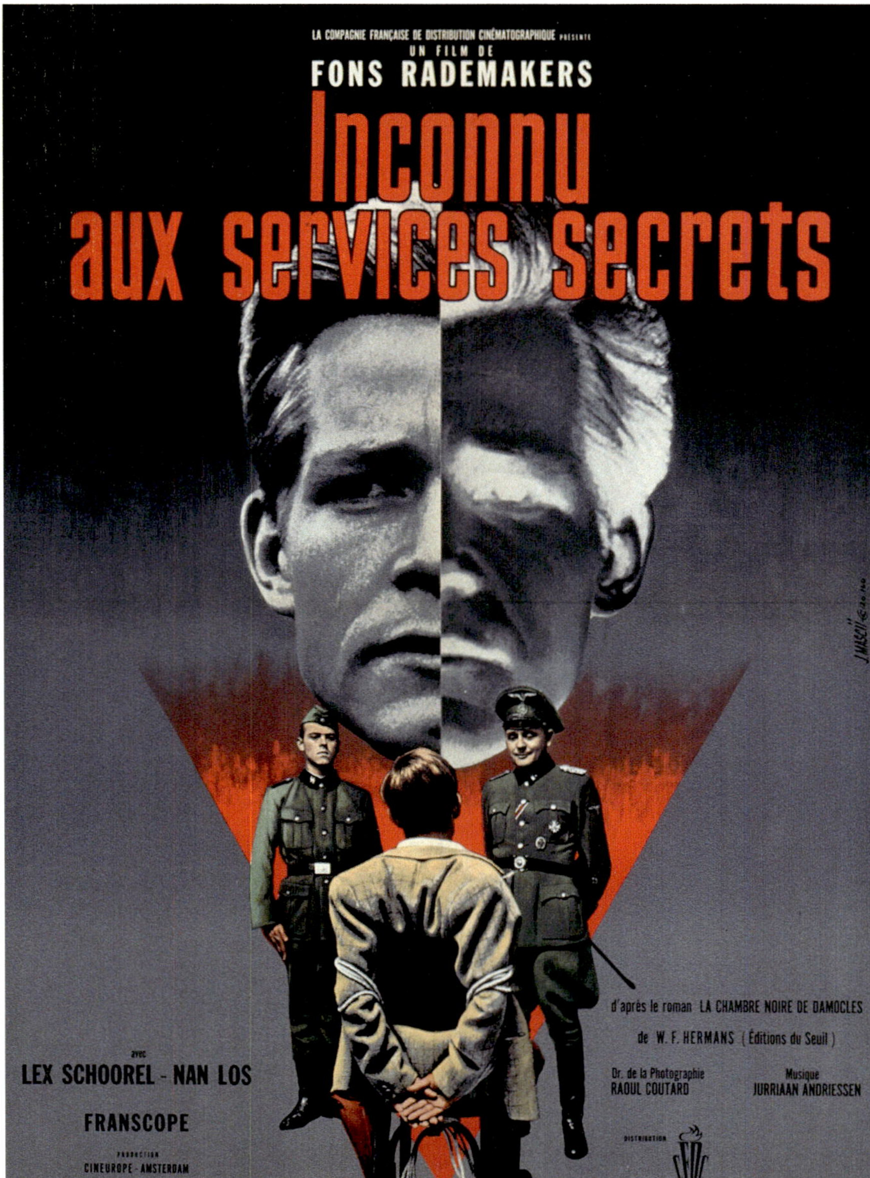

Plate 1
INCONNU AUX SERVICES SECRETS © Jean Mascii c/o Pictoright Amsterdam 2020. Collection La Cinémathèque française. Design: Jean Mascii (French poster ALS TWEE DRUPPELS WATER).

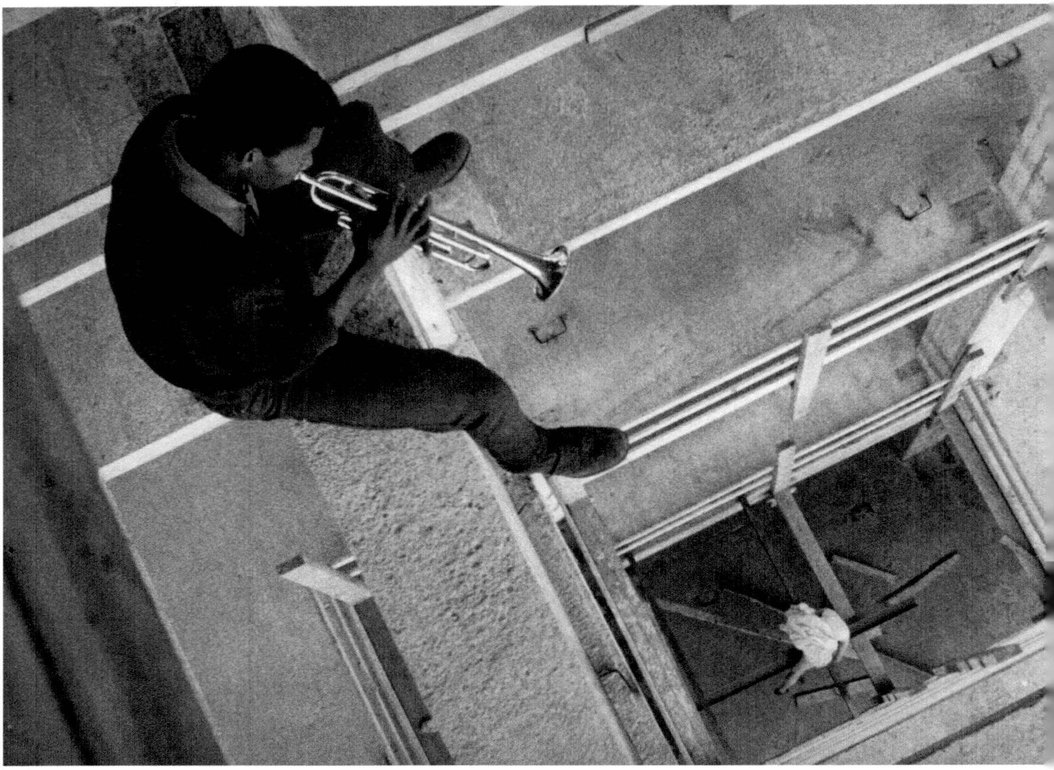

Plate 2
BIG CITY BLUES [René Deshauteurs] © Charles Huguenot van der Linden.
Collection Eye Filmmuseum

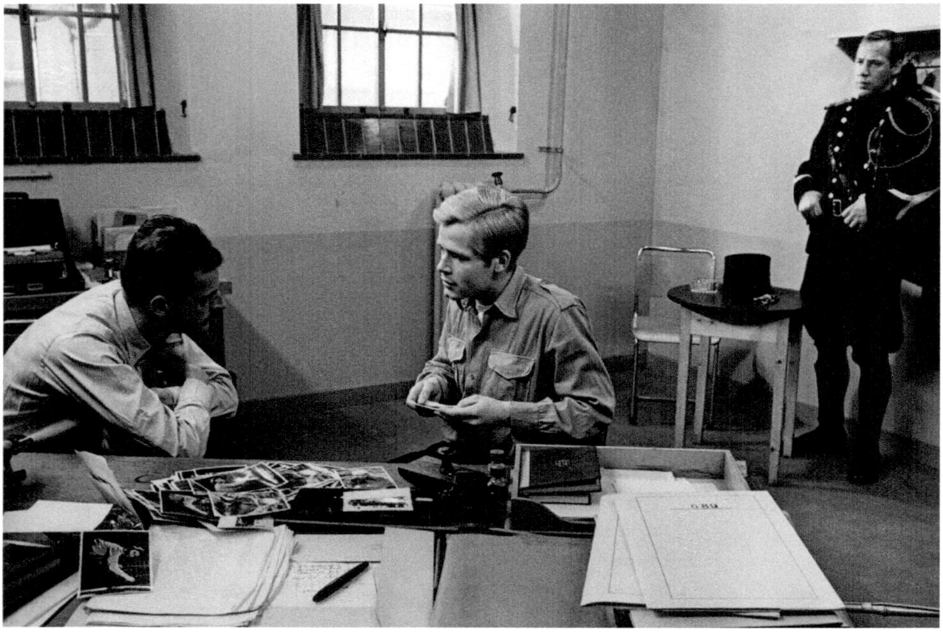

Plate 3
ALS TWEE DRUPPELS WATER [Van Doude, Lex Schoorel, Piet Römer] © Cineurope.
Collection Eye Filmmuseum. Photo: Ed van der Elsken

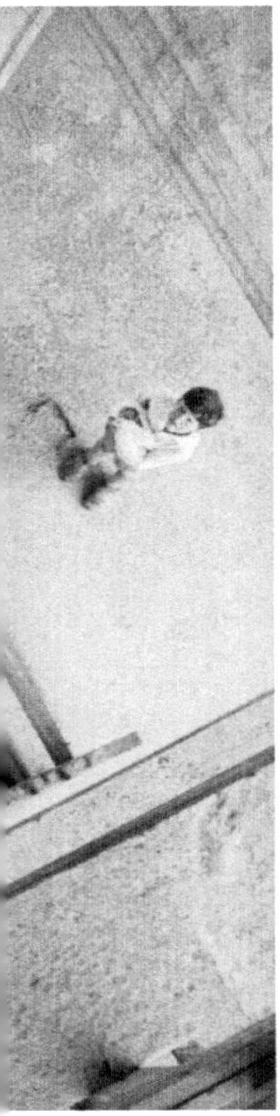

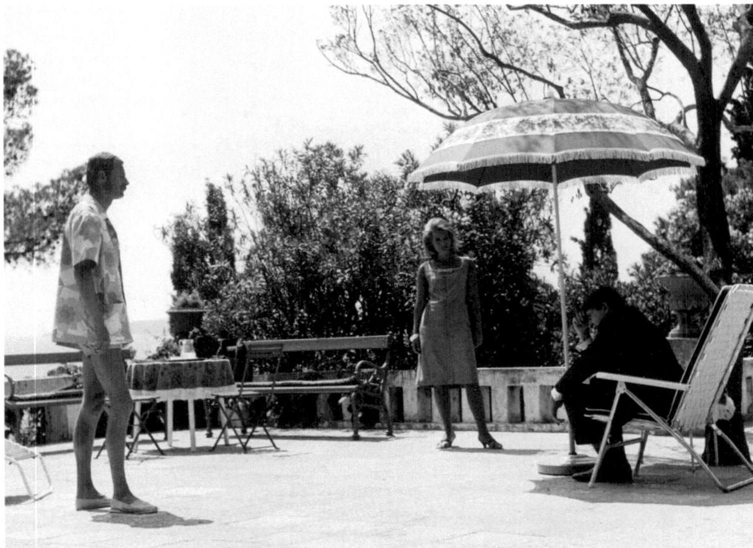

Plate 4
De dans van de reiger [Van Doude, Gunnel Lindblom, Jean Desailly] © Rademakers Productie BV. Collection Eye Filmmuseum.

Plate 5
De dans van de reiger [Gunnel Lindblom] © Rademakers Productie BV. Collection Eye Filmmuseum.

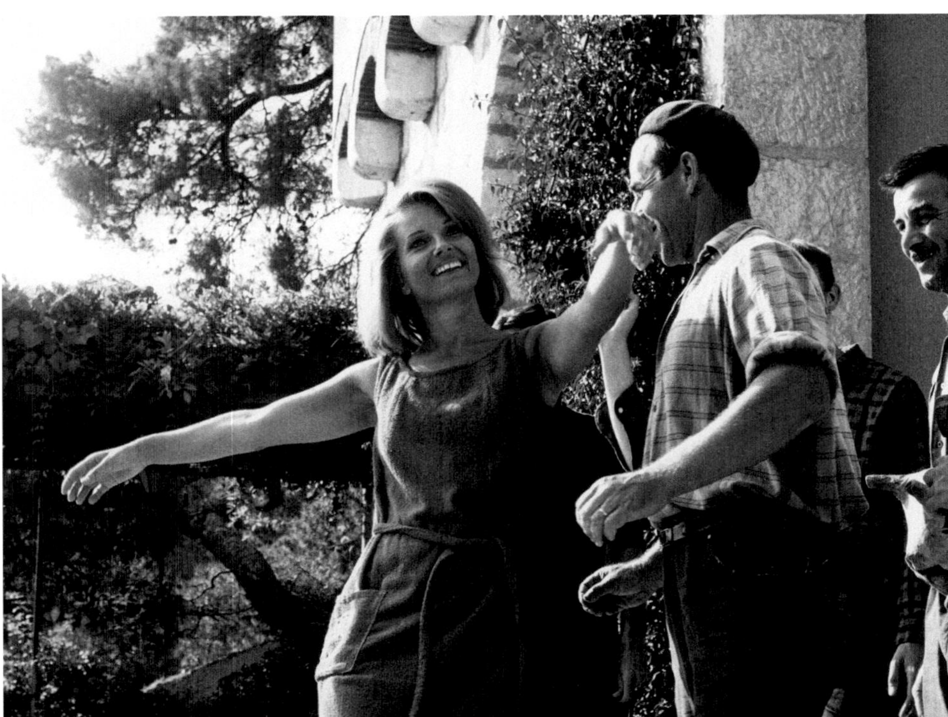

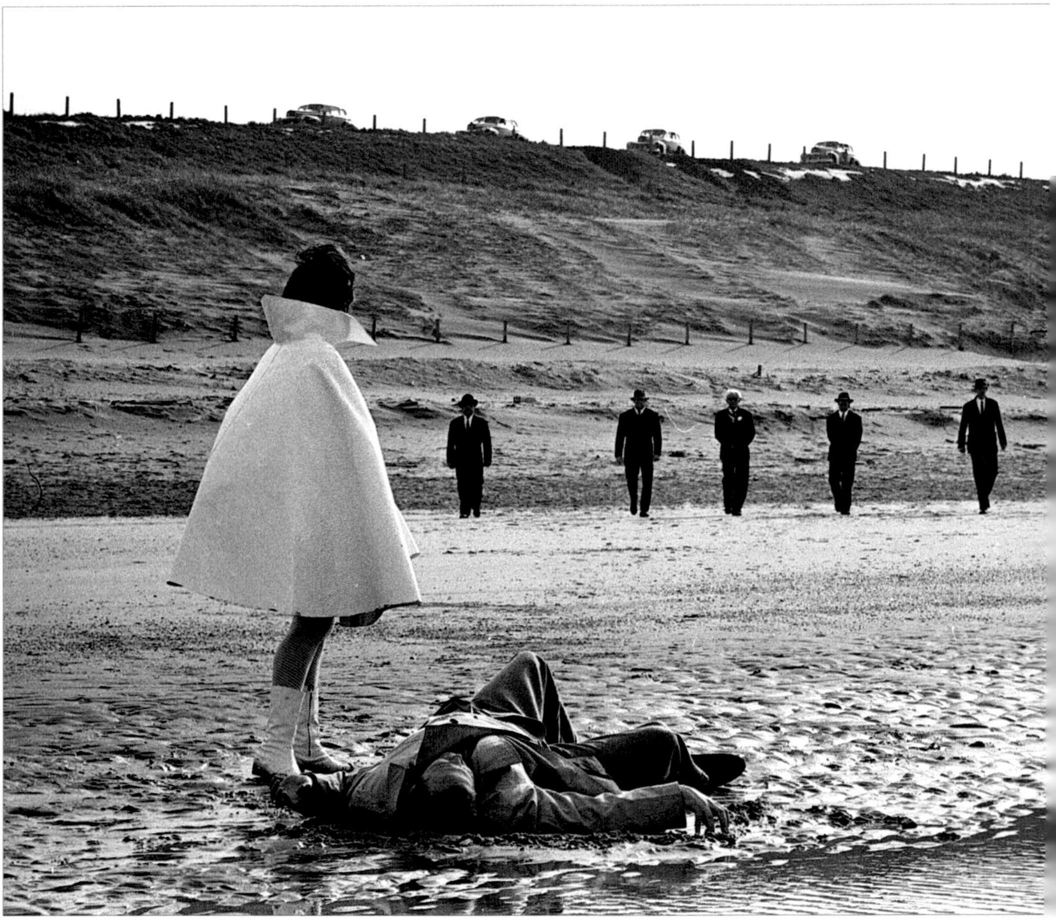

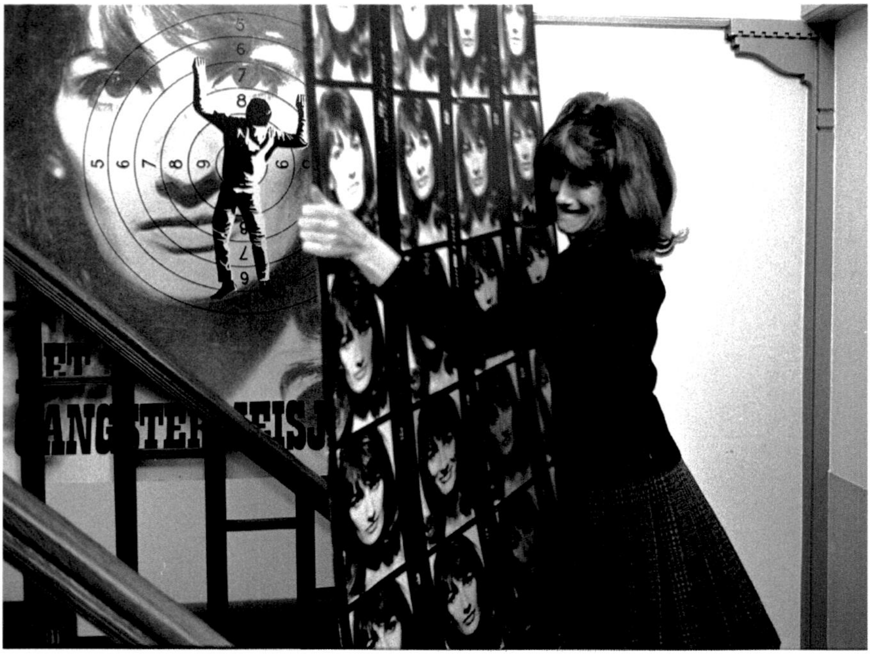
ET
ANGSTER EISJ

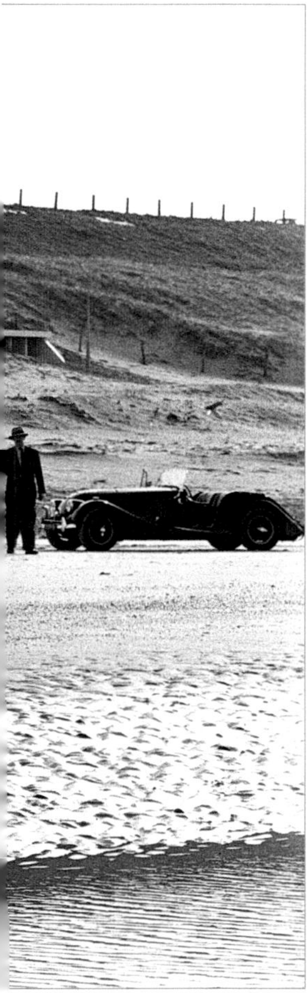

Left, top: Plate 6
HET GANGSTERMEISJE [Kitty Courbois (on the left)] © Jan Vrijman Cineproduktie. Photo: Eddy Posthuma de Boer

Left, bottom: Plate 7
HET GANGSTERMEISJE [Astrid Weyman] © Jan Vrijman Cineproduktie. Photo: Eddy Posthuma de Boer

Bottom: Plate 8
MONSIEUR HAWARDEN [Xander Fisher, Ellen Vogel, Hilde Uitterlinden] © Parkfilm. Collection Eye Filmmuseum.

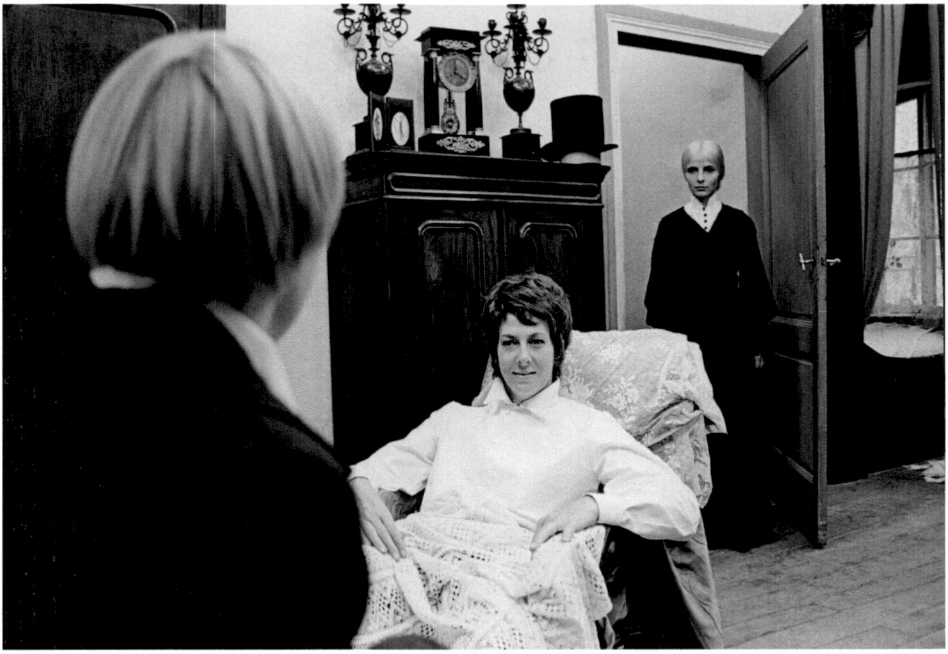

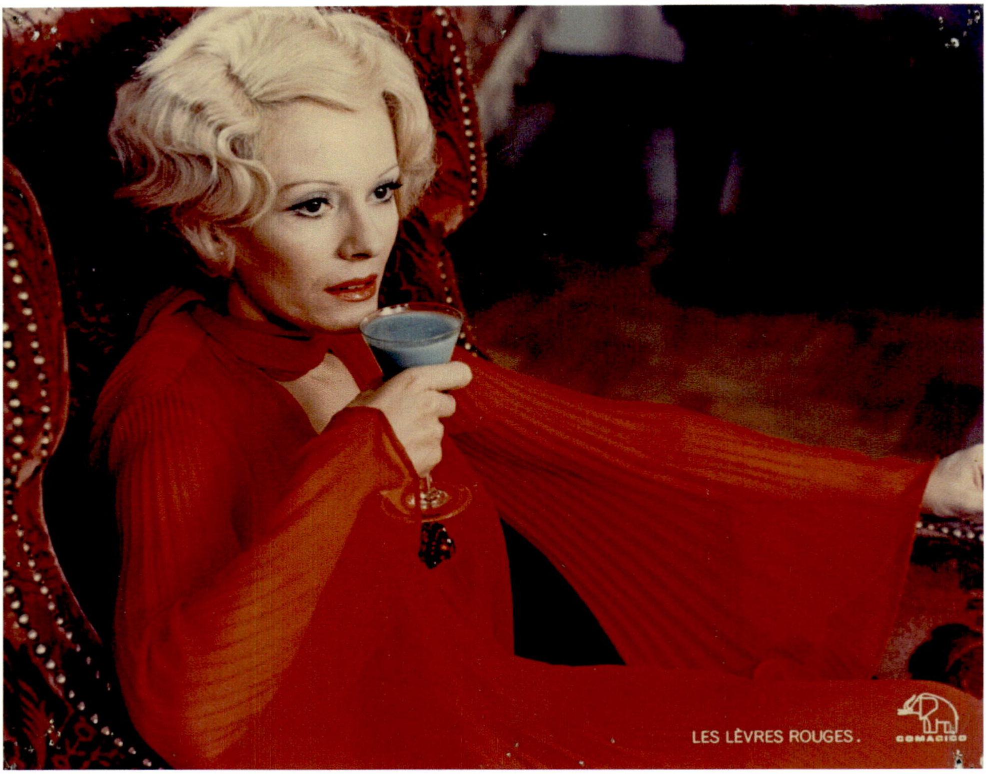

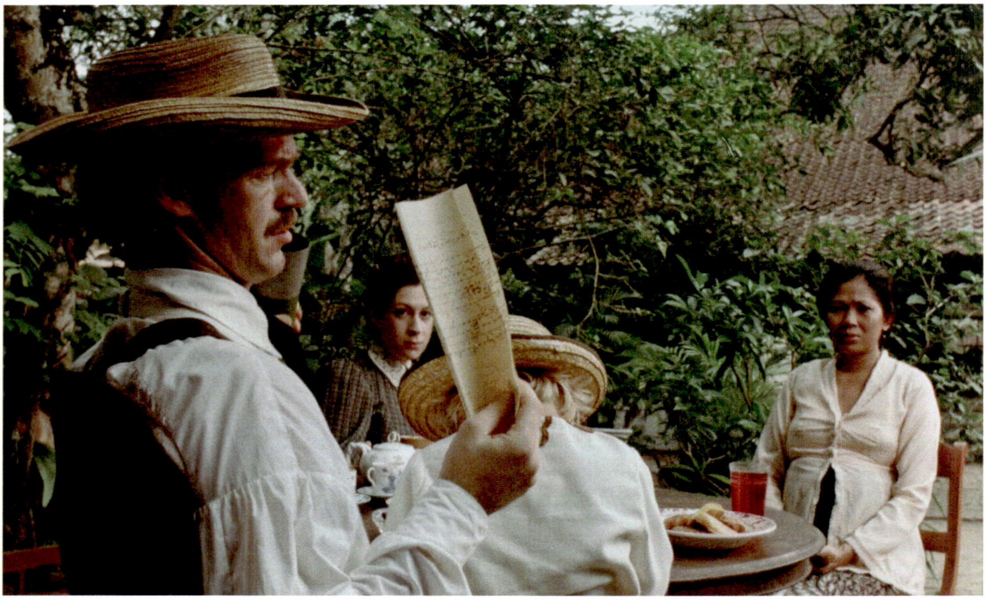

Top: Plate 9
LES LÈVRES ROUGES [Delphine Seyrig] © Maya Films. Collection Cinematek Brussels. Photo: Virginia Leirens

Bottom: Plate 10
MAX HAVELAAR [Peter Faber, Sacha Bulthuis, Rima Melati] © Fons Rademakers Produktie BV. Collection Eye Filmmuseum

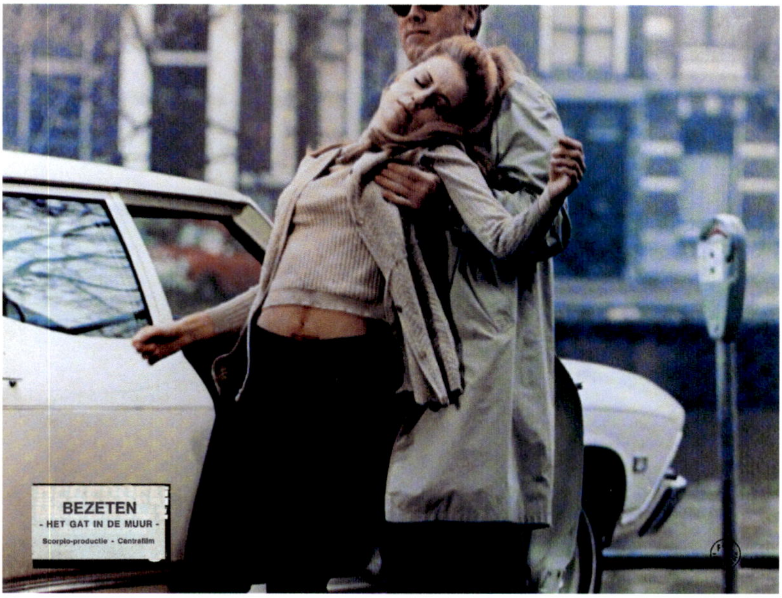

Plate 11
OBSESSIONS [Tom van Beek, Vibeke Løkkeberg] © Scorpio Films. Collection Eye Filmmuseum

Plate 12
BECAUSE OF THE CATS [Delia Lindsay] © Fons Rademakers Produktie. Collection Eye Filmmuseum

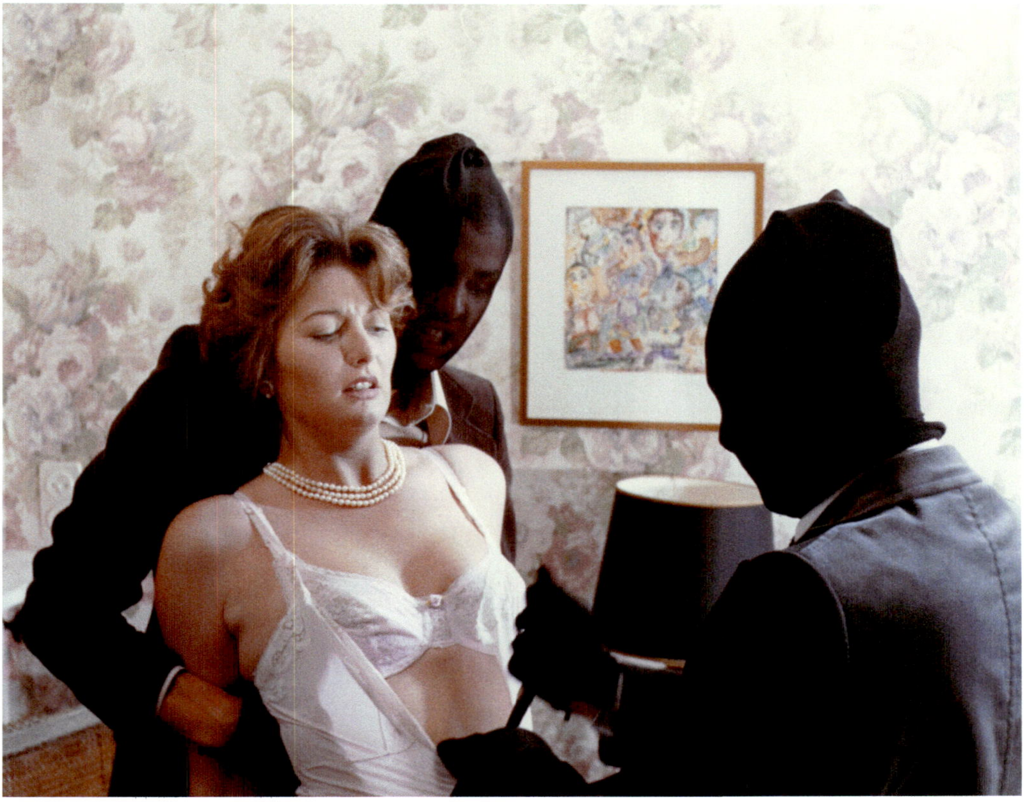

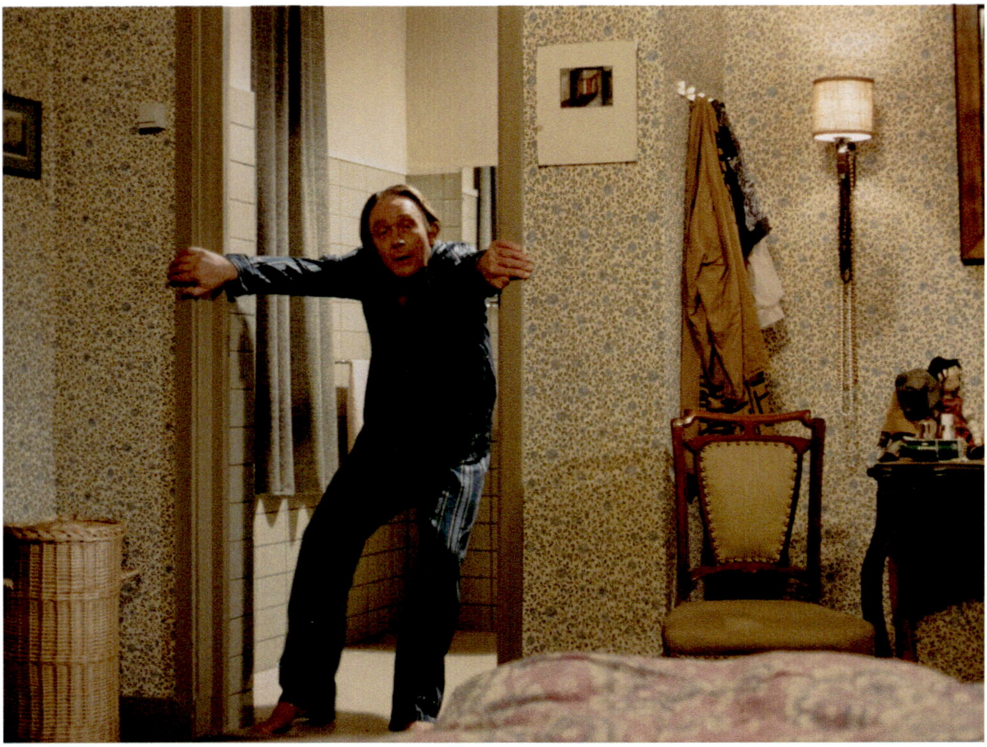

Plate 13
DOKTER PULDER ZAAIT PAPAVERS [Kees Brusse] © Bert Haanstra Films. Collection Eye Filmmuseum. Photo: Max Koot

Plate 14
MYSTERIES [Sylvia Kristel, Rita Tushingham] © Sigma Pictures. Photo: Sita Kaulesar Sukul

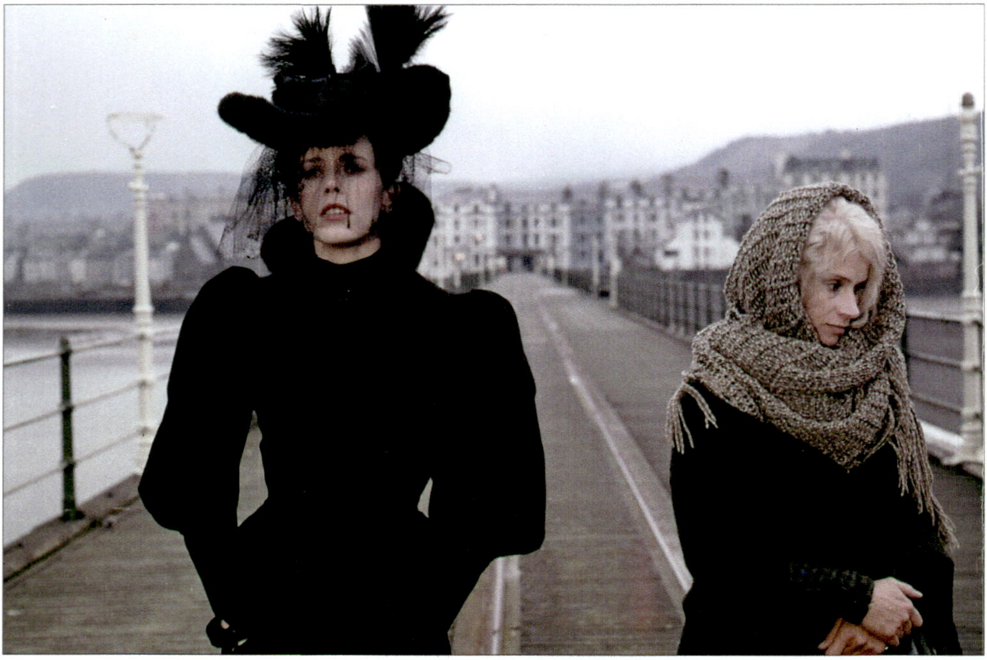

Plate 15
VAN DE KOELE MEREN DES DOODS [Derek de Lint, Renée Soutendijk] © Sigma Pictures. Photo: Anne Taverne

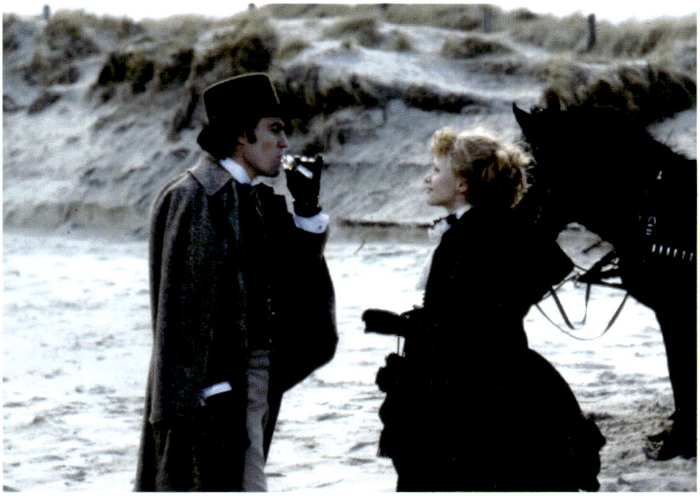

Plate 16
HET TEKEN VAN HET BEEST [Gerard Thoolen] © Cine/Vista B.V. Collection Eye Filmmuseum. Photo: Catrien Ariens

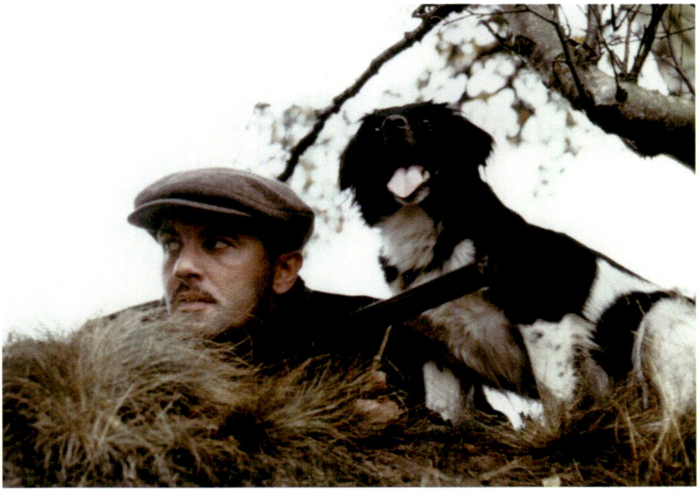

Plate 17
HET TEKEN VAN HET BEEST [Gerard Thoolen (in the background), an uncredited extra] © Cine/Vista B.V. Collection Eye Filmmuseum. Photo: Catrien Ariens

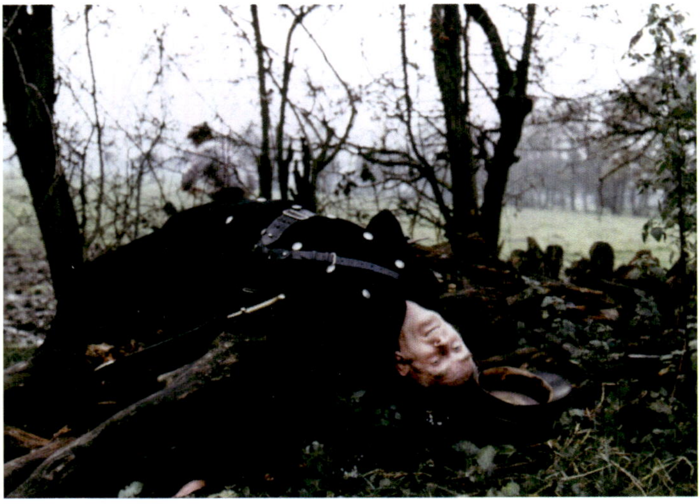

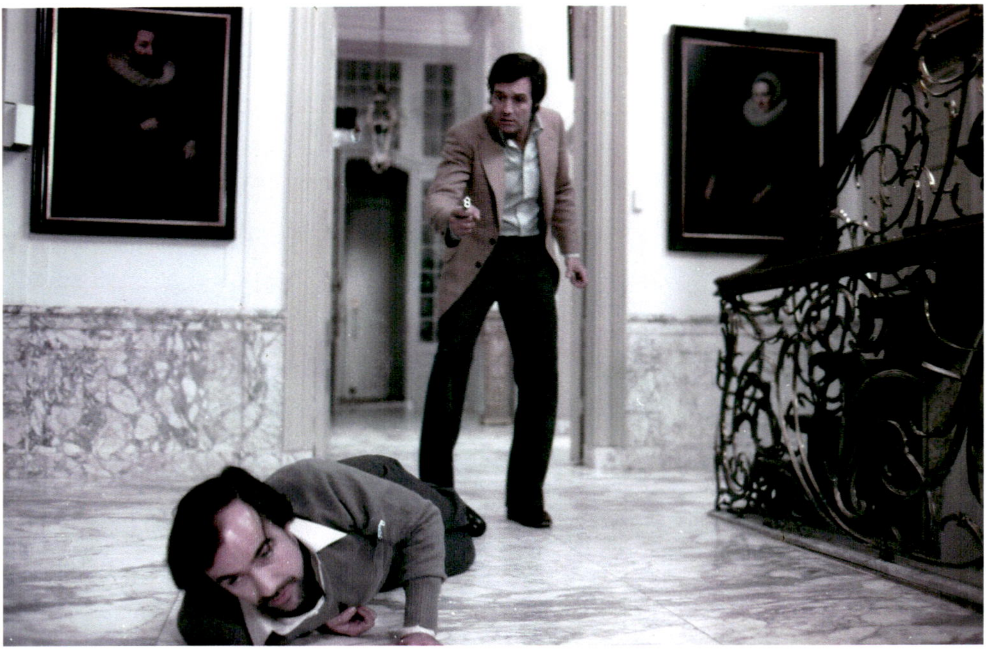

Plate 18
Flanagan [Guido de Moor, Eric Schneider (on the ground)]
© Sigma Pictures. Photo: Catrien Ariens

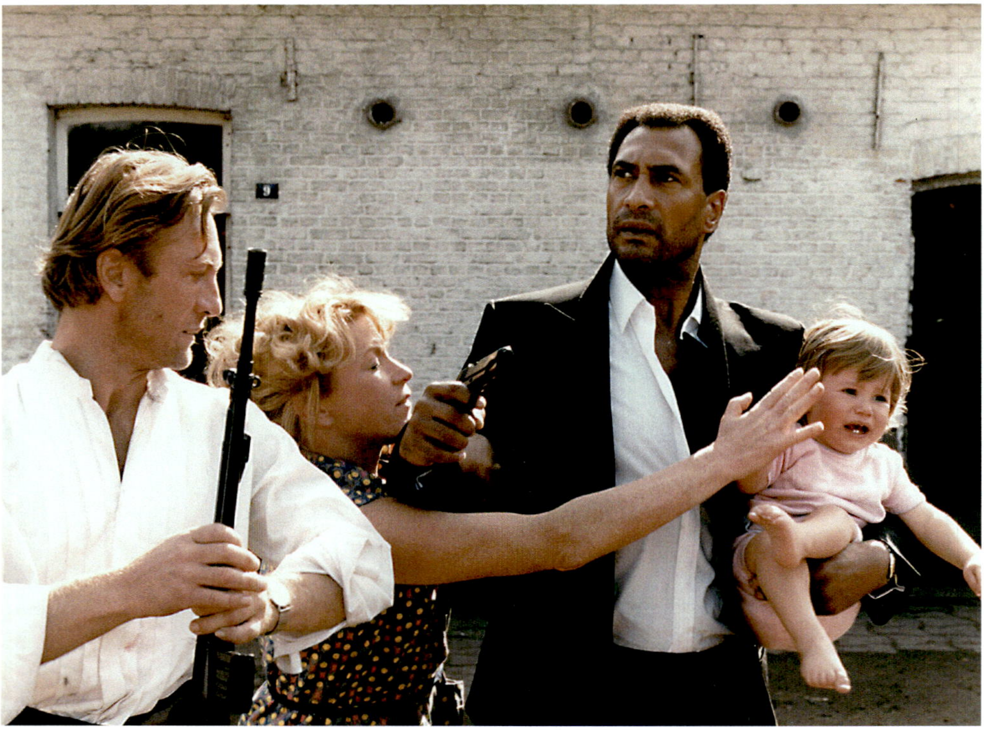

Plate 19
Wildschut [Hidde Maas, Chris Lomme, Jack Monkau, Bert Onraedt] © Cine/Vista B.V. Photo: Roland Minnaert

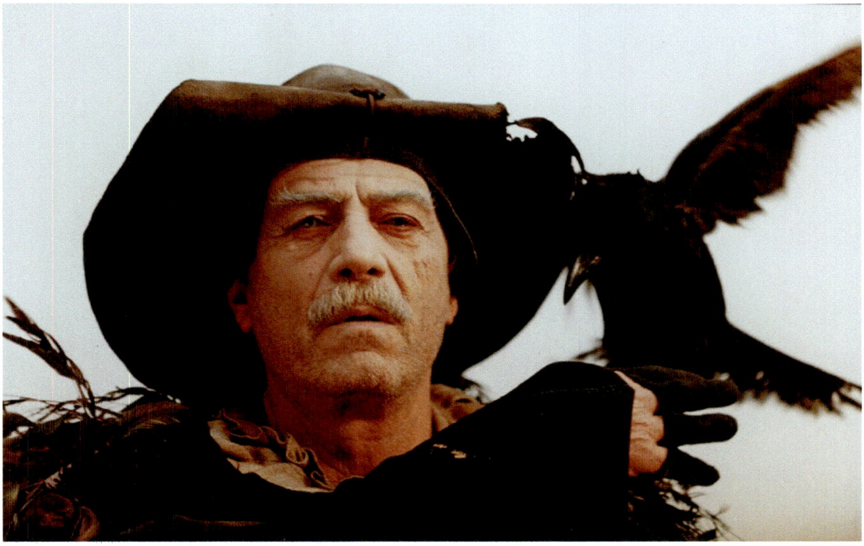

Plate 20
DE VLIEGENDE HOLLANDER [Nino Manfredi] © Jos Stelling Films. Collection Eye Filmmuseum. Photo: Michael Kooren

Plate 21
HET MEISJE EN DE DOOD [Leonid Bichevin, Sylvia Hoeks] © Jos Stelling Films.

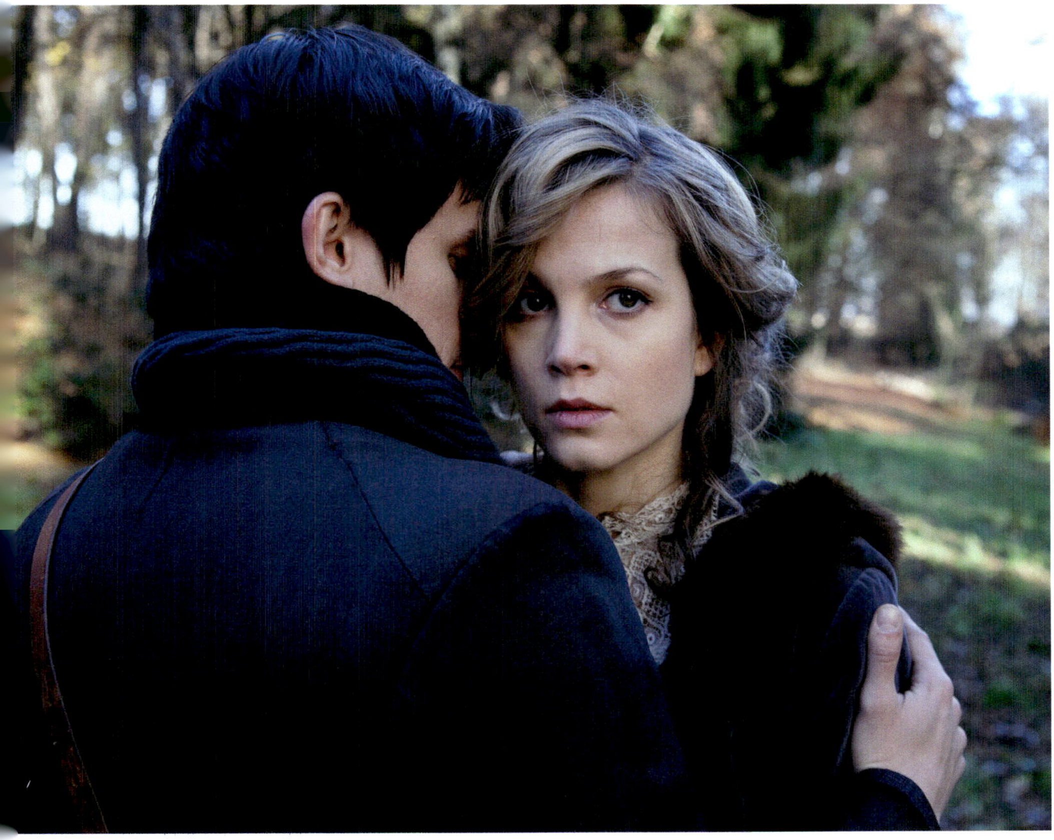

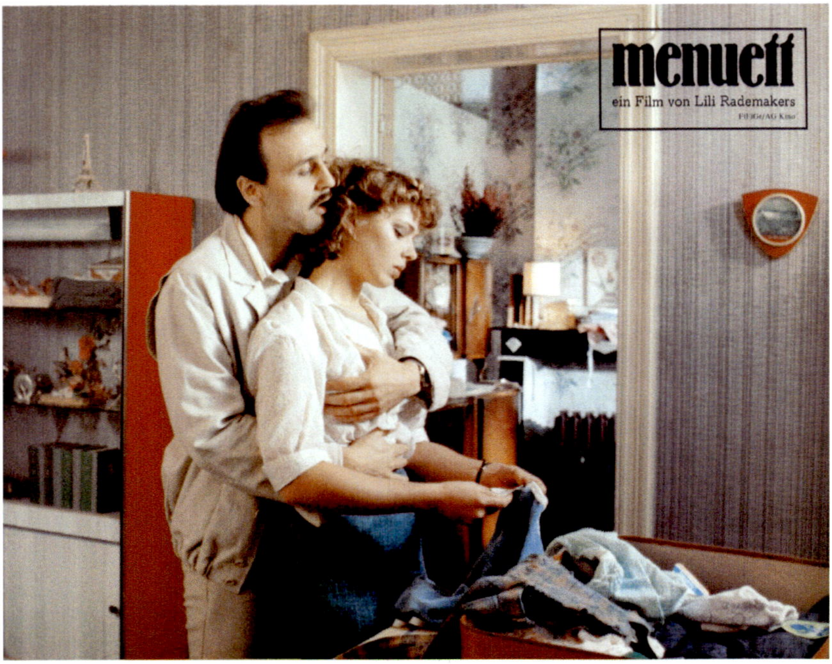

Top: Plate 22
MENUET [Theu Boermans, Carla Hardy] © Fons Rademakers Produktie. Collection Eye Filmmuseum

Plate 23
KRACHT [Theu Boermans (on the right)] © Sigma Pictures. Photo: Herman Poppelaars

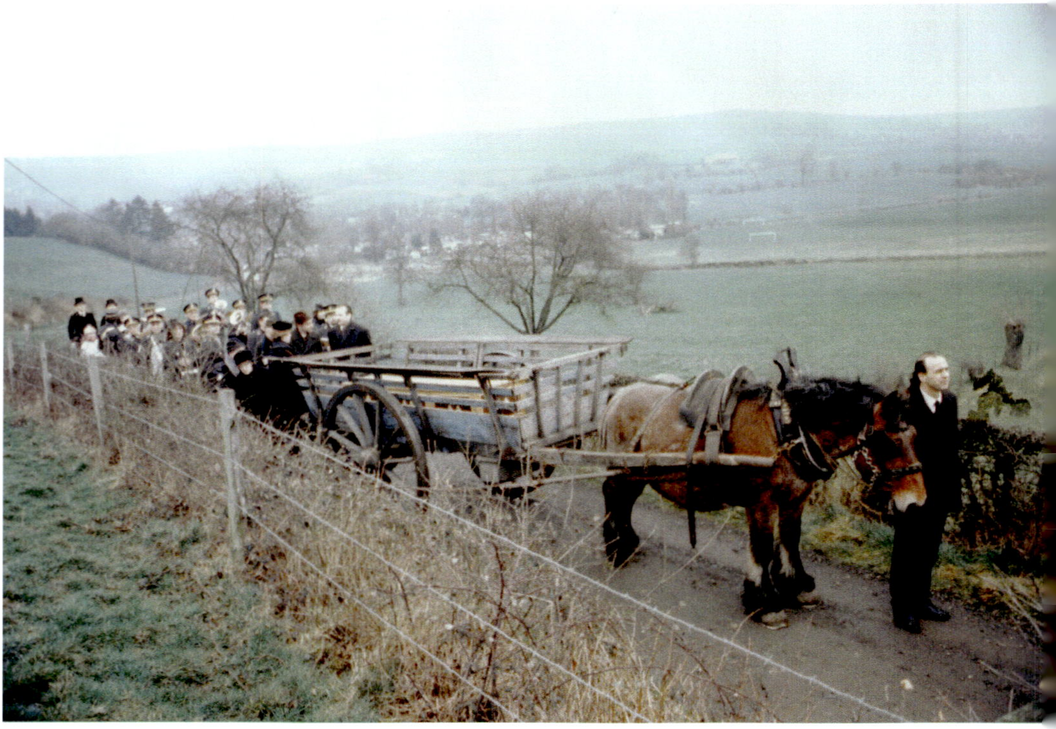

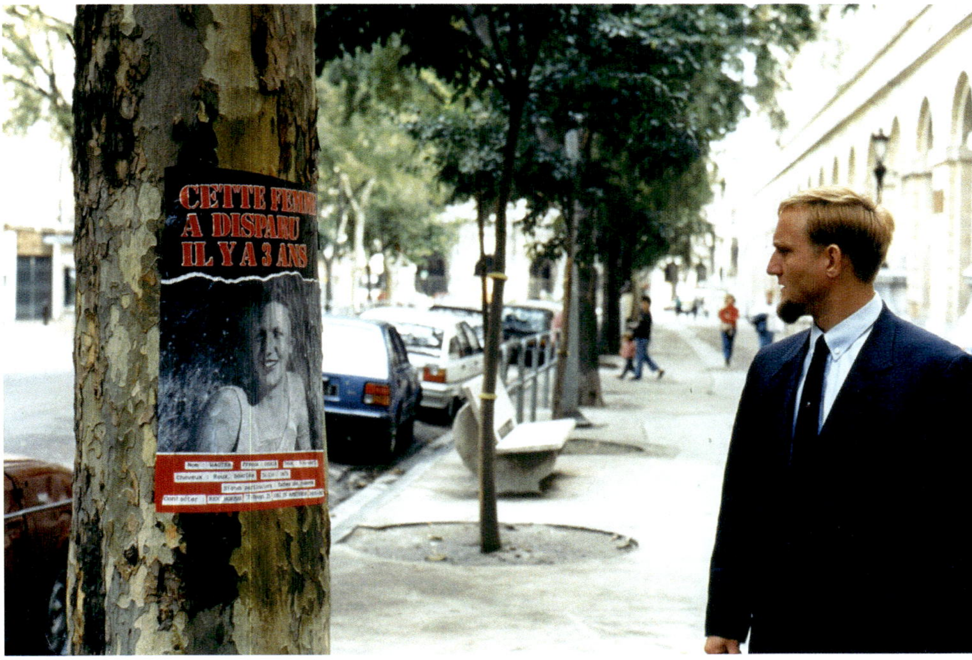

Plate 24
SPOORLOOS [Bernard-Pierre Donnadieu]
© Stoneraft Films BV. Photo: Jutka Rona.

Plate 25
GLUCKAUF [Vincent van der Valk, Bart Slegers]
© Bind Film. Photo: Ivo de Bruin

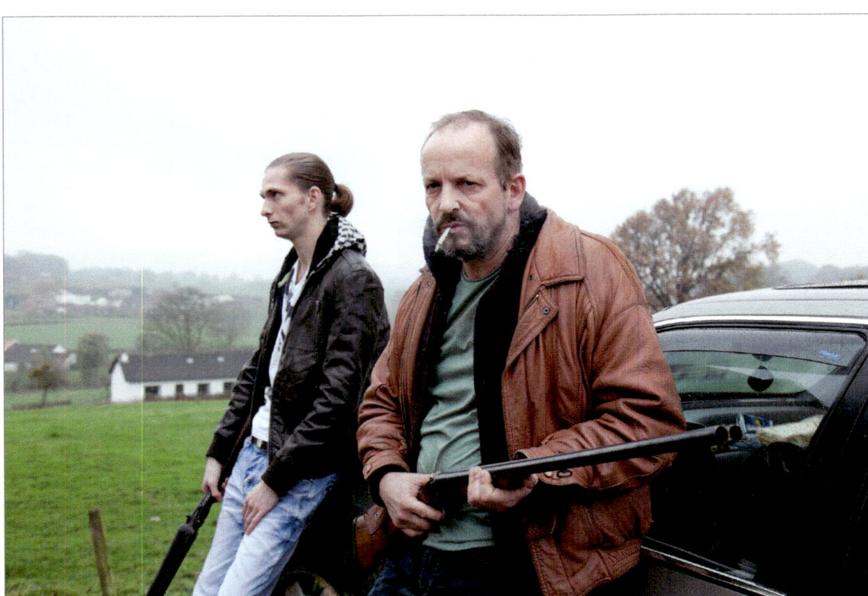

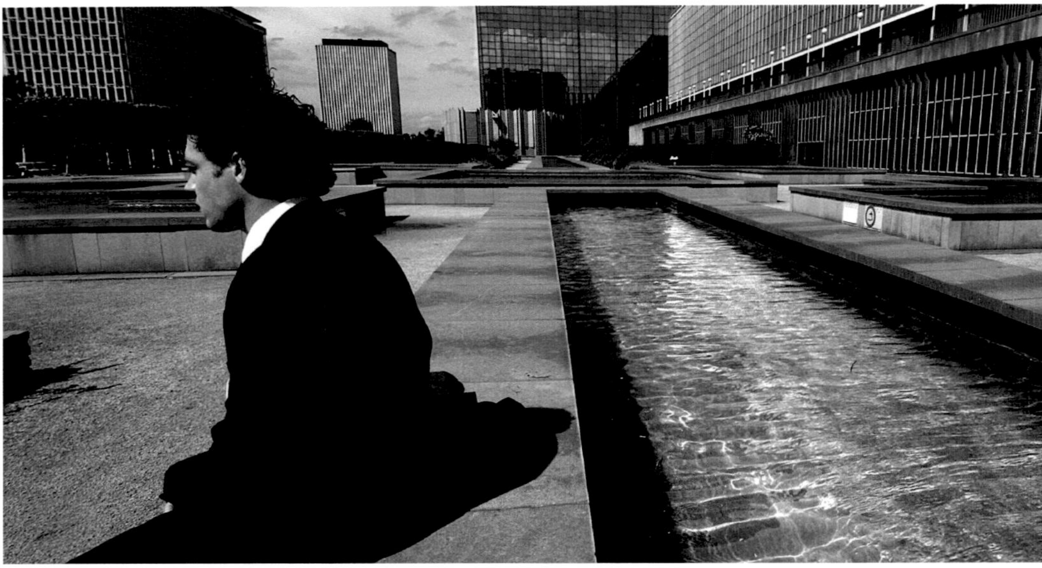

Plate 26
Wereld van stilstand [Fedja van Huêt] © Accento Films.

Plate 27
Wolf [Marwan Kenzari, Michael Knaap] © New Amsterdam Film Company.

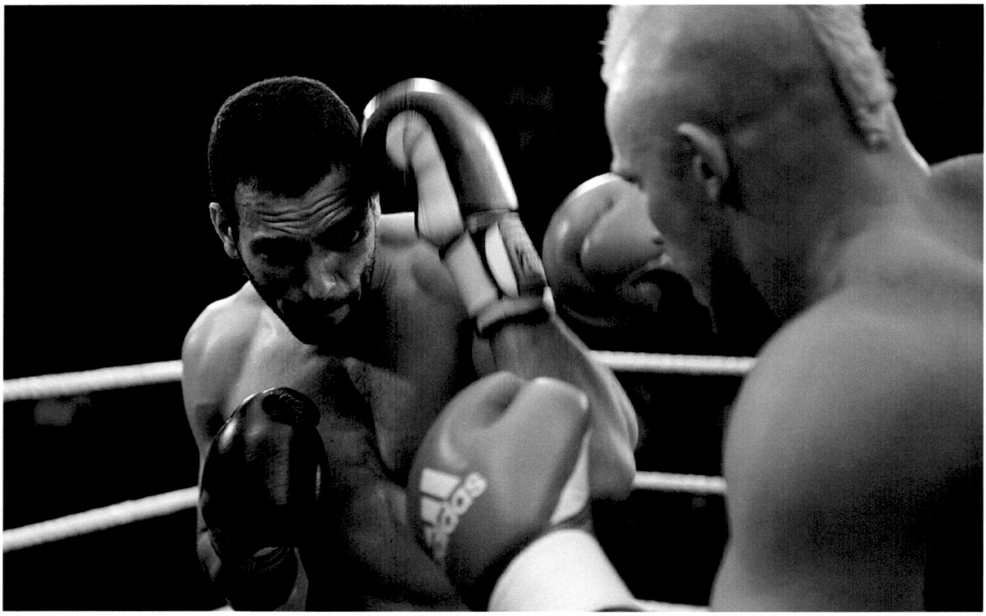

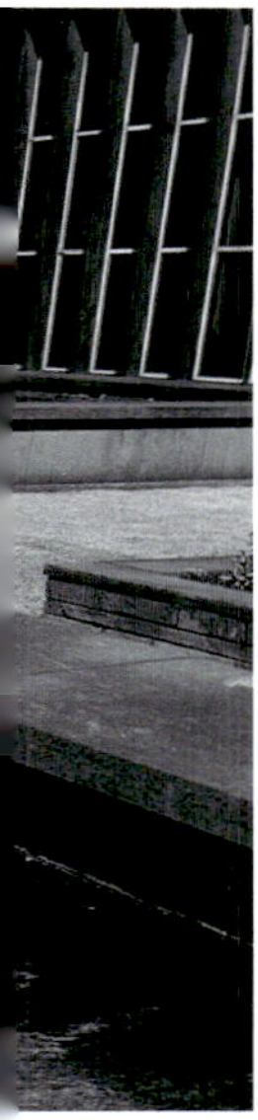

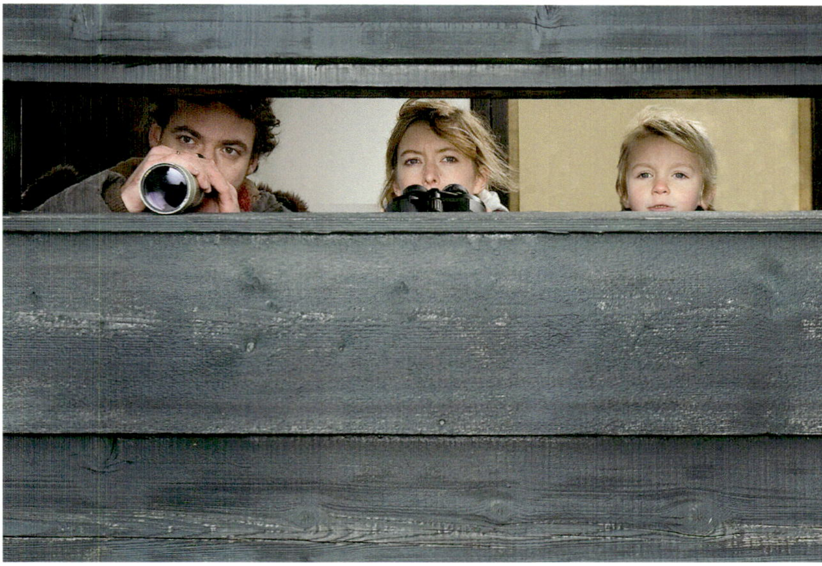

Plate 28
GUERNSEY [Fedja van Huêt, Maria Kraakman, Sonho Vischschraper] © Circe Films.

Plate 29
BOVEN IS HET STIL [Jeroen Willems, Henri Garcin] © Circe Films.
Photo: Victor Arnolds

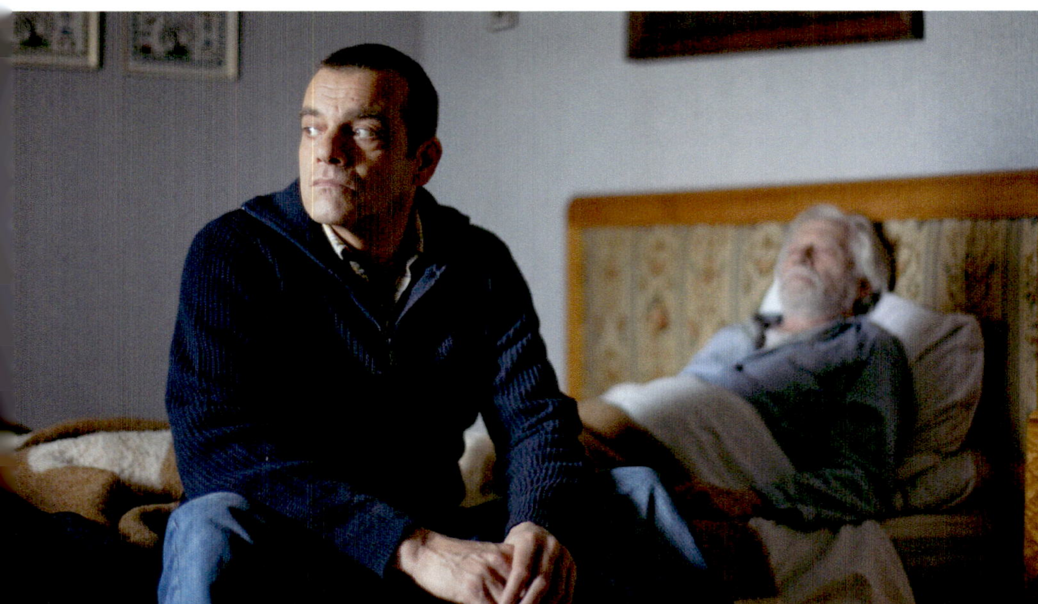

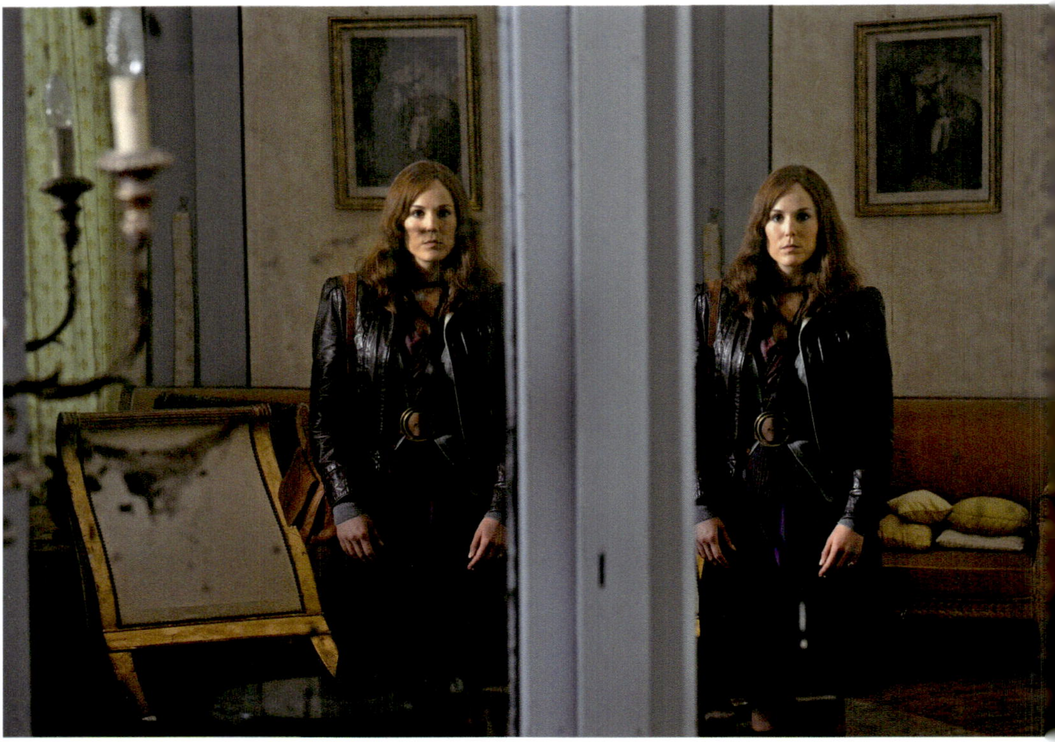

Plate 30
ZWART WATER [Hadewych Minis] © Accento Films. Photo: René de Haan

Plate 31
HET ZWIJGEN [Huib Broos, Vincent Croiset] © The Film Kitchen.

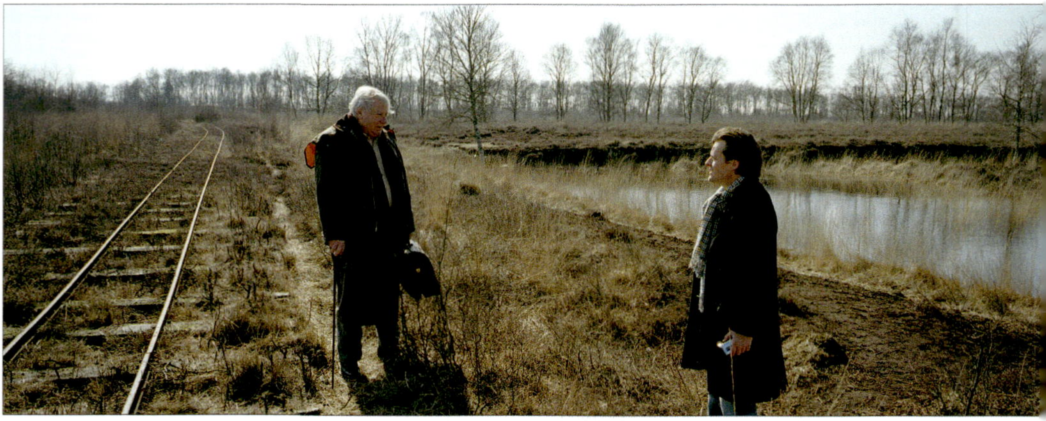

CHAPTER 5

Paranoia, Psychosis, The Horrific-Fantastic

Verstraten, P., *Dutch Post-War Fiction Film Through a Lens of Psychoanalysis*. Taylor & Francis Group, 2021
DOI 10.5117/9789463725330_CH05

ABSTRACT

The fifth chapter examines films in which characters no longer have a firm footing in 'reality'. It pits Rademakers' MIJN VRIEND against Maas's horror-thriller DE LIFT to claim how a story can benefit from a bit of paranoia. Whereas the protagonist in PARANOIA becomes deranged because he thinks he resembles a wanted war criminal, the woman in the early feminist classic VAN DE KOELE MEREN DES DOODS falls victim to an oppressive culture dominated by Calvinism and 'male wisdom'. Most of these characters ask themselves epistemological questions such as 'How can I interpret the chaotic world to which I belong?' Such a question tips over into ontological concerns: 'Does the world of which I think I am part, exist or not? Am I a figment of someone's imagination?'

KEYWORDS
Paranoia and psychosis – Hysteria – Epistemological and Ontological Questions – Todorov's the Fantastic – Nederhorror

At the very end of Mijn vriend: Het verborgen leven van Jules Depraeter [The Judge's Friend] (Fons Rademakers, 1979), the main protagonist Jules Depraeter looks into the camera and says triumphantly: 'They believed me.' Jules had just heard the verdict of the judge and the jury: he was sentenced to fifteen years in prison, but his 'good friend', the inquiry judge John Jenssens, was sentenced to no less than twenty years. Their accounts contradicted each other so completely that it was impossible for them both to have interpreted events accurately. 'They believed me' can imply that Jules' testimony was validated because it was closer to the 'truth', or it could mean his story was more convincing to the jury. I will refrain from any comparisons to the real-life case, widely covered in the Belgian press in 1978, but if one is to follow Rademakers' presentation of events leading up to the courtroom drama, the conclusion seems inevitable: Jules is a liar and a cheater, and the inquiry judge made some unfortunate choices, partly out of gullibility. Due to Jules' vibrant personality and his smooth talk, the sheepish judge was framed. The purport of Mijn vriend is unmistakable: the judicial system can do injustice to a suspect. The fact that there is a conflict between the letter of the law and the viewer's sense of justice has offered building blocks for many a fine tragedy.

Because of the huge media attention surrounding the actual sentencing, Rademakers had expected Mijn vriend, which premiered some 14 months after, to become an instant box-office success, perhaps not in the Netherlands but definitely in Belgium. It did not work out that way: the critical reception of the film can be summed up as lukewarm at best, and no more than 50,000 cinemagoers went to see the film in the Netherlands, which was disappointing for Rademakers. He and his scriptwriter Gerard Soeteman had attended the trial for six weeks, and the two were angered by the verdict that had put the blame on the inquiry judge. Nonetheless, the film did not end up an 'angry' picture; on the contrary, the entire court case is presented as so ludicrous that Mijn vriend is a comedy rather than a tragedy, much to the dismay of Soeteman, Bernink notes. Originally, Soeteman had written a script that made the viewer wonder whether the main character Jules is a pathological liar and knows this or whether he really believes in his own cunning scenarios. But since Soeteman's script was considered too lengthy, Rademakers omitted a number of scenes, which had the effect of changing the film's tone (Bernink, 121). Jules is represented as a cheerful guy who derives much pleasure from his role as master manipulator. The fact that his primary victim, the judge, is a prominent member of the bourgeoisie in Ghent only increases his pleasure. Due to Faber's flamboyant characterization of the main protagonist, Jules remains conscious throughout the film that he is deceiving other people. He is perfectly capable of distinguishing his fanciful fiction from the actual state of affairs. At no point in Rademakers' film does Jules give credence to his own fabrications. If, however, the film had followed the original script and Jules started to believe in his own fictions and thus display some features of a psychotic who had difficulty separating delusions from actual events, then MIJN VRIEND would have been a more intriguing—and perhaps also more successful—film.

One of the many things I like about DE LIFT (Dick Maas, 1983), a successful horror-thriller with some humorous moments, is when the protagonist, mechanic Felix Adelaar, meets with his predecessor Breuker, a man who used to work as an engineer for the elevator company Deta Liften. There have been several fatal malfunctions, because the elevator in an apartment building of fifteen floors has been going up and down inexplicably, resulting in several casualties. Felix wants to ask Breuker whether he has noticed peculiar details, but Breuker has been locked up in a psychiatric facility. Felix hears from Breuker's nurse that he is always sitting in a chair in the middle of a room, for he is 'afraid of walls'. The patient also injured both his hands, for he had tried to demolish the television screen with his bare hands. Breuker, who is on tranquilizers, does not utter a single word during Felix's brief visit but only stares at him with a puzzled scowl on his face. As soon as another patient throws a cup of chocolate custard against the wall, however, Breuker looks at the dripping custard in shock, his eyes wide open, in close-up. A next shot shows his hands trembling. After Felix has consulted a professor who explains to him that computer-driven machinery can go out of control due to the sensitivity of microprocessors, he goes to investigate the elevator at night. In the end, Felix discovers a transparent box containing a pulsating gooey silicon chip, and since this slimy stuff resembles the custard that was thrown against the wall, he understands that he must eliminate the box. Thus, his reading of a psychotic's physical reaction led Felix on the right track to neutralize the mischief. Or so it seems, for towards the end of the end credits, we hear the sound of the chip's beating again, as if it is still active somehow.[1]

In pitting the scene with the dazed and confused Breuker in DE LIFT to the portrayal of the sly chatterbox Jules in MIJN VRIEND, I aim to make a point about why the brief interlude in Maas's horror was so functional in terms of plot. The encounter with the paranoid former engineer was necessary for Felix to solve the enigma: he could gain control over the elevator because he was capable of reading Breuker's delusion in hindsight. Such narrative tension is lacking in MIJN VRIEND because Jules is like a puppeteer, pulling the strings until the very end: 'They believed me.' In short, the quality of a film is sometimes better served by a bit of paranoia than an excess of narcissistic desire. I hope to prove this by analyzing a number of films, including Adriaan Ditvoorst's debut feature, Nouchka van Brakel's fine adaptation of a fin-de-siècle novel about an unfortunate woman, a British-Dutch co-production on the life and times of the famous paranoiac Daniel Paul Schreber, and a grotesque *nederhorror* movie about deranged brothers in search of their little sister.

A KILLER IN THE CANALS: *AMSTERDAMNED*

Together with melancholia and schizophrenia, paranoia falls under the category of 'psychosis'. In his short essay 'Neurosis and Psychosis' from 1924, Freud claims that a neurosis is the consequence of a conflict between the ego and the id. Let us presume that a son wants to love his mother like his father does, but a cultural taboo forbids the boy this privilege. No matter how powerful, the son's ego has to refuse to accept this instinctual impulse. Commanded by the superego which is the container of influences from the external world, the ego defends itself by repressing the impulse, but any repressed element returns in a distorted form. This counterforce to the ego's defence creates an 'unwelcome' leftover—the symptom. In continually resisting the symptom as this substitutive compromise, the picture of a neurosis is produced. In the case of a neurosis, the ego has set a repression in motion, since it favours the demands from an external world over the impulses of the id: regardless of his love for his mother, the son will not engage in sexual intercourse with her.

Whereas the ego sides with the external world in the case of a neurosis, the ego's relationship with the external world is disturbed in the case of a psychosis because the ego is not able to silence the id but is overtaken by its impulses. When the id usurps the ego, the subject's relation to the external world becomes obscure, and hallucinations are given free rein. Judging from his changing terminology, Freud did not really know how to qualify psychosis: sometimes he spoke of repression and other times of disavowal or rejection. When Lacan elaborates on Freud's vision, he prefers the last term. According to Lacan, a psychotic has refused to accept the Name-of-the-Father as the master signifier that marks the entry into the symbolic order. This entrance implies that the forced choice between 'meaning' and 'being' has already been decided in favour of the former: One has sacrificed one's 'being' for a place in a field of signifiers. The price to pay for this subjection is the inability to express one's uniqueness. In answer to the question 'Who are you?', one has only a few poor words at one's disposal such as the term 'I', but this personal pronoun is interchangeable, for everyone else also uses this term to refer to him/herself. One's first name is not of much help either, for I do not share any essential feature with other people named 'Peter'. If one's first name is not totally arbitrary, it may have been given to you to honour some ancestor—and thus it has symbolic value. Like one's surname, it ensures that one is part of a family tradition.

Lacan examines the predetermined outcome of the choice between 'meaning' and 'being' in analogy to the choice between 'your money or your life': any rational person will give away the money, for if not, he will lose both (*Four Fundamental Concepts*, 212). The psychotic, however, hangs on to the illusion that he did not give up 'being' for 'meaning', and hence he is excluded from the symbolic circuit. His advantage is that he is not under the spell of signifiers, but this route is not as attractive as it may sound. The psychotic's stubbornness does not prepare him for a fortunate trajectory at all. By refusing to accept the 'bad' option of *le père* (the Name-of-the-Father), he is condemned to *le pire* (the worse) (Žižek *Enjoy*, 74-77). The word 'I' is irrelevant to him: in presuming that he is not symbolically castrated, for he does not lack in 'being', he has no need of 'I' as the substitute signifier for 'being'. As an outsider to the symbolic circuit, he does not have to acknowledge a number of cultural demands either: thus, the psychotic can come across as a loose cannon.

Without claiming that the perpetrator in the action-horror film AMSTERDAMNED (Dick Maas, 1988) should be diagnosed as a psychotic, this 'maniac' (according to the end credits) is nonetheless structurally positioned as one. He is present by his absence throughout Maas's movie: we have several point-of-view shots of him, usually taken just above the water in the canals. We can only surmise this from his heavy breathing and a musical theme. At one point the soundtrack suggests that he is approaching a salvation army soldier in a street of Amsterdam. When the woman suddenly looks over her shoulder, we expect to see him in a reverse shot, but there is no one. In a few other scenes, we presume he is near, but he occupies off-screen space and thus is never anchored as an 'I' in the film. The 'maniac' is an internal focalizor in several shots but not an object of focalization, which is a prerequisite for the viewer's identification. We only get glimpses of him during the spectacular speedboat chase in the canals, when he is pursued by main protagonist Erik Visser, but he is unrecognizable, wearing a diving suit with goggles.

It is only at the denouement of the film that we get some background information, but not from the psycho-killer himself but rather from his friend, the psychiatrist Martin Ruysdael. He tells the police that the man—a name is never given, as if to signify that he is no longer symbolically integrated—used to be a very experienced diver who had to salvage a ship three years ago. He was not told that there were barrels with chemical contents on board, and when one of them began to leak, the friend's face was severely mutilated. He became completely estranged from Martin, and moreover, the radioactive material had affected his brain. After a crosscut scene in which the diver unveils his gruesome face and stares at some pictures, the shrink continues his story. The police conclude that the man wanted to take revenge on society by making innocent people pay. Just as the police arrive at his place, he shoots an arrow through his head.[2] So, the only moments we see the killer alive on-screen are sandwiched between scenes in which he is being told about. Moreover, Martin has little more to say than that he has become a total outcast and that his actions are beyond any frame of comprehension, even for an experienced psychiatrist. And since the mutilated diver is never integrated into the symbolic network, as if he has not submitted himself to the order of 'meaning', he is labelled a 'maniac', a psychotic. The killer in AMSTERDAMNED has been transformed into a terrifying apparition who hides his gruesome face.[3] He is an external object, whereas PARANOIA (Adriaan Ditvoorst, 1967) presents a psychotic 'from within'. In this film, the symbolic network drives the protagonist crazy because he tends to over-interpret signs.[4]

EXISTENTIAL ISOLATION: *PARANOIA*

In the mid-1960s, Ditvoorst was considered the 'golden boy' of Dutch cinema. A promising future seemed to await this alumnus of the Film Academy, for he had received accolades from Jean-Luc Godard and Bernardo Bertolucci for his *nouvelle vague* inspired short film IK KOM WAT LATER NAAR MADRA [THAT WAY TO MADRA] (1965) at international film festivals. The successor to this 22-minute short, which was one of the sixteen titles included in the official Dutch film canon, was PARANOIA. This debut feature is one of those 1960s films that can be considered Dutch attempts to affiliate oneself with European art cinema. One can make specific pairs, as I already suggested in the Introduction: HET GANGSTERMEISJE and Fellini's OTTO E MEZZO; EEN OCHTEND VAN ZES WEKEN and Lelouch's UN HOMME ET UNE FEMME; DE DANS VAN DE REIGER and Resnais' L'ANNÉE DERNIÈRE À MARIENBAD. In the case of PARANOIA, its closest ally would be Roman Polanski's REPULSION (1965).[5]

PARANOIA was based on the eponymous story by W.F. Hermans. This may have seemed logical, for Ditvoorst greatly admired the one existing picture that had been inspired by Hermans' work (see Introduction). Though the initial friendship between Rademakers and Hermans had ended in bickering, Ditvoorst was apparently not disconcerted by Hermans' notorious reputation. This time, the influence of the novelist was relatively restricted. This was for the better, for Hermans considered Ditvoorst a 'pigheaded' director: if you gave him sound advice, Hermans told an interviewer, he only said that if he were to follow it, it would no longer be his film (qtd. in Verdaasdonk, 17).

In the eyes of Hermans, PARANOIA was a 'good' adaptation with 'stirring' parts and adequate acting, though its rhythm was 'tedious' at times (ibid., 17). Hermans' comment is worth quoting for the specific argument he gives to explain his problem with the film's prolixity. According to Hermans, a viewer tends to fall asleep when confronted with fragments in a film that are redundant to the story, whereas a reader does not bother about extensive and irrelevant passages. In other words, unlike a film, it is permissible for a novel to lack a clear narrative drive or to not be very suspenseful. Actually, Hermans' long story 'Paranoia', written in 1948, is a good example. Arnold Cleever believes that his landlord Gorraay wants to evict him from the rooms he is renting, and on top of this, after reading a police bulletin about an escaped SS man in a newspaper, he thinks the police are looking for him. He decides to hole up in his place and locks his girlfriend Anna in an adjacent room. When Gorraay threatens to throw Arnold's stuff out onto the street, Arnold shoots him on the staircase. He then jumps from his window onto the tramrails. This relatively simple plot is predominantly focussed on Arnold: the external narrator has made himself subservient to the vision of the character. The narrator does not tell what the state of affairs really is but only relates how Arnold sees events. In crucial passages, the narrator even uses the device of free indirect discourse: the narrator's phrasing is couched in the words of a character, or the narrator will paraphrase something the protagonist says or thinks without using quotation marks. When Arnold sees the photograph of the wanted SS man in the newspaper, for example, the narrator says: 'There was his own portrait! That was him! Those were his very own sad eyes, his own cruel and gloomy mouth!'[6]

We might surmise that the narrator is reading Arnold's deranged mind, but since we never get a clear external perspective, we never know to what extent it is deranged. The caption says that the escaped man is called 'C.D. van Maanen', with the narrator adding: 'One of the many pseudonyms he had used.'[7] This can be true, but it can also not be true. It can be a fact in the sense that Arnold presumes this is a pseudonym he has used in the past. In reading Arnold's thoughts, the narrator has omitted the fact that Arnold believes this and presents his ideas as mere fact. The newspaper item mentions that the wanted man 'can only speak with a whispering voice as a consequence of shellshock'.[8] Arnold was reading the article while waiting for his uncle to meet him. This uncle, who has not seen his nephew for a long time, is surprised by Arnold's hoarse voice. It is a consequence of the war, the latter whispers. But a few pages later, when Arnold's girlfriend Anna visits him, she asks him what is wrong with his voice. He does not reply, but the narrator observes: 'How odd she never had observed the peculiarity of his voice before! She always forgot about everything!'[9] It is highly likely that Arnold has started to speak with a whispering voice after reading the newspaper article to make it fit the description. Apart from his uncle who runs a business of gathering photographs as evidence in delicate affairs, he seems to believe the entire world is conspiring against him: his landlord, people outside talking about him, voices coming from behind a door. Objects are sizzling all the time at him: meat in a frying pan, the steam machine in a factory, a dripping drainpipe—they all make the sound of 'es-esser, es-esser' (Hermans 'Paranoia', 44). And even his girlfriend is not to be trusted because she was not there when he needed her the most.

In arguing that the plot of this 42-page-long story is too thin for an interesting feature-length film, Hermans did not understand that for Ditvoorst, the plot is subordinated to a film's style and atmosphere. The main storyline is similar to the book from which the film is adapted: Arnold's problems with the landlord, imagined or not, and his delusion that he is the lookalike of the man in the news are the key motivations for his idiosyncratic behaviour, such as locking Anna up in a room, shooting the landlord, and falling from his window into the street. In Ditvoorst's film, Arnold's paranoid interpretation of the photograph gains more emphasis. He goes to the mirror and combs his hair in a way that makes him resemble the wanted SS man a bit more. In a later scene, Anna looks for the paper to prove he is mistaken. Once again, we see the picture, but it is a slightly different one. This can only imply that in the first scene, we did not see the actual photograph but rather one that was envisioned by Arnold: he imagined that the picture resembled him.

As soon as we realize that all realistic shots might be tainted by Arnold's delusion, the entire film PARANOIA becomes ambiguous, and the many unorthodox devices contribute to this effect. In the prologue, there is a soldier on a train platform, the camera on the other side of the rail tracks. The camera pans with him as he walks; we only hear a rooster crow. In the second shot he keeps walking up and down the platform, but because the camera remains static, he is off-screen now and then. With every transition, the screen goes black for a very brief timespan. In the fourth shot, a lengthy one, the camera is at quite a distance from him, and the rail tracks constitute more than half of the shot. He is on the right in the upper part of the frame; he starts reading a book but then tears some of its pages. Most of the scene is in total silence: it is only after two minutes that we hear a church bell toll, the second sound after the rooster. After almost three minutes, music starts playing softly but increases in volume and becomes quite loud, when there is a shot transition, no black in between this time. With a swish pan to the left, the camera registers the arrival of a train. There is a transition to a book cover of *Robinson Crusoe*, while we hear the whistle of a train conductor. As soon as we hear the departure of a train, we see a postcard sent by 'Arnold' to 'Arnold Cleever', which is shown for

43 seconds, allowing us to read for ourselves the handwritten text. As we read about his fear and his uniform which smells like mothballs, we suddenly hear four rifle shots that disrupt the sound of a moving train; then silence again. We then see him a few years later enter a music store, from a high-angle. The music is loud, but suddenly it is silent again, whereupon Arnold says, while holding a record: 'May I listen to this?' His voice rings unnaturally clear in the absence of any surround sound. When he puts on the record and sits back to listen, we only hear automatic gunfire. Almost six minutes into PARANOIA, the opening credits start while the camera shoots through the window of a travelling train, accompanied by uplifting guitar music. This continues for about three minutes until it suddenly falls silent at a brusque transition to a closed door.

These first nine minutes of PARANOIA, with superb black-and-white cinematography by Jan de Bont, prepare us for many of the devices used in the remainder of the film: sound and image can be asynchronous; sound transitions can go from loud noise to silence; the framing can be deliberately awkward, such as when his head is at the bottom of the shot; we see a character, but the next shot can show her from the back, which comes close to a violation of the 180 degrees rule; the camera can switch from close to a high-angle shot; we see Arnold through a window, but this is like a superimposition, for we see the outside world mirrored in the window; at one point, there is also an overly lit scenery; and perhaps most striking, the camera makes a full circle in his apartment, and when it is about to make another circle, it stops at Anna. All these devices may give the impression of style for style's sake, but that would not do justice to Ditvoorst's film.

In his film, Ditvoorst relies on the principle of indirect 'point-of-view shots'. In the case of a literal, or direct, 'point-of-view shot', we see what the character sees: the camera coincides with his eyes. If he were to suddenly look around, the camera would do the same. The indirect version would have the camera imitate the vision of a character. Blurred contours, sudden shifts in focus, or awkwardly framed shots can then be taken as an expression of a confused state of mind. Strictly speaking, many shots are externally focalized since the protagonist is depicted on screen, but these shots are 'tainted' by character-bound focalization. That is to say, the external narrator conforms himself to the vision of the protagonist. In other words, the narrator restricts himself to the role of intermediary, and thus the viewer is sucked into the character's paranoid worldview. The cinematography in Ditvoorst's film serves to engage us with the delusory perception of the main protagonist who suffers from a maddening identification with a wanted SS man. Since there is no escaping from the idea that he is the man in the picture in the newspaper, he is in a downward spiral to lunacy. After Arnold shoots the landlord, we hear

Anna's voice, faintly from the adjacent room, calling his name. He puts on his cap and slowly opens the window. The light from outside is bright, and we see him fall over the ledge. He is shown lying on the ground in a top shot, whereupon the camera slowly tilts up and shows the canals opposite his house and its surroundings in a final turn away from the claustrophobic atmosphere in PARANOIA.

In an article on Peter Forgács's film SAJÁT HALÁL [OWN DEATH] (2008), Ernst van Alphen mentions that focalization when confined to one character (as is the case in PARANOIA) has a two-faced nature. On the one hand, it is relational, for when events are presented from a character's perspective, we see how he engages with his direct environment. The viewer is introduced to the protagonist's observation and interpretation of the world. On the other hand, it is striking that such a consistent focalization has all too often an 'isolating' effect'.[10] A character such as Arnold in Ditvoorst's film seems to be imprisoned in his own narrow perspective. In a film such as PARANOIA, the focalization by Arnold emphasizes that he is cut off from his surroundings, causing 'a kind of existential isolation' (Van Alphen, 260). We see the same effect in another great film adaptation, Nouchka van Brakel's VAN DE KOELE MEREN DES DOODS [HEDWIG: THE QUIET LAKES], which is based upon the classic novel from 1900 by Frederik van Eeden.

LADY IN THE LAKE: *VAN DE KOELE MEREN DES DOODS*

Adapting a text by Hermans was a bold move for Ditvoorst. Indeed, his entire career, which includes only five features and four shorts, was a series of bold moves. In my previous study, I briefly described several of his films to provide a context for his boldest step, DE MANTEL DER LIEFDE [THE CLOAK OF CHARITY] (1978) (Verstraten *Humour and Irony*, 311-317), perhaps the most bizarre film in the history of Dutch cinema. One of Ditvoorst's peers at the Film Academy, Nouchka van Brakel, also made only six features, and the four she directed between 1977 and 1987 can be taken as quite daring as well, mostly due to the themes she chose. Her first two pictures are about controversial love affairs: in HET DEBUUT [THE DEBUT] (1977), rated for an 18+ audience, a fourteen-year-old girl has a relationship with a 41-year-old man. In EEN VROUW ALS EVA [A WOMAN LIKE EVE] (1979), a mother of two children has a crying fit on Mother's Day, and her husband Ad arranges for her to go on a train trip to France together with her best friend Sonja. During her holidays, 'Eefje'—the hypocorism Ad uses for her—is enamoured by the lesbian Liliane who lives in a commune in rural France. She introduces herself as 'Eefje, meaning little Eva', but Liliane only wants to call her 'Eva'. When she tells Ad she has fallen in love with a woman, he considers it merely a 'passing fad'. After she actually sleeps with Liliane, Ad becomes furious, and from that moment onwards Eva begins to receive condescending looks not only from him but also from her environment. She responds to the prejudices by saying that one cannot stop an avalanche. Her husband claims custody over the two children, and the final verdict is in his favour.

In EEN VROUW ALS EVA, the husband seems generous and open-minded, at least at first: if his wife feels depressed, she deserves a holiday, and he tells her he will take care of the household. The problem, however, is that he expects Eefje to return as her 'old self'. As Liliane's lover, however, she wants to explore a new-found freedom, and the more her immediate surroundings attempt to confine her desires, the more stubborn Eva becomes in pursuing her personal happiness.

Whereas Van Brakel's first two films focus on contemporary situations, her third feature—VAN DE KOELE MEREN DES DOODS (1982)—was set in the past. This film about a nineteenth-century woman from an upper-class background is the crowning achievement of her career because the film functions as a projection screen for the dilemmas that the contemporary protagonists from Van Brakel's other pictures have to face. Dutch films from the 1970s are marked by a certain bluntness—characters who talk straight, who curse, who yell at each other—that can make viewers cringe, but in VAN DE KOELE MEREN DES DOODS, Van Brakel decided to use the ornate and archaic language of Van Eeden's novel from 1900. In an interview she said: 'Because one is confronted with the linguistic music of the past, with a stylized detachment, it is easier to feel sympathy for the characters and their emotions.'[11]

VAN DE KOELE MEREN DES DOODS starts in Merwestee in 1882 with a woman, clad in a dark dress with a shawl over her head. She is in the woods near a lake caressing a tree when a solemn text is printed on screen: 'How she searched for Death's cool lakes, where salvation is ... and how she found it.' The camera zooms in to a close-up of her face, and in a reverse shot we can discern a villa, partly covered in fog. In a subsequent shot, she casts her eyes down, and the fume above the land—this time created by torches—evaporates, showing the very same villa thirteen years earlier, during a garden party. The atmosphere seems joyful, but at one point, a young girl in a white dress runs into the woods slightly exasperated and starts to caress a tree with her eyes closed: 'It's me ... Hedwig ... Hedwig ... Marga ... de Fontayne.' She repeats her first name once more, but then she has a nauseating look all of a sudden and starts to puke. It is a puzzling start to a long flashback that will last almost the entire film, for it is only near the very end that we return to the older Hedwig walking towards the lake.[12] The opening is so enigmatic because her subdued ecstasy turns into immediate sickness after she slowly pronounces her own name to no one in particular. It seems an affirmation of her insertion into the symbolic order, and as the daughter in an upper-class family, she is supposed to behave according to a strict etiquette. Cut to a long travelling shot through a large room illustrating the family's wealth that ends with Hedwig in bed behind a white, transparent veil. She has typhus, just like her mother who is now in the comforting company of God, her father tells her. The camera moves around the veil, showing Hedwig frontally, and we see her lingering over the thought of her mother being with God. She has closed her eyes and without any cut, we see a shadow loom over Hedwig's bed and caress her forehead. While the camera zooms in, we see her mother near her bedside reading from the first chapter of *Alice in Wonderland*, in English. The brightly lit scene ends with the words: '*... Alice had begun to think that very few things indeed were really impossible.*'

Insofar as Hedwig's mother teaches her daughter to identify with the inventive Alice, the next scene shows that the mother's premature demise cuts short any realm of imagination. During dinner in a dark and gloomy room, her father tells Hedwig that she has to obey the governess who is opposed to sinful novels such as *Alice in Wonderland*. This prohibition against reading Lewis Carroll sets the stage for the tragedy: Hedwig has inherited her mother's free-spirited nature, but due to her mother's death she has been confined to the devout rules of Calvinism. Hedwig is unable to cope with conflicting demands. She is too naïve to acknowledge how much the artist Johan is in love with her, but still the governess calls her coquettish and sensual. She thinks it will please the family if she marries Gerard, a student of law, who has a decent and prosperous career ahead as a notary. But as a repressed homosexual, Gerard cannot perform his masculine duties. She then has a romantic liaison with the piano player Ritsaart who calls himself Richard Delmonte, and as often in a melodrama, no one but a musician knows how to interpret female desires. After a first kiss, she is confused because they have disgraced 'the holy illusion' of matrimony. Soon she switches from the symbolic to the imaginary: the affair implies that the 'mystery' has revealed itself, as she tells herself while naked in front of a full-length mirror: this is the dreamt-of unity between man and woman, to be enjoyed in private. Richard reactivates symbolic values, however. She may deny her marriage because it has never been 'consumed', but legally and in the public eye, she is Gerard's wife and an artist's lover.

A most interesting shot ensues. There is a pan to the right, and we see Hedwig writing a letter. In her voice-over, we hear that it is a farewell note to Richard because it is her duty to remain faithful to Gerard. While the camera keeps panning to the right without a cut, showing a caged canary along the way, we hear Gerard's voice. We first see Hedwig in the mirror and then Gerard reading another letter written by his wife and addressed to Richard: I hope you will keep our bond sacrosanct and that I may die soon. The combination of sound and image neatly comments upon Hedwig's restricted freedom of movement. Initially, she expresses herself in her letter, but while the camera continues to pan to the right, her words are soon recited by her husband in a disapproving tone. Hence her writings become embedded in a narrative determined by a culture of men. Gerard thinks it is a silly note, but if she wants to enjoy this pure and spiritual friendship, he has no problems with that. She replies, however, that he is mistaken: she belongs to Ritsaart because he has introduced her to the mystery of marriage. Her words of desire are superseded once again: upon hearing this confession, Gerard considers it his duty to kill his rival. Face to face with Ritsaart, Gerard hesitates to shoot, but at that moment the housemaid shouts that water is coming down the wall: Hedwig has cut one of her wrists in the bathtub. The two men both cooperate to save her life, and when Hedwig then whispers Ritsaart's name, Gerard decides to leave for three days so the two have sufficient time to disappear for good.

Richard's reputation as a pianist grows and Hedwig joins him on a concert tour, where she meets people from the ranks of the aristocracy. She then commits the 'greatest folly', according to Richard, when she discloses to a gossiping lady that she is not Richard's wife but only his mistress. After this confession by Hedwig, Richard fears he will no longer be invited to play at concerts. In the next scene, about a year later, they are married, Hedwig is pregnant, and Richard is feeling nervous because he will finally perform again after a long and unplanned break. Rather than a period of happiness, this is a prelude to impending disaster. While her husband is away, a baby girl is born, but according to the doctor, Charlotte is too weak to survive. Hedwig herself suffers from childbed psychosis, and after she has tidied herself, she takes some jewels and puts her baby in a travel bag, on her way to Holland. The moment she steps outside her residence, the screen turns totally white for a few seconds. We hear the sound of waves, and when the camera pans to the left we see Hedwig on the back of a ship, bathing in blinding light.

This overwhelming whiteness marks that by leaving home—departing from both Ritsaart and the doctor—she is at the mercy of the people she meets on the way. At the quay in Calais, France she throws herself at the feet of a total stranger and asks him for forgiveness: 'Would you like to take the poor sinner back?' The men at the quay do not understand her Dutch and think she is drunk. But the stranger, whom she mistakes for Gerard, decides to take her to a brothel. Upon arrival, the place elicits a laugh from Hedwig: this must be a funfair in hell. She thinks she is about to make love to Gerard and she calls his name repeatedly, but the man is only keen on taking her travel bag after having robbed her of her money already. As soon as the man gets hold of the bag, Hedwig becomes so furious that the brothel's madam requests him to put her on the train. Hedwig believes that 'Gerard' is to join her on her trip to Holland, but when the train starts to leave, he jumps out with the travel bag in his arms. Hedwig screams out loud: 'Charlotte!' as the train to Paris departs into a still overwhelming whiteness.

When the camera shows her from the back, we suddenly hear voices we have heard before: the priest, the governess, the doctor, Johan. It is clear that Hedwig hears these voices in her head, for she turns around and is cornered in the seat of her compartment. Tears well up in her eyes, for the comments are accusatory. While we still see Hedwig in medium close-up, Charlotte's cries are heard. Hedwig's face suddenly floods in white light, and she covers her eyes with her hands. The screen goes black for about eight seconds, with the sounds of a train on the soundtrack, and in the next shot she is put in a straitjacket in a mental institution. She is then stripped naked in her cell, and while the camera looks through the small window of the door like the doctor, Hedwig, who we see now has closely cropped hair, has a hysterical outburst in a shot that lasts about 90 seconds. The doctor tells the nurse that he is amazed that such a fragile beauty still has so much energy after six weeks. He adds that though she has had a good upbringing, she does not behave accordingly. This scene is key to VAN DE KOELE MEREN DES DOODS, for in the so-called 'melodramas of the unknown woman', a medical gaze is seminal to the woman's recovery. In films like NOW, VOYAGER (Irving Rapper, 1942), POSSESSED (Curtis Bernhardt, 1947), JOHNNY BELINDA (Jean Negulesco, 1948), or CAUGHT (Max Ophuls, 1949), as Mary Ann Doane has argued convincingly in *The Desire to Desire*, there is always a doctor or psychiatrist who is able to read the symptoms of the female body. He is able to interpret precisely what is ailing the woman. The mother in NOW, VOYAGER treats her daughter as an ugly duckling, whereas the psychiatrist encourages the daughter to explore her beauty in order to resist her mother's repressive regime.[13] In VAN DE KOELE MEREN DES DOODS, however, this particular psychiatrist is incapable of making a correct diagnosis of Hedwig. She comes from a decent family background and thus her deranged behaviour is a sign of a depraved nature, as if she is a strange anomaly. We come to realize, however, that her hysterical outbursts are precisely the result of her so-called decent family background: this woman, living in the 1870s, has been made into a hysteric, determined by a culture of religious fanaticism and 'male wisdom'.

After the psychiatrist dismisses her from the mental institution, she is far from cured. She had told him her name was 'Jeanne', that she has no past, except that she delivered a baby called Charlotte. She becomes addicted to morphine, and after she is paid for having sex with a man whom she initially took for Ritsaart, she continues to work as a prostitute. She has a brightly lit memory of Ritsaart after another injection with morphine, but that is about the only positive scene before she is hospitalized. The scenes in the hospital do not constitute the final episode of the film, because thereafter she returns to Holland to visit the mortally ill artist Joop, a friend of both Johan and Ritsaart, who always used to describe Hedwig as a 'sphinx'. She sees Ritsaart one more time and says to him: 'I will never be able to break away from you, but I never want to see you again.' Before the flashback ends, she cuts the umbilical cord with her class, for she starts working the land and cooking meals for a farmer's family.

But this final episode in Holland shows that the hypersensitive Hedwig is unable to conform to the strict conventions of a patriarchal society ruled by a Calvinist God and therefore chooses a life on the periphery. This alternative route is suggested in the hospital, where she has a flashback of her mother reading from *Alice in Wonderland* as nurse Paula reassures her that she is now in the midst of great turmoil but that quiet waters will be ahead of her. This nurse, who teaches her that God has not given up on her, is played by the very same actress, Claire Wauthion, who performs the role of Hedwig's mother! The fact that Hedwig takes Paula's persuasive advice seriously should not be taken as a conventional conversion in which His Name is honoured. If her psychosis was the consequence of her refusal to be symbolically anchored in a male-dominated society, we have to see 'God' here as a signifier, putting her at ease with the imaginative domain of Alice 'in which very few thing were really impossible'.

It deserves to be emphasized that this alternative route in VAN DE KOELE MEREN DES DOODS is suggested thanks to the casting of Wauthion in the double role of both nurse Paula and Hedwig's mother. As a consequence, the nurse becomes the mediating character between mother and daughter, creating a chain of female solidarity, but at the same time we should not overestimate this bond. It is a utopian trajectory that prevents Hedwig from committing suicide right away: she has discovered a way—if only temporary—to cope with oppression, but this path in no way announces a new society or world order.

It is tempting to read Van Brakel's next movie, her fourth feature EEN MAAND LATER [A MONTH LATER] (1987), in tandem with VAN DE KOELE MEREN DES DOODS, despite its contemporary setting. EEN MAAND LATER can be regarded as the ultimate experiment in female solidarity. Responding to an advertisement in a newspaper, housewife and mother Liesbeth, married to a psychiatrist, swaps life with the bachelor-journalist Monika, who is 'anti-marriage' but has several lovers. They have agreed that their groundbreaking experiment will last for one month, and after a slow start with some mishaps, the women start to enjoy the change more than they had expected: Liesbeth is free from household obligations, starts singing backing vocals in a band, and meets a number of interesting guys; Monika falls in love with Liesbeth's husband Constant. They decide to extend the period by one more month, but now some tiny cracks reveal themselves. Liesbeth is skiing with Hugo, her rich French lover, but she starts to miss her three children; Monika is still attracted to Constant but is annoyed by her 'motherly' duties. By this time, the children have started to rebel, and daughter Judith in particular is fed up with that 'horny bitch'. Monika goes back to her own place and tells Liesbeth that it did not take her twelve years but only one and a half months to end up in an 'identity crisis'.

Wondering where to go from here, Liesbeth, Hugo, Monika, and Constant meet up for dinner at a restaurant. The two men suggest conservative scenarios: Constant suggests that Monika marry him and get pregnant. Hugo wants to add seven more children to the three kids Liesbeth already has. She can only say: '*Seven more? Over my dead body.*' Then Hugo, who is meeting Monika for the first time, makes a flirtatious remark by offering to bring the journalist home. Monika can only sigh in contempt: '*No, please, that is so cliché: Hugo brought her home and they consoled each other.*' Liesbeth turns away from her lover and asks her husband: '*And what about us?*' It is a key moment in the film. Constant asks Liesbeth to visualize her idea of the future, and she tells him: '*You establish your practice at home, and I became the manager of let's say, 26 antique shops.*' In a medium close-up, Monika immediately replies, with a smile, that all's well that ends well. Over the table, she toasts a glass with Liesbeth, who confirms that the outcome is happy, indeed. In a final shot before the end credits begin to roll, there are fireworks in the dark night.

Van Brakel's entire film can be seen as leading up to Liesbeth's visualization. It is a peculiar scene because the scenario she outlines has an unmistakably utopian dimension for several reasons. First, the men who are both smooth talkers have fallen silent, and the final shots are cut in such a way that they are visually excluded as well. Second, Monika's reply is very prompt. She has no second thoughts and supports Liesbeth's idea unconditionally, even though it means that she will have to sacrifice her current relationship with Constant. Third, the fireworks in the final shot punctuate the fact that the suggested ending is excessively happy and thus unrealistic, since it is only possible if the men were to take on many more domestic obligations than they do right now. Due to the abrupt shift to the fireworks, the men are robbed of the opportunity to respond to Liesbeth's scenario. The oddness of the final scene in Een maand later is interesting because its utopian dimension prevents us from believing in progress: if the situation for women in the 1980s seems better than for women in the 1880s, that change is not fundamental, only cosmetic. Reading Een maand later in tandem with Van de koele meren des doods, Liesbeth's existence is shown to be different from Hedwig's but only slightly so; the parallels are more striking. And this is emphasized even more by the casting, for both Liesbeth and Hedwig are played by Renée Soutendijk.

MEMOIRS OF A NERVE PATIENT: *SHOCK HEAD SOUL*

A psychotic has refused to choose 'I', that is, refused to take up a position in the symbolic order. He (or she—the main protagonist in VAN DE KOELE MEREN DES DOODS was a good example) has renounced the Name-of-the-Father, the fundamental signifier which has no signified. The Name-of-the-Father is strictly symbolic and is not connected to an object but is the 'empty' guardian of the social network. It functions as a guarantee that one has a certain position within the symbolic order: you are known as the son of; at school, you are the brother of; if you have the same surname as a famous cyclist, they will ask whether you are family related, etc. However, in renouncing *le père*, in cutting loose one's ties with the social network, one has no other option than *le pire*. One is no longer an 'I' within a social field, but this 'I' has been exchanged for (objet petit) *a*, the object-cause of desire. Refusing to compromise, the psychotic installs in his delusion a sort of quasi-Name-of-the-Father. In some films, such a fake authority can be relatively conventional, as in VAN DE KOELE MEREN DES DOODS, but in other films, the substitute takes more peculiar forms: the title hero in DONNIE DARKO (Richard Kelly, 2002), diagnosed with paranoid schizophrenia, follows the instructions of a giant rabbit; the nameless protagonist-narrator in FIGHT CLUB (David Fincher, 1999), suffering from insomnia, is mesmerized by the hypermasculine macho Tyler Durden, who will be his guide in life.

The best-known case of an exaggerated quasi-authority in psychoanalysis is the notorious case of Daniel Paul Schreber (1842-1911), formerly the *Senatspräsident* of an Appeal Court in Dresden. Freud had never met Schreber, but he wrote an extensive analysis based on the judge's autobiographical *Denkwürdigkeiten eines Nervenkranken* [*Memoirs of a Nerve Patient*] (1903). Paranoid patients are marked by the habit to reveal '[things] (in a distorted form, it is true) [which] other neurotics keep hidden as a secret' (Freud 'Psycho-analytic Notes', 9). For that reason, Freud considers it legitimate to base his interpretation on the autobiographical account of a patient he had never encountered.

Schreber writes that he had nervous disorders twice as a result of work-related mental overstrain. During the first nervous disorder, he spent six months in professor Flechsig's clinic, a professor who was held in high esteem by both the judge and his wife. Schreber writes of his wife's heartfelt gratitude: she revered Flechsig as the man 'who had restored her husband to her, and hence it was that for years she kept his portrait standing upon her writing-table' (qtd. in Freud 'Psycho-analytic Notes', 12). Some eight years later, he started to suffer from visual and auditory illusions and had to be treated at the clinic again, this time diagnosed with 'hallucinatory insanity'. He thought he was the 'only real man left alive' among the dead (68), and because of this quality, he exerted an attraction upon God, who can only communicate with corpses and who is blinded by His ignorance of human nature. Schreber believed he was able to redeem the world, but this task required him to transform into a woman so that God could impregnate him with divine rays. Enormous numbers of 'female nerves' had already passed over into his body, and 'out of them a new race of men will proceed' (17). God, who Schreber described as 'ridiculous or childish' (27), demands a '*constant state of enjoyment*' from him, and Schreber regarded it his duty to provide Him with this (34, emphasis in original).

In his analysis, Freud explains the crucial role of Flechsig, which is at odds with the detailed account in the official medical report. This professor is the 'first seducer' to whose influence God as his ally has yielded (39). Flechsig, so adored by Schreber's wife, becomes the object of a 'feminine (that is, a passive homosexual) wishful [f]antasy', but due to an internal resistance, the person he longed for turned into his persecutor (47). The professor was then replaced by God, and since a process of decomposition is characteristic of paranoia, further duplications take place. Flechsig recalls the memory of Schreber's late older brother, and God is related to the patient's late father, who was known as an 'eminent physician' (52). He wrote popular textbooks in which his recommended methods of childrearing were widely adopted and used in Germany. Antoine Mooij mentions that Schreber's father was a strict man who demanded his son's respectful submission. He was a narcissistic tyrant who issued orders to be obeyed, and due to his rigid parental techniques, he had been an imaginary father, in the spirit of the obscene father from *Totem and Taboo*, rather than a symbolic father, a fair and just spokesperson of the law (Mooij, 161).

At the root of Schreber's delusions of being impregnated by divine rays is an 'infantile conflict with the father whom he loved' (Freud 'Psycho-analytical Notes', 55), for in a paranoid scenario, an instinct is first fixated and then repressed before it returns in a necessarily different form. The mechanism of Schreber's paranoia can be taken as various 'contradictions of the single proposition: "*I* (a man) *love him* (a man)"' (63). Freud distinguishes four types of contradictions, starting with delusions of persecution: I do not love him—I hate him, because he persecutes me. The second type of contradiction, erotomania, can be summed up as: I do not love him—I love her, because she loves me. The third type consists of delusions of jealousy: It is not I who loves the man—she loves him. And the fourth kind of contradiction is the sexual overvaluation of the ego: I do not love at all—I do not love anyone.

Simon Pummell's SHOCK HEAD SOUL (2011) is not based on Freud's analysis but on Schreber's autobiography. If the film had told the judge's case history, it may have been a 'commendable adaptation', a 'quality film', in the pejorative sense of Truffaut. Pummell's film is a fictional account, but its story is intercut time and again. What is most striking are the talking heads, such as film historian Ian Christie, psychoanalyst Andrea Sabbadini, and psychiatrist Roger Kennedy, who live in current times but are dressed in formal clothes of a bygone era as if they are Schreber's contemporaries. They comment upon the importance of the memoirs but also about the enigmatic chapter three that is removed, allegedly at the request of Schreber's sister. At several points, actors in the role of their character ask questions directly into the camera, and in frontally staged shots, the specialists respond to them. The experts are seated in the very same bench that is used to reconstruct Schreber's case in court. He was called to court to plead for '*his freedom as a psychiatric patient*', as a text in the film mentions, and this plea is based upon his manuscript, about to be published. His idea to write a book was, as he reads aloud in a prepared statement, to '*give the reader the chance to judge whether his so-called delusions are in fact revelations of God's work*'. Schreber is convinced that history will agree with him, and to underscore this conviction, the film inserts quotes from a letter exchange between Carl Gustav Jung and Freud in which the latter suggests that the judge should have been made a professor of psychiatry, indicating that what is presumed to be madness can also be a form of higher wisdom. Moreover, Schreber claims that his notes are his '*private religious beliefs*' and as such do not legitimize confinement, for everyone is entitled to freedom of religion.

Because of all the interruptions, the narrative scenes in SHOCK HEAD SOUL appear to be presented as separate episodes: we see how Schreber's wife Sabine unconditionally supports her husband; we see there is a mutual affection between Sabine and Dr. Flechsig; we see scenes of Schreber in the clinic; upon his return home in the winter of 1902, he meets the adopted teenager Fridoline who is rumoured to be Sabine's illegitimate daughter; and there are also several flashbacks, shot with anamorphic lenses, indicating how harshly Schreber's father treated his son. Sabbadini emphasizes that the father had developed all kinds of devices to control his children: there was '*a sort of torture machine*' to make sure that children would sit up straight, and we see how the young Schreber is subjected to them; the boy is also supposed to recite the prayer of Our Father properly; in another scene, he is forcefully fed in the company of his extremely authoritarian father. This last scene is inserted between fragments from the clinic in which Schreber is fed in the company of Dr. Flechsig, which capitalizes on the analogy between the father and the doctor. In the clinic, Schreber constantly spits out his food while shouting repeatedly

'A Leper Led by Lepers'. Significantly, at the end of SHOCK HEAD SOUL, Schreber's sister visits him after he has been declared cured. She admonishes him to get some rest: '*Your organism is poisoned, toxic.*' She compares this to the condition of their 'poor' father who had worn himself out with his books and his plans for reform, to which Schreber replies: '*But he certainly left his mark on the world. A life devoted to others.*'

Pummell's formal film techniques constitute the nature of the psychotic protagonist. On the one hand, the film has a very calm, almost thoughtful rhythm. In the opening scene, the camera slowly circles around Schreber and his wife for some time while snow falls down in slow motion. The judge tends to speak in a slow manner; his oral presentation is very steady, suggesting that he has a reflexive nature. Ample room is given to the experts to explain the historical relevance of Schreber's case clearly. On the other hand, this apparent tranquillity is alternated with brusque interruptions and distorted representations of space. The structure of Pummell's film is atemporal. Several inserts are a repetition of previous shots. The performance of the actors is interrupted by texts on the screen—such as Schreber's own writings, which includes deletions ('un-manned') and corrections ('sacrificed')—about the sixth miscarriage of his wife, about his severe insomnia, and about his blackened and impure nerves. There are many jump cuts, e.g. when the movements of a circling camera are cut off, picked up again, cut off again, et cetera, or when Schreber is shown in his isolation cell in top-shots. Moreover, his image multiplies itself during his solitary confinement so that at one point we have four Schrebers in one shot. Several scenes are shot with a wide-angle lens, distorting the viewer's sense of space: as a consequence, the benches at the court have an enormous curve, and the distance between Schreber in the front seat and his wife behind him is exaggerated. Further, a great number of shots have a change in focus or have a foreground but more often a background that is not sharp, presenting characters as a vague apparition. So, despite the calm camerawork and the occasional use of slow motion, most of the techniques—the out-of-focus shots, the jump cuts, the duplications—emphasize a sense of restlessness. Schreber has clearly fallen victim to an unparalleled confusion, especially since he feels waylaid by the so-called Writing Down System.

This System '*contains every word in every language known to Man*', as one text mentions. First, we see many spheres with mobile keys that float in the air while they have been cut in half. We then see that the divided spheres have long glowing strands. Meanwhile, letters drift downwards. Schreber is staring intensely at the spheres with keys. A written text announces: '*Words and voices fell on me, dictating every thought.*' Then we have an overhead shot looking down upon Schreber writing. This is followed by another text: '*Yet the miraculous ability to draw down God's nerves to my soul gave me power over God himself.*

I was chosen.', after which the '*to my soul*' is replaced—by handwriting—with '*to my body*'. It is significant that Schreber's 'I' is as much active as passive. On the one hand, he is an instrument of God's nerves, but on the other hand, he is privileged and exalted. The text hints at the possibility—not uncommon for a psychosis—for personal pronouns (I-you-he) to lose their grounding, which is symptomatic of his difficulty to comply with the symbolic order. There is a clear visual analogy in Pummell's film: Schreber is an object of focalization (a third person), for the camera is focused on him when he ducks skittishly. We then see why he ducks: he feels besieged by the spheres. But these spheres are the product of his observation: we can only explain the presence of them to his subjective vision, turning Schreber into an internal focalizor (first person). Visually, Schreber oscillates between the grammatical position of a 'he' (an object of our look) and an 'I' (the bearer of the look); in the latter case, the film narrator conforms to Schreber's perception. This mechanism is confirmed by the frequent change in focus: now Schreber is in sharp focus and the spheres are out of focus; then in the next moment it is the other way around and Schreber is out of focus. Thanks to Pummell's concern with depth of field, Schreber is a protagonist, permanently changing back and forth between the first and third person. The linguistic shifts from 'I' to 'he' and vice versa are also expressed at the audio-visual level in SHOCK HEAD SOUL.

A CYBORG MESSIAH: *ROBOCOP*

One might consider RoboCop, the cyborg police officer from Paul Verhoeven's eponymous Hollywood debut feature, a modern-day version of Schreber. Like this nerve patient, RoboCop has difficulty articulating his 'I': on his first patrol for the police squad in Detroit, Agent Alex J. Murphy is shot and killed. His body is then resurrected and adorned with cybernetics by the megacorporation Omni Consumer Products (OCP). The result of this operation, named RoboCop, is presented as a cyborg law enforcer who can clean up the city. But instead of a completely blank memory, he still has some remnants of his former existence as 'Murphy'. ROBOCOP (1987) is an action science-fiction spectacle in the vein of mid-1980s American blockbusters, but Verhoeven has the ability to add sardonic humour to such fare. This sci-fi hit can be called satirical for a number of reasons. First, the film's excessive violence follows the style of comic books: the villains shoot at the 'good cop' Murphy until they have run '*outta ammo*', which is accompanied by their raucous laughter. In addition to this excessive violence, it also has a particularly gory showdown: the scene in which Emil, one of the villains, is totally disfigured after being covered in toxic waste is given ample screentime. Second, ROBOCOP is a 'darkly comic media satire', as Christian McCrea asserts, with 'shit-talking executives' who lack all moral concern and are only interested in sales and money (*'I'd buy that for a dollar'* is a repetitive slogan). Verhoeven presents a mediatized environment in which there are screens everywhere, in a postmodernist critique that one cannot escape being affected by representations. Even the news items are intercut with 'bad television ads' (McCrea): the publicity for the family board game 'Nukem' (*'get them—before they get you!'*) can only be taken as a crude joke.

Third, Verhoeven likes to state that for him, ROBOCOP is a 'cyborg Messiah', a retelling of Christ's resurrection. Given the brutal violence, this American version is in blatant contrast to Pier Paolo Pasolini's neo-Marxist adaptation of the life and times of Jesus, IL VANGELO SECONDO MATTEO [THE GOSPEL ACCORDING TO ST. MATTHEW] (1964) which Verhoeven admires as the most accurate rendition of the gospels. Bearing the Italian black-and-white film in mind with Jesus as a pacifist defender of the poor amidst rural surroundings, the parallel between Christ and RoboCop seems satirical. Nonetheless, the parallel is serious as well, for ROBOCOP critiques a greedy consumerist culture to such an extent that it has affinities with Pasolini's neo-Marxist Jesus film. Fourth, and most relevant to my aim, Verhoeven has described ROBOCOP as the first in his 'psychosis' trilogy (Van Scheers, 380). His use of the term 'psychosis' is loose (Williams *The Erotic Thriller*, 167) and can best be explained by looking at the second film in the cycle, the dystopian science-fiction TOTAL RECALL (1990). Douglas Quaid never knows whether he is a construction worker who has implanted memories of a trip to Mars in the guise of a secret agent or whether he was actually an agent-turned-rebel at Mars who was transformed into a terrestrial. *'If I am not me, who am I?'* he asks himself, but the enigma remains unsolved until the very end. Quaid is for Verhoeven a psychotic subject because he cannot decide which reality is true—and neither can we, the viewers.[14]

ROBOCOP, on the contrary, offers us an inverted scenario of psychosis, so to speak. As the initiator of the cyborg project, the young executive Bob Morton of the firm Omni Consumer Products says about RoboCop: *'He does not have a name. He's got a programme. He's a product.'* He is programmed to serve the public trust, to protect the innocent, and to uphold the law. And, as we will find out, he will mercilessly use force if necessary. There is a so-called *'fourth directive'*, which Dick Jones, the senior vice president of OCP, adds to RoboCop's psychological profile: *'Any attempt to arrest a senior officer of OCP results in shutdown.'*

This specific directive ensures that Jones is installed as a quasi-Name-of-the-Father. RoboCop can neither reject nor turn against this authoritarian figure: no matter how strong RoboCop is, he will collapse in the case of revolt.

There is nonetheless a glitch in the programme, for the cyborg cop is not supposed to have any memories of his former identity. But in several point-of-view shots, we see some brief fragments from his past, though he cannot make sense of the clips. One of them has a young kid asking: '*Can you do that, dad?*' as T.J. Lazer does a trick with his gun on television. RoboCop's incoherent remnants of Murphy's past appear to him as strange delusions, but the point, of course, is that they are not. In the case of a psychosis, presumed fantasies that come across as strikingly real are mental fabrications, but in this inverted case, the sudden scenes that involuntarily bombard RoboCop refer to real past experiences. RoboCop only gets a hunch of his erased identity when the Detroit police officer Anne Lewis—who was with him during the fatal shooting—recognizes RoboCop's imitation of T.J. Lazer's gimmick with the gun as Murphy's signature trick.

Evil is beaten when Dick Jones is eliminated. Because of the fourth directive, RoboCop was only able to kill the senior vice president at the moment that the president, his superior in rank, said: '*You're fired, Dick.*' These words have a performative function here: by speaking these lines, Jones is no longer a senior officer of OCP, and thus RoboCop can get rid of the excessively dominant father who had falsely assumed a position of symbolic authority. When the president thereupon asks RoboCop: '*What's your name, son?*', he can finally say his name '*Murphy*', which is the last word in the film. Throughout Verhoeven's picture, it was impossible for Murphy to take up his symbolic identity; he was prevented from speaking 'I', which usually brings a subject close to psychosis. He had flashbacks from his past, but he was not able to recognize them as 'my' memories until he killed the evil quasi-father who obstructed his access to the symbolic order.

DUTCH EXISTENZ: *DE MARIONETTENWERELD* AND *WERELD VAN STILSTAND*

In RoboCop, the cyborg was a product that was subject to the laws and whims of father figures. The charm of De marionettenwereld [Marionette] (1993), Elbert van Strien's graduation film from the Film Academy, nominated for the Student Academy Award, is that the situation is reversed, or at least it seems so: a psychiatrist who is in the position of 'the subject supposed to know' is told that he is the figment of a young boy's imagination. The six-year-old Chris claims to his analyst Rogier van Zanten that he can make things happen. He reveals that he has invented Rogier, who has just started working at a new office, after his predecessor, Mr. Verdoorn, was hospitalized due to a heart attack. Later that day, a long-haired woman suddenly steps into Rogier's car at a gas station. He is flabbergasted by her frankness, but when she continues to make both bold and flirtatious remarks—'I only do this with weak males'—he starts to feel more at ease with her company, and ultimately, they kiss. He has good hopes of meeting her again at the gas station, but Julia does not show up.

Meanwhile Chris makes some correct predictions such as 'there is a gun in your drawer'. When the boy draws a picture of a woman, named Julie, drowning in water, Rogier asks whether she should be saved, and he answers 'no'. Then the psychiatrist accidently knocks over a glass and the liquid spills over the drawing: now Julia is definitely drowning. During a visit to his predecessor in the hospital, Mr. Verdoorn asks Rogier whether the kid drew anything, and then suddenly collapses. Waiting in the corridor, Rogier sees a corpse covered with a sheet: judging from the hair, he thinks it might be Julia. He goes to Chris's house in the night and takes the boy by force. While Rogier says that the man 'is about to die because of your stories', Chris uses the moisture on the window to draw a diagram that ends in a horizontal line. Soon the news arrives that Mr. Verdoorn has passed away. The next day, Rogier pulls a gun at the kid, who calmly says: 'When you shoot, everything stops existing.' When the boy adds: 'I know you won't shoot me', we get a high-angle shot from the staircase: we see Rogier shoot, but Chris is off-screen. There is an immediate transition to a frontally staged wide-angle shot of Rogier, with whispering voices off-screen, some singing, and the slowed-down ticking of a clock. When the clock stops, it seems as if Rogier is falling into a black hole, but suddenly he stands up in an impeccably white space, again in a frontally staged wide-angle shot. He is surrounded by five doctors; one of them diagnoses him with a distorted sense of reality. He takes the doctor by his collar: 'He's still playing games with us.' In the background it seems as if Julia is at the porter's desk. When the doctors are gone, Rogier panics: 'I'm right', he keeps telling himself. We then hear: 'Of course you are right. They don't know any better.' An extreme close-up of Rogier's eye shows a faint reflection of Chris, dressed in angelic white. Chris's voice repeating 'Everything will be fine' closes the film.

DE MARIONETTENWERELD is very much a conceptual film.[15] Initially, Rogier thinks his client has a problem and that he is supposed to help and preferably cure the kid. Chris, however, turns Rogier into the object of his problem: the boy presents himself as the psychiatrist's mastermind. Gradually, the scenario gains in credibility, and the idea that the kid is the deity he claims to be turns Rogier into a madman. But if Chris is indeed a mastermind, the kid must take on the responsibility that goes with that. When the child refuses to do so according to Rogier's standard, Rogier shoots Chris. The status of the world is now very much unclear, underscored by the wide-angle lenses. Is Rogier a deranged man who has invented a kid he believes can determine the fate of people, such as Julia, Mr. Verdoorn, and ultimately Rogier himself?

In that case, Rogier is a paranoid man who suffers from a 'distorted sense of reality', as the doctor diagnosed. There is another possibility, just as credible, that Chris is a young puppeteer who is pulling the strings, since Rogier, with whom the viewer identifies, is convinced of this. When the doctors are out of sight, the kid presents himself again, first as a voice off-screen and then as a reflection in one of Rogier's eyes. On the one hand, the final sequence might confirm the authenticity of Rogier's scenario, but on the other hand, it casts doubt on the kid's existence, for he is not shown directly, only as a faint image.

In three imaginative shorts, Van Strien elaborated upon his preoccupations in DE MARIONETTENWERELD. VERBODEN OGEN [FORBIDDEN EYES] (2002) is about an adolescent who looks 'normal' but is actually of alien descent. Once his eyes meet the eyes of the girl of his dreams, he will disintegrate, and at the end, he cannot resist the temptation. In HET VERBORGEN GEZICHT [THE HIDDEN FACE] (2004), a young girl does not interpret her grandmother's strange behaviour (a weird voice, her fall to the ground) as a sign of illness, but she thinks her grandma is no longer her grandma. And if her grandmother is bewitched, perhaps the house is too, with its eerie wallpaper. But these two shorts are topped by the third one, DE WERELD VAN STILSTAND [ARRESTED WORLD] (2005), which is clearly a tribute to LA JETÉE [THE PIER] (Chris Marker, 1962).

Like Marker's film, DE WERELD VAN STILSTAND is in black and white, has a length of almost half an hour, consists of a chain of freeze frames, and makes extensive use of voice-over. This voice tells us about a journalist who attributes the success of a mediocre writer he meets to a dirty conspiracy. According to the journalist, the taste of the masses is valued over originality. He gradually becomes paranoid and no longer recognizes his own face in the mirror. He grows a beard and a moustache. He tries to trace K who has sent him a note, ordering him to investigate the authorities. But wherever he goes, all the time someone seems to have preceded him. When he finally meets this K at his editorial office, he sees his exact look-alike, albeit without a beard and a moustache. He points a gun at K, but he ends up with a hole in his own forehead, and slowly the bearded man dissolves. He regains his identity at that moment: 'He was the man of arrest who has put the world into motion', the voice-over says. Back home, we see how his hand caresses the face of his girlfriend Betty, and for the first time in the film—at the end—we see a shot that is in motion.

As a medium, photography is split in time: it portrays a moment that immediately becomes the past. Whereas film positions us into the 'now' because of the stream of moving images, photography inevitably remains within the past. One always lags behind in time. This belatedness exactly corresponds with the experience of the journalist: he follows the traces of someone who has been where he arrives, and he cannot remember whether he himself may have been the predecessor. This effect legitimates the choice for photography as a stylistic means in Van Strien's film, to illustrate that the protagonist is split in time.

Moreover, the photographic style contributes to the oppressive atmosphere of the film. We often see the journalist amidst impressive buildings or huge pillars or among a crowd. Shot in extreme long shots, he seems to drown in the space that encapsulates him. The framing is typical as well: his head is behind a window or he is shown between the doorposts of his bedroom. When he is shot closer, he is usually in sharp focus while his environment is out of focus, or the other way around. At times, he switches from sharp depiction to a total blur within the very same photo shot. These procedures with shot composition, framing, and focus affirm that he has difficulty in interpreting his immediate surroundings.

In addition to the lack of a solid ground, he suffers from the feeling that two men are pursuing him. Looking down from his window, he sees both of

them on the street. In and of itself, this shot is not remarkable, but it recalls a similar scene from UN CHIEN ANDALOU (Luis Buñuel, 1928). From a high angle, the characters observe peculiar events. Buñuel's film sticks to the conventional grammar of cinema, since it basically relies upon eyeline matches and shot/reverse shots. We see a character looking, and in a subsequent shot we see the content of the character's vision. The content of this vision is what makes the film properly bizarre. When ants crawl out of someone's hand, this does not mean that there are 'really' insects, but that is the way the character perceives it—or rather hallucinates it. Similarly, the journalist in Van Strien's film sees two people crop up out of nowhere, even in the guise of doctors. When travelling by metro, their bodies are reflected in the windowpane, but their reflection gradually dissolves. This slow disappearance strongly suggests that they are a permanent hallucination.

After the bearded double of the journalist has disintegrated following the shooting, the voice-over mentions that the journalist has rediscovered himself. Despite this optimistic statement, the images problematize a presumed happy ending. Once again we see him as a small black figure on an immense square. When he comes home, we see him from a high angle and sitting in his bedroom: he is once again framed by the doorposts. These shot compositions imply that nothing has changed. Nevertheless, the world starts to move as we see how his hand touches Betty's face in close-up. This very moment clearly references LA JETÉE, since the one scene with moving image in Marker's film shows a woman's face in close-up. The protagonist had been wondering whether she existed for real or whether she was born out of his imagination. The fact that she is moving seems to confirm the first option—she actually is alive—but within the context of LA JETÉE, the option that she is a fantasy woman remains valid. The moving image is in soft focus and hence connotes romanticism. Moreover, the man acts as if he himself thinks he is dreaming. Since the final shot in Van Strien's film refers to an image that possibly has the status of a dream, the protagonist is probably still stuck in a world of delusions, notwithstanding the optimistic voice-over. And thus, the 'photo novel' WERELD VAN STILSTAND presents itself as an enduring hesitation between illusion and a sense of reality.

DARK WATER: *DE POEL*

In his classic study on the fantastic, Tzvetan Todorov distinguishes the uncanny from the marvellous as neighbouring genres of the fantastic. If there is a fiction film that depicts a world as we know it, there is neither a devil nor a vampire. When someone claims he has met a hobbit, he may probably be having a hallucinatory vision: the supernatural encounter is explained as a misperception by the character. The natural order remains intact, and the fanciful apparition belongs to the category of the 'fantastic uncanny' for Todorov. But when the natural order is short-circuited and we accept the apparition as truly supernatural, we enter the realm of the fantastic marvellous (or fantasy): confronted with hobbits, goblins, elves, and wizards, the usual 'laws of reality' are no longer applicable; a reader/viewer has to figure out the mechanisms of this supernatural universe (why does the ring give magical powers to its bearer?) and the features of the characters: Can they change into animals? Are they not able to stand daylight? Can they put a spell on others? The genuine fantastic is defined by Todorov as a particular case of the category of 'ambiguous vision' (33). The viewer/reader incessantly hesitates between the options of 'the imaginary' or 'the real': it is impossible for the viewer (and usually, but not necessarily, for the character as well) to decide whether an apparition is an illusion of the senses or a 'real' supernatural being. The fantastic 'occupies the duration of this uncertainty' (Todorov, 25).[16]

Most genres are characterized by specific narratives or iconography. In a western, for example, there is a cowboy riding the saddle, there is a town with a saloon in the midst of a wide-open prairie, and there is a man-to-man showdown, but in the fantastic, the viewer's position is the most important condition. This also means that the generic label can suddenly evaporate once the status of a mysterious apparition is revealed to the viewer.[17] If the mystery regarding the identity of an enigmatic figure is not solved, however, a possibly agreeable atmosphere can convert into horror, as we see in DE POEL [THE POOL] (Chris W. Mitchell, 2014).

After both Rob and Lennaert are fired as bank employees, they decide to go on a hiking trip with their families in the woods. Rob, recently divorced, takes his teenage daughter Emilie; Lennaert is married with Sylke and they have two teenage sons, Marco and Jan. Lennaert persuades everyone to set up camp beyond a 'no trespassing' sign in a nature preserve near a pool. The first evening they have a pleasant meal, but then Rob tells the company a spooky bedtime story about four guys who never returned from a scavenger hunt, and the local people presumed this was due to a creature in the pool. At that very moment Emilie shows up from the dirty pond, and the two boys have the fright of their lives, to the delight of both Rob and Lennaert. But they stop laughing very soon, for Murphy's Law starts to operate. Anything that can go wrong, will go wrong: the meat is rotten; there is no telephone signal; the camping gas burner no longer works; Lennaert finds out that Sylke is having an affair with Rob but keeps his discovery silent; after being assigned by Lennart to find something fit for consumption, Rob returns with a rabbit that has been dead for days to show how he thinks it's a 'stupid game'; Rob throws the animal into the pool to the anger of Lennaert, for he pollutes the water supply; a dead rabbit in Rob's tent is a bad joke as well as a bad omen; Lennaert and his son Jan try to find a supermarket but despite a compass they end up walking in circles; Rob catches a few eels from the pool with a rabbit's head as bait, but apart from Lennaert who refuses to eat the fish, everyone gets an upset stomach; Rob becomes so ill that he asphyxiates on his own vomit—or did Lennaert perhaps strangle his rival at night and blame it on the vomit, as a brief insert suggests; Lennaert must amputate one of Marco's fingers due to blood poisoning.

The question that looms over DE POEL is whether Lennaert is acting so deranged out of frustration with his wife having cheated on him with a good friend and with the bad turn his holidays took, or whether he is triggered by an external force. The cuckolded Lennaert has a stronger connection with Jan than with Marco. The latter is erotically interested in Emilie and considers her his future conquest, but Jan is the sensitive type who allows Emilie to teach him how to knit. After Rob's prank with the spooky story, Jan is lured into the pool by a voice he thinks belongs to Emilie. A person is faintly visible in the background. Someone grabs his leg, but it is his father who wakes him up: it was all a dream, in retrospect. But, inexplicably, Jan's feet are covered in clay as if he had been outside after all. The very next night, Jan shines a light over the water, and just when a face shows up, his father asks him whether he is sleepwalking. He then dreams about a shell, and in the morning he has a shell in his hand and a voice whispers 'Take me with you'. A few scenes later, the camera pans behind Lennaert's back, and we get quick dissolves with fragmented shots of a red-lipped woman with wet hair and red nails. Once again we hear a voice whisper 'Take me with you'. When Jan joins his father, the apparition is gone. It is from this moment onwards that Lennaert seems to go mad. Marco tells his brother that their father did not blink his eyes when he cut his finger, as if he enjoyed doing it. On top of that, Lennaert burns Rob's corpse, arguing that the dead body is a 'source of putrefaction'. He knocks Sylke down when she throws the shell that he had taken from Jan into the pool. As she recovers, she starts yelling at him, and humiliated, he walks into the woods, and then there is once again a series of brightly lit dissolves with fragmented shots of the same girl who encourages him to start anew and to take action. No action is required towards Sylke because she is so dazed and confused due to a nasty wound at the back of her head, so he only leads her away. But there is a female voice urging him to run 'faster, faster', and he sees that Marco is kissing Emilie, which Lennaert had forbidden for the duration of their holidays. Lennaert and Marco get into a fight, and then Jan intervenes by pulling Marco away. Lennaert uses the opportunity to slit Marco's throat, to the horror of Jan and Emilie. Jan runs away until he falls down from fatigue. A soothing voice reassures him to sleep, but he wakes up with his mother beside him, her throat slit as well. He hears Emilie scream and runs towards the sound. Jan arrives in time and knocks his father down; he then ties him up in a sleeping bag and drags him into the pool. Lennaert yells that it does not make sense, for 'the sacrifice has to be pure': Emilie is supposed to be the victim, the father explains, just before he drowns. Under water, Lennaert briefly sees the girl before she swims to the surface. Only Jan and Emilie are left, and when they try to leave the woods, they get lost and end up back at the pool. Jan hears Emilie say 'And now?' While we see him at the back near a highway, he looks over his shoulder. Apparently, Emilie is next to him, wearing her coat. But when she takes his hand and turns her face to Jan, we see she is not Emilie but the mysterious girl from the pool.

Up to this point, the viewer can believe that this girl was only a figment of the characters' imagination. Rob had made his daughter Emilie appear from the water to scare the two boys, but any other creature from the pool belongs to the domain of mythmaking. Hence, this girl seemed either a product of Jan's imagination or a product of Lennaert's hallucinations. This would make it logical that the father gradually went crazy and lost all control. His apparently imaginary encounters with the girl and her whispering voice functioned as a beacon of rest amidst all the turmoil he could no longer manage. Lennaert and to some extent Jan had become so paranoid in the woods—best signified by their impossibility to find an exit—that the viewer assumes that the girl has a fictional status rather than a realistic one. Her apparition was too brightly lit for the darkness of the woods, but the final shot tips the balance in favour of a 'real' girl. She might, of course, simply be Jan's fantasy, or it could be that she has replaced Emilie in a typical twist ending of a film playing with the dividing line between reality and fantasy. Because of the plausibility of both options, the horror of De poel becomes an example of the fantastic.

ONE SISTER-BRIDE FOR SEVEN BROTHERS IN A DUTCH SLASHER: *DE JOHNSONS*

In DE JOHNSONS (Rudolf van den Berg, 1992), a girl's dreams are scary forebodings of the existence of creatures that come to haunt her and her mother. Since their existence is never questioned in the film, DE JOHNSONS is a full-blooded horror picture and, without a doubt, my personal favourite among the so-called 'nederhorror' films. DE LIFT and AMSTERDAMNED by Maas, mentioned at the beginning of this chapter, are predominantly psychological in nature, thrillers featuring some horror scenes. Some kind of danger terrorizes people, and we only become aware of its source when it is too late. DE JOHNSONS, however, is about a mother-daughter relationship, but this is embedded in 'anthropological humbug' (in the words of the director in the documentary XANGADIX LIVES!, made to memorize the legacy of DE JOHNSONS). One of the reasons the film gained a cult following is that it is a fairly unique and isolated attempt in Dutch film history. If it bears comparison to any other films, then American pictures from the 1970s come to mind: CARRIE (Brian de Palma, 1976), because of the girl's indisposition; DELIVERANCE (John Boorman, 1972) for the encounter with psychopaths in an unpopulated area; and slasher films like HALLOWEEN (John Carpenter, 1978).

According to Carol Clover, in the majority of slashers, the male perpetrator starts a killing spree for failing to turn into a 'real' man. Regardless of his age, the killer's identity remains that of a 'mama's boy', and as a consequence of his attachment to his mother, he usually is 'sexually inert' (Clover, 80). His frustration at not having killed his father is successfully projected onto his female victims. It is the choice between 'sex or the saw', as the oldest son Drawton Sawyer tells his brother Leatherface in TEXAS CHAIN MASSACRE II (Tobe Hooper, 1986). The so-called 'Final Girl' in slasher films, however, stands apart from other girls. She is often quite boyish in character and look and does not flaunt her sexuality. She is able to resist the male psychopath all on her own; no last-minute rescue by a man is required. The Final Girl is the reversed mirror image of the killer, but her consistent victories in slashers imply that the 'combination masculine female repeatedly prevails over the combination feminine male' (86).

At the start of DE JOHNSONS, a text is written over a photograph of a man. A voice-over reads aloud that in 1934 the man wrote about Xangadix, an embryo in a crystal ball who shall impregnate a cobalt blue-eyed woman with evil. Two days later, the man died. Cut to Doctor Johnson who, totally exhausted, receives applause after presiding over the delivery of a septuplet. But soon thereafter he goes into a dark forest, begging for salvation. While he puts yellow mud over his face and shouts in desperation: 'Appear, whatever thy shape or name ... God .. beast .. mystery .. come ... COME.' He briefly stares at the apparition of Xangadix before the screen turns white.

We move 21 years forward in time: the blue-eyed Victoria Lucas is working as a news photographer, taking pictures of a garbage strike. The image of many bags of garbage in Amsterdam is a striking one in this film, put to great use in one of the later scenes when Victoria rescues herself by jumping from a building into a huge pile of garbage bags. Victoria gets a well-paid assignment to take a picture of a night heron in De Biesbosch, a national park in the south of the Netherlands. Daughter Emalee, who is about to turn fourteen, is eager to join her mother in a tent. This plot is crosscut with a story about Winston Keller, a professor of anthropology of Surinamese descent who is alerted to unique film material by Angela, one of the staff members. In the cellar of his faculty, there are moving images of Vidal Makay's expedition to the Indians in 1934. Angela explains that Vidal stole the embryo Xangadix and then went raving mad and committed suicide. On its return home, the ship of the expedition collapsed, as if it had been cursed. Winston's father enters during the screening of the film fragments and panics: he insists that they destroy the material. While a shot of Xangadix is projected over both father and son, there is a transition to a close-up of Emalee who has the same bad nightmare she has had before about the Xangadix sign and much blood (although she is not familiar yet with Xangadix or its sign). She later mentions to a psychiatrist that her nightmares could be an announcement of her first menstruation, but we know better, since her scary dream is followed by a further explanation about the myth by Angela. The box with the film came from the widow of Doctor Johnson who was one of the few to survive the shipwreck following the expedition to Latin America.

The next day, Winston is taken by a representative of the ministry of education and science to a remote prison in De Biesbosch in which seven psychopaths are being kept. They were responsible for a bloodbath in an orphanage fourteen years ago. At the age of only seven, the seven brothers—who had never uttered a sentence—killed sixteen people. The ministry produced fake reports at the time to keep the drama a secret. On video footage, Winston sees how the bald brothers cruelly tear a doctor apart in the shower and then make a sign with the man's blood on a wall. By now, Winston recognizes this as the Xangadix sign. His visit to De Biesbosch is alternated with Victoria and Emalee's trip to the national park, and at one point they pass each other on the water just as Winston says that he requires information about the mother of the psychopaths who, as it later turns out, were the first test tube babies in Holland. Winston is immediately distracted by Victoria, whom he calls a 'beautiful woman' out of her earshot.

During his research into the former orphanage, Winston discovers the

Xangadix sign again and learns that eternal night will come over earth once the seven brothers fertilize their younger sister. Winston thinks this is nonsense, for he is not as superstitious as his father (who burned much of the material on his own initiative), but the professor nonetheless advises the ministry that it would be best to kill the septuplets. Owing to the crosscutting, it has been clearly spelled out that Emalee is the younger sister who has her first period that very day. When she takes a walk at night, she sees the prison, which she remembers from one of her dreams, though she had never set foot in De Biesbosch before. When she recognizes some other details, Emalee realizes that her repetitive dream is a foretelling to warn her of danger. Her mother remains sceptical, but Emalee insists they get away from the park as quickly as possible. In the meantime, the brothers have sensed the vicinity of their sister and break loose one night on a full moon after creating a short-circuit that makes all the screens go dark.[18] It will lead to a scene that is as horrific as it is humorous. When visiting the prison, Winston asks a guard whether he was the 'head of custody', whereupon the man turns a swivel chair around and reveals a severed head on its seat: 'No, this is it.'

From here onwards, DE JOHNSONS develops into a slasher, and each of the bald-headed brothers with their clay-like monstrous faces will eventually be killed in various ways: a head cut off, a pin through a door that cracks a boy's skull, via electrocution. Victoria and Emalee are responsible for the executions, but Winston comes to their assistance, once he has tracked down the mother of the seven brothers. Emalee comes under the spell of the last remaining brother who gives her a plastic bride's gown. She is about to be ritually wed in a subterranean vault as he leads the barefoot girl in the direction of the embryo Xangadix, but Winston eliminates the psychopath with a pressure washer. Winston's father yells at Victoria that the embryo cannot bear the warmth of a mother. Victoria embraces the ugly creature and Xangadix subsequently explodes. Accompanied by baroque music, we see in slow motion how mother and daughter are covered in litres of blood.

In 2017, 25 years after its original release, a documentary called XANGADIX LIVES! was made by Bram Roza and Yfke van Berckelaer who considered the film incomparable to any other Dutch film. Fanboy Roza had been spellbound by the film from an early age because it was so outrageous, but he became even more intrigued when he found out about its curious production history. Originally, the script was written as *The Johnson Blues* for the American market with actors Glenda Jackson and Oliver Reed in mind, and it was intended as a 'DELIVERANCE meets CROCODILE DUNDEE meets STRAW DOGS' with a couple of hillbillies roaming New York City. When the project failed to get off the ground, it became a Dutch production. With Ruud van Hemert as director, who had made a reputation with two successful black comedies, the idea was to turn it into a darkly humorous horror picture. But Van Hemert, nicknamed 'Ruud de Bruut' due to his aggressive outbursts, was fired three weeks before the start of shooting. When Van den Berg heard about a movie that was already financed but had no director, he joked that he was available. Reading the script, he realized it was uncharted territory for him, since he was known for arthouse psychological dramas—his latest film was DE AVONDEN, based upon a literary classic (see chapter two). But the writer Leon de Winter, a good friend, offered to rewrite the material, and after ten drafts within three weeks, it had become a completely different film. There was a huge premiere in the famous Tuschinski movie theatre in Amsterdam, but Van den Berg was nonetheless criticized by several reviewers for lending his name to a film of questionable value. Dutch critics were not used to genre pictures let alone horror films with superstitious motives, and Van den Berg was initially apologetic in interviews, claiming he had to earn a living. But when DE JOHNSONS raised some 'unexpected enthusiasm' over the years from horror fans, he liked to stress that thanks to the 'operatic' finale and to the psychology between the mother and the daughter, it nonetheless had a bit of a 'Van den Berg signature'.

CONCLUSION: STRANGER THINGS

The characters in this chapter lose a firm footing in 'reality' (whatever that may be): they are not under the spell of the signifier, for they have refused to accept the Name-of-the-Father. Instead of *le père*, which enables them to address themselves as an 'I', they have chosen *le pire*, the impossible path of desire. The symbolic order has no consistency and has at best an alternative universe for them in store: the traumatized mechanic Breuker in DE LIFT has become apathetic, only reacting upon seeing a meaningful sign in the chocolate custard dripping from the wall; Arnold in PARANOIA sees a conspiracy in everything and thinks that everyone can identify him as the wanted SS man. Following the premature death of her mother, who could have facilitated an entry into an imaginative domain, Hedwig in VAN DE KOELE MEREN DES DOODS falls victim to an oppressive culture, dominated by Calvinism and 'male wisdom'. After her own daughter dies, Hedwig is no longer able to separate fact from fiction, seeing former husbands where they are not. Schreber in SHOCK HEAD SOUL is the famous paranoid man who has delusions of being impregnated by divine rays, and Pummell's film alternates between a rhythm of tranquillity and brusque interruptions, between Schreber as a first person (internal focalizor) and a third person (object of focalization), thus punctuating his hallucinatory visions. Similarly, the 'cyborg Messiah' in ROBOCOP is psychotic, since he alternates between his identity as the robotic law enforcer and his former existence as the dead cop Murphy.

The characters in this chapter struggle with epistemological questions that are typical for a modernist mindset: Who am I in the world I am part of? How can I interpret this chaotic world? In the case of the films by Van Strien, these epistemological questions tip over into ontological ones: Does the world I think I am part of exist or does it not? Am I a figment of someone's imagination? The films by Van Strien belong to the fantastic because they make us doubt incessantly. Similarly, the status of the girl in the pond in DE POEL is never resolved: she could be a hallucination or she could be genuinely supernatural. Whatever her status, her apparition drives father and son crazy, turning DE POEL into a horrific-fantasy film. By contrast, in DE JOHNSONS, the girl's scary dreams about strange things materialize into an actual assault by outrageous creatures born from a supernatural legend.

NOTES

1 DE LIFT was sold to many countries, but non-Dutch viewers are perhaps better acquainted with the remake DOWN (2001), featuring Naomi Watts. Unfortunately, this film about a series of disastrous events occurring in a skyscraper had in retrospect an unlucky date of release, four days preceding 9/11. Whereas DE LIFT had been a success in the Netherlands, DOWN was a total flop in Maas's mother country.

2 The police inspector in AMSTERDAMNED is comically ineffectual: he never intervenes successfully, because his conclusions always come too late. In his book *Buurman, wat doet u nu?*, Dick Maas writes that he regretted the ending of the film, saying that instead of the killer's suicide, there should have been a stand-off with the inspector (53).

3 Very comparable to the black comic thrillers of Dick Maas is BUMPERKLEEF [TAILGATING] (Lodewijk Crijns, 2019), which is also heavily influenced by DUEL (Steven Spielberg, 1971) and FALLING DOWN (Joel Schumacher, 1993). When Crijns's film failed to attract many viewers despite positive reviews, Maas made a public statement telling people to go and see BUMPERKLEEF. He said it was a shame that these kinds of films were underrated in the Netherlands. In the prologue of BUMPERKLEEF, a race cyclist runs through a field with his bike on his back, clearly in panic. A man next to a white van in the background calls out to ask whether he wants his phone back, but the cyclist's panic only increases. When he is on the road again, we see that he is deliberately hit by the white van. The driver puts on the white uniform with a yellow apron of a pest control expert, and before he sprays insecticide

into the cyclist's mouth, he tells him: 'The time for excuses is over.' The film itself is in fact the longer version of this prologue. Hans is on his way to his parents by car together with his wife Diana and two daughters. Knowing that his mother is always annoyed by late arrivals, Hans gets frustrated when a white van on the highway is driving too 'slow' in the left lane, with a truck on the right. Slow is a relative term here, since the van driver is driving at the prescribed speed limit. Diana warns him to keep a distance, but the cocksure Hans overtakes the van on the right and makes a condescending gesture to Ed, the man from the prologue. When the family makes a stopover at a gas station, Ed catches up with them and tells the daughters a nasty story about rats that sacrifice their children to get to the other side of a water. Hans acts arrogantly but refuses to apologize. As he notes that the van is following them, he keeps this silent to his wife and kids, whose images are now out of focus and whose voices are drowned out. Hans then decides to confront Ed but is robbed of his phone. When he ultimately says sorry, Ed calmly replies: 'The time for excuses is over.' He puts on his uniform and uses a pressure sprayer with insecticide as a weapon. When they get away, Hans is on the brink of paranoia, seeing white vans everywhere. While Hans and his family contact the police after a crazy rollercoaster ride in a sleepy village, Ed visits Hans's parental home, asking the mother whether she thinks she is responsible for her son's upbringing and behaviour. Many eventful situations later, the police come to the rescue of the entire family. Whereas they think Ed is gone, he lets the two daughters know he is still around but that they are not to blame. In the final scene, Hans brings his kids to school, which they consider very 'uncool'. Despite his warning, the daughters bike through the red traffic light because they do not want to be late. This scene suggests that Hans has learned a lesson from his terrible humiliation: he has become much more cautious. In the eyes of Crijns, this is a crucial distinction between BUMPERKLEEF and the films by Maas such as DE LIFT and AMSTERDAMNED, for in these latter films, protagonists do not undergo any psychological development (qtd. in Van der Burg, 'Ik neem'). Unlike the middle-aged citizen William Foster in Schumacher's FALLING DOWN, who transforms into an angry avenger one hot morning in a traffic jam ('*I* am the bad guy?'), Hans from BUMPERKLEEF, changes into a coward who will pay his dues, a path less travelled in such movies. The final shot of Crijns's film is ominous: Hans does not see when a white van rides over the pavement behind his back. As the screen goes black, we hear the sound of a crash.

4 In DE VERGETEN MEDEMINNAAR [THE FORGOTTEN RIVAL LOVER] (John Korporaal, 1963), paranoia is not the result of an over-interpretation of signs but of repression. Since the protagonist suffers from amnesia, he resides in a psychiatric institution. At one point he believes he was a landscape architect. He is permitted to design the garden of the institution and later sees the very same design in front of his house, where his former mistress Marie lives. She does not call the police, because her new lover is afraid the amnesiac might remember that he had caused

an accident and gotten rid of the body. The protagonist is persecuted not only by the new lover but also by a bearded man with a razor in his hands. It turns out that this man is a hallucination: the protagonist was running away from his former self. The hallucinatory shots in Korporaal's B-picture are particularly remarkable and a jazzy score contributes to a nerve-wracking atmosphere at times.

5 It is also tempting to draw parallels with a later film by Polanski, LE LOCATAIRE [THE TENANT] (1975), because Arnold was a tenant himself. In addition to many of the unorthodox devices utilized in Ditvoorst's PARANOIA, LE LOCATAIRE efficiently uses zoom lenses to articulate that the male tenant comes to identify with the previous tenant, an unfortunate woman, to such an extent that he even seems to become her. The final scene in LE LOCATAIRE is a repetition from an early moment in the film: he has now taken the place of the hospitalized woman and he sees himself visiting himself.

6 'Want daar stond zijn eigen portret! Dat was hij! Dat waren zijn eigen droevige ogen, zijn wrede, mismoedige mond (...). (Hermans 'Paranoia', 46).

7 'Een der vele schuilnamen die hij had gebruikt' (Ibid.).

8 'Ten gevolge van shellshock kan hij slechts spreken met fluisterende stem' (Ibid.).

9 'Of zij de eigenaardigheid van zijn stem nooit eerder had opgemerkt! Zij vergat altijd alles!' (Ibid., 57).

10 Van Alphen mentions that a consistent use of character-bound focalization is exemplary of modernist literature. Virginia Woolf's novel *The Waves* (1931) employs the narrative technique of this 'radical perspectivism'. In separate sections, we read the observations of six characters, but instead of seeing connections, we are confronted with 'the discrepancy between the characters' perceptions as well as between characters' perceptions of themselves and the ideas others have of them' (259). DE GOLVEN [THE WAVES] (Annette Apon, 1982) is an adaptation of Woolf's novel, but in this film the perceptions are conveyed by lengthy voice-overs. Though the characters interact with one another in one room and are in search of the harmonic bonds from their childhood, the effect of an 'existential isolation' is as striking in Apon's debut feature as in Woolf's novel.

11 'Doordat je geconfronteerd wordt met de taalmuziek van het verleden, met een gestileerde afstandelijkheid, wordt het je gemakkelijker gemaakt om met de personages en hun gevoelens mee te gaan' (qtd. in Anonymous 'Nouchka van Brakel').

12 The film ends here, in 1882, but Van Eeden's novel mentions that she dies in late 1888 of pneumonia at the age of 32.

13 NOW, VOYAGER ends with an astonishing deadlock. Charlotte Vale starts a relationship with a man who is father to a daughter. Like Charlotte at that age, this Christina/Tina is also an ugly duckling because of a 'bad education' by her mother. Hence Charlotte recognizes herself in Tina. When Tina's father proposes to Charlotte, she declines the offer, with the film's final sentence: 'Don't let's ask for the moon. We already have the stars!' If she were to marry Jeremiah, she would become

a 'mother' to Tina. Given her own problematic history with her mother, the idea of 'motherhood' as such is so fraught for Charlotte that she prefers the role of a good companion of Tina to that of 'mother'/stepmother.

14 In the neo noir thriller BASIC INSTINCT (1992), the third of the 'psychosis trilogy', police detective Nick Curran is driven crazy by Catherine Trammell: she presents herself so obviously as a treacherous femme fatale and potential killer that he cannot believe she is the cunning perpetrator of the crime he is investigating. Despite her provocative retorts that Nick is a 'bad' cop, unable to control his emotions, he comes under the spell of the risk she represents and fails to see the ice prick under her bedside in the final shot.

15 For years, Van Strien had been trying to turn his 30-minute film into a feature, and he finally succeeded. In October 2020, MARIONETTE was finally released as a 112 minute film, set in Scotland and entirely spoken in English. This time, the boy Emmanuel ('Manny') Craig is traumatized by the premature death of both his parents, whereas the female psychiatrist Marianne Winter has lost her husband in a car accident. After she shoots the boy—who had warned that the world would cease to exist upon his death— Marianne kills herself as well. She then enters an alternative universe in which her husband is alive again. Since she is convinced that her period in Scotland was not a dream, she returns to Aberdeen, and the boy comes to haunt her again. The end is ambiguous. Marianne tells Dr. Carlson: either '*we all exist in the mind of a ten-year-old boy*' or she is the voice in the boy's head that helps him to come to terms with his trauma of being an orphan.

16 Todorov also mentions another variety of the fantastic in which it is difficult to separate the real from the illusory: something has occurred, but we do not know whether our interpretation of the event was correct. He calls this possibility the 'error of perception' (36).

17 ZOEKEN NAAR EILEEN [LOOKING FOR EILEEN] (Rudolf van den Berg, 1987) is such a film in which the status of an enigmatic woman is revealed. After the death of his beloved Marjan in a car accident, Philip takes over her store in antiquarian books because he cannot accept her death. One day, a miracle seems to occur: 'Marjan', with a different hairdo, enters the shop with a 59-day-old baby in her arms. Philip's assistant is as flabbergasted by the resemblance as Philip is. The woman later states that her name is Eileen W. (she does not give her full family name) from the vicinity of Belfast, Northern Ireland. At one point she vanishes, apparently because a certain Marc has shown up who claims he is her husband. It turns out that Eileen is in hiding in Amsterdam, staying with a prostitute girlfriend. After Philip has been knocked unconscious, he is interrogated by an inspector, who advises him to bury his wife. And in the next scene, he visits Marjan's grave for the first time. ZOEKEN NAAR EILEEN is in fact the obverse of Hitchcock's VERTIGO (1958). In this latter masterpiece, Scottie Ferguson suffers from 'acute melancholia' after the suicide of the blonde Madeleine. Frenetically, he searches for her and he often thinks

he spots a look-alike. He then sees the brunette Judy, who does not really look like Madeleine. Nonetheless, he persistently believes that she is Madeleine, and after he has transfigured her into a spitting image, the necklace she is wearing reveals that Judy *is* Madeleine. He discovers the truth of a terrible deceit thanks to the fact that he could not accept that he had not been able to prevent her death. By contrast, Philip's obsession with Eileen evaporates in ZOEKEN NAAR EILEEN once he reconciles himself with the idea that she really is not Marjan. The moment he visits the grave, he is able to bury her mentally and come to terms with her absence. After a renewed encounter two years later in a very lengthy epilogue that functions to fill in the gaps of Eileen's backstory, it is suggested that they have a future together. Philip even utters the false cliché 'wounds heal', which is false in the sense that psychoanalysis presumes that traumas endure. ZOEKEN NAAR EILEEN had the potentiality of a fantasy as long as doubts remained about the status of Eileen: is she Marjan masquerading as another woman, or is she perhaps a delusion, a figment of Philip's imagination? In the end, she is neither. Since she has become a woman without a secret, there is little risk for Philip in starting a romance with Eileen. It is as if Scottie had become interested in the real Judy and not in the fact that she ever posed as Madeleine. If that were the case, VERTIGO would probably not have been the masterpiece it is rightly considered to be.

18 The prison guards had been watching Laurel and Hardy's performance of 'Shine on Harvest Moon' when the seven psychopaths in DE JOHNSONS prepared their escape.

BIBLIOGRAPHY

Anonymous, 'Nouchka van Brakel over het kleine opdondertje', Vrij Nederland (16 September 1995), https://www.vn.nl/nouchka-van-brakel-over-het-kleine-opdondertje/ [Accessed 17 May 2020].

Bernink, Mieke, *Fons Rademakers: Scènes uit leven en werk* (Abcoude: Uniepers, 2003).

Broeren, Joost, 'BEYOND SLEEP: Dwalen in een slapeloos moeras', *De Filmkrant* 384 (February 2016), https://filmkrant.nl/recensies/beyond-sleep/ [Accessed 10 October 2019].

Clover, Carol J., 'Her Body, Himself: Gender in the Slasher Film', 1993, ed. by Mark Jancovich, Horror: The Film Reader (London and New York: Routledge, 2002), 77-89.

Doane, Mary Ann, *The Desire to Desire: The Woman's Film of the 1940s* (Bloomington and Indianapolis: Indiana University Press, 1987).

Freud, Sigmund, 'Neurosis and Psychosis', *The Standard Edition of the Complete Psychological Works of Sigmund Freud, Volume XIX (1923-1925): The Ego and the Id and Other Works*, 24 vols. (London: Vintage, 2001), 147-154.

—, 'Psycho-analytic Notes on an Autobiographical Account of a Case of Paranoia (Dementia Paranoides)', *The Standard Edition of the Complete Psychological Works of Sigmund Freud. Vol. XII (1911-1913): The Case of Schreber, Papers on Technique and Other Works*, 24 vols. (London: Vintage, 2001), 9-79.

—, 'Totem and Taboo', *The Standard Edition of the Complete Psychological Works of Sigmund Freud. Vol. XIII (1913-1914): Totem and Taboo and Other Works*, 24 vols. (London: Vintage, 2001), 1-161.

Hermans, Willem Frederik, 'Paranoia', *Paranoia*, 1953 (Amsterdam: G.A. van Oorschot, 1985).

Maas, Dick, *Buurman, wat doet u nu? Films maken in Nederland: Tips, trucs, anekdotes, roddel & achterklap* (Amsterdam: Parachute Pictures, 2017).

McCrea, Christian, 'Fascism for Liberals: RoboCop (Paul Verhoeven, 1987)', *Senses of Cinema* 83 (June 2017): http://sensesofcinema.com/2017/cteq/robocop/ [Accessed 17 May 2020].

Mooij, Antoine, *Taal en verlangen: Lacans theorie van de psychoanalyse* (Meppel: Boom, 1975).

Todorov, Tzvetan, *The Fantastic: A Structural Approach to a Literary Genre* (Ithaca, New York: Cornell University Press, 1975).

Truffaut, François, 'Une certaine tendance du cinéma français', *Cahiers du cinéma* 31 (1954): 13-17.

Van Alphen, Ernst, 'On the Possibility and Impossibility of Modernist Cinema: Peter Forgács' Own Death', *Filozofski vestnik* 35, 2 (2014), 255-269.

Van der Burg, Jos, '"Ik neem het op voor de brave burger: Lodewijk Crijns over Bumperkleef"', *De Filmkrant* 425 (November 2019), https://filmkrant.nl/interview/lodewijk-crijns-bumperkleef/ [Accessed 12 May 2020].

Verdaasdonk, Dorothée, 'Interview met WFH: Een fantasie waar geen romancier tegenop kan', ed. by Dorothée Verdaasdonk, *Fons Rademakers: Literatuur en film* (Utrecht: Uitgeverij Cambium, 1984), 8-21.

Van Scheers, Rob, *Paul Verhoeven: Een filmersleven* (Amsterdam: Podium, 2017).

Verstraten, Peter, *Humour and Irony in Dutch Post-war Fiction Film* (Amsterdam: Amsterdam University Press, 2016).

Williams, Linda Ruth, *The Erotic Thriller in Contemporary Cinema* (Bloomington and Indianapolis: Indiana University Press, 2005).

Žižek, Slavoj, *Enjoy Your Symptom! Jacques Lacan In and Out of Hollywood*, 1992 (Revised Edition. New York and London: Routledge, 2001).

CHAPTER 6

Passages à l'Acte

Verstraten, P., *Dutch Post-War Fiction Film Through a Lens of Psycho-analysis.* Taylor & Francis Group, 2021
DOI 10.5117/9789463725330_CH06

ABSTRACT

The sixth chapter addresses so-called *passages à l'acte*, when characters lose their symbolic consistency as a consequence of the violent outbursts they have committed. The chapter starts with the notorious opening scene in Rademakers' BECAUSE OF THE CATS, which recalls Kubrick's A CLOCKWORK ORANGE. There are many more examples of violent acts in Dutch cinema as a result of an uncontrollable urge, ranging from a more or less calculated blackout to the dark impulses of well-to-do citizens, from the mechanisms of group pressure to irrational outbursts. Several of these films are deliberately atemporal, and in the most intriguing one, VAN GOD LOS, the internal narrator exists in the gap between his symbolic death and his biological death, punctuated by his posthumous voice-over.

KEYWORDS
Passage à l'acte – Murderous acts lacking proper actors – (No) chances for redemption – Atemporal films – Posthumous voice-over

In August 1967, Freddy Heineken—who had financed Rademakers' ALS TWEE DRUPPELS WATER—wrote to the director that he did not want to invest money in an adaptation of Nicolas Freeling's detective novel *Because of the Cats* (1963), since he preferred 'de stille kracht' [the hidden force] to 'de stille verkrachting' [the hidden rape].[1] The brutality in the novel did not put off other potential investors, such as Paramount's Bud Ornstein, but the production history of this international picture would turn into a litany of postponements and aborted negotiations. Hugo Claus had already suggested in 1967 that the novel be shot in the vein of TOUCH OF EVIL (Orson Welles, 1958), and Welles himself confirmed that he was highly interested in playing the protagonist, Inspector Piet van der Valk.[2] In addition to his enthusiasm, Welles worked in mysterious ways, however; to cut a long story short, the collaboration between Rademakers and Welles came to a dead end. Instead of shooting the film in the late 1960s, Rademakers had to curtail his ambitions, and so he went back to Claus in 1972 to ask him to write a screenplay for an English-spoken Dutch-Belgian production. When BECAUSE OF THE CATS premiered in March 1973, this was bad timing for two reasons. First, in the Netherlands, Rademakers' film was totally eclipsed by Verhoeven's TURKS FRUIT, an unprecedented box-office success that had opened one month earlier. A failure in his home country, Rademakers' seventh feature was much better attended abroad, making a decent profit in the end (Bernink, 96-97). Second, BECAUSE OF THE CATS might have become a *succès de scandale* if it were not for a film like Stanley Kubrick's A CLOCKWORK ORANGE, released in 1971.[3] For present-day audiences, Rademakers' tough police procedural definitely has a cultish appeal, but at the time BECAUSE OF THE CATS was predominantly regarded as a run-of-the-mill picture.

The most notorious scene in Rademakers' movie takes place in the first ten minutes. Inspector Piet van der Valk is called late at night: in the rich suburb of Bloemendaal, Bob Maris had been robbed by a couple of '*bastards*' once again. Though Bob wants his wife to keep silent because he is worried about her mental state, Mrs. Maris tells Van der Valk the burglars were extremely efficient. There is a sudden insert: a man with a black stocking over his head grabs her by the throat and puts his gloved left hand over her mouth which has just uttered a yell. This insert lasts less than two seconds and we are back in the present, with Bob pacing up and down. Only then does the flashback properly start. We see the couple return from their regular bridge night to find their porcelain crashed and pictures stolen. While Mrs. Maris walks in the direction of the camera, she is suddenly taken from behind in a repetition of the earlier brusque and brief insert but shown from a slightly different angle. While she is gagged by a man, Bob is surrounded by four other burglars in dark suits with ties and black stockings over their faces. As soon as he says: '*I demand* ...' he is taken by his nose so fiercely that he sinks to the ground on his knees. After Mrs. Maris offers them all the money in the house, a hand goes down her knee-high dress and lifts it up. '*No, please*', the anxious wife begs, whereupon the kneeling man says: '*You won't get away with it.*' They allow Bob to stand up and he proposes a deal: he will give them the money and he will give them half an hour head start before he calls the police.

As soon as he finishes speaking, the burglar holding his wife gives her a push and makes her stumble. A low-angle shot shows that all the burglars have turned their backs on Bob. One of them puts a shoe between her legs and says '*Open your legs*'. He repeats himself, this time with a harder tone. The camera is close to Mrs. Maris, who is lying on the rug. She is now surrounded by the burglars: we only see their trousers because of the low position of the camera. Bob yells that they must leave her alone, but visually he is eclipsed, hidden behind the backs of the burglars. When he wants to come to her rescue, he is hit on his nose. They drag his wife onto the bed, and we hear Bob say in the present: '*I couldn't do a thing. They would have murdered me.*' While Mrs. Maris is struggling on the bed, Van der Valk asks whether they were armed. Bob's affirmation is illustrated by one of the burglars holding out a knife towards Mrs. Maris. She now stops resisting and the scene is practically—and uncannily—silent for about thirty seconds. Two men take off her dress, and we see them cut her bra in close-up. Bob looks over at his wife with an expression of infuriation, but neither he nor she makes a sound. After some moments, she utters 'Bob, do something'. One of the men kneels down and takes off her underpants, then looks in the direction of Bob and says calmly: '*Yeah, Bob, do something.*' She is thrown onto the bed, entirely naked, her pubic hair visible as well. In the next two minutes she is gang-raped by two guys, sometimes shown in long shot, sometimes in a medium close-up a bit above her head. An insert shows that Bob is looking on, paralyzed, but then one of the rapists tells him: '*Well, you like watching, Bob.*' When another guy is about to rape her doggy-style, he challenges Bob, who has been reduced to passivity, by saying: '*Don't you want to defend your wife's sweet little honey pot?*' One of the guys then asks number six: '*And what about you?*' But he does not want to take advantage of the woman: '*The cats won't like it.*' One of the invaders takes a vase and throws it towards the mirror, breaking all the glass. '*Oh, shut up.*'

Back in the present, the inspector realizes that the phrase 'The cats won't like it' will be key in solving the crime. He discovers that the cats refers to a group of girls in Bloemendaal, whereas the boys are called the Ravens. During his interrogation, Van der Valk guesses correctly that Erik, the one who uttered the phrase 'The cats won't like it', is the only one among the '*whole lousy bunch who is man enough to face the facts*'. Erik explains that the boys and girls have come under the spell of a guru, Hjalmar Jansen, who has created his own commune: '*The smaller the group, the more important the rules, the stricter the discipline.*' Embedded in Erik's account is the performance of a ritual, including a display of sex by a couple that is spattered with cat's blood. Visiting Hjalmar's place, the inspector has a man-to-man fight with the guru. When Van der Valk is down, Hjalmar promises to break all 24 of his ribs, but then Feodora, a call girl whom Van der Valk has just recently met, intervenes and shoots Hjalmar. Van der Valk hopes he is still alive, but he has breath for only one last sentence, addressed to Feodora: '*I only wanted to fuck you, that's all.*' Van der Valk assures her that he will take the blame by telling his superior that he shot his opponent out of '*self-defence*'.

The parallel between the infamous opening scenes in A CLOCKWORK ORANGE and BECAUSE OF THE CATS is obvious: we are witness to scenes of graphic violence in which an older married couple is turned into victims. In both cases, the man is reduced to a helpless onlooker. In Kubrick's film, brutal torture and harassment are shown in the present while Alex and his droogs perform 'Singing in the Rain' in predominantly long shots and a few wide-angle closer shots; in Rademakers' film, brutal rape and harassment are embedded in a flashback in a classic shot/reverse shot pattern. Apart from the fact that the latter scene did not arouse as much controversy as the highly theatricalized scene by Kubrick partly because of its later release, what is perhaps most significant is the sudden and brief insert in BECAUSE OF THE CATS that precedes the actual telling of the gruesome events by Mrs. Maris. This brief insert is atemporal in every regard: the flashback has not even started, but we are unexpectedly confronted with a snippet of random violence. In defying a narrative order, the insert signifies the rape's traumatic impact on the couple. The intrusion was so shocking that it obstructed the coherence of their story, as illustrated by the brief insert.

The opening scene in A CLOCKWORK ORANGE was so notorious because the theatrical terror was presented to us as a shocking performance. Whereas the torture by Alex and his friends seemed to be a preconceived plan, the violence and the ensuing rape by the boys from Bloemendaal seemed spontaneous, as indicated by Erik's refusal to join in as well as by his phrase 'the cats won't like it'. As we learn later from Erik's account, the guru teaches his pupils that people should have the freedom to explore what they really want to do without being restricted by '*pathetic legal fallacies*'. This may be read as an invitation to random violence, as practiced by the boys, but this contradicts the actual lesson of the guru. In his confrontation with the inspector, it becomes clear that Hjalmar does not target ordinary citizens such as the Maris couple; instead, he wants to challenge those who are supposed to uphold the law. Democracy is a '*grotesque joke*', according to the guru, because an inspector should defend a perpetrator of a crime rather than beat him up. For that reason, Hjalmar starts hitting Van der Valk in the stomach with the aim of unleashing an extra-legal violent energy in him: the '*sheer force of pure destruction*' will become his '*heart's desire*'. In short, an inspector, as bearer of the law, is a worthy opponent, but the violence enacted upon the helpless citizens Maris is no more than a display of destructive power: it is a travesty of the guru's theory.

Earlier I associated the brief insert with the traumatic impact experienced by the Maris couple, but here is a second irrationality: the assault committed by the boys is a pointless excess of Hjalmar's lessons, and via the insert it is presented as a crack in the narrative. The name for such a meaningless outburst beyond the forces of our control is a *passage à l'acte*, committed in the moments of a blackout. Such a *passage à l'acte* can be distinguished from 'acting out'.[4] In *Seminar X*, Lacan compares acting out to an audience member who jumps on the stage, begging the public to interpret his uncommon deed. Acting out always implies an address to the Other: do you see what is bothering me? The *passage à l'acte* 'is when an actor jumps from the stage into the audience'. He goes from the limelight into the darkness, and 'as such the Real appears behind it' (Hewitson). An outburst—violent or otherwise—becomes a *passage à l'acte* when the person loses his own symbolic consistency and cannot translate his impulsive deed into speech and thought (Žižek *Violence*, 65). In fact, he himself also becomes a victim of his uncontrolled behaviour. This chapter will register some remarkable manifestations of a *passage à l'acte* in Dutch cinema—from a revengeful *vaqueiro* in JOÃO AND HET MES to deranged psychopaths in SCHEMER and VAN GOD LOS.

A CALCULATED BLACKOUT: *JOÃO EN HET MES*

A meaningless violent outburst usually implies that one is mentally incompetent while acting. However, George Sluizer's highly recommendable film JOÃO EN HET MES [originally: JOÃO A FACA E O RIO] (1972), acknowledged as a 'Cannes classic' in 2018,[5] introduces us to the oxymoron of a calculated blackout. Sluizer's debut feature, entirely spoken in Portuguese, is set in a rural region in Brazil and is centred around a trip through the jungle along the Amazon river. Its many landscape shots are often a bit low-angle to emphasize the magnificent, rugged nature and the sky above. The aged *vaqueiro* [cowboy] João has been a widower for many years, and since his eight daughters are adults, his house is empty and cheerless. Only the eighteen-year-old Deodato, an adopted son whom he rescued from a flood eight years ago—shown in the film's opening—still lives with him. João discusses with a befriended judge the possibility of marrying the nineteen-year-old Maria, whose late father he had helped in the past. When the judge mentions their difference in age, he simply replies: 'When I buy a horse, I always buy a young one.'

Sluizer's film depicts the masculine codes that João lives by: he lassoes young bulls; he kills jaguars with a knife; and at one point, we get a close-up of a deer's eye right before João slits the animal's throat. When he burns his hand palm, he does not cry out. The harsh environment prepares us for the strict delineation in gender roles: a man has to earn money to give his wife a good life; a wife has to respect her husband; a man has to respond when someone speaks ill of his wife; and flirts are unacceptable. When João sees from a distance that Maria and Deodato are laughing together, this results in a quarrel ('You are no longer my son, for you conceal things from me'). There is one manly thing João is not capable of: Maria does not get pregnant, and even a pilgrimage does not help. He tells the judge that he wants to go to the Amazonas and aims to return within a year, loaded with gold. He will get very rich indeed, but it ultimately takes him four years.

When João is about to return home, he visits a tavern with his friend Zeferino. When the latter hints at the possible infidelity of Maria during João's absence, the old cowboy cuts Zeferino with a knife. This results in a huge brawl, and the local judge admires João for resisting his opponents single-handedly. Since Zeferino, 'strong as an ox', recovers miraculously and does not file a complaint, the verdict is restricted: João no longer has access to the Amazonas area. Since Maria had gone to her mother's place, he meets her there, dressed in an impeccably white suit and fancy shoes. When he lays eyes upon his wife, she is holding hands with a three-year-old girl. He is told that Maria is simply taking care of 'Luisa's child', but he illustrates his disbelief by buying an expensive knife, foretelling her: 'This knife will bring you death.'

After Maria tells the black Doña Ana about her worries, this older woman challenges João: 'The devil's got into you ... You are killing your wife like you kill jaguars.' João has to appear before the Governor, but he says the woman is spreading lies, and during another interrogation, he says it was no more than a 'bad joke'. The attitude of the authorities against the charges of Doña Ana is that they cannot condemn a man on the basis of his 'intent'. Maria runs to the house of the befriended judge, but he is not at home. João takes her for a ride on horseback, and Maria asks him whether she can go to confession. He agrees, for one cannot refuse this to a Christian, he says. The priest reassures Maria: 'He will not harm you; a woman's duty is to accompany her husband.'

Man and wife continue their trip on horseback, and Maria's relief is underscored by romantic music. They start making love in an idyllic spot, and as Maria visibly enjoys the sex, the music intensifies. But suddenly João takes his knife, and while his face turns red from jealous rage, he cuts her. He starts running, a dark silhouette in the dusk, and then he rides to the judge's house, yelling: 'A terrible thing has happened. I've killed my poor Maria.' Sluizer's film ends with a voice-over by the judge: João will be sentenced to twenty years in prison, but he is permitted to pass in freedom on the condition that he does not carry a weapon. He will die during a fight after another prisoner slanders Maria.

On the one hand, João seems temporarily insane, for he kills his wife during the happiest moments we see the couple having together. And this insanity is confirmed when he confesses to the judge that a most dreadful thing has happened, as if it was an act he did not commit on purpose but one that befell him. On the other hand, João is not that mad, for he uses the pronoun 'I', taking responsibility for the murder: 'I've killed ...' In fact, his violent act is a logical extension of the cultural codes regarding gender: if a man has reason to believe that his wife is not faithful, he must set things straight and punish her. Moreover, João had already announced that he would kill his wife with a knife. Both Maria and Doña Ana took his threat seriously, but the male authorities, such as the Governor and the priest, downplayed it. And in the end, he is given a mild sentence: he is sent to jail but does not have to spend his time in prison. This verdict serves to fuel the idea that João's killing was not totally illegitimate but in line with unwritten codes of machismo: by stabbing his wife, he did what a man had to do.

MURDEROUS ACTS WITH OR WITHOUT ACTORS: *ROOIE SIEN* AND *HET TEKEN VAN HET BEEST*

The first twenty minutes of ROOIE SIEN [RED SIEN] (1975), Frans Weisz's fourth feature, have their antecedents in some extremely popular films in Dutch cinema. Just like the box-office success CISKE DE RAT (Wolfgang Staudte, 1955), it is about a child whose mother is a prostitute and whose father is away at sea. This time, the child is a girl and not a boy, and in ROOIE SIEN, any confrontation between mother and child is missing. Just like Verhoeven's WAT ZIEN IK!?, another great box-office success discussed in the introduction, ROOIE SIEN portrays the routine of a prostitute, Sien Breman, working in the red-light district of Amsterdam. These scenes are set in 1912, however, and not in the 1970s, and drama has replaced the comic situations of Verhoeven's debut feature. These parallels are definitely cut short the moment Sientje's father Ko comes to visit his wife 'at work'. We know then that the nine-year-old Sientje, as red-haired as her mother, is raised by Ko's parents. We know that Ko's mother advises her son to stay away from his wife, for Sien is extremely disdainful of her husband who could offer her no more than potatoes with grease because he made too little money. We know that Ko had beaten her up because in his eyes she would lose her decency once she started working again in the red-light district. And we know that Sien prefers her pimp, 'beautiful' Frans—a 'real man'—over Ko, who happens to be her husband, a pitiful creature in her eyes.

About twenty minutes into Weisz's film, Sien is trying to please a male customer. While 'beautiful' Frans is about to steal the man's wallet, Ko suddenly appears in the background, out of focus. As Frans tries to sneak away, the camera cuts to a shot behind Ko, positioning the latter as an obstacle. Frans, this presumed 'real man', meekly hands over the wallet to Ko, who returns it to the alarmed customer. Alone with his wife, Ko is stunned to hear that Sien is disgusted by him and that Frans has made her feel like a woman again. He puts his hands over her throat, and we get a series of close-ups: of his face, of her face with her mouth agape, of his face again, of her hand that glides down his shoulder, of her throat, of his face with a blank expression. We get a last shot of her face whereupon the screen turns black. Strictly speaking, this black screen marks a transition to Sien's funeral, but it also signifies his blacking out: he committed an act that he did not want to commit at all. The killing of Sien was, as the definition of a *passage à l'acte* runs, an act without an actor, for the father is so lost he cannot verbalize his mischief.

The film continues to chronicle Sientje's career, starting in Rotterdam in 1923. She declines a marriage proposal by Gerrit and chooses a more adventurous life: the balladeer Jan Meijer predicts she will have a great future as a singer. There are some ups and downs, but the couple has quite some success, particularly thanks to her talents. They get married, she has a baby, but then Jan starts being unfaithful to her and encourages her to amuse a rich baron, to her dismay. He blames her 'silly virtue' for their split-up. By way of farewell, Sien eventually sings 'Telkens weer' [Over and over again] on stage, a song that has become an evergreen. Though the plot focuses on Sien's whereabouts, my main reason for including ROOIE SIEN in this chapter is the role of her father Ko, who is no more than a marginal character.

Sien refuses to read the letters her father sends her, for she considers him a bastard. She hates his excuse of mitigating circumstances based on her mother's bad reputation. One evening, Ko enters a café to listen to her: not knowing who he is, she flirts with him. When he introduces himself, she is much too flabbergasted for a proper response. Jan follows them to her grandparents' place, but Sien insists that her companion put his knife away, for 'my father is a killer'. The scene is shot in rack focus: first Jan is in sharp focus, then her father. Either one or the other is always out of focus to indicate that they cannot be a part of Sien's life simultaneously. When the camera shows Sien, the camera pans to the right, revealing Ko's mother in the background. 'If you badmouth my mother's name once more, I will kill you', Sien warns her father, who then confesses that her mother was already pregnant before the two of them met. 'My only objective was to make her quit her work. But it worries me that she started exactly like you do, in a bar.' Sien ignores his words by retorting that he is a total stranger to her and that she will choose her own way, 'even if it kills me'.

It is striking that Ko speaks his lines in a very flat and monotonous tone; his performance is devoid of any expression. He is unable to raise his voice, and it seems as if the act of strangling has alienated him from his own personality, as if he is the living dead. He has lost practically all his social ties: biologically, he is not Sien's father, as he has confessed, and even if he were, Sien has renounced his paternal claims. At best, Ko is still a son, for we have seen his mother in the background of one of the shots. At the very end of ROOIE SIEN, after Jan and Sien break up, Ko comes to visit her again. She says she does not want his help but, speaking once again with little inflection, he makes it clear that he needs her help. She embraces him at the very moment her own daughter enters the room. She introduces Ko to the girl: 'Sien, this is my father.'

This utterance marks the moment of his symbolic acknowledgement, which is the precondition for Ko's recovery. By calling him 'father', a bond that has once again become possible thanks to her separation from Jan, this opens up the potential for Ko's reintegration into society. This is confirmed by the final tilt-up shot of the three of them walking down the street. Ko has been the walking dead, a symbolic outcast ever since the death of his wife. Sien has offered him an escape route to redemption.

There is no such redemption for the protagonist in HET TEKEN VAN HET BEEST [THE MARK OF THE BEAST] (Pieter Verhoeff, 1980), a film set on the border between Friesland and Groningen, based upon a notorious case that took place in 1929. The opening lines explain that IJje Wijkstra wanted to become a musician or to explore Buddhism, but he never had it in his mind to commit an evil deed. The first seven minutes are a constant reminder, via a voice-over by IJje, that something terrible is about to happen but that it is beyond his will or intention. He is a 33-year-old single man pursuing freedom but, he wonders, was his fate perhaps already sealed? A bit later, he muses that he was caught in a 'web of circumstances', in a 'labyrinth from which I had tried to free myself'. And again a bit later: Did this fate befall him because he was 'born under the mark of the beast, the scorpion, about whom it is written that no one can make war with it?' Time and again, the voice-over indicates that IJje could not influence or alter what awaited him. It would have been better had he never been born, he even sighs. IJje's voice-over commentaries, spoken in retrospect, are meant to prepare us for the ultimate disaster near the end of Verhoeff's film.

When Hendrik Botter, father of six young children, is arrested, his wife Aaltje seduces IJje. He has to take care of his old mother, but at one point, he starts living at Aaltje's place. From that moment onwards, they become the object of nasty gossip, and IJje's brother Dirk takes their mother under his care. IJje asks Aaltje to live at his home—first as his 'maid', then as his wife—and to have her children put under the protection of the Board of Guardians. Even the reverend comes to visit them and predicts that 'the house of the wicked will be destroyed'. After IJje's dog has been hanged, four constables arrive at his place to take Aaltje away. She starts to panic, and his reaction, in blind rage, is to use his guns against the intruders, killing all four. Then he sets his own house on fire. The final text mentions that he is sentenced to prison but dies at the age of 46.

LICENCE TO RIDE A CAB: *NACHTRIT*

The protagonist in HET TEKEN VAN HET BEEST is provoked into violent actions: if the police had not come to his house, no killings would have taken place. Similarly, cab rider Dennis in NACHTRIT [NIGHT RIDE] (Dana Nechushtan, 2006) acts out of despair, since he feels cornered. The violent events in NACHTRIT are set against the backdrop of the so-called 'taxi war' in Amsterdam in 2000. Until the late 1990s, taxi licences were quite scarce in Amsterdam, so a taxi driver was willing to pay a large sum of money for an official licence, sometimes obtained on the black market. In an attempt to stimulate more competition among taxis according to neo-liberal principles, the government decided that the expensive licences were no longer required. Many taxi drivers were angered by the huge drop in value of their official licences , and there were violent incidents in the streets of Amsterdam directed at Taxidirect, a new taxi company, including burnt cars, blockades, and intimidations. Policemen had to intervene, but Taxidirect went bankrupt in 2002. Nechushtan's film starts just before the liberalization of the market: Dennis is eager to obtain a licence, for he dreams about starting his own limo-taxi service together with his brother Marco, or 'Co', a car mechanic. Dennis is introduced to the boss of the one and only taxi company, 'Uncle Jan', who likes Dutch sentimental ballads as much as the brothers do.

Ignoring rumours about an imminent change in rules, Dennis does not get suspicious when he suddenly encounters little difficulty in buying a permit. The conditions for the loan, however, are still unfavourable: the interest he must pay is ridiculously high. Too late, Dennis realizes that he has been set up: his licence becomes worthless overnight, and he is in serious debt. When Dennis's payments are behind, cage-fighting twins hired by Uncle Jan come to threaten him. His brother reproaches him for being a gullible lambkin, but Co's wife Elize tries to comfort Dennis, to the chagrin of Co who thinks that the two of them have always been too close together. But as befits good brothers, they make up with one another. That is the starting point for sheer drama: one evening Co offers to take over from Dennis as a taxi driver, and while Dennis has sex with Elize, Co is beaten up so terribly that he ends up in hospital, seriously handicapped.

Having lost his permit since his payments are overdue, Dennis feels so depressed that he decides to create 'chaos'. He goes behind the wheel of a rivalling company, and this provocative act makes his colleagues aggressive: they demolish his car, smashing all the windows. He gets a note telling him that Uncle Jan's men might take revenge on Co's wife and daughter. He brings them to safety without delay, and then rides his wrecked cab into Uncle Jan's car. One bodyguard dies, and Uncle Jan is wounded. Confessing his crime at a police station to an officer who is well acquainted with Uncle Jan, he is told that the police cannot protect him. Since Jan has survived, he will settle accounts with Dennis, the corrupt officer foretells him. Back on the street, Dennis takes his bedridden brother into the limo and makes sure that Elize drives the limo, with husband and daughter, to Morocco, where there is 'lots of parking space'. In the final scene, Dennis is making his coffee when someone enters off-screen. We see a look of resignation on his face before the screen goes black: we then hear three bullets being fired.

Comparisons between taxi driver Dennis and Travis Bickle from TAXI DRIVER (Martin Scorsese, 1976) who also works night shifts, are inappropriate, for the latter film has set a standard for quality classics, which NACHTRIT has not.[6] Apart from the ominous (background) noises on the soundtrack of both films there is an obvious common denominator, nonetheless: the protagonists both go crazy. Travis is a paranoid protagonist who makes it his mission to clean up the 'dirt' of the streets in New York. The pimps who have authority over the young girl Iris become his main targets, but killing them equals suicide. According to Žižek, this suicide is already announced in the famous mirror scene. While addressing his own image, he says: '*You talkin' to me?*' He seems to practice a possible situation in which he meets an unsympathetic subject, but here the despicable 'you' is visualized as himself, as his mirror image. After Travis is wounded, leaning against a wall after the bloodshed, he mimics a gun with his fingers and mockingly shoots himself. Žižek argues that Travis seems to say by way of this mock gesture: 'The true aim of this outburst is myself', as if Travis himself is an inextricable part of the dirt that has to be eradicated. Instead of the self-reliant hero who solves problems by triumphing over evil, Žižek describes Travis's 'irrational' outburst of violence as an 'implicit admission' of an 'impotent *passage à l'acte*'. If Travis were just to kill himself, it would have been plain suicide, with a personal motive. Travis can only 'triumph', however, by removing himself with a big bang: he has to publicly expose himself as scum (Žižek 'The Act').

Dennis's outburst is similar to Travis's mission, but not quite, and this is the paramount reason NACHTRIT cannot approximate the impact Scorsese's film had. Whereas Travis is a ticking time bomb throughout, Dennis is a likeable guy in principle: he is good with Co's young daughter, he gets along with his colleagues, and he can make a damn good cup of coffee. When people compliment him on his great coffee, he explains his method: put mineral water on the filter coffee, but this water should not be boiling, only hot, and add a pinch of salt. But Dennis is not very smart, at least he is not smart enough to see through vicious tricks—or, in the words of a union leader: 'A taxi driver has the IQ of a dead dog, and none of your colleagues will help you' (once you are in serious trouble).

Unlike Travis, who was a natural born lone wolf, Dennis is much more gregarious. The lack of solidarity among his colleagues frustrates him, and this adds to his anger because he has every reason to feel duped and cornered. Whereas Travis causes murder and mayhem because he sees the city as such as filthy, Dennis takes violent revenge because Uncle Jan and his entourage have been fooling him. As in the case of Travis, Dennis's use of violence can be called 'impotent': he exposes himself to Uncle Jan as the man who injured him, and, as the corrupt policeman implies, with this action, Dennis has more or less signed his death warrant. Travis's violence can be considered a *passage à l'acte* because he has been battling his own demons, but Dennis attempted to kill Uncle Jan and his bodyguards out of sheer bitterness. If they had not treated Dennis so unjustly, he would never have considered such an outrageous crime. In that sense, his use of violence is not a true *passage à l'acte* because it is somehow excusable according to the logic of many a western film. Forbidden by the letter of the law, his revenge is nonetheless presented as a kind of justice: you have done me wrong, so there is an excuse for my outburst.

Because of this logic, NACHTRIT is a psychological drama-thriller that does not transgress mores as rigorously as TAXI DRIVER does. Whereas Travis declares himself '*God's lonely man*' as a sign of his mental breakdown, Dennis is, all in all, a sympathetic big galoot. On the surface, the middle-aged Jörgen Hofmeester from TIRZA (Rudolf van den Berg, 2010) is akin to Dennis from NACHTRIT: Jörgen may seem like a reasonable and average citizen, but he eventually goes ballistic. On closer examination, the reasons for Jörgen's vengeance are quite different. Dennis becomes an unfortunate victim of corrupt circumstances, whereas Jörgen imagines he is a victim due to a cocktail of circumstances. He uses the new boyfriend of his favourite daughter as a projection screen for all his worries. His illegitimate outburst is so horrible that it can only be represented obliquely.

EACH MAN KILLS THE THING HE LOVES: *TIRZA*

In the opening scene of TIRZA, Jörgen is at Schiphol Airport. First, we see him at the back waving farewell, then we see him amidst the crowd, still waving. In the car he tries to contact his daughter Tirza, because she has left her iPod on the passenger's seat, but her phone is on voice-mail. The first of the three narrative strands concerns an explication of Jörgen's current situation: his oldest daughter Ibi has moved to France; Tirza has gone to Windhoek, Namibia; he has become 'superfluous' at the publishing house; his money has evaporated on the stock market some years ago due to some bad advice he received; and his ex-wife pays him an unwelcome visit. She complains about Tirza, that 'little witch', and she tells Jörgen that she still despises him because he never gave her an orgasm. She claims it took much effort for her to 'wake the beast from hibernation'. Much later he discloses in a sort of internal monologue that after his wife had left him, he had sex every Thursday afternoon with the cleaning woman from Ghana, always in the same position in the living room. A second strand concerns his attempts to track down Tirza in Namibia because he never hears from her: no phone calls, no e-mail messages. This second part can be considered a road movie because he ends up at the Big Mama sand dunes in the desert of Namibia in the company of the nine-year-old black girl Kaisa. A third strand concerns a number of Jörgen's flashback memories—though many of them could also be dreamlike hallucinations—in which it becomes clear that while he was not on good terms with Ibi, he idolizes Tirza, his 'highly gifted Sun Queen'.

Some of these flashbacks are relatively brusque, as when he hits the German tenant who is dating Ibi, clearly angry at her father for interfering with her affairs. The smoother flashbacks are usually related to Tirza, and it is even unclear whether all these memories actually happened or not. It is highly probable that the first flashback—in which Tirza is suddenly back at the kitchen table asking her father advice about how to lose her virginity—consists of mental images he has entirely made up himself. He tells her that she has to put boys at ease, touching them gently and telling them: 'I'm Tirza and I'm in love with you.' She first whispers this sentence and then embraces him, repeating the words once more as if he were her lover. In another scene, she asks her father to see her as a woman, with breasts, a belly, and 'very long legs', but he insists that she is not yet a woman, to which she replies: 'I am the only woman you have.'

Jörgen's ex-wife condemns the overly symbiotic relationship between father and daughter. Tirza had an eating disorder in the past, and her mother reproaches her former husband for putting too much pressure on his 'highly gifted' daughter: she had to swim, had to play the cello, had to take ballet lessons. Because Jörgen turned her into his project, there was no space for any intimacy between mother and daughter. The bond between father and daughter is so close that any boyfriend is envisaged as an intruder by Jörgen. During her graduation party, she introduces her Moroccan boyfriend Choukri to her father. And though Choukri is a great cook with no interest in politics, Jörgen

finds reason to disqualify the Arab lover: because Choukri has the 'same face, the same hair, same eyes' as 9/11 terrorist Mohammed Atta, he will probably have the same thoughts and the same hate against the Western world. Jörgen claims to be a 'good judge of people', but Tirza believes that this is poor basic dog psychology. Due to the physical resemblance to Mohammed Atta, Choukri is projected, in the distorted mind of Jörgen, as the source of his downfall that had set in after the Twin Towers crashed.

Most intriguing in TIRZA are the few incoherently brief inserts in which we see that crumpled pages are put in someone's mouth. The narrative in Van den Berg's film is a lengthy prelude to prepare the viewer for the symbolic articulation of the inserts. It will turn out that Jörgen has killed both Tirza and Choukri in a cottage even before the couple was to depart for Namibia. He may perhaps think he is waving farewell to his daughter in the opening shot, but she is already dead by then. He apparently has repressed the memory of murdering the couple, and the incoherent flashes of the pages in someone's mouth are some mental leftovers. He might sincerely believe that he is searching for his daughter in Namibia, and his horrible mischief only gradually begins to dawn on him. While lying under a starry sky, he discloses the details to the young girl Kaisa from the slums of Windhoek who has kept on following him during his journey in the expectation that the white man is in desperate need of company.

In flashback, we see through a rainy window that Choukri is lying atop Tirza. The camera tilts up and a glass reflection reveals that Jörgen is watching. He recounts in a relatively flat tone to Kaisa that it was 'no love but fury', and that Tirza, his 'dearest Sun Queen', suddenly looked at him, surprised. We then see him enter the room in slow motion, the camera focused on his face. 'And then I picked up a poker and hit her on her head.' We never see the poker actually hit Tirza, but the camera shows the blank space right behind Jörgen. We only see parts of his head when his body comes erect to beat her with extra force. Then we are back in the present, and he continues the narrative: 'She collapsed immediately. I hit her again and again. I kept on thinking: you are my own darling Sun Queen.' In comparison, Choukri's torture is more explicitly visualized. After beating him with the poker, he forces Choukri to pray because he wants to see whether Allah will come to rescue 'Atta'. 'If you don't pray, you shall eat.' He tears pages from the Quran and puts them, crumpled, in the mouth of Choukri—which we had already seen twice before in a fragmented presentation. As a token of his insanity and his moral depravity, he then takes a chainsaw, and from a canted low-angle, we hear him say: 'Let's see who is stronger: Allah or the MX 190.' We then hear the voice-over: 'And then I pruned him', and back in the present we first see Kaisa's eyes in close-up. She lies next to Jörgen, while he continues: 'I pruned him, like a sick fruit tree with dead branches.'

It is highly significant that he comes to confess his crime to Kaisa of all people. First, Jörgen confesses to her in his native Dutch tongue, while the earlier conversations he had with Kaisa were in English. So the words he utters have no meaning at all to her. Second, it is likely that Kaisa is only a figment of Jörgen's imagination: a few scenes preceding the confession, Kaisa and Tirza were interchanged with one another via crosscutting: hugging Kaisa equalled hugging his beloved daughter. Third, as he had told Kaisa earlier in Dutch, he had lost everything to 'Mohammed Atta'—his wife and daughter making love to 'hunky Arabs', and his hedge fund having evaporated due to 9/11. Kaisa, however, has lost nothing at all, because no one can take anything from her. He has to pour himself glasses filled with medicines against shame, but she has no shame either. He asks her, in Dutch: 'It's great to be a nobody, isn't it?' And he concludes from this: 'In fact, you're already dead.'

By choosing the 'already dead' Kaisa as his listener who cannot make sense of his story, his confession falls flat and is not symbolically integrated. Of course, it is addressed to the big Other, but he does not have to expect a reply or retribution. His story has no internal audience, just as the visualized parts of his flashback do not show the killing of Tirza, for that is the traumatic kernel of his story that resists display. Throughout the entire film, Jörgen is confronted with his impotence (by his wife) and his superfluity. The only object of affection that he had left—Tirza—was about to cut the cord with her father. Jörgen was turning into a man without qualities who could only kill the thing he loved. He had repressed the non-visualized event of Tirza's death, and his search in Namibia was a prolonged acceptance of the fact that he was, like Kaisa, already dead himself. His ex-wife leaves a message on his phone that Tirza has been found; Jörgen had buried her in the garden of the cottage, but we never see him listen to the voice-mail. At the end of the film, he brings Kaisa back to her poor shanty in the slums, but her mother has died in the meantime. The final shot of Jörgen is of his body lying on a bed in the shanty, covered with flies. It is a fitting conclusion to the film, for if he were to understand the full impact of his violent *passage à l'acte*, as illustrated by his confession story, he would be too guilt-ridden to identify himself as a 'father'. So, as a sign of his self-erasure, death awaited him in a setting in which he is a total nobody. But, as he told Kaisa before, 'It's great to be a nobody, isn't it?'

TIRZA is shot in an atemporal manner: the memory is so overburdened by guilt that it can only be repressed. The film narrative necessarily defies conventional causality. It requires quite a few conditions for Jörgen to remorsefully face his dreadful deed: he can only tell it to a non-understanding girl, while the reminiscence is only visualized partially, for the slaying of Tirza is off-screen. Whereas the non-chronological order of TIRZA is pretty obvious after a

few minutes, the atemporality of ONDER ONS [AMONG US] (Marco van Geffen, 2011) is cleverly disguised. We do not recognize the pre-credit sequence as a foreshadowing of the danger lurking underneath the small town in which everything seems so normal on the surface.

IT'S OH SO QUIET: *ONDER ONS*

Van Geffen's ONDER ONS starts with a crane shot in which the camera tilts down from the sky to the water and the reed. The camera pans to the right, and as the screen goes black, we read the title. We are introduced to a 'normal' family in a new housing estate: Peter and Ilse are a couple with a young boy, Stijn, and a second child on its way. Because of Ilse's pregnancy, the Polish girl Ewa is hired as a nanny. In their house, the colour blue is dominant, for as Ilse likes to say, it '*is always bright, not too heavy-handed*'. Formally, the film is not that 'normal', however: ONDER ONS is shot in wide-screen, and its framing is meticulous.[7] All the environmental shots of the houses or the playground are static, and their impression is 'clinical'. The first shot of Ilse we see her between two doors, as if she is trapped. It is also an indication that spontaneity is not one of her assets. Raising a family seems just another one of her projects. We never see Stijn have an intimate moment with his mother, only with Ewa, who is later blamed for spoiling him too much. Ewa has also good contacts with Aga, another nanny from Poland, but suddenly she wants to keep her compatriot at a distance. Ewa's behaviour is increasingly unpredictable: she stays out late with Stijn, in spite of the cold weather; she laughs hysterically while there is vomit on the floor. At one point, Stijn's father Peter brings her to the parking lot of the Eurolines buses: she is going back to her home country, and Ilse has insisted that Ewa is given two months' extra pay. Ewa has a cuddly toy for Stijn, but once the bus is out of sight, Peter throws it in a garbage can.

Halfway through the film, we suddenly go back in time, and this part will cover the period from the first encounter between Ewa and Aga at the playground until Ewa's return to Poland by bus. Aga's wishes are strictly materialistic: she is adamant that she will never go back to Poland, and for that reason she has broken up with her Polish boyfriend. She makes a casual remark about a rapist in the neighbourhood who has killed his female victim. She is flirting with many a Dutch guy, to the slight embarrassment of Ewa. Aga takes Ewa to the place where she is staying, and while they are recording how they are dancing in the garden, Anton, Aga's employer, shows up. Anton offers to film them, but the camera is suddenly inside the house: we see how Aga goes to the toilet, but through the garden door Anton is visible. From the next scenes onwards, Ewa refuses to respond to Aga's attempts to contact her. When Aga asks 'Why are you acting so foolishly?', Ewa's only reply is: 'Leave me alone' (in Polish).

In a long static take, Ewa apologizes for her behaviour to Aga. We see the two of them dance, and after that, there is a sudden transition to a long take of Ewa at the Eurolines bus. Aga shows up to say farewell, and Ewa asks her, a bit agitated: 'Is Anton here?' Aga is talking to the bus driver as Ewa has already stepped into the bus, halfway the vehicle. Aga is walking to the door but it has been blocked by Anton and it closes before she can address Ewa. Aga waves at the bus, while Anton is out of focus in the background.

Cut to Ewa in the bus, but this is meant to put the viewer on the wrong track. Judging from the conversation by a drunken boy, this is her trip to Amsterdam, which is then confirmed by the intertitle 'Ewa', and her introduction to Peter and Ilse who are now reduced to off-screen voices (*'I hope you like blue'*). From here, there is a cut to the dance scene in the garden. Anton is no more than an off-screen voice, but as soon as Aga goes to the toilet, he walks into the frame, close to Ewa. With a soft voice, he asks her to dance, and then he says: look at me. He touches her hair and has the mobile phone close to her face. Ewa turns around and walks away.

Anton once addresses Ewa when she is outside with Stijn, but her face turns numb. She tries to avoid him, and the camera is on her heels as well. We now understand why she is a failure as a nanny: she locks herself indoors despite Ilse's commands for her to go outside with Stijn. Once she does go away with Stijn, she returns home very late, much to the chagrin of Ilse. Ultimately, she decides to put herself to the test and stands near Brasserie Bakboord in the dark, while Anton is in the brightly lit space. In an extremely long shot, accompanied by ominous sounds, they face one another at each end of Anton's car. After some time, Ewa steps slowly into the car; the camera zooms in on her motionless face through the windshield. No one utters a word, and

Ewa seems puzzled that nothing happens, even after he has made her step out. The next scene we have seen before: Ewa and Aga dancing in the disco, and their laughter is cheerful.

The final scene is once again at the Eurolines bus station but from yet another slightly different angle. Ewa is already on the bus when Anton, blocking the door, tells her: *'Ewa, you're a very smart girl. I would never touch you. Not you.'* Aga is too late to say farewell, as we already know, for the door closes. While Aga starts waving, Ewa is screaming in the bus: *Stop the bus*, but to no avail. She starts crying on the back bench. Cut to Aga who is still waving enthusiastically, but in the background we see Anton out of focus. This is the last we see of Anton; rather than seeing him abuse Aga, we get silent shots of the neighbourhood, with all houses and trees identical. Peter comes home by car, Ilse is already inside. Then three more shots of the new housing estate, without characters, followed by a repetition of the opening shot. The camera tilts down into the water and then pans to the right. Since there is no cut to black this time, we see Aga's body floating in the water, head down without briefs, from right to left. While there is classical music on the soundtrack, the camera tilts up, beyond the reed, to the sky, while we hear the singing of birds.

The key moment is the transition from the last shot of both Aga and Anton to the silent shots of the neighbourhood. At that very moment we become aware of Anton's horrendous crimes, we see a series of empty landscape shots. If we were to assume a conventional causality, it would be logical to show Anton's atrocious rape and murder, but Van Geffen chooses a different option. Although ONDER ONS is about a serial rapist and killer, the film does not show any violence at all: there is a news report in the background about the murder of a girl named Melissa; Aga once asks Ewa what could be the fun of a rape and a subsequent murder; and we see Aga's body in the water as an aftermath effect. One may conclude from this that ONDER ONS represses violent representations, but by giving us the empty landscape shots of a bourgeois environment instead, it suggests what is at the root of this exceptional violence. In an environment of outward normalcy and uniformity, Anton is required to be an average man—and he certainly looks like one—but in fact he is the odd man out. It is ironic that Aga describes Anton's wife Veerle as a bitch, not knowing that he, of all people, hides his dark impulses behind a friendly face. Just as Anton represses his vile instinct by pretending that he is one of us (similar to Patrick from Paul Verhoeven's ELLE, see chapter nine), ONDER ONS represses any depiction of horror and violence: it only shows its gruesome aftermath.

ONDER ONS shares with SCHEMER [DUSK] (Hanro Smitsman, 2010) the structure of overlapping scenes presented from a different perspective, and like Van Geffen's film, SCHEMER moves back and forth in time. In this way, the central event, which was inspired by a widely reported murder that took place in the vicinity of Bemmel in 2003, is postponed in Smitsman's film.

CHRONICLE OF A DEATH FORETOLD: *SCHEMER*

SCHEMER starts with five adolescents waiting in a car near a home. Their girlfriend Jessie has disappeared, and her mother comes outside to ask whether they have heard anything. Caesar answers: 'No, nothing.' Cut to Caesar walking in a field of tall grass, participating in a search party for Jessie's body. The camera pans to the right, then to the left, depicting the five friends from the opening scene: three boys (Caesar, Mick, Rico) and two girls (Frauk, Ilse). Frauk wants to quit, for people have been searching the entire week, but her friends think that's a bad idea. Then she stops and looks off-screen; the camera now focuses on Caesar who looks her in the face and then walks on to the bank of a small lake. The camera is behind Caesar's back, and in the distance we see vaguely what could be a body. Given Frauk's words, it seems an unexpected discovery. Cut to a zoom-in on a flabbergasted Frauk, while on the soundtrack we hear her say: 'Jessie, Jessie.' Some three minutes into Smitsman's film, these words belong to a flashback, which shows Jessie suntanning on the grass.

SCHEMER shows how each of the five friends have a reason for disliking—if not hating—Jessie. These reasons are explained in episodes that start with the name of a character, announced by a black screen with white letters. Frauk starts to suspect Jessie of trying to steal her boyfriend Rico, but when scenes are shown told from Rico's perspective, we see that he himself is actually aiming to seduce Jessie. They even start to kiss, but then Jessie pushes Rico away and she leaves in distress. A bit later, the scene is repeated, but this time from Jessie's perspective. When they kiss, Rico starts to feel her body, and she panics. In a subsequent shot, Jessie inspects her body in a mirror, and she turns out to have a skin disease. She writes Rico's name on a piece of paper, an indication that she is in love with him but simply afraid he might discover her skin problem. The only one who actually finds out, because she is drying her wet clothes in the bushes, is Caesar ('I find it sexy'), but his surplus knowledge does not help him to persuade her to love him. Ilse, Jessie's closest friend, is officially dating Caesar, but when Jessie tells her that her boyfriend kissed her, Ilse immediately confronts him, to his dismay. Finally, in order to hide that he actually fancies Caesar, Mick at one point wants to disavow his homosexual desires by starting to kiss Jessie in public. Since she reacts angrily, Mick feels humiliated. And so the film shows us the seeds of distrust towards Jessie that are sown. When Mick mentions to his friends that he could murder Jessie, they start to think of ways of killing her. Caesar even practices how he would strangle her on Mick until the latter really starts to choke. Jessie then suddenly arrives to intervene: 'Stop it, you deranged psychopath.'[8]

Caesar concocts a plan: Rico should ask her to go to the floodplain, and Ilse should give her a cola with a sedative. When Jessie is still in doubt as to whether she really wants to go, Caesar offers her the car's seat upfront. Ilse stays at home, and Frauk asks to step out together with Rico, but Caesar decides the latter has to stay. So Jessie is together with the three boys. SCHEMER suddenly jumps forward in time: Frauk is waiting for Rico's return. He is in shock and cannot really talk, whereas Frauk wants to reassure him by convincing him that it is not their fault. Ilse acts nervously when Jessie's mother asks her about her daughter's absence: 'I had to lie for her.' In a reversal of cause and effect, we see first the aftermath of Jessie's murder for a couple of minutes before we get to see the reconstruction of the fatal evening. But this reconstruction is presented after another detour, for first we see how Ilse remembers the evening: she did not put pills in Jessie's cola, as she was supposed to do, and then there is the telephone call from Caesar: 'Guess who we are wrapping up in plastic?' When she starts crying, her mother presumes that Caesar has broken up his relationship with Ilse.

The scenes of the aftermath function as a chronicle of a death foretold. Frauk asks permission to leave the car once Caesar seems about to strangle Jessie. After Frauk's departure, Caesar's eyes are downcast, but suddenly he puts a rope over Jessie's head. There is quite a number of shots, mainly close-ups: a struggling Jessie, an obstinate look on the part of Mick who has come to Caesar's assistance. The few times we have a two-shot of the boys, one of the faces is out of focus. There is only an extreme long shot in between, of the car at the small parking lot near the lake. At the end, there is a rack focus from Caesar to Mick, and they both start laughing, apparently to release pent-up energy. Rico walks back home after Jessie has been wrapped in plastic; Mick and Caesar make sure the corpse drowns in the lake. The two boys embrace, and with a longing look Mick says to Caesar: 'Fuck it, we did it.'

We see the friends visiting Jessie's mother; Caesar trying to comfort her, albeit quite awkwardly; Mick being congratulated on a 'nice speech'; but also Caesar in tears and wanting his girlfriend Ilse to leave. A bit later, we see Ilse at the police station and Caesar is handcuffed: apparently she has made, or is about to make, a confession. We go back to the scene in which Caesar wants her to 'get the hell out' of his house. He then goes to the lake, pulls the body onto the banks of the lake, and then the scene with the search party from the beginning is repeated. Caesar arrives at the body first, and pulls her shirt down so that no one will see her skin disease.

The key moment of SCHEMER is obviously the killing of Jessie, emphasized by the slow build-up to the murder. Significantly, this build-up is presented in an atemporal mode to underscore the outrageous nature of the violence. Because of the atemporality, we already know that the murder has taken place before we see its actual unwinding. Thus, we become painfully aware of Caesar's dilemma: once he has set the ball rolling, there is no point of return without a loss of face. His facial expression is one of hesitance, but he nonetheless puts the rope over Jessie's throat. Mick starts supporting him, but by this time, we know he is basically motivated by his repressed fondness for Caesar. To kill a girl together with his best friend is extremely exciting for him, as the aftermath illustrates, precisely because it has to be kept a secret.

The final part of SCHEMER is dedicated to Caesar's attempts to come to terms with his *passage à l'acte*.[9] But he can only pay for his crime once the body has been found, so he makes sure that the corpse is put on the banks. The overall strategy of SCHEMER is to show main scenes twice in order to make the viewer realize that every first viewing of a scene is based upon a misinterpretation. The ultimate discovery of Jessie's body, shown in the very beginning of SCHEMER, was a surprise to the people involved in the search party, but at the end, we know it had been set up by Caesar as a precondition for his redemption: an official verdict (not part of the film) will be required for his reintegration into the symbolic order.[10]

I'M DERANGED: *VAN GOD LOS*

Redemption comes too late for Stan, the internal narrator in VAN GOD LOS [GODFORSAKEN!] (Pieter Kuijpers, 2003), but we only understand this once we realize, relatively late, that the film has a cyclical structure. Stan recounts the tragic events in retrospect, depicted in a picture that was hailed with favourable reviews. VAN GOD LOS is loosely based on the notorious 'gang of Venlo' whose members committed a series of violent crimes between Carnival in 1993 and Carnival in 1994. It was Kuijpers' debut feature, and it remains his very best film, if we take him at his word that RIPHAGEN (2016) is his last film as director. VAN GOD LOS offers a clear motivation—a bit too clear, perhaps—for the deranged behaviour of the two main characters. Both Maikel Verheije and Stan Meijer are marked by the traumatic absence of a respectable father figure. Maikel refers to his father only once, when he apologizes to his friend Stan for an inappropriate remark about the latter's father. Maikel mentions that the only time he has ever seen his own father, 'the bastard' had a pile of presents for his son's birthday, but when his father discovered he had the date wrong, he took all the presents back with him to his own place.

Since the events depicted in VAN GOD LOS are often brutal, the style of the film is dovetailed with the content: grainy images, jittery camerawork, bleached colours, relatively fast-paced editing. Kuijpers makes abundant use of voice-over, which always risks being considered a weakness according to the slogan 'show, don't tell', but here it works effectively. The story is consistently narrated by Stan, a relatively average adolescent who due to a combination of circumstances makes a series of poor choices. One of these choices is his decision to become friends with the long-haired Maikel, played by Tygo Gernandt as a bigger-than-life character, which makes him an object of both fascination and repulsion. He promises a life full of adventure, but he is also a loose cannon. Since Maikel's actions are focalized by Stan, we recognize this ambivalence in his facial expressions. Stan's emotional response ranges from awe and excitement to embarrassment and repressed anger, for he cannot rein in Maikel's behaviour.

The first twenty minutes of VAN GOD LOS narrate how Maikel has come to substitute for Stan's biological father who was a key point of reference for him, despite—or perhaps due to—his absence. When Stan was six years old, his mother married the dentist Herbert. In his first voice-over Stan expresses his dislike of the upper echelons of society via a reference to Carnival, the most important celebration in his hometown. While we see extreme long shots in slow motion, partly sharp, partly out-of-focus, of a crowd cheering during a parade, Stan explains that the inhabitants of his town only show their true colours during the three days of festivities when they wear masks on their faces. In other words, the citizens give in to their impulses only in disguise, but without a mask they behave like cold-hearted hypocrites, pretending to be civilized people. He sees his mother as an ostrich who has no sense of what might bother her son. After she tells him to take off his cap and proposes to go on holidays in an expensive hotel, we hear in voice-over: 'If she didn't like what she saw, she pretended it wasn't there.'

This remark is followed by a flashback in which we see a young Stan, wearing a cap, waiting at a gas station. The flashback is more colourful than the rest of the film, implying that it triggers happy memories. Slow motion shots of a man who comes his way with a big smile on his face are accompanied by a voice-over in which Stan explains that it took quite some time before he found his real father, but that he never told his mother that he had had contact with him. According to his mother, the man was a 'failure'. This judgement is never explained, but Stan's father earns his money as a truck driver, a low-class occupation, which was perhaps beneath her means. Anyway, the minute Stan sees his father, he knows it is him right away, which emphasizes that he resembles his father (or at least he thinks he does). In recognizing his similarity with his father, however, he accentuates how much he does not identify with both his mother and her current husband. It is to Stan's great annoyance that everyone in his relatively small community, upon hearing his name, says 'Ah, the dentist's son'. This misrecognition, of course, implies that he is expected to display behaviour befitting a boy from a well-to-do upbringing. If he is more like his low-class father, as he thinks he is, he must be a 'failure' too.

While his mother is packing the suitcases for their holidays, Stan leafs through the paper and sees an article about a dead truck driver. In the obituaries, he finds a name that shocks him—Bert Mulder—emphasizing that he, Stan Meijer, does not carry his father's family name. There is a transition to a scene in the past, apparently one week after his first encounter with his father. Stan had asked him whether he could come and live with him, but his dad avoids giving a clear response and instead proposes they meet again next week. Before Stan goes back to his mother, his father gives him his watch as an object to remember him by. In the second flashback, after reading his father's name in the paper, Stan refuses to join his mother on holidays, and we see him leaving a letter behind, 'for mom, confidentially'. While walking along the road with a suitcase, an elderly couple takes him in his car and brings him to the gas station where he is expecting to meet his father. He waits for quite some time, until dark, and while recounting in voice-over that he never saw him again, the very same couple passes by and takes him back home. Instead of acknowledging that his father was a coward, he keeps his confidence in him as a character and invents a series of excuses: perhaps the old man was held up at the French border or even arrested in Germany, for they are very strict over there. But this missed encounter leaves a scar nonetheless. From this particular incident, he draws the following lesson: 'I should have known that one should not let anyone get close.' The important point here is that he does not acknowledge that his father was an untrustworthy bum or a failure; instead he concludes that humankind as a whole is depraved: once you care for someone, you will be deceived, period.

Upon his return home, his stepfather, dressed in his dentist's outfit, passes him by without noticing him. He does not question where he has been the last couple of hours. What's more, throughout VAN GOD LOS, there is never any conversation between this man and Stan; we only hear his voice off-screen. Apparently, his mother did not miss him; the envelope is still on the table, and has not been opened. We never see her offer him affection, which is affirmed when Stan attends his father's funeral, while his mother is conspicuously absent. We see Stan from the back at a distance from the crowd, and when the camera tracks forward, it goes over his head. Then the camera zooms in on him from a reverse angle, until medium close-up. He is contemplating in voice-over: 'Would he have ever mentioned me? What was I doing here? I hardly knew him. I looked like a fool.' But when Stan looks to the right, he sees a dark shadow approach him in slow motion, and gradually it becomes clear that Maikel is coming his way. He had known Maikel only briefly, but he feels so comfortable with him that he even tolerates the company of the 'junkie' Sef who considers himself an 'occasional user' but who, according to Stan, 'uses on every occasion'. The three of them participate in some small crime, and when they are arrested with a considerable amount of money, Stan explains to the police that what he had on him was simply pocket money. The 'dentist's son' is allowed to go home, but the other two are taken into custody for quite a period. When Maikel visits Stan at the funeral, he had just been released from prison. Stan is amazed: 'It beats me how he knew', but the slow motion arrival of Maikel punctuates the impact upon Stan. Mentally, this scene seals Stan's pact with Maikel, for the latter stood by him at the right moment. In the absence of a father, Stan chooses the mesmerizing daredevil Maikel over his disinterested mother and stepfather. It shows that Stan could put more trust in a psychopath rather than in his bourgeois mother.

Out of disgust with the mentality of the bourgeois, Stan starts to sympathize with Maikel. This long-haired guy leads his life as if it is Carnival the entire year, without wearing a mask. At the same time, Stan is valuable for Maikel in his contact with Anna Sprengers, a girl who could have dated any boy but had chosen Maikel. Since the latter would not be acceptable for her parents, Stan functions as a useful go-between. He can visit her place and act as her so-called boyfriend, for he is the 'dentist's son'. He is permitted to take her out, so that Maikel can have sex with Anna in his car.

A chain of criminal events is set in motion when Maikel and Stan think they can commit a simple burglary: they intend to rob the hash dealer Johan Schreurs, but it drives Maikel crazy when things do not go as planned. They have difficulty tying up Johan, and Maikel shoots him in the flank. Shocked by Maikel's action, Stan takes off his mask unintentionally. While he is guarding the hurt dealer, Maikel ruins the place, looking for money, but to no avail. In a blind panic, Stan starts hitting the victim with a baseball bat. Maikel takes over from his buddy and shoots the dealer ('Sorry, Johan') in the head. Stan has to vomit afterwards, but Maikel tries to reassure him by saying: 'It was a stupid accident. If he had cooperated, he'd have been alive. We have to trust each other. What happens to you can happen to me, too.'

I already mentioned that VAN GOD LOS uses slow motion frequently to accentuate key moments in Stan's life: the meeting with his dad; Maikel's arrival at the funeral; the shot when Stan first lays eyes on Anna, Maikel's girl, or later when he is preparing to get away with Anna. The brutal killing of Johan is, however, too atrocious, and this is not only indicated by Stan's vomit. First, there is a discrepancy between the execution itself and Maikel's account. When Sef runs into the two boys, Maikel boasts about the killing: 'You should have seen his face, those eyes, when he knew I'd shoot him.' But

Maikel had his own eyes averted before shooting Johan who moreover was lying motionless and face down on the ground. Second, the actual moment of firing itself is rendered obliquely. As Maikel is about to shoot, the camera cuts to a huge framed photograph on the wall, but the contours of the portrait are vague. In the glass of the photograph, the killing is mirrored. Due to the superimposition, it is pretty vague as well, but the sound of the shot is clearly audible. After the shot, the focus shifts and we can discern the framed picture: Johan Schreurs is dressed up as Prince Carnival, which is a honorary position in the south of the Netherlands. Upon leaving, the glass is shattered with the baseball bat.

The oblique representation, marked by the superimposition and the shift in focus, is an indication that a limit has been trespassed, especially if we consider that this killing, which Maikel euphemistically attempts to call an 'accident', is embedded in Stan's account. From this first murder onwards, a point of no return has been reached. When he hears that Johan was a provider of hash for the influential Turk Osman Sukur, he fears he has to run for his life. But the gangster boss proposes that they can escape revenge by becoming his hired killers. Stan's line of reasoning is symptomatic of a survival mode: the victims had to be killed anyway. They had to pull the trigger at men who in fact were already dead. Stan decides to shoot Hassan, the first man on the list, remembering Maikel's line 'What happens to you can happen to me, too.' After he has executed Hassan, there is a cut to a blurred shot. There is a stain in the middle, and on the outer edge of the frame we see the wall of what is probably a church, for a statue of the Virgin Mary can be discerned. There is a shift in focus once again: the stain in the middle becomes sharp, and it is Stan who takes his cap of his head; now the background becomes out of focus. There is a transition with Stan in a mirrored position but now sitting in a café, which suggests that the church must have been opposite the café. Visibly crestfallen, Stan attempts to recuperate himself: you have to ban your emotions, keep people at a distance, don't let anyone get too close, 'that's all'. His rationale is visually translated in the depiction of subsequent killings. In one lengthy darkly lit panning shot, we then see a series of men being executed, and the lack of a cut here signifies that it has become a sort of routine for the boys. We see Maikel and Sef scream at the victims, but we do not hear a sound except for Stan's deadpan commentary and a choir singing Gregorio Allegri's 'Miserere Mei Deus'. Whereas the first two murders were examples of a *passage à l'acte*—throwing Stan off balance—the lengthy pan accompanied by solemn music suggests that the victims mean 'nothing' to him, as he told himself. By this time, Stan has apparently become devoid of emotions: the executions have been symbolically integrated by him, for he is capable of saying that they have numbed him.

Problems arise when Osman stops asking them to kill. Maikel is in desperate need of a constant flow of money, and when he goes over to Osman's coffeehouse Ishmir to obtain compensation, he feels put off by an unsatisfactory explanation.[11] Once outside, there is an out-of-focus shot, with Ishmir in the background. Maikel walks towards the camera, but we can only see him in sharp focus when his face is in close-up. He is breathing heavily in frustration. There is a cut to Osman's granddaughter who brings the boss a cup of tea, in slow motion. A crosscut to Maikel who goes back to the coffeehouse and shoots twelve bullets through the glass door, the last part of the segment shown in slow motion. The cup of tea falls to the ground, also in slow motion, and, as is later confirmed by the police, Osman's granddaughter is among the victims. What is remarkable here is that Maikel is not out of focus while he is shooting nor in the aftermath when he is making a phone call to Stan, but only preceding his action. In other words, he is blackened out when he has not killed yet; in Maikel's case, it seems as if the shooting is required to bring him back to his senses. This is what distinguishes the 'accidental' criminal Stan, who has to recover from the act, and the raving maniac Maikel whose mind only comes to rest by killing. A *passage à l'acte* does not derail Maikel; it gives him energy.

In the climactic event of VAN GOD LOS, the distinctions between the two are articulated most clearly. Stan wants to help Anna, who by now is convinced of Maikel's furious whims. He sells some stuff, including his father's watch, so she can get away, but Maikel is already waiting for them. Stan thinks they can escape unseen because Carnival enables them to be dressed as gorillas and Anna in a rabbit suit. It is only when they are in the car, with Sef as the fourth passenger, that Stan hears that they are going to rob an elderly couple who according to Sef has plenty of cash hidden in jars—'junkie crap', according to Stan. Sef and Maikel will do the robbery, but Stan joins them because he cannot bear the thought that Sef might molest them. While Mozart's 'Lacrimosa' sets in, everything goes wrong. The guys do find many jars but no money and Stan gets increasingly nervous due to the violence inflicted upon the elderly couple.

Maikel gives the gun to Stan and encourages him to shoot the old woman. 'I know her', Stan tells him, because this was the couple that gave him the lift years ago when he was searching for his father. Maikel takes off Stan's gorilla mask, but the woman does not recognize him (because he was only a kid back then). Stan shows his 'friends' the money in the hope of calming them down, but their anger is only increased because they think he wanted to betray them. Stan puts the gun to Maikel's head who challenges him repeatedly: 'Shoot, Stan!' At that moment, the woman seems to realize who he is: 'Stanny?' Stan is distracted for a moment, and Maikel slits her throat in a slow movement.

While slow motion is used often in this film, the performances by the actors are also deliberately slow on a number of occasions. Maikel can be very energetic, but he can also act in a very restrained manner. While he has a gun pointed at his head by a totally freaked-out Stan, who does not pull the trigger, he shows off a cool demeanour. The slitting of the woman's throat amid a situation of high tension becomes a matter-of-fact act on Maikel's part: I can do this in a calm manner because it does not affect me.

Initially, Stan is too stunned to even move, but once outside, he shoots an unguarded Maikel in his chest, witnessed by Anna inside the car. Stan tells Anna to go, and he himself kneels down with Maikel. He now repeats a sentence, twice, that Maikel had mentioned to him before: 'What happens to you happens to me, too.' The shooting of Maikel point blank is an outrageous moment: in fact, given the mantra of 'what happens to you happens to me', it is a suicide in disguise. This is illustrated by an atemporal dissolve to a shot in which the camera scans a body lying in a coffin, from toe to head, revealing it is Stan. After this brief insert, which is a flashforward, we go back to the present. Stan throws away his gun, and in voice-over we hear him say: 'Regrets? No. Not for one moment.' With his hands in the air, Stan gives Sef the opportunity to stab him, shown in slow motion. Sef takes Maikel in the car, and Stan is left behind, bleeding to death. On the verge of dying, we hear a final contemplation: 'What you love, you lose.' Life could have been different, and there is once more a flashback to the one meeting with his father in the truck, but, as Stan realizes, 'appearances are deceptive'. At the same time, death has an advantage too: Stan's voice-over mentions that no one can get near to him anymore. The film then ends with a blinding white screen before the end credits roll.

Though I have gone to quite some lengths to describe the plot of Kuijpers' VAN GOD LOS, this does not explain yet why this is a much appreciated Dutch movie. First, this history of violence is consistently mediated by the 'reflexive' voice-over of Stan, the sanest character among the perpetrators. In the absence of father figures, Maikel can take the place of a big brother, and their bond is sealed by the identical ring with a number of death skulls he buys for Stan. The voice-over is to a great extent contemplative, and this is justified by the remarkable status of the narrated text. The images in the prologue of the carnival parade where people are 'alive' behind their masks before they return to their dead old selves, according to Stan's voice-over, are juxtaposed with the cleaning of a dead body: we never see a face, but we see that blood is being washed away, and on repeated viewing, we recognize the death-skull ring. Just before Sef stabs Stan at the very end of the movie, there is, as I mentioned, a brief flashforward insert: after a dissolve, we see the camera tilt up, starting with the shoes and ending at Stan's head, lying in a coffin. He is wearing the very same suit as the headless corpse at the beginning. So, whereas Stan is lethally wounded at the end of the film, the flashforward insert reveals that he was already dead from the very beginning, thanks to the parallel with the prologue scenes. The voice-over is posthumous and clearly told with hindsight, for sometimes Stan anticipates events: 'I had better ...' 'I should have known ...' Thus, the voice-over originates from the living dead, a literal living dead, which makes him more or less equal to the townspeople for they are the living dead in a figurative sense, except for the three days they wear a mask during Carnival, according to Stan.

Second, one of the assets of Kuijpers' film are the slowed-down movements of characters, which, when used inappropriately, can be the most worn-out of devices. This is a cheap trick for a spectacular effect, but in this film, it is used during those moments when Stan—this average guy—is thrown off balance. Annoyed by his mother and stepfather, he makes the choice to hang out with Maikel, despite the fact that he considers Sef a nuisance, but from then onwards he is caught up in a turmoil of events. Every slow motion underscores that he is on board an unstoppable train. I already mentioned the shot when Maikel approached him as a dark shadow at the funeral of Stan's father: mentally, this sealed Stan's pact with Maikel, for the latter stood by him at the right moment. Another example is the first time Stan lays eyes on Anna, which is punctuated by a slow motion presentation of her movements as he immediately falls under her spell. He is fascinated by her, not only because of her appearance but also because she is Maikel's girlfriend. Since she belongs to this 'bad boy', she can never be his girl. When she tries to kiss him, he is hesitant, not because he does not like her, but because he is worried about Maikel finding out. At the same time, conscious of Maikel's whimsical behaviour, he is very protective of Anna: he thinks it is his self-acclaimed duty to save her, but his attempts to help her weaken his own position, for ultimately it makes Maikel suspicious. Slow motions are also used when Stan realizes that his plan of going away with Anna is obstructed and Maikel forces him to join him.

Even though the slow motions stand out, VAN GOD LOS also uses the cinematic devices of time-lapse photography (when time seems to be moving faster), rack focus (change from sharp to out-of-focus and vice versa) and blinding white light. Each of these devices indicates in their own ways that Stan is derailed by the events, as if he is no more than a marionette amidst a series of irrational violent outbursts. The only way he can make any sense of what has happened to him is via a posthumous voice-over, hovering between symbolization (proved by his narration) and its beyond (his death). Hence, VAN GOD LOS has a cyclical structure: bleeding to death at the end of the film, Stan is shown, as we realize with hindsight, as a headless corpse in the prologue.

REQUIEM FOR A CHAMP: *WOLF*

The success of VAN GOD LOS resulted in an eponymous television series that has aired since 2011 on national television, somewhat irregularly.[12] Each and every episode of 50 minutes is a dramatization of a real-life crime, and so far, BEVERMAN & ZN. (Michiel ten Horn, broadcast on 18 September 2017) is the crowning achievement. In cinema, WOLF (Jim Taihuttu, 2013) is the film par excellence to equal the rawness of the violence in VAN GOD LOS, especially when the protagonist gets caught up with a criminal gang.

Shot in black and white, WOLF opens with a scene shot from inside a shopwindow at night. Majid and his friend Adil are in doubt whether to steal the black Asprilla motorcycle or the grey one. Once they have decided, the window is smashed before our very eyes. The scene is emblematic of Majid's existence, marked by petty crime and hanging around with his friends. He is on bad terms with his father; his older brother is the 'good' son, but he is terminally ill; his younger brother is too young to speak up. Majid is given the opportunity to work at a flower auction to help him integrate into mainstream Dutch society, but he looks down upon this work. He has one particular talent, though: when he visits a kickboxing school, he breaks his opponent's jaw in a test fight. He is too undisciplined, however, to build a career in sports. His trainer gets mad when he continues hitting after the referee has ended the match; he behaves brutally toward his Dutch girlfriend Tessa and even more violently against anyone who dates her.

But the worst is yet to come. The Turkish Hakan, head of a criminal organization, is interested in Majid because of his strength. Hired as a security guard, Majid has to pull a gun during a deal. He starts using cocaine as a means to release his tension. A big match in the ring potentially awaits him, but he neglects his trainer's demand that he train twice a day. His trainer tells him: 'Well, walk away again. Do what you do best, disappear', adding in a dismissive tone: 'Your father and brother will be proud.' When his braggart pal Adil suggests robbing an armoured car, Majid, knowing that the plan has been concocted by Hakan, does not want to participate until Adil says: 'I told those Turks you're in as well.' In the heist, Adil kills two men, but his friend Vleermuis is fatally wounded. They make money, but the loot is not as big as expected. Majid, downcast about Vleermuis's death, decides to keep a low profile for a while, but then Adil seduces Tessa, who is furious and hits him. When Majid asks about Adil's black eye, the latter says he interfered when 'that filthy Turk' Baris, one of Hakan's gang members, was flirting with Tessa. Predictably, Majid's revenge induces more violence: on his way to the dressing room for a kickboxing match, he is seriously hurt by Baris and his friends. Hakan says: 'If you go down in the second round, we will forget about this.' When he sees after the first round that his father and his younger brother are among the audience, he forgets about the deal and knocks out his opponent in the second round. We see Majid in close-up in the dressing room, recovering from the physical effort. The door opens—end of movie.

A Dutch film like WOLF was unheard of in Holland[13] because, as Taihuttu himself explained, Dutch distributers are not inclined to invest money in a film that is a 'checklist for politically incorrect movie-making' (quoted in Linssen, 2013): shot in black and white, containing nasty violent scenes, paced slowly at times, and taking as its subject non-sympathetic foreigners who appear hopeless (underscored by the choice of black and white). And Wolf as the one character who has the chance to improve his position does not succeed, leaving it a matter of debate whether he fails because of his environment or his own lack of spine, or perhaps both. Whatever the reason, the problem with Wolf is that he is caught up in a cycle of violence because he postpones any reflexive moments. Adil acts as a good friend, but Wolf does not see that Adil misuses their friendship. He stands up for Adil too unconditionally because Wolf has the irascible nature and the strength to do so. And his support for Adil results in hard-hitting blows and violent scenes in which Wolf gets involved.

In many American movies, such as several Clint Eastwood films, violence is used in a desire to 'get even': revenge is justified via the unwritten rules of compensation because the 'bad guys' deserve punishment. Violence helps to distinguish the morally good from evil. By contrast, the Korean director Park Chan-wook is often criticized for the sadistic violence in his movies such as BOKSUNEUN NAUI GEOT [SYMPATHY FOR MR. VENGEANCE] (2002) and OLDEUBOI [OLDBOY] (2003), since reviewers tend to take it as an expression of the director's 'morally bankrupt' worldview . This is a misinterpretation of Park's cinema, Steve Choe argues, for his films present an 'unforgiving logic': it may seem 'cool', but it only results in a terrible and bloody mess. In an interview, Park stated that 'revenge is an endless circle of evil' (quoted in Choe, 96). The characters are caught up in an 'implacable compulsion toward vengeance' (95): driven by revenge, they must kill, but in the end, there is retribution for no one. Films like WOLF and VAN GOD LOS respond to a similar logic: there is a paradox in the violence in these films, for the characters think it will ward off what haunts them, but it only ends up bringing their inner demons in closer proximity.

CONCLUSION: WHERE IS MY MIND?

In this chapter on *passages à l'acte*, I have described some acts that lack proper actors: a character such as Ko in ROOIE SIEN seems temporarily out of control when he strangles Sien, whereas IJje in HET TEKEN VAN HET BEEST and Dennis in NACHTRIT are pushed to such extremes that they commit violence beyond their control. In SCHEMER, the murder is executed as a consequence of the mechanisms of group pressure rather than a calculated arrangement. The irrational outbursts in the atemporal films TIRZA and ONDER ONS are represented obliquely: Jörgen has repressed the memory of his deed, and only some mental leftovers hint at the inevitable return of the repressed; in ONDER ONS, it is suggested that the disquieting calmness of a bourgeois environment can be a cover-up for the dark impulses of a 'normal' citizen on the condition that he conforms to the conventions of domestic life. VAN GOD LOS uses many cinematic techniques—such as rack focus, slow motion, and time-lapse photography—to indicate that narrator Stan is derailed by the events: he is carried along by the daredevil Maikel who uses violence to feel alive; the moment Maikel uses it, he is brought back to his senses. He is only affected by it afterwards, though he prefers to deny this. Stan's posthumous voice-over is an indication that he can talk about it but only belatedly, from an afterlife perspective. He is a narrator who exists in the gap between his symbolic death and his biological death: it is only because he has already paid for everything with his life that he can comment upon the use of violence. The character of Wolf in Taihuttu's movie is a mixture of both Maikel and Stan: in theory, Wolf is a good guy with a difficult relation with his father (like Stan), but he is too easily inclined to violence and crime, and that ultimately does not pay.

NOTES

1 *De stille kracht* was a canonical novel by Dutch writer Louis Couperus. Rademakers had expressed the wish to adapt the book, which was set in the Dutch East Indies, into a film. In 1974, DE STILLE KRACHT was shown on television as a much-praised four-hour-long mini-series, directed by Walter van der Kamp.

2 In TOUCH OF EVIL, Welles also played a detective, albeit a corrupt one.

3 Whereas BECAUSE OF THE CATS was a bit too late, the twenty-minute short BIG CITY BLUES (Charles Huguenot van der Linden, 1962) was premature. This title has only very few spoken words, was nominated for an Oscar in the category of 'Short Subjects, Live Action Subjects', but the film has been practically forgotten. It was shot in black and white with remarkable camera angles and had a frenet-

ic jazzy score. At times it was deliberately overexposed to create a grainy look. A teenage delinquent is sitting in the backseat of a police car. His black companion is taken out of the building and exchanges looks with a young boy, who holds a white rabbit in his arms. The screen goes entirely white. A young girl in a white dress takes the boy's rabbit and he starts chasing her. She runs into a run-down building and two teenage boys cast eyes on her. One of them goes after the girl out of boredom, and the lengthy chase sequence results in her fatal downfall. The young boy finds his rabbit back and hears the black teenager play the trumpet. A few moments later, we are back at the beginning: the one delinquent already in the police car, the other on its way. The boy lets his rabbit walk around as in the beginning, and then a girl in a white dress arrives. She grabs the rabbit and the boy chases her into the building, end of the short. The topic was considered too explosive and therefore Huguenot van der Linden was not given the opportunity to turn his short into a feature-length picture. To his sorrow, Huguenot van der Linden saw how Stanley Kubrick achieved success with a similar topic, nine years later: A CLOCKWORK ORANGE.

4 I already used the term 'acting out' in chapter one, but then as it was defined by Sherry Turkle.

5 During the 2018 edition, the prestigious Cannes film festival presented a full 4K restoration of the original 35 mm Techniscope camera negative of Sluizer's film.

6 Another clear reference to one of Scorsese's films: During a party at Uncle Jan's place, a tense atmosphere arises when one of Jan's bodyguards, the cage fighter Ruud, thinks that Dennis is laughing at him. This scene is reminiscent of the tension between protagonist Henry Hill and the unpredictable Tommy DeVito in GOODFELLAS (Martin Scorsese, 1990). Dennis tries to make a funny remark, which Ruud finds insulting, but when the bystanders start to laugh, the situation is resolved.

7 For ONDER ONS, cinematographer Ton Peters worked with Christian Berger's Cine Reflect Lighting System. During a workshop at Rialto in Amsterdam on 19 February 2010, the Austrian director of photography Berger explained the benefits of CRLS, which he had used to shoot the critically acclaimed DAS WEISSE BAND [THE WHITE RIBBON] (Michael Haneke, 2009).

8 This of course recalls the scene in STRANGERS ON A TRAIN (Alfred Hitchcock, 1951) when Bruno wants to show two elderly women during a party how to commit the perfect murder. He puts his hands around the throat of one of them, but as he sees Barbara, the girl who is wearing the very same glasses as the woman he had killed, he loses himself and the elderly woman nearly chokes.

9 At the end of SCHONE HANDEN [CLEAN HANDS] (Tjebbo Penning, 2015), the young boy Yuri kills his father Eddie. Normally, a parricide is the most horrible of crimes, but the film legitimizes the shooting as the best of actions at that moment. Unbeknownst to his naive wife Sylvia, Eddie had earned his income by drug dealing.

Once she finds out about her husband's unscrupulous nature, she tries to flee with her two children to a foreign country. Eddie becomes so deranged by her 'betrayal' that he puts the lives of every family member at risk. At the peak of the danger, Yuri shoots his daddy. As their happy and sunny existence in Spain shows, this killing was to the advantage of Sylvia and her two children. The epilogue suggests that the kid has committed a crime with 'clean hands'.

10 Like SCHEMER, Smitsman's SKIN (2008) was also inspired by a notorious incident that had received widespread media coverage. SKIN was based on the famous murder by stabbing in 1983 of a fifteen-year-old black boy (Kerwin Duinmeijer) by a sixteen-year-old skinhead. At the time, it was reported as being racially motivated in the press, but in Smitsman's film, this motivation is downplayed. The kid became a skinhead only as a reaction to unfortunate personal circumstances: his Jewish father was still marked by Holocaust experiences and his mother had just died from cancer. The stabbing followed obnoxious behaviour, and the victim's 'skin' was irrelevant. By suggesting there was only a slightly excusable or understandable reason for the killing, the murder in SKIN is not as radical as a *passage à l'acte*.

11 The Turks have started to regard Stan as untrustworthy because he had been seen at the police station. Stan had never told Maikel that he went there to meet Anna who had been interrogated after she had spread the rumour that Johan Schreurs was dead due to an 'accident'.

12 The television series VAN GOD LOS had nine episodes in 2011, ten in 2012, six in 2013, and six in 2017.

13 Though a Dutch film, WOLF basically derives influences from foreign films. Taihuttu's picture recalls the sense of frustration evident in Kassovitz's LA HAINE (1995), also shot in black and white and set in a poor urban area; it is reminiscent of several Martin Scorsese pictures, recalling the street mentality of MEAN STREETS (1973), the boxing scenes in the black-and-white RAGING BULL (1980), and the tracking shots behind the back of the protagonist in GOODFELLAS (1990). The confrontations between a young Arab and a gangster boss seem to be inspired by UN PROPHÈTE [A PROPHET] (Jacques Audiard, 2009).

BIBLIOGRAPHY

Bernink, Mieke, *Fons Rademakers: Scènes uit leven en werk* (Abcoude: Uniepers, 2003).

Choe, Steve, *Sovereign Violence: Ethics and South Korean Cinema in the New Millennium* (Amsterdam: Amsterdam University Press, 2016).

Hewitson, Owen, 'What Does Lacan Say About ... Acting Out?' *Lacanonline.com*,https://www.lacanonline.com/2010/12/what-does-lacan-say-about-acting-out/ [Accessed 13 March 2020].

Linssen, Dana, 'Jim Taihuttu in zwart-wit: Checklist tegen politiekcorrect filmmaken', *De Filmkrant* (August 2013), https://filmkrant.nl/interview/jim-taihuttu-in-zwart-wit/ [Accessed 13 May 2020].

Turkle, Sherry, *Alone Together: Why We Expect More From Technology and Less From Each Other* (New York: Basic Books, 2011).

Žižek, Slavoj, 'The Act and Its Vicissitudes', *The Symptom* (2005):http://www.lacan.com/symptom6_articles/zizek.html [Accessed 17 May 2020].

—, *Violence: Six Sideways Reflections* (London: Profile Books, 2009).

CHAPTER 7

From Historical Discomfort to Historical Trauma

Verstraten, P., *Dutch Post-War Fiction Film Through a Lens of Psychoanalysis*. Taylor & Francis Group, 2021
DOI 10.5117/9789463725330_CH07

ABSTRACT

The colonial history of the Netherlands was the subject in Rademakers' adaptation of MAX HAVELAAR. Together with DE SCHORPIOEN, it is a clear example of a film that registers attempts to cover up a dreadful state of affairs. HET ZWIJGEN is centred around a local mystery on audiotape, whereas DE BENDE VAN OSS shows how Catholics run a small-town community. These accounts of 'historical discomfort' will shift to 'historical traumas', with characters increasingly affected by gruesome events. This results in a protagonist's repressed childhood memory, as in DE AANSLAG, whereas a mother in LEEDVERMAAK is caught in a cycle of never-ending repetitions. In the case of CHARLOTTE, the protagonist's horrific life story can only be presented in cut-up fragments, addressed to a 'beloved you'.

KEYWORDS
Historical discomfort and historical trauma – Aural temptations – Transgression of rules – Repressed memories – Past as eternal present

There is much to be said to the credit of Fons Rademakers' courageous enterprise of MAX HAVELAAR (1976). To start with, it was nothing less than a bold ambition to adapt *the* all-time classical novel in Dutch literary history written by Multatuli in 1860. There were some obvious laments, voiced by those critics who took the novel as a point of reference: the focus on the dramatic events was necessarily at the expense of an attention to style, and the film was not as stratified as the book's polyphony might have required. Although Rademakers' film lacked Multatuli's motivation to bring about a revolution, the attempt to shoot MAX HAVELAAR in the vein of a David Lean epic in Panavision was nonetheless daring for the standards of Dutch cinema: there was a reason that MAX HAVELAAR with its budget of 6 million guilders was the most expensive Dutch film at the time. The film attracted 727,000 filmgoers in the Netherlands, but at least as important, MAX HAVELAAR won a few international awards such as the special Jury prize at the Teheran film festival and a Bodil Award for best European film.

Apart from a comparison between novel and film, as usual favouring the 'original', the film could possibly end up in a hornet's nest because Indonesians might suspect that a Dutch director would excuse the role of Dutch colonization, which was so critically discussed by Multatuli. The nineteenth-century writer was highly esteemed in Indonesia because of the accusatory tone in his novel. Due to its potentially controversial theme, the film had to walk a tightrope in both the Netherlands and its former colony Indonesia. In addition to the tenuous relationship between the two countries, Rademakers and his predominantly Dutch crew shot the movie in a country that was totally foreign to them. And indeed, the shooting of MAX HAVELAAR was fraught with difficulties. Schedules were obstructed time and again: some actors did not show up; locations had to be cancelled; set dresses disappeared; horses that had been ordered did not arrive in time; a tiger had escaped; the cutter was not fit for his job; Indonesians were angered by a Dutch flag on the set (Bernink, 104-105). And, on top of that, a work print of the film was stolen at Cinetone. The fear that the Indonesian ministry of communication might censor parts of the film turned out to be unfounded, but a first official screening of MAX HAVELAAR only took place in Indonesia in 1987, some eleven years after its initial release.

The troublesome shooting period and its turbulent aftermath were reflective of the film's content: the adaptation made its viewers once more aware of what is a key concept in this chapter: historical discomfort. The term historical discomfort is appropriate for a film like MAX HAVELAAR or DE SCHORPIOEN [THE SCORPION] (Ben Verbong, 1984): the protagonist is witness to questionable colonial practices but in trying to rectify the deplorable injustice, he becomes relentlessly active while everyone around him tries to reduce him to passivity. In the course of this chapter, discomfort will shift to 'historical trauma'. In that case, a subject has suffered from such terrible experiences as war violence that he/she is doomed to repeat them, although it renders the subject 'hyperbolically passive' (Silverman, 59), as we will see in the analysis of LEEDVERMAAK [POLONAISE] (Frans Weisz, 1989).

'THY PATHS OF RIGHTEOUSNESS': *MAX HAVELAAR*

In her reading of T.E. Lawrence's autobiographical account *Seven Pillars of Wisdom* (1926), Kaja Silverman discusses how the writer—better known as 'Lawrence of Arabia', after the famous Lean epic from 1962—incorporates 'Arabness' (338). It is common for someone from an inferior class to identify with the cultural standards of the superior group, but the encounter the British officer Lawrence had with Arab rebels in the years 1916-1918 had given 'rise to an inverse desire' (Silverman, 299). His writings indicate that he felt increasingly uneasy with British imperialism, because the Westerner tried to 'batter and twist' an alien people 'into something which they, of their own accord, would not have been' (qtd. in Silverman, 311). Though Silverman goes to great lengths to analyze Lawrence in terms of both reflexive masochism and the desublimation of homosexuality, for my purpose her quite concise explanation of 'double mimesis' is most helpful.

Lawrence's strategy is to 'beat the Arabs at their own game'. He does not just imitate the Arab habits, he attempts to surpass them. 'If you wear Arab things', he advises, 'wear the best'. As Silverman argues, Lawrence adopts their attitudes, customs, and dresses, prompting the Arabs to imitate him back as a presumed 'ideal'. On the one hand, a colonial paradigm is at work, for the Arabs identify with him as a member of a superior group: they want to be like Lawrence. On the other hand, he turns this paradigm topsy-turvy, because the Arabs want to be like someone who has stylized himself as a perfect representative of 'Arabness'. Via this double mimesis in which the white man mimics the colonized other, who in return imitates him, the Arabs in fact become 'that which they have always been' (Silverman, 312).

Even though Lawrence's cultural masquerade will in the end benefit the rewriting of his subjectivity rather than serve the Arab cause, Silverman claims, the political potential of double mimesis seems clear-cut: if a 'white skin' idolizes a 'brown mask', can this propel a desire among the other to treasure one's own mask? One is inclined to say yes, but on the basis of both the novel and the film adaptation of MAX HAVELAAR, the answer would be yes, it could have worked this way had Havelaar at a crucial point judged the situation differently. Rademakers' film has a double framing story to illustrate that reality is obstinate. The first story concerns the paternalistic attitude of the Netherlands, illustrated by an embarrassing contrast between the Dutch bourgeoisie and the situation of the poor peasants in the Dutch East Indies, as Indonesia was called during the colonial era, from 1816 to 1949. The film opens with a text from the throne of King Willem III in 1850 on the importance of bearing fruit from the colonies, followed by Dutch soldiers marching through the fields. Then we see the courageous boy Saidjah and his double-crowned buffalo Pantang. Panic erupts when a tiger threatens the community, but the buffalo saves the day by killing the animal. Pantang is worshipped as a hero, but the Regent comes to visit them and requests, as usual, a gift. Since the community has nothing but chickens and rice, the Regent demands the buffalo. A farmer mentions that they will be unable to plough the sawahs, but the Regent turns a deaf ear to him. When Pantang is taken, a boy who stands up to protest is shot instantly. While the camera still lingers on the dead body, we already hear the voice of the Dutch reverend Wawelaar before we see him address the churchgoing crowd from his pulpit. The essence of his sermon is that God in His infinite wisdom has granted to a country small in size the power over the lost sheep in the far-away islands of the Indian Ocean. By distributing bibles to the people of Java, Wawelaar preaches, those poor souls can be saved from damnation.

By combining a shot of the boy's corpse and Wawelaar's voice, the two entirely different scenes are connected. It clearly suggests that the Dutch religious community, consisting of 'decent citizens', is totally blind to the disgraceful exploitation of the local inhabitants, while the official word is still that the population in the colony benefits from the presence of the Dutch. Unlike Multatuli's novel, MAX HAVELAAR returns in its final scene to the church, and the solemn singing about 'Thy paths of righteousness' drowns out the protagonist's desperate indictment of the abuse and the murder of natives, perpetrated 'in your name', as Havelaar says repeatedly to the portrait of King Willem III on a wall. The 'righteous' believers have still neither a clue about the situation nor has the king, the film's end implies.

The second framing story starts after the opening credits, some twelve minutes into the film, when Havelaar addresses his former classmate and coffee broker Batavus Droogstoppel [Dryasdust] on the streets of Amsterdam in 1860 and asks him whether he wants to publish the thick manuscript he is carrying with him. Havelaar assures him it also has parts on coffee. That raises the interest of Droogstoppel, this exemplar of short-sightedness and petty bourgeoisie. While all the papers are scattered over the floor, his wife is disgusted because she reads the chapter title 'On Prostitution in Marriage', but Droogstoppel is delighted to find fragments on coffee auctions, which is followed by a dissolve to the regency of Lebak on the island of Java, 1855. We then see for more than two hours the actual content of the manuscript, which of course is meant to give substance to the powerless words Havelaar addressed to the portrait of the king. Once he realizes to what extent the natives are being mistreated and exploited, he expects the Governor-General who had appointed him to be prepared to listen to him. Havelaar presumes that this highest officer simply was ignorant of the situation ('he must have been badly advised'), for the man had spoken dearly of the local population to Havelaar before: 'They are people like us, with the same abilities and the same destinations.' To his shock, these words appear to have been hollow, for the Governor-General simply does not want to receive Havelaar. Out of anger that a man of authority refuses to listen, Havelaar 'wants to be read' so that the general public will learn about corruption by both the Dutch dignitaries and their native stand-ins, such as the Regent. Havelaar hopes that he can use the naïve coffee broker Droogstoppel for his political project but realizes that he can only persuade him to publish the text by pretending the book is about coffee culture.

The very long embedded story concerns the sudden death of the Assistant-Resident Pierre Slotering of an 'acute liver abscess' after a visit to the Regent. Havelaar is happy to hear he is appointed as Slotering's successor, for he considers it an 'important mission' to work in the 'poverty-stricken' area of Lebak, where there is hardly any trade and agriculture. Havelaar regards it as a challenge: he presumes that the Governor-General wants to test his qualities, though Havelaar's wife Tine thinks—correctly—he only got this tricky post because her influential brother-in-law interceded for him. Havelaar delivers a speech full of promises to improve the situation for the poor, but for them it is just talk. Gradually, Havelaar realizes that there is a vicious circle that ignites corruption. The Regent is a tough old bird who has to support a large family and staff. Since the Dutch rulers do not pay the Regent properly, he can only fulfil his familial duty by selling the harvest of his starving subjects and by appropriating the pauper's buffalos. One day Havelaar sees a crowd of natives working at the Regent's place and he encourages them to go to the rice fields to make their own income. The peasants are too docile, however, to be sent away by Havelaar for they are supposed to be 'happy to help the Regent to feed his family'. The tactic of the Regent is to propose a gift in return: when Havelaar has the inconvenience of many snakes in his garden—probably a cunning trick from the Regent himself to prevent another intervention by Havelaar—he should ask the natives to help him. But Havelaar refuses the offer because he does not want assistance from people he cannot properly pay. He wants the population to speak up; he wants to teach them to give up their submissive attitude.

Havelaar wants to file an official complaint about the Regent's behaviour. The last straw that breaks the camel's back is the account by the widow Slotering that her husband, Havelaar's predecessor, was poisoned because he was critical of the Regent's practices. The complaint, however, requires that peasants are prepared to testify. At this point, the concept of 'double mimesis' is relevant, for Havelaar has tried to stylize himself in deep sympathy with the natives. He is not like the peasants in terms of his clothing, for he is, as everyone knows, appointed as Assistant-Resident, but he equals them in his humbleness. He lives a relatively modest life, mostly out of necessity because of their limited means; he is trying to monitor the circumstances among the population; he addresses the peasants directly, asking about their situation. By being inquisitive, he hopes they realize that he is seriously willing to improve their existence. Soon after the young Saïdjah and Adinda start to put their trust in him, Havelaar is dismissed with ignominy. Since he thinks it is a huge misunderstanding, he leaves by carriage. Adinda steps inside as well, but when the carriage stops when peasants want to give Havelaar a respectful send-off, the girl insists on getting off: 'I want to act. I want to look for my friends in the Lampongs.'

Had Havelaar gone 'underground' like Adinda, he could have become their Lawrence, but he assumed that the Governor-General was a man of common sense with an ear for his grievances. By making the trip to the Governor-General, Havelaar's rebellious stance is neutralized by the colonial system. Enraged by the injustice committed in the king's name, the only option left for him is for his manuscript to be read.

Rademakers' film chronicles Havelaar's attempts to have his manuscript—considered by Droogstoppel to be the 'parcel of Shawlman'—published, but it does not refer to the outcome, the actual existence of the novel, let alone its influence. Havelaar's desperate cry to the king's portrait at the end changes into the happy choir singing of the Dutch churchgoers, and it is highly significant that Droogstoppel—whose reading of the manuscript started the flashback to the period in Lebak—loudly sings along as well. Whereas Multatuli's major aim was for the colonial system to be reorganized to minimize the exploitation of the local people, the ending of the adaptation is quite pessimistic: Havelaar can yell at the portrait, but his accusation will be drowned out by religious backstabbers. In highlighting the idea of a successful cover-up of the injustice in the Dutch East Indies, MAX HAVELAAR implies that corruption will persist.

Though Havelaar as a character is righteous and good-hearted, it is striking that the film adaptation also presents him as naïve and megalomaniac. His wife Tine calls him, with some disdain in her voice, 'My Napoleon' on his way to the meeting with the Governor-General, for he takes irresponsible risks. When his son's dog falls into the sea, he jumps after the animal, despite the presence of sharks. He responds to the anger of his wife by saying that he cannot be killed for he presumes he was selected to do important things. And whereas he tends to identify with the natives, he is overjoyed that he can eat 'real Dutch cauliflower' preserved as canned food. In endowing the protagonist with such character flaws, it makes sense that Rademakers' film does not end on a positive note and downplays the political effects of the novel.

Max Havelaar undeniably had an impact, not only as a literary text but also as a political pamphlet (Pattynama, 171), even if its effects were not immediate. In the long run, Multatuli's indictment contributed to a growing nationalism in the Dutch East Indies that accelerated the process of decolonization in the late 1940s. This process has remained a sore spot for the Dutch. When Indonesia declared itself independent from Holland in 1945, the Dutch government responded by sending military troops, for the Dutch believed that if they were to lose the Dutch East Indies, disaster would strike the Netherlands. After four violent years, the Dutch realized in late 1949 that the battle was fruitless. The military action resulted into nothing less than an inglorious retreat without any positive or corrective follow-up. This black page in Dutch history provides the background for DE SCHORPIOEN [THE SCORPION] (Ben Verbong, 1984), a highly odd but most intriguing feature film. It is odd because the actual plot seems for much of the film far removed from the situation in the former colony. But is it not the intriguing point of DE SCHORPIOEN that this historical episode is so charged that it requires an exceptionally lengthy detour to address the improper behaviour of the Dutch colonists? Is its history so repressed that it can only return in a tale with a seemingly forced and frenetic preamble?

A CONSTITUTIONAL HABIT OF STINGING: *DE SCHORPIOEN*

Verbong's picture starts with what Garrett Stewart calls a series of 'liminal shots': in the prologue, eleven black-and-white photographs are shown for the duration of two minutes, but it is difficult to make heads and tails of them. A body with blood on the floor? Is this murder? A plane on the water, then a man who waves his arm and apparently yells? Does the plane come to his rescue? Dissolve to a subsequent picture: the plane is at quite a distance and also a bit above the water. If we assume chronological order, then the plane is leaving the man behind. After the seventh picture of soldiers wading through a river, we suddenly have filmed footage in colour: a man stands at his bedside packing things, the camera tracks forward towards him, and a shot is fired. The man looks up, straight into the camera, which becomes a black-and-white freeze frame for a couple of seconds. The three subsequent pictures concern the aftermath of the execution, including a blood-tiled floor. It is to be expected that these enigmatic pictures of violence will return in the remainder of the film, but the first hour of the 98-minute feature film does not make even the slightest connection.

Netherlands, 1956. A truck driver named Lou Wolff walks into a café and participates in an illegal roulette game. When he later goes to his boss Karl Wissing, he tells him he cannot yet give him the 6000 guilders. Back in his truck, there is news on the radio about the Hungarian Uprising. When he rides into town, two soldiers are bothering a woman, and he comes to Helma's rescue. To her colleague Anna, she says: 'I need the money.' Lou is invited by the two night hostesses to drink in their pub. He is told that if he wants a place to stay, Anna's mother runs a pension, and all rooms are vacant. He has in mind to sell his truck at a garage, but his boss is on his tail already. Karl wants to make him an offer: Lou will receive a great sum of money if he gives him his passport so that Karl can have a Hungarian engineer come over to the Netherlands. Karl will deliver a new passport to Lou and tickets for a trip to America as well so that he can visit both his ex-wife and his child. Lou has no choice, for Karl can go to the police, and with a criminal record Lou cannot enter the US.

Standing in front of a mirror, he starts practicing: '*My name is Wolff, Lou Wolff, I come from Holland*.' He suggests to Anna that they go on a date before his departure, and she accepts on second thought. She tells him about her failed marriage before they have sex in a car. As he is about to check out at the pension the next morning, he reads in the paper about the death of the driver 'L. Wolff'. There is a picture of a burnt car. The camera zooms in to his face in close-up while he is reading. The camera then zooms in slightly from behind, while we zoom in to his face in profile. He asks whether he can take the newspaper and whether he can stay for a couple more days. At the mortuary, he is shown a totally burnt corpse by the pathologist who tells him: 'I wouldn't wish such a death on anyone. The guy had taken the money. His boss has identified him.'

In a tunnel, he has a meeting with Karl, but the tone of their conversation is snappish: 'You were supposed to leave, that's why I paid you.' 'I met a woman.' 'If you do not leave, I cannot be blamed for the consequences.' Intrigued by the sinister words of his boss, Lou starts to search for the man whose identity he has taken, William Kemp, and visits his house. An Indonesian woman, Njai van Kemp, is not permitted to open the door for anyone unless he is Mr. Ducroo. So, within a few minutes of screen time, Lou takes on a third name.

It turns out that William wanted to tell Ducroo 'everything', but the woman can disclose only a few cryptic lines. 'He frequently said: "They used me; they will pay for it." But I warned him that some forces, which we do not know, are stronger than us. Let bygones be bygones.' Njai adds to this: 'I did not clean up anything.' When Lou leans forward to take a close look at a picture of William on a desk, we see Lou's own face superimposed via a glass reflection.

From this point, mysterious characters persecute Lou. His room is turned upside down and he is beaten up. He searches for Ducroo, an investigative journalist, for he guesses that this man can tell him who is threatening him. Ducroo refuses to tell him anything until Lou shows him his passport, i.e. a passport with William Kemp's name. 'That is the name of a man who killed three people in the former Dutch East Indies. I'm going to Indonesia for some additional research, but meanwhile you could contact Colonel Snijder of the ministry of war.' Ducroo dies, however, of cerebral haemorrhage that very evening, but Lou doubts the correctness of this diagnosis.

Lou tracks down the colonel, a strange and reclusive man at some remote spot in the ministry. Snijder's hobby is to collect insects, because each species has a perfect aesthetic form. 'Take a scorpion, that is a mechanism rather than a living creature—and it can be hidden under every stone.' Since the meeting with the colonel offers no valuable clue, Lou breaks into Ducroo's office at the newspaper. And while he starts reading some writings by Ducroo, after more than one hour into the film, there is a first transition to the former colony, to a scene featuring William Kemp who is putting poison in an alcoholic beverage. When a man is about to drink, lying in an easy chair, the camera tracks forward, a bit shaky. Soon thereafter, he lies on the ground, and this colour scene is exactly like the third black-and-white photograph in the beginning. After a shot of Lou still reading, a plane lands on water—similar to one of the photographs in the prologue. A man is left behind at sea in a small boat, but then he finds out it is leaking. He yells at the plane—we remember this from another photograph at the beginning. After these briefly fragmented representations of murder, there is a conversation between a man named Vaandrig and Karl Wissing. Vaandrig says he has found out that someone from the troops is selling weapons to the enemy, and he wants protection for he has proof. Karl advises him to take shelter at Kemp's place for the time being. When Vaandrig spies on an actual transaction of weapons, he recognizes to his fright that Karl is involved and takes a few pictures, shown in black-and-white freeze frames. We see that Karl contacts Kemp and says that the two previous ones went excellent as well and that he has nothing to fear, for his chief in Bandung will cover him. Kemp suggests that this time it will be a stray bullet during a hunting party.

Vaandrig does not want to participate in a hunting party, however, for as he says: 'I have rather grown scared of our own people than of those terrorists.' Then we see a repetition of a brief scene from the prologue: a shaky camera tracks towards Vaandrig packing his things near the bedside, but this time we get the reverse shot which shows that Kemp is firing a gun. He pulls Vaandrig away and we see blood on the tiled floor. Kemp orders his wife to clean it up and she starts reluctantly using a wet mop. Back to Lou who murmurs twice the phrase Njai had uttered at Kemp's place: 'I did not clean up anything.'

To Anna, Lou says that he has evidence of crimes dating from the year 1949, but she wants him to stop it. He contacts Karl who says he will reveal who gave the assignment to eliminate Kemp. But as he is about to meet Karl in the tunnel, there is a tracking jump cut forward to a body halfway. Lou picks up the gun next to the dead Karl and starts running. He goes to Kemp's place, and the woman repeats her mantra 'I did not clean up anything.' But Lou only wants to know who Kemp's superior was. She says she does not know but that, once, her husband received a framed scorpion as a present from his chief.

When Colonel Snijder pretends he does not recall the name of Kemp's superior, Lou puts the man's hand in a box with scorpions ('you were the chief'), and while Snijder is yelling out loud, the camera pans along stuffed animals: buffalos, a giraffe. Lou goes back to his place, but a mysterious man with a hat is waiting for him. Thanks to Anna's scream, Lou gets away in time. He decides to surrender to the police, because he has all the information to incriminate others. But as Anna already predicted, they will not believe him. And indeed, their next meeting is in prison, for Lou is being made to pay the price for the events while everybody else gets off scot-free. In the meantime, we hear a telephone call by a man whose shadow is projected onto the wall to the police: he says that the man may be released, but if he causes trouble, we will make certain that he will carry the can for Karl's death. 'And that shebang with his name has to stop. He is named Wolff, and nothing else.' Upon his release from prison, Lou is given his things back. The receptionist says: 'A good ending, isn't it, Wolff?' But meanwhile he has signed the document with 'William Kemp'. Anna is waiting outside, and when they start to embrace, the camera tracks backwards. After some seconds, the camera zooms in on his face to a close-up and there is a slow dissolve to the headline of the newspaper *Trouw*: Dutch army vindicated after all. Then the paper is caught by the wind.

Although it may seem paradoxical, the merit of DE SCHORPIOEN resides in its uneven structure. During the first hour, Verbong's film has a quite conventional pace, but as soon as Lou starts reading Ducroo's writings about the violent events in Bandung, the tempo accelerates considerably in the last 35 minutes. Suddenly Lou—and the viewer as well—becomes caught up in a whirlwind of developments. We go from one murder scene to another murder scene to a third. And back in the present, Lou first comes across the dead body of Karl, then he has a violent encounter with Colonel Snijder, followed by an attempt to kill him. Thereafter he ends up in prison and is set free. Lou has the idea that he understands the conspiracy, but there are too many incidents and too many secretive deals. The problem is not that the past is shrouded in mystery but that there is *too much* coherence. Because of this excess—and that is the crucial lesson of the overloaded final part of DE SCHORPIOEN—a clever manipulator who is in the powerful position of being able to pull the strings can turn any nosey parker into a scapegoat.

There is a chain of coincidences that reveals a connection between small-time crook Wolff and an episode in Indonesia. It requires the perseverance of a thorough journalist to discover hidden details, and after his unfortunate demise (probably murder), it additionally requires the impertinence of a resolute 'nobody'—a truck driver with gambling debts—to break into Ducroo's office to read the documents. In terms of storytelling, it may seem like an unnecessary lengthy prelude to the heart of the matter, but by postponing the narrative unrolling of the opening 'liminal shots', basically consisting of photographs, it becomes clear how deeply concealed the traumatic Indonesian fight for independence was for Dutch soldiers. But once Lou has access to the documents, there is such an accumulation of horrific incidents that any attempt to entangle the actual happenings not only leads to a trustworthy scenario, the very same trail of horrors can also be used to create a counter-narrative. Precisely because DE SCHORPIOEN shows us an excessive cocktail of conspiracies and revelations in its final part, Verbong's film indicates how such a dark page of history can continue to be repressed.

DE SCHORPIOEN is not unique as a Dutch fiction film about the years of decolonisation in Indonesia. The most notable companion pieces are GORDEL VAN SMARAGD (Orlow Seunke, 1997)—in which the history of the East Indies is used as a backdrop for a love story (see chapter three, note 10)—and OEROEG (Hans Hylkema, 1993),[1] while Jim Taihuttu's delayed 2020 movie DE OOST [THE EAST] about the infamous contra-guerrilla of the Dutch Captain Raymond Westerling in the late 1940s is not yet available at the time of writing. DE SCHORPIOEN is such a fascinating movie because the entire film is centred around a historical void: it shows how a repressed history can return, but as soon as it pops up, this history is unscrupulously swept under the carpet again as if it had never returned in the first place. In short, the history of Bandung can be downplayed as no more than a fanciful story by a truck driver.

SONG TO THE SIREN: *HET ZWIJGEN*

The state of affairs is different in HET ZWIJGEN [THE SILENCE] (Adri Schrover and André van den Hout, 2006), for in this film the people in the village of Koekange (in the province of Drenthe) know about a violent incident that took place on 4 November 1927, but no one knows—or at least everyone pretends not to know—its exact details. 'Oh horror piece, so unprecedented' is the title of the so-called murder song of Koekange: 'its melody is a consolation, their words a curse', according to the opening lines of HET ZWIJGEN. The throat of the sheep trader Hendrik Bakker had been cut, and thereafter his maid and a retarded shepherd boy were murdered as well.

HET ZWIJGEN is a fiction feature, but it is based upon an actual murder. One of its attractions is that the film is interlaced with old archival footage—most of it authentic—and thus the cinematography can be taken as an ode to the mysterious if not surreal atmosphere of that footage. Especially, the contemporary scenes with the sulky ferryman give the impression of a pre-modern community, with its sawmill and old cemetery. The main protagonist Victor Dreisen is a city boy who works at the Meertens Institute for folk culture, and after inheriting a small, deserted, and neglected cottage amidst the peatlands of Koekange, he proposes to his boss to conduct research on popular songs in Drenthe. His real reason is that he wants to refurbish his cottage, but he keeps silent about this to his boss. His work-related reason to spend time in Koekange is that he will investigate why a crucial tape, D49, is missing in the Institute. This tape contains the remainder of the so-called murder song.

Victor meets a few strange fellows: a young, mute shepherd; the elderly Mr. Wiegman who collects old stuff; and the aforementioned ferryman. And he is witness to strange events, but people act as if he has hallucinated them. He sees a baby in a basket in the water, but no one confirms it; later, the police comes to ask whether he is clairvoyant because they have found the corpse of a baby; he makes a photo with his mobile phone of a small funeral procession, but there is nothing to see on his screen. 'A Polaroid always works', a policeman tells him. In an archive, searching for what happened in 1927, he sees some old footage featuring Wiegman. But perhaps the man is Wiegman's father. He comes to realize this because the bargee Geesje, with whom Victor gets romantically involved after he hears her mesmerizing voice singing the first part of the murder song, is an exact look-alike of her mother.

When Victor visits Wiegman, the man gets mad when he hears about the Meertens Institute, since Victor's employer had sent him a letter back in 1979 that they were not interested in his collection. Victor sees the missing tape D49, however, and is able to secretly copy fragments of it. The singing continues with the lines 'Where is my baby? Where is its cradle?', which is remarkable because the legend does not mention a child. Victor is asked to attend a *grand guignol* performance, with masks, of the local theatre company replaying the murder. But Geesje's uncle Lambert, acting as the killer, is quite drunk and says after the performance: 'There was also a baby, but I am not supposed to tell you that.' In another meeting with the mute shepherd's boy, Victor insists he give him information because he is sure he knows everything. At the graveyard, the boy indicates that, contrary to common wisdom, the maid named Rietje Stolk was murdered first and the sheep trader only second. The boy does not respond when he is asked about a baby.

Meanwhile, anonymous villagers try to scare Victor away by pinning a sheep's head to his door, apparently because they consider him an intruder in a local mystery. The second time he receives a sheep's head, it is wrapped in a newspaper dated 17 February 1977, and it mentions an accident at a lock of a nearby canal. On footage in the archive, Victor sees that a young Geesje has candy in her hand but gives it to a man, probably Wiegman. Still more
intrigued by this man, he finds out that D49 is incomplete. He then asks Wiegman whether he is the son of Doctor De Vries, because Victor saw Wiegman at the man's tomb. Yes, Wiegman admits, and 'my mother's grave is nearby. She was Rietje Stolk—it's not a secret, but no one ever mentions it.'

Once he is made part of the circle of connoisseurs who know the village's secret, he keeps humming the murder song's melody. Having refused to wear the earphones the shepherd's boy has given him, he at one point hears Geesje's voice from afar, singing. He steps into a rowing boat but gets stuck in swampy water. While the singing continues to mesmerize Victor, we see that the ferryman has made a coffin.

The traumatic event from 1927 seems to have set a few rules: the local inhabitants know about it, but they are not supposed to talk about it, at least not to strangers. And insofar as they mention it, they keep silent about Rietje Stolk's baby. But as soon as Vincent, a stranger in town, is informed about the identity of the baby by Wiegman himself and can probably guess the motive for the threefold murder, the melody of the murder song becomes an earworm that he cannot get out of his head. But if every inquisitive outsider is to die once they come to know about this historical trauma, the events can continue to be shrouded in silence. Put this way, it seems as if the people in Koekange belong to a close-tongued rural community that cooperates to keep strangers at bay, but there is another side of the coin to their silence or their *zwijgen*, to refer to the film's title.

Sometimes, the welfare of a community is better served by a certain amount of secrecy, especially when any additional information can aggravate rather than shield an open wound. The city boy may think that he can submit a full account of the incident for the archive of the Institute, which aims to preserve folk culture, but the community itself seems to realize that knowledge can be a burden, too. So many years after the event, the perpetrator is dead anyway, and any publicly known development might encumber the next of kin in an unwelcome manner. Even though Victor tries to integrate into the community of Koekange, he is still a city boy who has set himself the task of discovering details that will be officially documented. Whereas the cinematography highlights the mysterious beauty of the rural environments, Victor remains the odd man out, who is accepted for his interest in Koekange and its inhabitants but who had better not find out too much.

SMOOTH CATHOLIC CRIMINALS: *DE BENDE VAN OSS*

De bende van Oss [The Gang of Oss] (André van Duren, 2011) is the 'Catholic' version of a film about crime in a closed community—and that 'Catholic' nature makes all the difference. The film starts with a brief scene in 1945 in which a huge amount of paperwork on corruption and excessive crime in Oss, a city in the south of the Netherlands, is brought to a department, but the Roman-Catholic minister of justice does not want to make a case of it, arguing that it is too complicated. He allows the incriminating files to be thrown away. There is an immediate transition to 1938, and a voice-over by Johanna van Heesch explains in a nutshell the nature of the corruption: there are a 'bunch of misfits' led by self-appointed leader Wim de Kuiper who steal from the rich and give to the poor ... at least, sometimes; the local cop looks the other way when he is paid off; the priest sins while taking confession; and several local fires are started to rip off the insurance companies. The central government located in the north of Holland, which is predominantly Protestant, sends the military police to Oss to re-establish order, but this only increases solidarity among the inhabitants of Oss. They may not be 'devout' Catholics, but they all hate Protestants. Johanna works in a meat factory, but in the night she works in a bar that has no licence to sell liquor. Johanna's mother has no idea who the fathers are of her two daughters, and Johanna's behaviour is as sexually uninhibited as her mother's. She has the ambition of turning the bar into a modest restaurant, and at the beginning of Van Duren's film, her husband Ties is soon to be released from jail.

In monochrome colours, De bende van Oss meticulously chronicles the nature of corruption. Unlike Het zwijgen, which takes an outsider as a point of reference, Johanna—who bears the nickname 'the slut'—is an insider: the bar-restaurant is a centre of activities. When a guy who is temporarily 'dazed' stabs a man in the stomach, Wim simply orders everybody to go outside. Problems are solved without any intervention of authorities, for they are deeply distrusted. Johanna is an accidental witness to the brutal murder of a protestant sergeant of police, executed by Wim and one of his accomplices. He then goes to Johanna's bar-restaurant and gives her a great amount of money, apparently for the third time. 'You can either pay off or shoot a witness', he tells, 'but there won't be a fourth time'. To underscore the fact that it is the 'gang of Oss' that runs affairs in the city—and not the military police—the grave of the dead sergeant is dug up and his coffin is exposed in the street, without a lid. The crude joke is meant to suggest that he is 'resurrected', just like Jesus.

The key event of the film is the result of a plan concocted by Harry den Brock, Wim's counsellor, and Johanna. Harry, one of the regulars at Johanna's place, sees how she suffers from her husband's domineering attitude, aggravated by her pregnancy. Ties wants her to get an abortion, particularly because it is doubtful that he is the father. Harry proposes a plan whereby Johanna takes out an insurance policy on Ties's life, after which the young Jan Greeven, who has prospects of becoming a professional cyclist, will shoot Ties on a trackway. Jan is prepared to do so because he hopes to leave Oss together with Johanna, who has her brown hair dyed blonde. Then Harry is pressured by Wim to reveal the name of the culprit, for 'nobody gets shot in Oss without my permission, least of all my cousin'. Harry has no quibbles about giving the name. When Johanna complains about his complacency, he replies that he has betrayed no one, since 'Wim is with us'.

In the Protestant community of Koekange, portrayed in HET ZWIJGEN, the enigma is structured around a conspicuous void: there is a murder song, but it is incomplete; a baby is part of the story, but no one mentions it; most of the characters prefer an existence as hermit (the shepherd's boy, the ferryman, Wiegman). It is no wonder that the outsider Victor is gradually driven mad. By contrast, the entire 'Catholic' community in Oss is engaged, with Wim as the key figure. What is crucial is the public dressing down of Jan. A great number of inhabitants of Oss have gathered near the forest when Wim gives a speech to a terrified Jan, who is forced to admit that he has shot Ties. Wim then gives him a pat on the back: 'It's just like church, if you confess, we can forgive you. Then we never talk about it again. We keep our mouths shut.' This ritualized display of a secret and its subsequent confession is what fundamentally separates the Catholic from the more tight-lipped Protestant mentality. The overt atonement of Catholicism is highlighted in an exemplary manner in the forest scene in which Jan is put in his place. The consequence of Jan's penance is that he is re-integrated as a 'friend' within the community, which is totally averse to the military police force consisting of Protestants from the north. Later, when it suits his purposes, Wim betrays Jan to the police after all, and it turns out that Jan is happy to confess everything because the murder had plagued his conscience.

DE BENDE VAN OSS makes us privy to many clandestine activities via the film's 'inside' characters. People are allowed to know and see everything on the condition that they keep the code of silence, for 'silence, that's what has made Oss great'. During the final 40 minutes, Wim overplays his hand when Johanna's half-sister Trees is misused during an orgy with the mayor, a factory boss, and some clergymen. Ultimately, Trees is found dead. Holding Wim responsible for Trees's drowning, Johanna takes revenge on the man who claims that he banged her mother so often that she is probably his daughter.[2] In terms of the story, Johanna's refusal to live by the code of silence is crucial, but for the sake of my argument, Wim's unsavoury practices are particularly intriguing. The inhabitants of Oss have no other option than to stoically accept the way Wim runs things. To the detriment of Johanna, her mother agrees to accept Wim's explanation that Trees died of an unfortunate accident. In Johanna's mother's eyes, the death of daughter Trees is collateral damage. Because of this 'Catholic' mentality, any unlawful actions are covered by the cloak of charity. Hence, DE BENDE VAN OSS has no *passage à l'acte* because it strictly speaking cannot have one: if everything is potentially condoned, then nothing can be too outrageous. Wim is unpleasantly surprised when Johanna accuses him of Trees's death by drowning, for he is not used to this kind of retort. Van Duren's film illustrates that due to a Catholic attitude, atrocious vice crimes have remained unpunished, but they leave scars, and for Johanna who has become fed up with the 'Catholic' attitude, a limit has been trespassed. In the end, she grabs the opportunity to step on board the Holland-America line.

STRATEGIC MASQUERADES: *ZWARTBOEK*

'Houdt het dan nooit op?'[3] ['Will It Never End?'], uttered by Rachel Steinn in ZWARTBOEK [BLACK BOOK] (Paul Verhoeven, 2006), is one of the best-known quotes in Dutch film history, but it is not necessarily a good sign when it is quickly subjected to parody in poor films such as SNUF DE HOND IN OORLOGSTIJD [THE DOG SNUF IN WARTIME] (Steven de Jong, 2008) and in SPION VAN ORANJE [SPY OF ORANGE] (Tim Oliehoek, 2009). This particular quote is symptomatic of an ambivalence surrounding ZWARTBOEK, the first Dutch film Verhoeven made after DE VIERDE MAN [THE FOURTH MAN] (1983), 23 years earlier. The film, which premiered at the Venice Film Festival in 2006, can be called 'vintage Verhoeven'. SOLDAAT VAN ORANJE had already been tailored to American taste, but after Verhoeven's Hollywood successes such as ROBOCOP (1987), BASIC INSTINCT (1992), and STARSHIP TROOPERS (1997), it should not surprise anyone that he was capable of shooting an energetic Hollywood-style movie in Holland. With ZWARTBOEK, he lived up to these expectations, for it has fast-paced action, such as resistance fighters trying to free prisoners, followed by a German counterattack since the operation had been betrayed. It also had gruesomely spectacular scenes: after the liberation the female protagonist is presumed a collaborator and as such is stripped naked, beaten up, and then covered a bucket full of excrement. Its violence is visceral at times: the murder of many Dutch Jewish citizens trying to escape to the marshes of De Biesbosch on a barge is particularly graphic and, as is typical of Verhoeven, 'unnecessarily' prolonged.

ZWARTBOEK is also 'vintage Verhoeven' because of the Jewish protagonist Rachel Steinn who as a double agent succeeds in infiltrating a German headquarter by transforming herself into a Marlene Dietrich-like blonde singer by the name of Ellis de Vries. Patricia Pisters observes correctly that Rachel/Ellis continues the tradition of Keetje from KEETJE TIPPEL (1975), Fientje from SPETTERS (1980) and Agnes from FLESH+BLOOD (1985): they are 'quite intelligent', they follow their 'instincts for survival' and they 'use their bodies to get what they want' (184). Verhoeven's heroines share a certain opportunistic behaviour with the leading females in the films from Rainer Werner Fassbinder's latest period, such as Maria in DIE EHE DER MARIA BRAUN [THE MARRIAGE OF MARIA BRAUN] (1979) and the title characters of both LILI MARLEEN (1981) and LOLA (1981). I mention this not only to recall that Fassbinder's work ethic on set was as frenetic as Verhoeven's but also because Fassbinder had the ambition by this time to shoot a 'Hollywood film' in his home country.

Despite the fact that ZWARTBOEK won three Golden Calves and has a more than decent IMDb score of 7.7, Verhoeven's film was lambasted in a famous—or notorious—interview that colleague-director Alex van Warmerdam gave at the Nederlands Film Festival. To the amusement of the public, he comically criticized several details, and he was entitled to it, for Van Warmerdam himself is known as a director very keen on details. He mentioned the 'too large outfits' of the Germans, whereas the Nazis were always sharply dressed. It did not make sense to him that Rachel would be dyeing her pubic hair blonde while talking to a stranger. Moreover, the Jews who are about to escape are too joyous and they wear their fur collars and jewels much too visibly—it is no wonder they are mowed down, for they 'asked for it'. Since Van Warmerdam had not planned to disparage Verhoeven, he ended by saying that SOLDAAT VAN ORANJE, Verhoeven's war film from 1977, was 'ten times better' than ZWARTBOEK. Even though I agree that the 1977 film—one of the very best in Dutch history—is superior to the 2006 one, I will make an argument in favour of ZWARTBOEK via an odd detour.

In the early 1930s, before the Motion Picture Production Code was enforced in mid-1934, gangster films were tremendously successful in the United States, as exemplified by the reception of LITTLE CAESAR (Mervyn

LeRoy, 1931), THE PUBLIC ENEMY (William A. Wellman, 1931), and SCARFACE (Howard Hawks, 1932). Eighteen years after his role as Tom Powers in THE PUBLIC ENEMY, James Cagney played Cody Jarrett in WHITE HEAT (Raoul Walsh, 1949) in what could be considered a parodic performance of his earlier role. A classic gangster usually has a close attachment to his mother, but Cody is a psychopath whose terrible headaches can only be cured when his mother consoles him. Halfway through WHITE HEAT, Cody has a lengthy hysterical outburst in prison when he hears the news that his mother has died. At the end of the film, he stands on a gigantic gas storage tank. When he sets this tank on fire, he shouts amidst the flames: 'Made it Ma, top of the world!' The narrative structure of WHITE HEAT still conforms to the conventions of the gangster film from the 1930s, but at the same time, Walsh's film exaggerates these conventions to the point of ridicule, owing to the manic but also superb acting by Cagney.

This mechanism of cleverly walking the line between convention and parody can be applied to ZWARTBOEK as well. Verhoeven's film teaches us that in times of war, as Pisters explains, nobody is transparent and everybody is to be distrusted (185), but ZWARTBOEK hammers this point home. There is the elderly reliable notary Wim Smaal, but he is the 'unexpected collaborator' (Burke, 208) who collects in his 'black book' the possessions of rich Jews and passes their names on to the Germans. Another example of the 'chilling ordinariness of collaboration' (Burke, 208) is Van Gein who arranges the passage for Jews on a barge, but he is in cahoots with the Nazis as well. The most crucial denouement in ZWARTBOEK is that the courageous resistance hero Hans Akkermans turns out to be a vicious schemer. When the Germans are almost defeated, it seems just for Hans to retrieve the loot from the nasty Obersturmführer Günther Franken who hoped he could get away with all the valuables he had robbed from the Jews—until it becomes clear that Hans had always been Franken's companion in this dirty business. The entertainment girl Ronnie was the darling of Franken, but near the end of the war she quickly changes sides and becomes the sweetheart of a Canadian soldier, thereby escaping the punishment of a shaved head that all traitors received. In her role as double agent, Ellis has to play-act that she falls in love with the Hauptsturmführer Ludwig Müntze and then, as the convention from Alfred Hitchcock films tells us, the two of them really fall in love. Burke concludes that 'ZWARTBOEK's characters inhabit a grey zone of moral ambiguity more readily than earlier films' on the Second World War (208), but this is even put too mildly, for the film is so eager to turn the distinction between good and bad inside out that it borders on incredibility. This is a problem if one considers ZWARTBOEK a 'serious' war picture only, but Verhoeven has always had a habit of ironically overdoing conventions. Much in the way that Walsh's WHITE HEAT is a classic gangster film that also includes its excess, ZWARTBOEK is a war picture that invites its viewers to read the film also as a parodic extravagance.

If there is nonetheless a problem with Verhoeven's film, it is due to the way the war adventures are embedded, for the framing of the war period in ZWARTBOEK seems to disavow the impact of historical trauma. The famous quote 'Houdt het dan nooit op?' is a reaction to a most tragic series of events that befall Rachel. While nearby, the Germans bomb a farmhouse, which was her hiding place, killing the entire Dutch family, several children included. Unexpectedly reunited with her parents and her brother during a crossing on a barge in the large company of other Jews, a German patrol boat takes them by surprise: Rachel is the only one to survive by diving underwater. While giving a performance as a singer, she is accompanied on piano by Franken, the man whose face she remembers from the patrol boat. Moreover, because Franken is involved in a rivalry with Müntze, he makes the Resistance group believe that Müntze's mistress Rachel is to be suspected of treachery. She is only able to face their leader Gerben Kuijpers, whose son has been killed due to the treason, after she has discovered the identities of the actual collaborators. And a final blow that provokes her aforementioned outburst is the news that a firing squad has executed Müntze.

Considering their traumatic impact, this accumulation of disasters is something Rachel deals with quite acquiescently. She is the epitome of a pragmatic woman, very adept at adjusting herself to situations, however awkward the occasion. When Gerben asks her whether she is capable of fulfilling a dangerous job—playing a double agent—she replies rhetorically: 'What do I have to lose?' His answer—'Your life'—is met by silence from her, as if her life is worthless anyway. Her realization that her existence is an empty shell does not result in total passivity or *aphanisis* (the topic for the next chapter); instead, she understands that her life can be filled with new experiences, and since she has nothing to lose, risky adventures are no big deal. Remarkably, there is no breakdown on Rachel's part during the entire film; she has to vomit when she sees Franken because his sight brings back the memory of the barge, shown via brief flashback inserts, but she quickly recovers since she is supposed to sing a happy song about 'naughty Lola'. Except for these inserts, there are no flashbacks on Rachel's part during the depiction of the war itself, an indication that at least for her, life went on, despite its emptiness. In favour of the fast-paced film, one can say that the developments took place so quickly that there was hardly time for reflection and that Rachel is caught up in the turmoil of events.

But here is the catch: the entire episode of the war, from September 1944 to a few days after the liberation, is couched as a flashback. The film begins when Ronnie visits Kibbutz Stein in Israel as a tourist and recognizes Rachel, who lives by the name of Rachel Rosenthal and works as a schoolteacher. After Ronnie has left again, Rachel sits by a lake, slightly distressed, and the flashback starts. So the actual main story is a recollection by Rachel, but there are no incoherent parts, there are no scenes that seem tinged by her subjectivity. At the end of the embedded story, she also sits at a lake as Gerben waits for the traitor Hans to suffocate in a coffin, and then there is a shot of the water itself to create an imperceptible transition to Rachel still sitting by the lake in Israel in 1956. Still looking slightly distressed as at the start of the flashback, she quickly cheers up when her husband and her two children find her: 'Hello, my darlings!' Her husband asks what she had been thinking about, and she keeps her answer very vague: 'The past'.

The opening suggests that it is the meeting with Ronnie that triggered the unpleasant memories, as if Rachel had practically forgotten about it. This suggestion is confirmed by the final scene: she has built herself a happy family life in Israel, and the way her husband asks what she had been thinking does not sound as if he was expecting her thoughts to have gone back to that bloody war again. Rachel seems to have been able to block the remembrance of these life-determining months: the memory of the war is not on her mind daily or regularly, as is the case with trauma survivors. The fact that her flashback is coherent and without ruptures underscores that for Rachel, it is something she can recall pretty clearly: the depiction of the past is neither a blur nor is its temporality out of joint, as is often the case with trauma. In addition, despite the film's smooth transition from 1945 to 1956 via the shot of the lake, for Rachel the war has become a thing of the past, closed off from the present. This may be tailored to suit the action-packed drama that ZWARTBOEK clearly was meant to be, but it goes against the traits of trauma survivors mentioned in any textbook. The key problem for traumatized people is that past and present cannot be separated from one another and that the horror of the past endures into the present. A person who suffers from traumatic experiences returns to them constantly and involuntarily. It is only by bearing in mind the ease with which Rachel learns to put on an act for tactical reasons that we can argue that she also has a certain ease in repressing her memories of the war. Contrary to the theories on trauma, flexibility has become her nature to such an extent that Rachel can forget the horror but also recall the events in a quite coherent manner.

Despite these critical remarks, I would like to end in defence of ZWARTBOEK. As mentioned above, key characters opt for 'inauthentic' positions and strategic masquerades. Wim seems a trustworthy notary (but he is not); Hans a courageous resistance fighter (but he is not); Van Gein a reliable chap (but he is not); Rachel/Ellis switches roles repeatedly, and to save her skin, she hides her Jewish background. The many strategic masquerades in ZWARTBOEK have set the tone for a number of subsequent war films I already discussed in previous chapters: Walter Süskind plays a role as subservient to the Nazis in order to save his family in Van den Berg's 2012 picture; Riphagen acts as Mr. Nice Guy but he is a dirty rascal in Kuijpers' 2016 film, and to escape his opponents, he even plays dead—the best of strategic disguises—thanks to a false certificate. One of his opponents, Jan van Liempd, a member of the resistance group led by Gerrit van der Veen, infiltrated the German police and had a false SD pass to organize a raid on the State Printing House. OORLOGSWINTER [WINTER IN WARTIME] (Martin Koolhoven, 2008), based upon the eponymous 1972 popular youth novel by Jan Terlouw, has not been mentioned so far but is another case in point. Set in a snowbound small community in January 1945, the fourteen-year-old Michiel van Beusekom favours his Uncle Ben, who has joined the resistance, over his own father, who is the local mayor. Michiel, whose perspective we share consistently, believes his father behaves too obediently towards the German occupants. In the course of the film, in which a cold blue light prevails and the redness of the Nazi flags stand out, the boy is forced to change his mind. Ben turns out to be a traitor, whereas the father stoically accepts his execution for a murder of a German soldier he did not commit. His father's courage becomes clear to the son afterwards when Uncle Ben tells him that his father had refused a remarkable offer: the Germans were prepared to let him go in exchange for another innocent citizen. And on top of these deceptive appearances, Michiel finds out that his nasty neighbour Schafter was not so bad after all because his sympathy for the Nazi cause was a red herring to prevent them from suspecting that he had a Jewish woman in hiding.[4]

Characters in Dutch war pictures of the 21st century often adopt a false pose, and with hindsight, we can say that the 1986 film IN DE SCHADUW VAN DE OVERWINNING was a precursor to this tendency to show Dutch citizens masquerading themselves in World War II movies. Peter van Dijk is a typical resistance fighter who is prepared to die a martyr's death, but at the same time he acts as the leader of a pack of collaborators, with many members dressed up as Nazi officers, in order to fool the Germans. Moreover, Van Dijk impersonates the non-existent 'Baron Van Tuyl', a product of Blumberg's imagination; in turn, the Jewish Blumberg plays a game of deceit throughout by inventing not only the baron but also the German general Von Spiegel.

By contrast, in other Dutch war movies from the twentieth century, the protagonists usually assume a straightforward, 'authentic' role: the few schemers and traitors—such as Robbie in SOLDAAT VAN ORANJE and Mies Evertse in PASTORALE 1943—are relatively marginal characters.[5] If the protagonists do use masquerades, these are occasional and random rather than structural and imperceptible. After Dorbeck takes away Ducker's clothes in ALS TWEE DRUPPELS WATER, Ducker has no other option but to travel in a nurse's uniform. Although he himself thinks the disguise is ridiculous and unconvincing, it hurts his masculine pride that everyone behaves courteously toward him and addresses him as the 'sister'. He easily gets through to the liberated part of the Netherlands, and even a German officer gives the 'sister' a lift. When Erik in SOLDAAT VAN ORANJE goes from London back to the Netherlands, he receives a British naval uniform. He is puzzled by this choice but is told '*it is exactly the same as what the Jerries wear, you can't tell the difference ... from a distance*'.[6] When Erik asks if they have any '*tails*' for him, he gets the not very reassuring answer that with a naval uniform the Germans '*will treat you as a prisoner of war; it's better than being shot as a spy*'. Upon seeing Erik in the uniform, one German soldier will remark to another that it is a peculiar outfit, but they guess it belongs to the *Kriegsmarine*, the navy of Nazi Germany. Although Erik does briefly attend a German party—in tails—it is always clear

that he has joined the Resistance unconditionally. Schults and his men in PASTORALE 1943 are also committed to the 'good' cause, but unfortunately they are no more than well-meaning amateurs. Each time they use a masquerade, it discloses their clumsiness, as mentioned in chapter four: during a raid on a distribution office, one of them is immediately recognized; and when pretending to be German soldiers, one of their moustaches is clearly hanging loose.[7]

To illustrate my point that the main characters in twentieth-first-century war films are more skilled and professional in strategic masquerades and deception than those in twentieth-century pictures, let me briefly compare Rachel in ZWARTBOEK with Hannie Schaft in HET MEISJE MET HET RODE HAAR. Rachel dyes her hair blonde in order to penetrate the enemy as a double-crosser, with success. By contrast, Hannie does not try to infiltrate the Nazis and is always firmly on the side of the Resistance. She dyes her red hair black near the end of the movie for the sole purpose of remaining undetected by the Germans. This proves to be in vain, for the roots of her hair reveal her identity after all. This minor detail illustrates that Hannie was more talented as a reckless member of the underground than in the role of a daring imposter. Hannie's 'authenticity' is only rivalled by another 'pure' resistance fighter in Dutch cinema, Cor Takes from Rademakers' triumphant DE AANSLAG [THE ASSAULT] (1986), the first Dutch feature to win an Academy Award for Best Foreign Language Film. Despite Cor's relatively minor part in the film, the episodes between him and protagonist Anton are regarded as particularly impressive.

A DUTCH *RASHOMON: DE AANSLAG*

After a deadly assault on the collaborator Fake Ploeg in a street in Haarlem, the twelve-year-old Anton Steenwijk is brought to a prison cell of the police station in Heemstede that evening in the so-called hunger winter of January 1945. The body was found in front of the house of the widower Korteweg and his daughter Karin, but before the police can get there, they carry the corpse to their neighbours, Anton's family. Anton's older brother Peter gets angry and wants to move the body to the house of the old couple Beumer, but alas, the Germans have arrived. From behind a window, Anton sees Peter take the gun of the dead collaborator and run away.[8] While he himself is taken into a truck, Anton witnesses that the Germans round up many people, including his parents and the Kortewegs. In prison, he has a conversation in the dark with a female resistance woman: she whispers about a married man who perhaps did not realize that she loved him. She touches Anton's face with her right hand. Anton only sees her clearly for a brief moment, when a flashlight reveals her face. Later the Germans take him away because he is not supposed to share a cell with a 'saboteur'. He is brought to the Ortskommandantur, which used to be an old hotel, and the next day to a German headquarters. While eating some delicious sweets at the headquarters, he overhears the news that his parents and a number of hostages were killed as a reprisal for the murder of Fake Ploeg, but he is too young to be greatly affected by it and his life goes on when an uncle from Amsterdam picks him up.

Anton becomes an anaesthetist, which is a symbolic profession here, for his attitude is to forget about the war. The only time he goes back to the empty area where his parents' house used to be, now covered with weeds, is in 1952. He briefly visualizes a body on the streets and then is called inside by the old Mrs. Beumer for a visit. She speaks highly of Peter, for in her interpretation of the event, he tried to help the severely wounded Fake Ploeg, while Anton knows that Peter was in fact trying to move the body so that the Beumers would become the focus of attention for the Germans. And even though Anton tries to keep the memories of that evening in January 1945 at bay, De aanslag shows that the past comes to haunt him, inevitably. A voice-over in 1956 mentions that Anton's memories of the assault are stored away in the 'fog of time', but he will be increasingly affected by it from the 1960s onwards. He dates several girls until he meets the stewardess Saskia de Graaff, whose father belonged to the resistance. The moment Anton sets eyes on Saskia, he recognizes a startling resemblance to the woman in the prison, which is emphasized by a flashback insert.[9] They get married within a year after their meeting, and soon thereafter a daughter (Sandra) is born. The story then jumps forward to the film's key encounter in the post-war period: one of Saskia's father's former comrades is to be buried, and during the reception after the funeral ceremony, he overhears a man talk about the assault. Anton's subsequent conversation on a bench with this Cor Takes—whose code name is 'Gijs' among the resistance veterans—is the pinnacle of DE AANSLAG.[10] Anton mentions that he is doing fine: happily married, great daughter, nice job. But Cor distrusts this statement: 'Why did you address me? You could have remained silent', implying there is an urge on Anton's part to open up the wound.

Cor tells Anton that he was responsible for the killing of Fake Ploeg, together with Truus Coster. The collaborator committed the worst possible torture practices, so he had to be shot, though Cor and Truus knew that the Germans would take retaliatory action. Cor has no regrets for killing Fake nor does he feel responsible for the aftermath of that killing and its consequences for Anton. But the latter starts to cry because he realizes that at the age of twelve he had shared the cell with Truus, the 'saboteur' according to the Germans. This is shown via blue-tinted flashback scenes. She was executed in the dunes three weeks prior to the liberation in May 1945. Cor wants to meet with Anton again, for although Cor had his lips sealed when interrogated by the Gestapo, he has not stopped talking ever since the war ended. It is Cor's way of coming to terms with the traumatic history of the war. At one point, Anton's father-in-law says: 'It seems that it will all bubble up to the surface sooner or later, this disease ... for everyone.' When Anton replies 'It doesn't seem to have affected you', the thoughtful silence of the resistance veteran is telling.

When Anton visits Cor's apartment, his host immediately mentions the possible imminent release of the war criminal Willy Lages and how it is making all the resistance veterans sick to their stomachs, another indication that the war will not be over for them.[11] The scene in Cor's gloomy basement shows how his life has stopped since the assault: he has preserved Truus's gun, her bicycle, and a map of Europe with a lipstick kiss close to Wijk aan Zee. Significantly, the adult Anton remembers that he had a lipstick kiss on his forehead when he saw himself in the mirror in the Ortskommandatur, but the original scene only shows a blood stain on his forehead. Truus never gave him a kiss; instead she touched his face with her blood-stained hand. He then sees a photograph of Truus on the wall, and as he stares at it, Cor's face suddenly pops up in close-up, frontally staged: 'She is it, isn't she?' he inquires quite compulsorily. Then the assault is visualized: Cor/'Gijs' shoots Fake in the back; Truus stops to finish it off, but Cor sees that Fake has his gun out and while he shouts 'Watch out', she is hit in the back. ('I always presumed that Ploeg was shouting', Anton says). Cor finds a place for the injured Truus to take shelter, but due to a collaborator screaming, the Germans soon arrive and he has to leave her behind. Cor still has not recovered from his sense of guilt from having left her.

The voice-over announces that Anton finally knows the identity of the woman who has come to possess his life. He soon divorces Saskia, who was the spitting image of Truus. Liesbeth will be his second wife, born after the war, but they never discuss it. She gives birth to a son, Peter. But Anton starts suffering from nightmares and bouts of despair. In his holiday home in Lucca, Italy, he has a serious panic attack. Though no year is given, this happened probably in the late 1970s. The doctor gives him a recipe, but Anton tears it apart, for he refuses to be intimidated by chilling memories that have come to haunt him so belatedly.

Anton's initial position can be compared to Rachel's, albeit with crucial differences. Rachel was the axis of a number of gruesome events but is able to relegate them to the past. Anton was only an indirect witness: because the blinds were down, he only heard the gunshots and Cor's scream, but he did not see the actual shooting. He saw his brother run away with a gun, and he was able to repress the memory of his parents being rounded up. But the memories return, in some cases via an 'innocent' trigger. Did he fall in love with Saskia because she reminded him immediately of the woman in prison? When his second wife gives him a clove to alleviate his toothache, he remembers that his mother used the same remedy when she had a toothache that fatal evening. But ever since his visit to Cor, things have become worse: he is overwhelmed by feelings of unrest and even uncontrollable emotions. On what turns out to be his last night, Anton's father tells his son: 'He who does not know his past will not understand his present. Remember that, Tony.' This quote will reverberate like an echo throughout DE AANSLAG: the greater his emotional distress, the greater the need for Anton to solve the riddles of his past. The older he grows, the more urgent his desire becomes to find out exactly what had happened. His first father-in-law had told him that 'this disease' will manifest itself one day. Initially, the past is clearly separated from Anton's present, as it is for Rachel, but with the passing of time, the past and present get caught in an ever-tighter feedback loop for Anton. With each and every new piece of information, his perspective on that one decisive event is altered, even though the witness accounts are cumulative and not as contradictory as in RASHOMON (Akira Kurosawa, 1951), whose narrative structure functioned as a source of inspiration for DE AANSLAG.[12]

If Rachel's pragmatism represents one end of a spectrum (life goes on, the past is past), then Cor Takes is at the other end: for him, it is always January 1945 because he is still consumed by the tragedy and his feelings of guilt about Truus's fate. Whereas Rachel restricts herself to a brief and general answer—she was thinking about the past—Cor's strategy is to talk through the trauma in precise details. The way he talks about the assault at the funeral, it would not surprise us if we were to find out that he was describing the unfolding of events for the hundredth time. He has become an automaton, telling the same old story over and over again. As is the case with many more veterans, Cor has remained stuck in time. They are able to go on living as long as there is a status quo. The news that the Nazi Willy Lages might be set free is too disturbing a rupture for one of them, so he commits suicide. Cor can only talk about the deplorable fate of this comrade by staring out the window, keeping his back turned to Anton the entire time. Cor subjects himself to self-obliteration: he partakes in the symbolic network but not with his current self, for there is no future for him. Or he envisions a 'bad' future in which the Nazis are pardoned. And in that sense, it is not surprising that he does not introduce himself as Cor Takes but as 'Gijs', for that is the name people remember him by. Hence, his loss of self in the post-war period is signified by the eagerness with which he adopts this code name: after the assault, 'Gijs' has become the living dead.[13]

TIME OUT OF JOINT: *LEEDVERMAAK*

Cor Takes was introduced to Anton—and to us—during a funeral ceremony, but we meet the Jewish Ada from LEEDVERMAAK (Frans Weisz, 1989) during the most joyful of occasions, the wedding party of her daughter Lea. Based on a theatre play by Judith Herzberg, the film covers only a few hours and is set in one specific place, namely the residence of Simon and his wife Ada. In spite of the film's dramatic unity with its resolute adherence to the present, Weisz's LEEDVERMAAK constantly evokes the past and the future in terms of its content. Thanks to this discrepancy between content and form, the film has become an astonishing achievement.

Most of the characters are introduced because they are being recorded on film by Alexander who was the previous husband of Lea, the current bride. The guests are caught by surprise and must improvise a brief speech on the spot to express their hopes and wishes for the married couple. Whereas the atmosphere is cheerful, each and everyone's pose in the presence of the video camera is quite awkward. Moreover, the shots, in black and white, are frontally staged, and such a set-up always comes across as an 'aggressive' form of addressing the film spectator. The film is meant to be watched in the near future by the bridal pair, and Alexander's reason for making the recordings is that he regrets that no one had made any recordings during his wedding a few years ago. Lea's third marriage is to Nico, a doctor by profession, who has promised that he will quit smoking and work fewer hours a week, a prospect that makes her very happy. On top of that, her parents give her a holiday trip as a present, to which Lea's father Simon adds during his speech: 'My wife Ada insisted we should give a trip, because we ourselves were never able to ... well, we don't have to go into that.'

A wedding is the day par excellence of promises for a bright future: the bride and groom have a trip to look ahead to; not only Lea, but also Nico hopes that his second marriage will be more prosperous than the previous one; the guests wish them all the luck; the recordings are meant to commemorate this special day, to be rewatched ideally when they have grown old together. The master of ceremony, Hans, has bought white camellias for Nico to give to his bride. The only problem is that camellias were what Nico gave to his first wife Dory, who remarks sarcastically that it would probably be asking too much to expect a more original gift from Nico. The incident with the camellias is symptomatic of the film's temporality: as a symbol of purity, a bouquet is meant to represent good fortune, but here it immediately recalls a past that is better forgotten. Though Weisz's film addresses a number of problematic issues between a variety of guests (some of them minor such as Dory's refusal to give violin lessons to Lea any longer), I will restrict myself to those dreadful experiences the older generation had to suffer between the years 1940-1945 that cannot be covered by any promise of a better future. The various wartime memories pop up at irregular intervals in the daily lives of the characters and, regardless of how special the occasion is, the wedding is no exception.

There are three main approaches to their war experience that can be distinguished in the film. Nico's father Zwart has adopted a mask of humour. He introduces himself with a joke: 'I'm Nico's father, though there are no witnesses to prove that fact, it's a persistent rumour', and then starts laughing out loud himself. A bit later, he gives a brief and factual account of his life to Lea's parents on the basis of some old photographs: his Jewish wife and his oldest son Simon passed away during the war, the latter having died from an infection in a hospital; during those years, Zwart himself had quite a few things on his mind, 'resistance, etcetera, etcetera'; Duifje is his second wife. Duifje is the type who only tries to keep a conversation going. When Dory reacts somewhat sharply at one point, she replies: 'I only wanted to say something neutral.' Her social talk seems aimed at avoiding uncomfortable silences. She is the perfect companion for a man who wants to keep the atrocities of the past at a distance. She explains how she had a necklace with a Jewish star, which she inherited from Zwart's first wife, but that when Nico was an adolescent, he did not want her to wear it. She talks about it as if it were no more than a precious adornment for her, as if she were not really aware of its loaded meaning. The fact that her husband Zwart allowed her to have it offers food for speculation. It could be considered a crude joke on his part, as if he were saying: 'I can pretend that I have come to terms with my war memories, for I can accept that my wife is wearing a Jewish star as an ornament.' But it is clear that he is not free from painful memories, as detected by his remark to Lea that people like her who make music never seem to be sad.

The second position is represented by Aunt Riet, who is a single woman, but who owes her identity as 'Mamma Riet' to the war. When she introduces herself to Hans as Lea's 'safe house mother', she is delighted when he tells her that Lea talks more often about her than about her very own mother. After Lea's parents were taken away to Germany, the young 'Liesje', as Riet used to call the four-year-old girl, was under her care for three years. When Riet later narrates how happy they were for 'Liesje' when her parents returned safely, Lea remarks in a somewhat irritated manner: 'You tell this story on each and every occasion.' In the voice-over that gives us Riet's thoughts, however, it becomes clear that she regretted the return of Lea's parents, particularly that of mother Ada. 'My nipples always hurt when Liesje started to cry.' 'So many people did not return from Germany, but why did they?' 'Would he [Lea's father] ever think of me?' 'If she [Ada] were to die of electroshocks, I could marry Liesje's father.' These reflections indicate that the war gave Riet the opportunity to take up the role of mother, which she then had to surrender after the liberation, to her unspoken chagrin. This explains why she makes inappropriate remarks without realizing it. 'A theatre play with only Jews is an impossibility. For it would be anti-Semitic if one of them were to have an evil disposition.' Due to her sullen tone, this statement implies that Jews have gained an unjustified privilege due to their history as war victims: even if they were to do bad things, we are no longer in the position to put a blame on them for anything. Moreover, Riet refers to a French movie she had seen on television, for she always likes to watch war pictures. From her description, it must have been MONSIEUR KLEIN (Joseph Losey, 1976). It was the story of a man who is persecuted, later arrested, and put on a train to Germany. 'But he was no French Jew at all.' She presents the tragic irony of this Monsieur Klein with a certain malice, as if to indicate that the Jews do not have an exclusive right to suffering.

For Riet, the deportation of Jews had the advantage of allowing her to act as a mother, but in the post-war period she was reduced to the identity of a 'single woman'. In addition, she is envious of those Jewish survivors who are able to 'wallow', according to her, in victimization. Riet's perception of Jewish privilege is the polar opposite of the third position: that of Ada, the Holocaust survivor. In the beginning of LEEDVERMAAK, Ada is either silent or politely receives congratulations. But when Simon has the attention of most of the guests, he suddenly says: 'Did you hear of Ada's latest heroic act? She buys a child's dress, but then she remembers that Lea is no longer a kid. How does she return from the city centre? Not by tram, guess what ... no, no, by police car.' Ada then explains in a flat voice and a slightly incoherent manner:

> There were two guys with uniforms and boots, talking German, I thought. ... I presumed that I was not permitted to travel, tried to open the doors. I will buy an umbrella later. The guys with the boots were suspicious. They grabbed me, I screamed; I should not have done that. The two guys grabbed my arm. I was confused.

There is a painful silence, for it is clear to all guests that time is out of joint for Ada: it requires only a minor trigger and then she is back in the war. For Ada, there is a thin line between past and present, if any. 'Yes, they were only doing their work. Yes, *Befehl ist Befehl*.'

To underscore her temporal confusion, the camera zooms in on Ada at one point, and in a reverse shot, focalized by her blind stare, we see the guests dancing in slow motion, slightly out of focus, to 'Venus' by Shocking Blue. This diegetic song is drowned out by extradiegetic sounds that make it explicit that Ada is physically present but mentally absent from the cheerful festivities. At the very moment 'Venus' becomes audible again, Ada turns her back to the guests and walks away. There are several other scenes that indicate that Ada's perception of the wedding is crisscrossed with distractions related to her traumatic past. The most obvious one is when she is in her bedroom, packing her suitcase. She walks past a mirror on the inside of her wardrobe, and suddenly she sees herself transformed into a younger version with curly hair. She watches her mirror image and then picks up a photograph of a child, probably a young Lea, before she comes back in the present. The proximity of the past is also illustrated by the blunt question she asks Duifje: 'Do you ever wonder whose place you have taken?'—a clear reference to the guilt that the Jews who survived the war felt. It is a question that the happy-go-lucky Duifje simply does not understand, even accusing Ada of being a party spoiler: 'I think you are mean; you only pretend to be crazy in order to hurt other people.'

In spite of Duifje's inconsiderate remark, there is an acute crisis. When Simon puts his wife Ada in an embarrassing situation by disclosing her strange behaviour to the guests, his strategy was to reveal that Ada wants to commit herself to a psychiatric institution the following day. Simon cannot stomach the thought that she wants to put her faith in someone else than him. If she abandons him tomorrow, he tells his daughter Lea, he will leave tonight. So her third marriage coincides with the possible separation of her parents, which makes Lea doubt whether she can go on honeymoon. Husband Nico replies: 'So you want to save the marriage of your parents, whereas you cannot even manage yours.'

The marital crisis of Lea's parents reveals that not only the first post-war generation of Jews is tragically scarred by the Holocaust but also their children.[14] When her parents were transported to Germany, Lea was left behind with 'Mamma Riet'. 'If I were to have a child', Lea tells her father at the party, 'I would have taken it everywhere with me and I would have comforted it'. 'But,' Simon defends their choice, 'this way you had a bigger chance of surviving'. Lea's brief but chilling reply sums up her trauma: 'Dying does not matter, but being left behind does.' She adds that she envied Dory who ended up in an orphanage, whereas she had to deal with her traumatized parents. And the prospect of her father leaving her mother is more than she can handle.

In LEEDVERMAAK, there is a mysterious guest who is always in one of the adjacent rooms from the revelry and only has some one-on-one conversations with a few guests. This ghostlike character introduces himself as Daniel whose parents used to live in the house before the war; he refers to his past lives and mentions that he has arrived at his very beginning, for he lives his life backwards. He says a number of cryptic lines, but he is most explicit in his conversations with Ada and Lea. Whereas her closest relatives regret Ada's decision to go into an 'insane asylum', Daniel praises Ada for her bravery: 'You are prepared to give up everything; you try to find peace of mind in order to live the autumn of your years.' Although a total stranger to Ada, Daniel adds that he is the only one who will not forsake her: 'You will see me at every visiting hour.' Given that Ada suffers from hallucinations, these words confirm that Daniel is to be regarded as a spectral appearance. He acts as the moral voice that comforts Ada and helps her to stick to her decision. Saying farewell to her daughter who is still displeased with her choice, Ada echoes Daniel when she says that it requires courage to seek help, whereupon Lea apologizes to her mother.

Daniel considers it his most important task, however, to annul the marriage, as he tells Zwart, Lea's father-in-law. Upon meeting him on the staircase, Lea is irritated by Daniel who declares his love for her: 'I can only fall in love in this house. And I won't let you go this time.' This frank doggedness of Daniel may seem strange, for it implies an immediate divorce from Nico, whereas Lea is so fiercely opposed to the possibility that her parents might separate. It may seem inconsistent in the first place that they are celebrating Lea's third marriage this very evening, but it is significant at the same time that she has never lived on her own. Probably too fearful of being on her own, her previous two marriages were the result of hasty decisions. And she is already sceptical about her third attempt: as she reveals to her mother, she doubts she can offer Nico the 'safety and security' he longs. Moreover, as she tells her bridegroom: 'If I were to really fall in love with you, you would probably die.' In other words, she cannot fully attach herself to people due to her fear of being abandoned. Seen in that light, Daniel might indeed be the best alternative. He is a reassuring 'ghost' who will always be faithful, as is clear in his conversation with Ada. But whereas her mother is seriously attempting to cope with her trauma, Lea rushes into marriages with men whose expectations of matrimony are too high. At the end of the party, she walks outside all by herself and steps into the 'just married' car. While she is thinking things over—maybe reflecting on her uncertain future with Nico or on her mother's decision—the end credit song sets in: Mathilde Santing's 'There Will Never Be Another You'. This seems a fitting song to end a wedding party, for this 'another you' might refer to both bride and groom, and it is illustrated by objects that connote happiness, such as the wedding cake. But here it is quite an ironic gesture, for after the conversations with both Daniel and her mother, it is highly likely that there will in fact be 'another you' for Lea to replace her current husband Nico.

DEATH AND THE MAIDEN: *CHARLOTTE*

Weisz could not have directed LEEDVERMAAK, had he not made CHARLOTTE (1981). To emphasize the importance of this key film, he tends to characterize his career in two periods: 'before and after CHARLOTTE'. After his ambitious debut feature HET GANGSTERMEISJE did not meet his expectations due to its modest box-office result, he had some commercial successes in the early 1970s. DE INBREKER [THE BURGLAR] (1972) was a hugely enjoyable gangster film with car chases along the canals in Amsterdam, but by the time he made HEB MEDELIJ, JET [HAPPY DAYS ARE HERE AGAIN] (1975), Weisz felt very unhappy on the set: filmmaking had become merely a livelihood. He decided his next project had to be a film that was dear to his heart: co-scripted with Judith Herzberg, he made CHARLOTTE, a biography of the Jewish-German artist Charlotte Salomon, who died at the age of 26 in Auschwitz, as the text at the end of his picture discloses. Thanks to a weekend pass to 'visit' her grandparents who are in hiding in the villa of the American benefactress Ottilie Moore in Villefranche-sur-Mer, she manages to escape Germany in 1939. In the south of France, she starts to paint and draw frenetically in the years 1941 and 1942. The posthumous publication of *Leben? oder Theater? Ein Singespiel* [*Life? or Theatre? A Song-Play*]—a book with no less than 1,325 pages—contains almost 800 gouaches, often accompanied by text written directly into the imagery.[15] In addition to text and imagery, she incorporated music as written cues, which explains the subtitle 'A Song-Play'.

While the voluminous book tells the serial narrative of her own life, Weisz's CHARLOTTE is a biography told in an atemporal fashion.[16] It starts with a long take of a room with a woman in bed on the right and curtains moving due to the open window in the middle of the long shot. We see that the low sun and light enters the room from the outside, as in those famous Dutch interior paintings. Only when the woman walks towards the window does the camera zoom in, very slowly. There is a similar shot composition some fifteen minutes later, and towards the end, Charlotte opens the shutters to this very same window, whereupon she starts packing a suitcase, putting on top a paper containing the words *Leben? oder Theater?*. She will bring it to Doctor Moridini, with the simple words: '*Please keep this safe, it is my whole life.*' In terms of chronology, the latter shot in the room is one of the very last, but we have no clue of the earlier two shots: partly because they recall a painterly still-life, any date is indeterminate—somewhere between 1939 and 1942. And in fact, it seems as if the second shot is a repetition of the opening, but since the low sun is not as visible, it is probably just another bright day. Whether that is the case or not is not that important—these shots of a 'room with a view' seem to indicate that the temporality of Weisz's CHARLOTTE is wilfully indeterminate.

Weisz's film has some historical markers: the year 1939 is mentioned explicitly, we hear a kid shout in French that the war has started, Charlotte's year of death is on screen. At the same time, CHARLOTTE is structured around an ahistorical kernel, so characteristic of trauma. After she leaves Germany by train and arrives in the south of France, Charlotte hears her grandmother say that she is the spitting image of her mother who had died fifteen years ago. When she discovers that grandmother is deeply depressed, grandfather says that it is '*all just in her mind*', to which Charlotte gets angry: '*You're even madder than she is.*' At the sickbed of his wife, the heartless grandpa then bluntly reveals to Charlotte that suicide runs in her family: Grandma's mother as well as an uncle had killed themselves. Even more shocking to Charlotte is that her mother did not die of influenza, as she had always believed, but that she had also taken her own life, just like her sister, Charlotte's aunt, after whom Charlotte was named. After the catastrophic revelations that these deaths were suicides, Charlotte finds the body of her grandmother who had died by poisoning herself. These cases might well have unhinged Charlotte, as Griselda Pollock claims, but the film chronicles why she did not collapse, even though she admits in voice-over that '*deep down I felt the same disposition, the same tendency towards despair and death.*'

Early in the film, we hear Charlotte's voice-over address a '*beloved you*', and this 'you' is the reason she is able to resist her hereditary disposition. In the second scene, when we see her behind the window of a train—which we later realize is the train that takes her to France—we hear her say: '*... you are the only one who listens to me as I listen to you, with such absolute love*'. This 'you' is a man on the platform who stretches his arms high in the air to bid her farewell, but we are only introduced to this Amadeus Daberlohn ('penniless Wolfgang') much later in Weisz's film. After she discovers her dead grandmother, a lengthy voice-over explains that she had to start doing '*something insanely out of the ordinary*' to prevent her from taking her own life. '*And then the memory of you came back to me. I tried to recall your face and appearance.*' This attempt to remember this 'you' is underscored by an image of a blank sketchbook page in the grass that transforms into a cartoon image of Daberlohn, whose name has still not been mentioned. Charlotte's voice-over continues, stating among others that she would like to become '*the living model of your theory. "That to really love life, one must also comprehend and embrace the other side, death and suffering."*'

It will result in gouaches that are depicted in the background, accompanied by text, that relate the history of her parents, including the depression that befalls Charlotte's mother Franziska as well as her father Albert's remarriage to the celebrated singer Paulinka Bimbam four years later. Charlotte has a complicated relationship with her stepmother: she admires her, she is jealous of her because she has to share her father's affection with her, and she is annoyed with Paulinka because the stepmother takes Charlotte's education into her own hands. When she says she has the ambition to join the Academy of Fine Arts, Paulinka hires a teacher to test whether she has drawing talent. To Charlotte's frustration, she is expected to draw an exact replica of the cactus in front of her, but she falls short on accuracy. Her rivalry with Paulinka reaches a new level when Daberlohn enters the family residence.

When Charlotte, now in her late teens, returns home one day, she hears peculiar guttural noises. A man is rehearsing with Paulinka, but Charlotte only spots him for the first time from afar as she looks outside the window. While eavesdropping on the rehearsals and peeping through the door the housekeeper has deliberately left ajar, Charlotte hears the intimate exchanges of words between Paulinka and her singing coach as well as the latter's vision of life: '*To really love life, one must really comprehend the other side, death and suffering.*' This sentence reverberates because Charlotte had already cited this line in her voice-over. The quote becomes her guidance not just on the basis of its content but also because of who has uttered it. In one of her voice-overs, Charlotte remembers that upon seeing one of her drawings titled *Death and the Maiden*, Daberlohn had said: '*You and I are "Death and the Maiden"*.' Later in the film, the original scene is repeated, meaning that once again Charlotte's recollection is presented before the actual occurrence.

The fact that Daberlohn identifies himself as 'death' makes sense, for as Paulinka tells Albert and Charlotte, he had lost his memory in the Great War and his head is permanently in the clouds, for he '*laid in the trench for three days with his friends dying besides him. He was the only one still alive when they were found.*' Apart from the fact that Charlotte is intrigued by Daberlohn because she overhears his flirtatious conversations with Paulinka, he fascinates her because he has actually experienced the atrocities of a war. '*I often wondered what someone like that would look like*', and she herself gives her answer in his presence: '*Rather like you*'. Paulinka is so lurid as to guess that this can be considered a '*first declaration of love*'.

Daberlohn is the only character who acknowledges that Charlotte is eclipsed in every regard by her stepmother who tends to impose her '*exalted standards*' upon her. But she has '*true painter's hands*', according to Daberlohn; she can look like '*Botticelli's Venus*' if only her whole body gets a '*jolt*'. No wonder this man who sees her potential and her talent becomes a point of reference for her, though he can also be rude to her. But despite his instances of cruel behaviour, she keeps running after him, because, as Daberlohn scathingly and arrogantly discloses, '*your strength lies in that* [i.e., in running after me].' And she will continue to run after him, for once she has joined her grandparents, she will never ever see him again but he will be constantly on her mind. Her life's work *Leben? oder Theater?* can only be made while the memory of her '*beloved friend*' gives her the courage to persevere, as her voice-over explains.

Charlotte had to suffer a number of catastrophes: the absence of a mother since the age of nine; the rise of antisemitism during her adolescence; the belated revelation in her early twenties that suicides run in her family; the discovery of her grandmother's corpse; her grandfather passing away on the train in the seat in front of her (of which it can be suggested that he died of an overdose of barbiturates that the real-life Charlotte may have put into the man's breakfast omelette).[17] But instead of taking her own life, like her mother and aunt did before her, the recollection of the traumatic fate of Daberlohn, who had to play dead for three days amidst the dead and the dying, gave her the energy to continue and to paint. He became living proof that someone who had returned from the war as an amnesiac and voiceless adolescent could recover by embracing the 'Nietzschean proposition of joyous sex and death-defying singing' (Pollock, 232). Daberlohn is addressed in a voice-over as the '*beloved you*' throughout the film, as if she needs to constantly remind herself of him to keep the risk of a relapse at bay. Charlotte therefore uses the form of an apostrophe, a well-known figure of speech in poetry in which an absent person is invoked. This invocation gives structure to the film and prevents it from being incoherent. For Weisz's film, as befits a picture on trauma, could not but take some liberty to present Charlotte's life story via cut-up fragments as well as repeated scenes and phrases in reverse chronology.[18]

MARRIED TO THE MOB: *LAYLA M.*

Most Dutch films about World War II, especially those from the twentieth century, are rooted in psychological realism. The films by Weisz about the mental consequences of the war, however, tend towards theatricality. His approach seems to suggest that historical traumas defy 'realism'. Characters are cut off from actual situations, for their present consists of a doomed past, as in LEEDVERMAAK. Evoking poetry, painting, music and theatre, CHARLOTTE is told in a non-chronological fashion. Whereas the war period itself has been widely covered in Dutch cinema, the controversial historical periods or events since the war—such as the violent decolonisation of Indonesia (the Dutch East Indies); the train and school hijacks by Moluccans in the mid-1970s; the failure of UN peacekeeping in Srebrenica in 1995; the murder of Pim Fortuyn in 2002 and of Theo van Gogh in 2004—have resulted in only a handful of films, most of which have not been very noteworthy.[19] If there is a topic with a certain historical urgency, then it is the country's so-called 'multicultural tragedy' as proclaimed by Paul Scheffer in a famous essay from 2000. The Netherlands was a country divided into pillars, with several groups living in 'peaceful coexistence' (socialists, liberals, Catholics, and Protestants). Due to this pillarization, a growing number of immigrants were not offered viable prospects. The seemingly tolerant attitude of the Dutch, Scheffer argued, could also be taken as a startling indifference towards their fellow citizens who had roots in Turkey, Suriname, and Morocco. As I already mentioned in my previous study on Dutch post-war fiction film, the overriding attitude of the 'native' Dutch towards the non-Western newcomers might be summed up as follows: 'I tolerate your presence, but do not interfere with my stuff'. The integration of immigrants was further problematized by 'white flight': the native-born Dutch tended to send their kids to schools with few if any pupils of Turkish or Moroccan descent. Especially the second-generation children of immigrants came to regard themselves as victims of this policy of 'coexistence without interacting'. Although the basic assumptions of this 'multicultural tragedy' were widely contested, it became a popular catchphrase to advocate the idea that an unbridgeable divide separates the Dutch from the newcomers and their children.

A cinematic reply to Scheffer's analysis can be divided into two tendencies. In the first, the gap between 'native' Dutch and non-western Dutch is exploited in the form of humour. Several 'multicultural' comedies, examined in chapter two of my study on humour and irony in Dutch cinema, were released in a relatively short timespan with great success. These films tend to be strategically ambiguous: they both affirm and contradict hackneyed images. But in the best of these comedies, such as SHOUF SHOUF HABIBI! (Albert ter Heerdt, 2004), the low-budget road movie RABAT (Jim Taihuttu and Victor D. Ponten, 2011), and the vibrant DE LIBI [argot for 'life'] (Shady El-Hamus, 2019), the self-mocking clichés are exaggerated to such an extent that a critical perspective starts to prevail. These films humorously confront their viewers with the difficult if not impossible position of the second generation, of those sandwiched between two cultures. In the turbulent years between the production of these titles, comic acknowledgement was as good as it was going to get.

Second, a few dramas have been made in the aftermath of these comedies, and though the quality of some is above average,[20] they are not particularly challenging in terms of style and form—except perhaps WOLF, discussed in chapter six. LAYLA M. (Mijke de Jong, 2016) is the best-known of these 'multicultural dramas', for it was a Dutch entry for the Academy Awards, and it won Golden Calves for Best Actress and Best Male Supporting Role. Layla Moubarit, of Dutch-Moroccan origin and born in Amsterdam, alienates herself from her father, a moderate Muslim who has integrated himself into Dutch society: he has his own shop and he is coach of a football team. Her daughter, however, is a hothead and considers her generation 'the pariahs in Holland'. Father is angered by her random use of inflammatory quotes from the Quran, but in response to her dad's dismay, the stubborn Layla only becomes more dedicated to her rebellion. She persuades her younger brother Younes to join a protest against a ban on gathering. After Younes is released from an interrogation by the police, he tells Layla he will not participate in any future demonstrations, for his Islam is not political. His sister does not yield to any intimidation: when the house of her friend Zine is examined because he is suspected of recruiting jihadists, she says that the intruders are cursed by Allah.

The Skype conversations she has with the deeply religious Abdel only add fuel to the fire. She decides to marry him, which means not finishing her exams and therefore giving up her ambition—for the time being at least—to become a doctor. She envies Abdel for being born in Morocco, for it means that 'you belong in the place where you were born'. From this point onwards, she is no longer the choreographer of her own life. Her husband Abdel takes her with him to Belgium, to a Jihadist training camp, which is raided by the police. She then accompanies him to Amman in Jordan, and when she meets her neighbour, the young mother Oum Osama whose husband is away, Layla tells Abdel: 'I don't think she has a clue what she's doing here.' But the point, of course, is that Layla herself has no clue. She is restricted in her whereabouts, and she is forbidden to visit a refugee camp near the border. Abdel and Zine force her to watch a torture clip on the internet, meant to legitimize their actions. When she sees footage in which Oum Osama's husband bids farewell before his suicide mission, she yells at Abdel not to do anything similar. The confrontation is shot in a manner that is exemplary of LAYLA M.: we have two characters in one shot, in conflict with each other. The focus shifts constantly, first the one (Layla) is in sharp focus and the other out of focus (her father or Abdel), and vice versa. This way of filming already starts from the time of their car trip to Belgium, demonstrating that Layla and Abdel were never on the same page.

When she lands at Schiphol Airport, she is immediately arrested and interrogated by the police. She remains silent, but the police officer tells her that 'we know all about you' and shows photographic evidence of her activities. She is shown what could be 'the last picture of your husband'. The final shot is a long close-up of Layla's face, but the officer only says: 'It's a bit late for tears.' The cinematography of De Jong's LAYLA M. is used superbly to tell the story about a young adult who becomes an easy target for radical Muslims due to her stubborn resistance of her father's authority. The frequent shifts in focus illustrate that her anger has made her blind to the exploitation of Abdel and his friends. And thus, Layla Moubarit turns unwittingly into Layla M., the customary way in which the media in the Netherlands refers to suspects (the family name being reduced to an initial). Since her return from Jordan, Layla M. has become her name for the outside world.

CONCLUSION: WHAT TIME IS IT THERE?

In this chapter, I have addressed strategies to cope with dreadful historical episodes ranging from a single event—such as an assault during the war—to systematic exploitation, as in the case of colonization. One of these strategies was the cover-up, as in the unsuccessful attempts by the protagonists in both MAX HAVELAAR and DE SCHORPIOEN to reveal the dirty methods and crimes of the authorities. In HET ZWIJGEN, the main character is an outsider who becomes intrigued by a local mystery but succumbs to aural temptations. As a consequence, this film emphasizes that such a secret history can also unite a community against the intrusion by a man from the city. In the Catholic community depicted in DE BENDE VAN OSS, there is a local crime boss who runs all affairs in town in an illegitimate manner and everyone is supposed to accept his position: a transgression of the rules has become habitual, for the law in the eyes of the people of Oss is represented by the hostile Protestants. These films can be seen as expressions of what has been termed 'historical discomfort': anyone who aims to disclose secrets or wants to rebel against a status quo must be reduced to passivity. In fact, Johanna is the only character in all these films who has some success with her protest, for the crime boss will have his comeuppance. But in her case a particular incident—the death of her half-sister—is required to have her break the code of silence.

In the second half of the chapter, there was a shift to 'historical trauma', for in the films under scrutiny, the characters themselves were directly affected by events: in contrast to Rachel in ZWARTBOEK for whom the series of tragic incidents seems a nuisance from 'the past', Anton in DE AANSLAG experiences how a repressed memory comes to haunt him in increasing and unexpectedly distorted fashion as the years pass by. Rademakers' war film returns from a specific vantage point in time to that one event, but the film is surpassed in atemporality by the two films by Weisz mentioned here. LEEDVERMAAK has a clearly delineated notion of the present (the wedding party), but the characters are either focussed on the future or, much more dramatically, on an un-narratable past. Charlotte, the title hero of another Weisz film whose chronology is fairly chopped up, is still able to give some meaning to her burdensome family life only by imagining herself as someone who is spoken to by a 'you' that the voice-over refers to throughout the film. In comparison, LAYLA M. is a conventional film in terms of its narration and style, but if its protagonist were to fully realize—perhaps in a sequel—how she has been deceived, an atemporal mode of storytelling is quite likely.

NOTES

1 I like DE SCHORPIOEN because its uneven narrative structure turns it into a reflection on the writing of history. By comparison, Hylkema's OEROEG, based on Hella Haasse's eponymous successful novel from 1948, has a more traditional angle. The film chronicles how the friendship between the Dutch boy Johan and Oeroeg, the son of an Indonesian servant, is affected by historical developments. As kids, they become 'blood brothers' for life, unaware of the animosity between the colonial power and the colonized people. As adults, however, they come to oppose each other. In the postwar years, Oeroeg leads a group of rebels fighting for independence from Holland, whereas Johan is appointed as lieutenant in the Dutch army. The injustice permeating the relationship between the two countries only gradually dawns on Johan. His first inkling of this inequality was when he was able to watch TARZAN, THE APE MAN (W.S. Van Dyke, 1932) in a regular auditorium while Oeroeg and other indigenous people were seated behind the screen. Much later, Johan learns that Oeroeg's father Deppoh has died because following orders was in his blood. When Johan's father lost his watch, Deppoh instinctively dived into the water to save the family heirloom and drowned. Whereas Deppoh's death was caused by unequal power relations, Johan's father was murdered by rebels, and Johan is made to understand that the two deaths are alike. When Johan is taken hostage by Indonesians, he is released in exchange for twelve rebels, and he sees that Oeroeg is one of them. 'Are we still friends?' he asks him on a bridge, to which Oeroeg replies: 'Only when we have become equals', hinting at the fact that one Johan equals twelve Indonesian prisoners of war. Johan then gives Oeroeg the heirloom that Deppoh had rescued at the expense of his life, and Oeroeg's farewell, which in my view is too sentimental, is: 'Far away or nearby, we will always be brothers.' This final gesture falsely suggests that camaraderie can neutralize political injustice.

2 When the military police find the local bookkeeper Harry and examine his books, the code is definitely broken. But the government refuses to prosecute the 'crime-ridden den of thieves' in Oss (as they were described by the controversial MP Rost van Tonningen in March 1939), so the clergy, the mayor, and the businessmen get away with their vice crimes.

3 I once saw a truck with the slogan 'Het hout nooit op' [the wood is never out of stock], which can be taken as an 'answer' to Rachel's question 'Houdt het dan nooit op?' [Will It Never End?]. The slogan works as a verbal pun because 'hout' and 'houdt' sound similar in Dutch.

4 OORLOGSWINTER attracted quite a crowd: some 850,000 viewers in the Netherlands. By telling the film from the perspective of a boy who experiences the war as an exciting but also grim adventure, OORLOGSWINTER resembles a Spielberg film such as EMPIRE OF THE SUN (1987). Michiel is asked to deliver a letter, but before the addressee can receive it he is shot for allegedly killing a German soldier. Michiel tries to help a wounded British pilot, the actual killer of the German. He has to distract a dog to escape from Germans. He is saved from drowning under the ice by a Nazi. And in an operatic finale, reminiscent of a spaghetti western, he has to pull the trigger on his uncle.

5 I do not consider Ducker in ALS TWEE DRUPPELS WATER as a schemer or traitor, since he is 'sincere' in thinking that he worked for the resistance, even when others believe otherwise,

6 'Jerries' was British Army slang for Germans.

7 Miep Algera in PASTORALE 1943 is a minor character who is seriously misjudged by her environment: her affair with a German officer was a cover-up for her activities as a spy. Her role in the narrative, however, basically functioned to put the amateurish resistance to shame.

8 Many years later, in 1983, Anton is informed by Karin that Peter came to their house, threatened them with the gun, but was then instantly shot by Germans. This will be addressed in chapter nine.

9 Both Saskia and the woman in the prison are played by Monique van de Ven, so the resemblance is deliberate.

10 Burke mentions that the funeral in DE AANSLAG is a 'private reunion', for the Dutch resistance had been 'marginalized incrementally' in the 1960s; 'national public celebration of the Dutch resistance had dwindled significantly'. Regarding Cor's communist affiliations, Burke adds that 'there is more than a small suggestion that left-wing veterans by far suffered the worst marginalization throughout the post-war decades' (201).

11 Cor receives a telephone call during Anton's visit. With his back turned to his guest, Cor tells him that one of the veterans once said, in 1952, that if they ever were to release Willy Lages, he would kill himself. 'We were all laughing ... then.'

12 In RASHOMON, a samurai has been murdered, but every new account does not clarify the circumstances, instead it only makes them more enigmatic. In the end, it has become impossible to reconstruct the crime case.

13 In the new millennium, Ben Sombogaart made some films in which historical circumstances decisively and dramatically affect the lives of his characters. The emigration wave to New Zealand in the 1950s in BRIDE FLIGHT (2008), or the Arab Uprising in RAFAËL (2018) are used as a backdrop for stories about missed opportunities and emotional conflicts. The devastating aftermath of the terrible hurricane in 1953 in DE STORM [THE STORM] (2009), resulting in the deaths of 1,836 people in one night, is condensed in the tragedy of a woman who is desperately searching for her lost baby, and only finds him some eighteen years later. DE TWEELING [TWIN SISTERS] (Ben Sombogaart, 2002) is Sombogaart's most epic and successful picture, if only because it was nominated for an Oscar for Best Foreign Language Film. The German twin sisters Anne and Lotte undergo two traumatic moments of separation. At a young age, they become orphans and are raised in different families. German relatives take Anne, who they think can be a useful farmhand. Lotte, who is suffering from tuberculosis, is taken care of by Dutch foster parents. Due to the mutual animosity between the German and Dutch families, there is no contact, but at the age of about twenty, Lotte manages to track down Anne. Though the encounter can only be brief, they are happy to reconnect. The second traumatic separation is historical in nature and is the result of Lotte's short-sighted response to the outbreak of the Second World War. Lotte is in love with David, but when the Germans invade Holland, David is astonished when she says she wants to end the relationship. Her reason is that because he is a Jew and she is officially German, he will start to hate her one day. On another occasion, she suggests she might become a Jew to ensure they have a happy marriage, but David does not understand her: 'Why all the fuss?' Lotte's tendency to judge people as representatives of nations is at the heart of her brutal rejection of Anne who comes to visit her after the war. Lotte has just received the official news she had already dreaded for years, that David has died in a concentration camp. Anne became a widow a few years ago, for Martin had been killed in the line of duty as an S.S. officer. She disliked his dedication to the nation but was simply in love with the man himself. During Anne's visit, Lotte is still wondering whether she might give her twin sister the benefit of the doubt, but then she lays eyes on a portrait of Anne and her husband, the latter dressed in his Nazi uniform. Lotte brutally expels her guest from her house and tells her that she never wants to see her again. Lotte feels that Anne, as a German, is implicated in the death of her Jewish husband. Since loyalty to the nation presides over family bonds, Lotte will remain unforgiving until decades later, when Anne recognizes her twin sister at a spa. Typical for a melodrama, we are confronted with a 'too late', and a regret of time lost. The two elderly women spend the night together in a forest; Anne is found dead the next morning.

14 LEFT LUGGAGE (Jeroen Krabbé, 1998), based on Carl Friedman's novel *Twee koffers vol* (1993), can be considered the more sentimental version of the poignant LEEDVERMAAK. Mr. Silberschmidt, father of the twenty-year-old Chaja, is searching frenetically for two suitcases he has buried during the war which contain his tap-dance shoes, his violin, the family album, etc. But he does not know the address, now that Antwerp has been reconstructed. His wife complains that he is always mentioning the war and that he does not understand that she wants to bury the past '*under a pile of cakes*', referring to her cooking habits. Meanwhile, Chaja, a student of philosophy, is fed up with all this Jewish thing, but she undergoes a change when she takes a job as a nanny with a Chassidic family. Although she hates their strict rules, she takes a great liking to the middle of the five kids, the four-year-old red-haired Simcha, who does not talk and still pees in his pants. She takes care of him and goes to the pond with him regularly to feed the ducks. Thanks to her attention, he starts to speak—'quack, quack' being his first words—and she is so fond of him that she considers him her friend. While she has one week off, the boy goes to the park all by himself and drowns. One of the Chassidim blames Chaja for alienating the boy from his parents, but Simcha's mother thinks she is a brave woman. The point of LEFT LUGGAGE is that the events related to this orthodox Jewish family have such a devastating impact on Chaja that, by the very end of Krabbé's film she is seen digging together with her father for the two suitcases. The impossibility of finding them symbolizes, as the mother has made explicit, a loss of self, caused by the traumatic history of Jewish people. Due to Simcha's death, daughter Chaja has been burdened by history as well, albeit on a personal scale. LEFT LUGGAGE was criticized for its 'heavy-handed sentimentality', but according to Mikel J. Koven, this judgement is unfair. Krabbé's film can also be taken as a homage to the so-called *shund* dramas, 'overwrought melodramas', hugely popular throughout Yiddish-speaking communities (Koven, 236). The film's lack of subtlety is best taken as 'its greatest strength', for the lively Chaja, the bizarre mother, the obsessed father, the cute Simcha are all to be taken as hyperbolic 'embodiments of culturally specific ideas'—that is, 'Jewish ideas' (237).

15 In the first 220 pages, textual narrative overlays the gouaches on thin semi-transparent paper (Freedman, 4).

16 The art historian Griselda Pollock, an expert on Salomon, has problems with Weisz's film because CHARLOTTE treats her 'painted images as a potential storyboard for a film about her life' (208). Pollock thinks that any attempt to reduce her work to an autobiography or to a story of tragic events underestimates the uniqueness of Salomon's image-music-text.

17 Weisz had been informed about a dark family secret, but he had to promise the surviving stepmother Paula Salomon-Lindberg not to use the material in the feature. Thirty years after completing CHARLOTTE, Weisz made the documentary LEVEN? OF THEATER? that contains Charlotte's confession of having poisoned

her grandfather. It is clear she disliked this awful man, Pollock asserts, probably because she had more than a suspicion that the grandfather had sexually abused his daughters who both committed suicide.

18 If you make a film about a woman so bereaved, Pollock argues, it can only be very incoherent. According to her standards, Weisz's CHARLOTTE is much too coherent still.

19 There is a great documentary on Dutch soldiers who have been on UN missions called CRAZY (Heddy Honigmann, 1995). There has also been a television series related to the Dutch UN soldiers in Srebrenica: DE ENCLAVE (Willem van de Sande Bakhuyzen, 2002), a film about the assassination of politician Pim Fortuyn: 06/05 (Theo van Gogh, 2004), and a film about the murder of Theo van Gogh: 2/11 HET SPEL VAN DE WOLF (Thomas Korthals Altes, 2014).

20 I would like to single out the television movie DE NIEUWE WERELD [THE NEW WORLD] (Jaap van Heusden, 2013), for which the main actress, Bianca Krijgsman, won an Emmy Award. The film is set in so-called 'no man's land' at Schiphol Airport, the area where asylum seekers are kept in detention and where officials conduct interviews to check their data. The story is sandwiched between two moments in which protagonist Myrte, a cleaning woman in this area, says 'kssss' to Luc, a refugee from Africa. The first 'kssss' is her regular hiss: this curt signal means that an asylum seeker has to lift his feet or has to take a different route, for she has just polished the floor. Luc, however, crosses the wet floor and says 'kssss' back. And, of all people, this man will have an impact on her like no other. Myrte is presented as a grumpy and calculating woman: daily she is greeted by security with an ironic 'sunshine'. Time and again, she smuggles her mobile phone through security by wrapping it in kitchen foil. She makes deals with asylum seekers in the bathroom: in exchange for precious objects such as jewellery, they can use her phone. She insists that Luc give up his wedding ring instead of his watch, and she sells items like these to a pawnbroker. With two guardians she has a running bet on who will be sent home, and Myrte usually wins: she has a perfect eye for distinguishing fakers from 'real' asylum seekers. In her eyes, Luc is a faker. She secretly looks at him while he has hidden himself in one of the toilets; she cuts a piece of his frizzy hair, 'softer than an abrasive sponge', and puts it in a drawer. Her son takes it and uses it as a fake moustache: 'Do I look like my father this way?' When she takes her son to work once, Luc is like a father to the boy. She decides to print pages of a war in Ivory Coast and delivers the material to Luc in the bathroom. She instructs him to learn everything by heart and to tell the official that he has deserted from the army. The trick appears to have been successful, but then the guardian hands her the money and tells her that she had a perfect score. She refuses the money, for it means that Luc's request for asylum has been turned down after all. She asks a guardian whether she can take Luc out for three minutes so that he can actually set foot in the Netherlands, beyond no man's land. When Luc passes Myrte on his way

to the airplane that will bring him back to Africa, they hiss at each other as a tender farewell: 'Kssss'.

BIBLIOGRAPHY

Bernink, Mieke, *Fons Rademakers: Scènes uit leven en werk* (Abcoude: Uniepers, 2003).

Burke, Wendy, *Images of Occupation in Dutch Film: Memory, Myth and the Cultural Legacy of War* (Amsterdam: Amsterdam University Press, 2017).

Freedman, Ariela, 'Charlotte Salomon, Degenerate Art and Modernism as Resistance', *Journal of Modern Literature* 41, 1 (2017): 3-18.

Koven, Mikel J., '*Twee koffers vol* / LEFT LUGGAGE', ed. by Mathijs, *The Cinema of the Low Countries*, 231-237.

Pattynama, Pamela, '*Max Havelaar*, of de invloed van de populaire media op de herinnering aan Indië.' *Indische Letteren* 21, 3 (2006): 169-185.

Pisters, Patricia, 'Lili and Rachel: Hollywood, History, and Women in Fassbinder and Verhoeven', ed. by Jaap Kooijman, Patricia Pisters, Wanda Strauven, *Mind the Screen: Media Concepts According to Thomas Elsaesser* (Amsterdam: Amsterdam University Press, 2008), 177-187.

Pollock, Griselda, 'Crimes, Confession, and the Everyday: Challenges in Reading Charlotte Salomon's *Leben? oder Theater?* 1941-1942', *Journal of Visual Culture* 13, 2 (2014): 200-235.

Scheffer, Paul, 'Het multiculturele drama', *NRC Handelsblad* (29 January 2000), https://www.nrc.nl/nieuws/2000/01/29/het-multiculturele-drama-a3987586 [Accessed 12 May 2020].

Silverman, Kaja, *Male Subjectivity at the Margins* (New York: Routledge, 1992).

CHAPTER 8

Aphanisis

Verstraten, P., *Dutch Post-War Fiction Film Through a Lens of Psychoanalysis.* Taylor & Francis Group, 2021
DOI 10.5117/9789463725330_CH08

ABSTRACT

Aphanisis is the key concept in chapter eight. It concerns moments when characters are so overwhelmed, usually due to traumatic events, that they become speechless (temporarily or otherwise). This occurs to the war victim in Rademakers' THE ROSE GARDEN who can utter no more than the name of his enemy. Moments of self-obliteration also befall the twin brothers in AMNESIA, the woman-disguised-as-man in MONSIEUR HAWARDEN, and the city woman who marries a farmer in KRACHT. Characters try to come to terms with personal issues, and they try to do so in films such as BLUEBIRD, GUERNSEY, NOTHING PERSONAL, and VERDWIJNEN which, even more explicit than the titles in previous chapters, beg comparison to international arthouse pictures such as those by the Dardenne brothers, by Varda, and by Bergman.

KEYWORDS
Aphanisis – Problems with names / naming – Urge to break with old habits – Comparisons to European arthouse

Little did Rademakers know that THE ROSE GARDEN (1989), in his own words no more than a 'decent assignment picture', would be his last feature (qtd. in Bernink, 139).[1] He was able to make this film in the wake of the success of DE AANSLAG, for which he had received an Academy Award for Best Foreign Language Film in 1987. For THE ROSE GARDEN, he was able to assemble a 'stellar' cast with Maximilian Schell, Liv Ullmann, Peter Fonda, and Hanns Zischler. but he was quite sarcastic: the subject required a German-language film he thought, but because of the presence of Ullmann and Fonda, it was decided it should be English-spoken. Though the film lacks subtlety basically due to its dénouement which is too utopian, the quality of the film is not as average as Rademakers suggested.[2]

The narrative structure and cinematography of THE ROSE GARDEN are quite conventional, but the behaviour of the main character—an elderly man with unkempt hair—is puzzling, especially in the first 30 minutes. He seems confused from the beginning, apparently startled by every sound, such as the wailing of the fire siren. When he takes a cab, he gets out in front of a crowd, staring at the firemen who are about to rescue a cat from a high building in Hamburg. Although he is in their eyesight, the public looks beyond the man, which results in an estranging mise-en-scène when shot from his position.[3] In the following scene, he is standing motionless in the vicinity of an old school. Before an explanation is given of his being there, we get a cut to another scene, this time at the airport in Frankfurt where the man, still haggard, loses his wallet. The young girl Tina gives it back to him, but then her mother, the lawyer Gabriele Freund, calls her daughter. Then the man starts running and shouting incomprehensibly, attacking a grey, bespectacled old man who was queuing for a flight to Montevideo, Uruguay. The attacker is arrested but does not speak or react to anything. They only know he has a concentration camp number tattooed on his arm. Gabriele is asked to represent the man who is accused of aggravated assault based on the hope that he might trust her since he made a drawing of Tina. Gabriele accepts the case because her condescending ex-husband Herbert advises her not to, saying that Eckert, the lawyer of the injured victim, will '*eat you alive*'.

Mr X is in hospital after a suicide attempt and keeps on calling out the name 'Krenn', but that is the only word he utters. Meanwhile, Gabriele finds out that X was born as Aaron Reichenbach in 1930 in Poland and that he has

been living in Quito, Ecuador since 1948. She feels responsible for him, for she wonders why this *'peaceful citizen'* came all the way to Hamburg and then to Frankfurt to attack an old man, *'seemingly without reason'*. The journalist Georg Paessler has done quite some research and tells Gabriele that he has had contact with Aaron who, according to Georg, speaks German poorly. Aaron was in Auschwitz with his younger sisters Ruth and Rachel. The girls were taken away in 1944, and ever since then Aaron has been trying to find them. Georg recently published a list of children who had been hung in an old school at the Bullenhuser road near concentration camp Neuengamme after they had been used for medical experiments: Rachel was among them. Aaron had come over to visit her grave, but there was none for these children, all the traces having been extinguished. The only thing that remained was their names written in the notebook of a Danish doctor. In a memorial book, Gabriele and Georg read a message that they presume is from Aaron: the letters R A R, adorned with funny faces. As Georg knows from his conversations with Aaron, that is
the way their father taught them to write at a young age. The journalist thinks the text beneath the three huge letters says: *'Hear My Cry, Oh God'*, in Hebrew. Georg explains that Arnold Krenn, the old man attacked at the airport, was commanding officer of the field camps in Hamburg at the time. To keep the memory of the tragedy alive, a rose garden has been planted near the school.

During the first half of THE ROSE GARDEN, Aaron only uses a few words in English, such as *'don't trust'*, *'airport'*, *'he knows ... Ruthi'*, because according to Gabriele, *'those who have experienced the hell of the concentration camps may be unable to speak the language of their torturers'*. During the second half of Rademakers' film, Aaron comes to trust Gabriele and becomes less bewildered. He tells her he did not write *'Hear My Cry, Oh God'* but *'God, Thy Way is Holy'*—the non-Jewish Georg had probably mistranslated it. The second half emphasizes Gabriele's efforts to criticize the hypocrisy of the German judicial system for the fact that a war criminal like Krenn had been able to *'slip through'*. Even though Krenn will not be convicted because he is *'declared permanently unfit to stand trial'*, as the closing lines state, there is nonetheless some sort of a happy ending. Herbert does his ex-wife a favour by tracking down Ruth Levi, Aaron's missing sister, who is currently living in Toledo, Spain. Ruth discloses that on a recent visit to the memorial, she had written down their names *'like we always used to do when we were children'*. Contrary to trauma theories, Ruth then gives a highly consistent rendering of what had happened in April 1945 at the Bullenhuser road. She had survived because she had played dead when she fell off a truck. With her coherent testimony, things come full circle. When Aaron leaves the country with Ruth, he seems in a gay mood, waving goodbye to Gabriele and Tina, as if he has been more or less 'cured' from the trauma.

Gabriele became interested in Aaron's case because up until that moment he had had no track record of doing anything strange but had crossed the Atlantic Ocean to display totally irrational behaviour, only muttering the name 'Krenn' as a sort of mantra. Facing this Nazi commanding officer, the Jewish elderly man suffers from what Lacan calls 'aphanisis'. Normally, every subject has sacrificed 'being' for 'meaning': you are given a first name and a family name so you can tell 'who you are', though such signifiers, by definition, cannot express 'who you really are'. Somehow, we subjects have learned to cope with this inadequacy of language; we manage as best as we can. We are represented by signifiers; they stand in for us—but they do not equal our 'being'. In the case of aphanisis, this conventional procedure becomes exaggerated. A signifier gains so much emphasis that the subject manifests itself elsewhere as 'fading' (Lacan *Four Fundamental*, 218). To relate this to THE ROSE GARDEN: the signifier 'Krenn' overpowers Aaron and this results in the latter's self-obliteration: he cannot even utter his own name anymore and is therefore registered for some time as Mr. X. As Žižek explains, when 'I' approach the 'phantasmatic kernel of my being' too closely, and when symbolic fictions no longer work as a protection shield against the horror of the Real, the subject disintegrates (*How to Read*, 55). As soon as Aaron sees and names 'Krenn', all words become abracadabra. The fact that he is only able to utter that one word repetitively is an indication that Krenn is connected to the man's trauma. This name is the signifier around which Aaron's entire being is structured, and THE ROSE GARDEN gradually reveals why, for Krenn is responsible for both Aaron's separation from his two sisters and the unknown fate of Ruth. Aaron is so consumed by grief, or is rather beyond grief, that even after decades he is magnetically pulled back to that experience. In the vicinity of the bearer of that name 'Krenn', he goes haywire. The reason for running amok is strictly related to the presence of the former Nazi commanding officer, and it is an illustration that time does not heal all wounds. The mere sight of Krenn provokes Aaron's aphanisis, the loss of his symbolic consistency. In this chapter, I will scrutinize a series of Dutch films in which characters have had traumatic experiences resulting in a certain loss of self: they want to acquire another name; they yearn for another way of life; or they aim to reset their family ties.

GUILTY OF DESIRE: *AMNESIA*

Martin Koolhoven's second feature film, following the telefilm SUZY Q (1999), is called AMNESIA (2000), but aphanisis might have been a more appropriate title. We see 'AmnesiA' written in large letters on the gate of the parental home of the protagonists, the twin brothers Aram and Alex. They have not had contact since a year after the death of their father, some ten years ago, when they were still young adolescents. When Aram suspects their mother is severely ill, he rings Alex and asks him to pay them a visit. The twin brothers are still spitting images of each other, and even their haircut is practically the same, as Aram remarks.

AMNESIA reveals its information in bits and pieces. The two brothers used to think alike, or this is at least what Aram asserts: he always knew what was in Alex's mind until a dramatic incident caused their separation. Brusquely inserted fragments suggest that their lives have been decisively determined by something in the past: the snippets of Alex's flashbacks are related to low-angle tracking shots of trees and him walking with a photo camera in a forest with his brother and a female doctor; in Aram's flashbacks we see him push a car forward. The actual dénouement will be reserved for the final part, but it is clear that the two have become alienated from each other. Aram took over father's garage but stopped after two years. He is still living with his mother, but she has no clue what kind of work he is doing. He carries out some shadowy assignments for a certain Eugène, a man who claims he holds a 'respectable position'. The latest job, however, is a burglary gone wrong: according to Eugène's information, the place was supposed to be unguarded, but Aram's accomplice Wouter is shot in the stomach. Aram takes the injured man to his mother's house,[4] just as Alex arrives home with an unexpected guest as well: out of nowhere, a girl named Sandra was on the backseat of his car. She accompanies him throughout the film as Alex's girlfriend, but her background remains a mystery. She takes medicines to prevent attacks of epilepsy, and time and again she finds herself in the vicinity of fire or happens to set things on fire. Since she is new to this family of three, like us, we are in the same position as she is, trying to figure out the relationships between the mother and her twins.

Despite his long absence, Alex is the beloved son who makes his mother proud. She knows he is a prize-winning photographer, though she had hoped he would succeed her dead husband, who in her words was both the 'best car mechanic' and the 'best storyteller'. The link between the dead father and the prodigal son is so strong for the mother that she starts calling Alex 'Theo' and kisses him passionately when Alex steps into her bed during a game of hide-and-seek. Aware of his mother's preference, Aram—who is well-dressed but has the habit of walking around barefoot—behaves rudely: he reproaches his mother for not having any beer in the house and tells his brother that qualifications like 'disgusting Alex' and 'unmannered Alex' are pleonasms. He disdainfully observes Alex starting to repair cars and wearing his father's working clothes. He makes contemptuous remarks when Alex has a rabbit, for their father had one as well. His most serious taunt, however, is when he repeatedly accuses Alex of cowardice,[5] the background of which gradually becomes clear.

During a walk in the forest, Sandra suggests that Alex make a 'postcard landscape picture'. As he is about to push the button, all of a sudden, the female doctor from his flashback shows up in his viewfinder. Cut to an adolescent Aram who is walking besides the woman and pointing out a particular spot: 'Lovely background, isn't it?' The woman is then replaced by Sandra, which visibly upsets Alex. He tells Sandra about his phobia: that he gets distressed when a person crosses his lens. He explains: 'I once photographed a terrible accident. By accident. It happened while I pressed the shutter. I burned the film. I didn't even dare to develop it.' Sandra, however, has found photos in a drawer of a sideboard; Aram had probably left it open on purpose, for we see his face in a close-up insert. Later, Aram gives Sandra an envelope and requests her to return it to Alex. Upon seeing the content, the latter explains that he had followed his father because he suspected him of having a relationship with the doctor. The pictures are proof of the son's presupposition, but he lies to Sandra that the woman had probably moved at a certain point. The real reason for the end of the affair is that the twins took the mistress into the forest for a photo shoot about 'working women'. Aram points out the lovely background, and when Alex is about to take the picture, his twin brother sees a smudge on the doctor's face. She asks him to wipe it off, but at the very moment Alex pushes the button, Aram pushes the doctor downhill to her death.

The key to the animosity between the twins is that Alex has not fully taken responsibility for the drama, as Aram explains when they return to the scene of the tragedy. For it was Alex who had made the photos of their father with his mistress in the first place; 'I only did what you wanted; you were too scared to do it'. So they both have a murder on their conscience, Aram argues. Moreover, Aram tells Alex that they are equally guilty of their father's death by suicide. The old man had not driven his car into the water, as the official report has it, but Aram says he had made it look like an accident. 'You're lying!' Alex yells, and with a 'maybe', Aram lets himself fall backwards. Aram lands on exactly the same spot as the doctor. The flashback shows that her head is lying immobile near a large stone in a creek, but she is not dead yet. 'I pushed', Aram states while he stands close to her body, but Alex has no more to say than 'I can't do it'. So Aram picks up a rock, and then there is a cut to the present. Aram is not dead either, and after a close-up of his bleeding face, we are shown the conclusion of his flashback, without dialogue, only a soundscape and shown in a slightly decelerated rhythm. Aram had found his father in his car in the garage, already dead, with a suicide note in his breast pocket. He pushed the vehicle into a canal and tore the note into pieces. Back in the present, Aram sees that Alex is holding a rock this time, and that is the end of the scene. Before Alex is back at AmnesiA, their mother lies with her head on the table, a bottle of wine within reach—a good remedy against a weak heart, as she believed. She herself is convinced that she would die of a heart attack, but the doctor had informed Alex that his mother suffers from cancer. It is unclear what caused her death. Anyway, to conclude, Sandra lights a match, and once again, there is a scene with fire.

In Koolhoven's AMNESIA, Alex refuses to admit his share in the tragedy, making it seem as if Aram is the sole malefactor. Strictly speaking, Alex has committed no crime at all. He did no more than take pictures: first, to collect visual evidence of the affair, and second, the doctor had to position herself at a specific dangerous spot for a nice picture. But he did not give her the fatal push, and he did not hit her with a rock. Significantly, however, Aram says that he only acted according to Alex's wishes, and that makes Alex guilty of desire. If Alex felt he was innocent, he would have no trouble photographing people. His incapacity to do so can be taken as a tacit acknowledgement of his guilt. Aram functions here as his superegotistic command: I only did what you wanted to do but were afraid to do; all I insist on is that you take responsibility for your desires. Very much in the vein of Professor Cadell in Hitchcock's ROPE (1948), who is shocked when two of his students put into practice his theory of a superman's license to kill, Alex is horrified and wants to shrink back from the consequences of the visual evidence he has produced. He sees his desire realized but does not want to pay the price for it.[6] Aram could seem to be the bad brother, but from a psychoanalytic perspective, Alex is at least as 'bad', for he is a coward who refuses to face the fact that what has happened is what he wanted to happen. Near the end of the movie, Aram takes a plant and explains that a strong one is clean but a weak and sick plant will suddenly be covered in greenfly. The comparison is meant to indicate that Alex is weak because he is too chicken to admit his share in their crime, but the superego command, embodied by his brother Aram, works as a constant reminder: You are as guilty as I am.

AMNESIA has quite a few low-angle and high-angle shots and even canted perspectives. There are some instances of direct address, and the frontally staged shots of Aram, in particular, have a menacing impact. Insofar as this deliberate stylization is functional, it contributes to Alex's disarray. He was so traumatized by what happened that he had to cut all his family ties loose. Away from his mother and his brother, he can only continue to exist as rootless Alex, disavowing his own personal history. In the beginning of AMNESIA, there is a girl in his bed, and before he bids her farewell to go visit his mother, she says: 'By the way, what's your name?' which implies that introducing himself by name is not—or rather, no longer—a habit on his part. His vain hope to undo the tragedy or perhaps to turn back time has come close to self-denial. It is quite telling that, when finally back in his mother's home, he attempts to occupy the empty place of his father by wearing his clothes and taking up his line of work. On top of that, he does not mind at all that his mother calls him 'Theo' a few times, as if it is much better than being called by his birth name. Rather than an 'I', Alex carries the burden of a guilty conscience, but his posing as his father Theo cannot make up for this loss of self. Any attempt to fill the painful absence of his father's demise is a pathetic one: he doesn't have the talent to be a mechanic; Aram keeps calling him Alex, and his mother calling him 'Theo' is obviously an uncanny mistake and a sign that her health is deteriorating.

Alex's inability to escape from his 'I' results in sleepless nights. The one time we see him asleep is when he has collapsed from fatigue after the tiresome car trip at night. His sense of identity is consumed by his guilt, and the fact that his brother dies while reconstructing the crime will probably only aggravate his guilt, for a superego voice does not need an embodiment (here represented by Aram) in order to bombard a subject (Alex) with commands. The burning of his parental home does nothing to make this stop. While Alex attempted to reject his identity by ignoring his name or by masquerading as his father, it all turned out to be futile in the end. By contrast, the title character in MONSIEUR HAWARDEN (Harry Kümel, 1968) is much more successful in taking on another guise, but this offers no guarantee that one can run away from one's past.

GENDER TROUBLE: *MONSIEUR HAWARDEN*

Hidden in a coach, it takes quite a while before we see the title character in MONSIEUR HAWARDEN, a Belgian-Dutch co-production dedicated to the Austrian-American film director Josef von Sternberg who made a great number of films with leading actress Marlene Dietrich, such as SHANGHAI EXPRESS (1932), BLONDE VENUS (1932), and THE SCARLETT EMPRESS (1934). During the trip, we see Monsieur Hawarden's blonde-haired maid Victorine, but it is only when the coach arrives at the remote mansion of steward Deschamp that we get a glimpse of monsieur's black leather gloves before we see the man's elegant appearance. Monsieur Hawarden is cheerfully greeted by the steward and his staff, but he will behave like a recluse, which gives rise to speculations about the mysterious guest and his relation to the maid, who is fancied by two of the male servants. Meanwhile, Monsieur Hawarden only leaves his room to enjoy the company of the steward's thirteen-year-old son Axel, to the delight of Mrs. Deschamp. On the invitation of the steward and his wife, the monsieur and the maid have an exquisite dinner, but the good wine makes the esteemed guest chatty. The story is quite incoherent, however: he talks about his ill father, about a marquise, a dance with an officer in Portugal... or was it in Vienna? His words are visually underscored by mental shots, including a duel in a forest.

The monsieur gets distressed—and is even missing for a while—after a narrator comes to visit the mansion. Illustrated by a magic lantern show, the traveller tells the story of a princess who had someone's tongue cut off and another man's eyes burned out, just on account of addressing her as a woman. As the princess turns eighteen, two princes arrange a duel in a forest to fight for her love. With a dagger, however, she stabs the heart of the winner. The people are appalled by her blood-stained hands. Her mother warns the princess that death will await her. Since then, the princess is on the run, not even knowing whether she is a man or a woman.

The story will be a mise-en-abyme for the entire film: much later it is revealed to us that Monsieur Hawarden is not a man but a woman named Mériora Gillibrand, in hiding at this mansion. She is waiting for a letter from her mother in Vienna, but it has yet to arrive. When the extremely faithful Victorine gets jealous due to Mériora's/Hawarden's fondness of the boy Axel, she tells her in anger that this letter will never arrive, for Mériora/Hawarden is dead in the eyes of her mother. Victorine wants to leave after having protected him/her against spying eyes for some twelve years. Mériora/Hawarden begs her to stay, for Victorine is the only one who knows his/her identity. But while she is about to leave, the two servants start to fight over her: Victorine wants to interfere, but one servant fractures her skull accidently with an axe.

After this horrifying accident, the protagonist visits Spa as a woman and is seduced by an officer who advises her at the roulette table, to considerable success. While walking, the officer says that the setting reminds him of Resnais's film L'ANNÉE DERNIÈRE À MARIENBAD. They ride horse together and visit the opera, for music helps her to recall memories, she remarks. During their first kisses—at last, for time is precious at their age, as he said at one point—Mériora insists that he keep mentioning her full name 'Mériora Gillibrand' and that he adds to this 'woman'. As he continues his amorous advances , she tells the officer her tragic history about two young handsome officers in Vienna, one of whom killed the other out of jealousy, out of alacrity, because of her. She briefly interrupts her story by instructing the officer: 'Give me your hands, you do not have to listen, I am talking to myself.' She continues: she did not know whether she was afraid of the officer or whether she loved him. And when he called out her name—'Mériora'—she came out from behind the trees like a gasping animal and she stabbed, she stabbed, she stabbed. The camera now comes so close to her face that the shot is out of focus. There is a brusque transition to a regular sharp close-up of her face. She says: I have been a fugitive for fifteen years, together with a maid. I dressed myself up as a man: Mériora Gillibrand, who had never been a woman.

After she tells her story to the officer, who does not seem particularly interested in it, she goes back to Deschamp's mansion in the guise of Monsieur Hawarden again, soaking wet due to a thunderstorm. She/he writes a letter to her/his mother: 'Things have been so long ago that they are no longer truthful.' Frontally staged, monsieur speaks directly to the camera in a series of brief confessions, interrupted by brief black frames: I envy the servant who killed Victorine because he can remember everything... And: I am still expecting your letter, mama. After a brief white screen, we see Mrs. Deschamp running up the stairs from a low-angle: a letter from Vienna has arrived. Monsieur reads the letter, but its content is not disclosed to us. The reading is followed by a series of inserts: a shot of a wall, a shot of the stairs. She/he opens a window and calls Axel. When the boy enters, the camera makes a quarter-circle pan to the left around Axel and then Monsieur Hawarden comes into view but with long hair and in a dress. Several dissolves suggest an intimate bond between the two of them. After a kiss, Axel leaves the room, and after a close-up of the door handle, the camera tracks backwards. We hear a sound of what is possibly a gunshot, after which the credits start to roll.

As regards its position in Dutch (or Belgian) film history, MONSIEUR HAWARDEN fared quite poorly, just like other Dutch films from the late 1960s with artistic ambitions (see the introduction). Kümel's Flemish-Dutch coproduction combined magic-realistic influences with a sober mise-en-scène (as in shots of Monsieur Hawarden's room and the number of insert close-ups of objects) but also some *nouvelle vague* devices. Though its reception abroad was quite good, the film climate in the Low Countries was not favourable for these endeavours. The cinematography of these films, in this case by Eduard van der Enden who used chiaroscuro to great effect, was usually critically acclaimed, but their beauty was also considered quite 'pretentious', to cite Peter van Bueren's evaluation of Kümel's debut feature (qtd. in Van Gelder, 119). There are a number of wilfully alienating shots: Monsieur Hawarden running in the forest after the magic lantern show; Axel on a horse; the camera swinging with the dancers resulting in some blurry shots; a terribly shaky camera with Monsieur Hawarden in superimposition as she registers Victorine's death. And though these extravagant devices may be slightly pretentious, they are nonetheless functional as well, since the story is estranging for two opposite reasons.

First, even for those viewers who do not know the quite famous actress Ellen Vogel, it is all too clear that Monsieur Hawarden is a woman. Her features are too feminine to pass for a man, and there was apparently little effort put into changing this (which is as weird as it is sympathetic: once you introduce yourself as a monsieur, the characters in this film stop wondering about your gender identity). Second, while recounting her decade-long travesty act to a disinterested officer who is only interested in her body, the camera zooms in to a close-up of her face which becomes a blur due to its proximity to the camera before it jump cuts to a regular close-up. This zoom followed by the jump cut seems to mark her self-obliteration, especially since it is preceded by her insistence that the officer call her by her female name and to explicitly add the term 'woman' to it. But the officer does not feel like reinserting her into the symbolic network, apparently oblivious to what has traumatized her. After her story, all he asks, with a blank stare at the ceiling, is: What happened to you? Because of this disappointing love affair, Mériora will remain the woman who has vanished, and she returns as monsieur to her former hideout. Until Victorine's unfortunate death, Mériora/Hawarden was satisfied by her status as the travelling dead whose only weak link to the outside world had been guaranteed by the maid. That's why she is so desperate when Victorine threatens to leave, for then the silk thread is broken. To emphasize her almost total alienation from society, whereby to save her skin she has to be constitutively misrecognized as 'monsieur', Kümel's MONSIEUR HAWARDEN offers a great many mirror shots: she is not a woman; instead, she is an image of (a) man. The only way that a connection to the community can be re-established—the only way that the image can be converted into symbolic identity—is by a written message from her mother. After she has received the long-awaited note from Vienna, whose content we can only guess, she dresses herself up as Mériora and only presents herself to the young teenager Axel. She shows herself according to the identity that she had denied herself for many years. But we can suppose that her mother has de-legitimized her existence as daughter. The off-screen sound suggests that this leads to Mériora's self-chosen demise in the guise of a Madame.

FARMER SEEKS WIFE: *KRACHT*

While in hiding in a mansion in a rural landscape, MONSIEUR HAWARDEN is lost in a gender masquerade. In a variation upon this theme, the artist Roos in KRACHT [VIGOUR] (Frouke Fokkema, 1990) hopes to overcome the urban ennui by living in the countryside as the new wife of a farmer-widow, but she will find herself ostracized. We are only introduced to Roos relatively late in Fokkema's film, for the first half hour is dedicated to the hilly area in the south of Limburg with its bare trees. Farmer Bert is bringing his deceased wife to the funeral by horse and carriage, followed by a brass band, but the roads are so muddy that the hearse gets stuck. Due to the delay, the procession arrives so late that another ceremony is to take place, so Bert returns home to burn the coffin in his own hearth. The takes are relatively long, and the camera is usually at a distance from the scenery to emphasize that the people are fused with the harsh environment. In this landscape—unchanging except for the seasonal transitions—the inhabitants live according to strict customs and opinions. One such firm belief is that the future of a farm is in jeopardy without a spouse. Encouraged by the local priest, Bert visits an agricultural congress where he meets Roos, who is shooting photographs. She is attracted to his sorrow as well as to his shyness, for it is in agreeable contrast to the obtrusiveness of the men in the city.

Working in her studio, Roos is dissatisfied with the quality of her paintings, which faintly recall the raw and grotesque work of Francis Bacon. She calls Bert in the middle of the night and wants to visit him. When he announces her arrival to the family, Bert's mother has some suspicious comments: 'She's not from around here?' But nine-year-old son Thomas is enthusiastic because he thinks that the guest will be his 'new mother'. After she is taken from the station by Jeu and Jo, two men who speak dry-comic lines as if they are being featured in Samuel Beckett's play *Waiting for Godot*, Roos arrives at the court of the farmstead. When she says 'I don't see anyone', Jo replies: 'But they do see you.' And indeed, while Bert is still away, the other residents can be detected peeping through the windows, shown via long shots. Their attitude of misgiving is the anacrusis to a fatal episode of 'farmer seeks wife'. When Roos says that she paints for a living, Bert's family thinks she is a housepainter, which is a first example of a number of misunderstandings. At the market, Bert is about to buy a traditional painting because, as he untactfully explains to Roos, he can see what it represents. Moreover, Bert has the habit of talking about his 'Marie Louise' all the time because he regards Roos as a 'good listener', unlike the medical staff who had treated his wife so poorly. Jeu and Jo alert Roos to the urn on the mantelpiece with Marie Louise's ashes in it. When Roos says she still feels her presence, Jeu advises her to put 'her' on the land 'so she will start working again'. Roos reads an old diary of Marie Louise in which she writes about her terrible headaches, about her love for Bert and Thomas, about her prayers to God. She starts to style her hair after the deceased woman, puts on her clothes, and tells Bert that she is doing so in order 'to come closer to you'. And when Roos is enjoying sex on the couch, her eyes suddenly catch a photographic portrait of Marie Louise on the wall. She gets pregnant, but Bert gets angry because he doesn't want to have to feed another mouth. Frustrated, Roos takes the urn and throws it against the wall, just above Bert's head.

Roos runs away, but the clay ground is too heavy for her. In a reverse shot, we see Bert and four men come after her, or is she just imagining it? In the following scene, we hear the sound of crows, just like we had been hearing the mowing of cows, the grunting of pigs, and the noise of a tractor. To the priest she confesses that though Bert and she had sex everywhere, his 'eternal sense of guilt' troubled him. She transforms herself into Marie Louise's look-alike, and although Thomas notes the resemblance, he says she is nothing more than 'his father's personnel'. Whatever she undertakes, Roos pales in comparison to Marie Louise: she can only be second best. Bert starts ignoring her, and after sitting next to Bert's handicapped sister Maria for a while, Roos climbs the stairs of the hayloft. Maria starts making strange sounds, but no one knows how to interpret her restlessness. Roos hangs herself and falls amidst the pigs after the rope breaks. The animals start eating her, and when Bert discovers this, he gets mad and screams that she was the only one who listened to him. In the presence of a friend from the big city, Jeu and Jo bury Roos. The two gravediggers prefer a proper burial to the reduction of a corpse to ashes in an urn. 'This is a fine place for her', Jeu remarks, to which Jo adds ominously: 'That remains to be seen. ... That remains to be seen.'[7]

REWRITING BRUEGHEL INTO UTOPIAN FEMINISM: *ANTONIA*

To a great extent, ANTONIA [ANTONIA'S LINE] (Marleen Gorris, 1995) can be considered the 'optimistic' and belligerent version of KRACHT. Gorris's film starts with a voice-over, told by Antonia's great-granddaughter Sarah during the last day of the old matriarch, as the final sentence reveals. We then have a flashback in which a younger Antonia, in her forties, returns to the rural village she grew up in which she has not visited for twenty years. She is in the company of her daughter Danielle, to see her dead mother. To her surprise, her 'always difficult' mother is still alive and welcomes her as a 'creature of Satan', but soon thereafter she draws her last breath. Antonia decides to stay in the big parental farm, and though she is a 'black sheep' in the opinion of some rude men, she proceeds in her own way. The voice-over mentions that she is tolerated just as one would accept a bad harvest or a deformed child. The only one who truly opposes her 'impure spirit' is the conservative priest, but once she has caught him in the act of groping a girl in a confessional booth, he keeps a low profile. Thanks to her quite stoic attitude, the position Antonia has created in the community makes her home a safe haven for all sorts of outcasts: the single woman Letta who likes being pregnant; the Curate who has left his service; the mentally handicapped Deedee who was raped by her own brother. Her own daughter does not want a husband but only needs a man to fertilize her, a strategy Antonia approves of. After the birth of her profoundly gifted Thérèse, Danielle starts a lesbian relationship. Thérèse turns out to be on very good terms with the hermit-philosopher Kromme Vinger [Crooked Finger], another outcast whom Antonia and Danielle visit regularly, despite his habit of quoting misanthropic lines by Nietzsche and Schopenhauer.

ANTONIA is structured as a family chronicle: some 40 years are covered in 100 minutes. The internal narrator, Thérèse's daughter Sarah, highlights not only key events but above all the positive characteristics of the women in her family tree. Most important is Antonia's intransigence: she withstands her mother's hysterical tirades; she is not disturbed by gossip; and she declines the proposal of farmer Bas, though she accepts him as an occasional lover. This crucial characteristic of tenacity is inherited by her exclusively female offspring, and in the case of Thérèse, remarkable intelligence is added to it. The film is shot in an efficient, realist style, intercut with a few magic-realist scenes, since both Danielle and her granddaughter Sarah have visions. Danielle 'sees' how a stone statue hits the priest and how Antonia's mother rises from her coffin to sing Gene Austin's 'My Blue Heaven'. Looking down from a hayloft, Sarah 'witnesses' how some deceased people—Antonia's mother, Kromme Vinger—attend a big festive gathering outside. Antonia and the farmer Bas are dancing together, but Sarah sees them in their younger days, before she herself was actually born. Her eyes of imagination seem to be an extension of Antonia's foresight, mentioned by Sarah's voice-over at the beginning and at the end of the film: looking into the mirror, Antonia concludes that this will be the day she will die. She therefore instructs Sarah to gather all her loved ones around her deathbed.

In Fokkema's KRACHT, the past, represented by Bert's memory of his dead wife, was an unbearable burden to Roos, even after breaking the urn with Marie Louise's ashes in it. She could not acclimate herself with the farmer's soil; in a vain attempt to escape, she runs over the clay like Ingrid Bergman's unfortunate Karin tries to climb the volcano in Roberto Rossellini's STROMBOLI (1950). By contrast, the past in Gorris's ANTONIA offers us a series of happy and tragic incidents—for that's life—but, more importantly, the past is also presented as a continuum of female lineage, from Antonia to Sarah. Significantly, the flashback starts at the moment of the death of Antonia's irksome mother, and this last encounter between the two illustrates that the daughter rode roughshod over her, even in the latter's dying moments. Because of this quality, the past does not become a burden, despite the pessimistic life lessons of Kromme Vinger; instead, the past has helped to build a pedigree of which Sarah could be proud.

In her review of ANTONIA, Karen Jaehne claims that Gorris's film 'pits utopian feminism against masculine philosophy' (30). As a counterweight to the tenets of Schopenhauer and Nietzsche, taught by the gnarled but respected hermit whose house is like a dark cave, ANTONIA 'maps out the existence of woman as the world of action' (ibid.). In its depiction of labour in the field or the labour of producing children, Gorris's 'matriarchal passion play' abundantly borrows from the visual tradition of Flemish and Dutch painting, such as the landscape portraits of Jacob van Ruisdael (27). According to Jaehne, Gorris can even be called 'the artistic heir of Pieter Brueghel', for his 'quotidian realism' is recalled most prominently (27). Gorris, however, rewrites his visual tableaus into a form of a 'humanist feminism': since Antonia adheres to a 'live-and-let-live philosophy', she allows her family to expand, taking in the native and the foreigner, shown in overview shots with dinners at long tables outdoors (29). Even if Gorris may keep a distance from Brueghel's 'implicit sexism'—he also painted, among others, *Dulle Griet* [*Mad Meg*]—she shares with him a 'flat-footed joy in peasant life' according to Jaehne (28). Regardless of the seminal importance of sexual politics and feminist issues, the premise of both landscape paintings and Gorris's film is that 'the land outlives our politics' (28). So the main point for the female characters is how to adapt themselves to the harsh lowlands: well, the women fulfil their arduous agrarian jobs successfully. Insofar as the graffiti on the wall—'A Welcome to Our Liberators'—at the end of World War II makes sense, it suggests that the return of Antonia will be liberating. This seems to be acknowledged when in a processional, the villagers chant the names of the saints, 'only female saints' (30).

Whereas the fate of Roos in KRACHT complies with the script of *aphanisis*, I have referred to ANTONIA as its polar opposite. Gorris's film is about a tight symbolic network in which each of the women have occupied a solid place, to their full satisfaction. As a paradoxical sign of Antonia's strength, she knows upon waking up that this is a good day to die, and she does so, surrounded by her loved ones. By contrast, Roos has lost all ties with her background. At the end of KRACHT, she has packed her suitcase and is about to leave by train, but she makes up her mind on a bench. She then returns to the farm and hangs herself. The fact that only Sjors, a friend she had called on her final day, attends her funeral affirms the loss of Roos's symbolic consistency. Instead of contact with the living, her problem was the imaginary proximity of the dead Marie Louise, turning her into the second Mrs. Bollens.[8]

TAKE THESE BROKEN WINGS: *BLUEBIRD*

ANTONIA won the Academy Award for Best Foreign Language Film at a time when Dutch feature cinema was going through an extremely difficult time: movie attendance had been in decline for some years, and there were hardly any hopeful signs. One might have expected the unexpected international success of Gorris's film to have set an example, but hardly any Dutch films on inter-generational harmony among either women or men followed. Instead, a blueprint for subsequent projects was offered by the low-budget film ZUSJE [LITTLE SISTER], a debut feature by Robert-Jan Westdijk that was greeted as a welcome surprise when presented at the Netherlands Film Festival in 1995. ZUSJE was about a brother harassing his younger sister with a video camera, for the guy's life had been a fiasco ever since their mother had taken their intimacy for incest. Rather than the representation of close blood ties as seen in ANTONIA, troubled family relationships and/or the desire to break kinship bonds became part and parcel of the majority of Dutch films. Examples include the father-son animosity in KARAKTER [CHARACTER] (Mike van Diem, 1997), the portrayal of a dysfunctional family in SUZY Q (Martin Koolhoven, 1999), the frictions among three sisters and their homosexual brother in ZUS EN ZO [HOTEL PARAISO] (Paula van der Oest, 2001), and many more.

But as suggested in the book *De broertjes van Zusje*, which documents film production in the Netherlands in the period from 1995 to 2005, there was a modest revitalization of Dutch cinema. Some of the uplifting features have already been discussed, either in this study (DE POOLSE BRUID; LEK; VAN GOD LOS; CLOACA) or in my previous one on humour and irony (ALL STARS; WILDE MOSSELS; JA ZUSTER, NEE ZUSTER; SIMON; SHOUF, SHOUF, HABIBI!). One of the very best is BLUEBIRD (Mijke de Jong, 2003), a so-called telefilm made to be broadcast on television.[9] Merel is a thirteen-year-old girl whose younger and handicapped stepbrother Kasper has been adopted by her parents. Merel does a lot with and for her brother: she walks him to the water in his wheelchair, she reads him stories, she takes him to the bathroom, and she cleans his bedsheets. Despite her efforts to take care of Kasper, her brother also steals the limelight within the family. One evening when they are only back home after dark, Merel's parents give her a dressing down because they think the late hour is too chilly for Kasper. In several shots, Merel seems isolated from her father and mother—for example, when she is in the foreground in focus, they are in the background and out of focus. It also indicates that they are blind to the true tragedy in Merel's life: apart from the fact that she is disappointed that she is not chosen to take over the lead role of an injured classmate in the school musical, they do not see that she is being bullied. It is not surprising that her father and mother are blind to this, since Merel tries to cover up all traces of her peers' behaviour. Her parents are kind and well-meaning, but she hardly gives them an opportunity to intrude upon her life, making up excuses for a bruised lip or a lost skateboard.

Merel is a bit of an introspective loner. She is good at gymnastics, and unlike her disinterested classmates, she usually has an answer to the teacher's questions. Though a particular reason seems to be missing, it just so happens that some pupils who consider themselves 'popular' choose her to direct their nasty remarks at, and others join them out of indolence. Her teachers want to be strict on bullying, but they only make it harder for Merel. Someone pins a note on Merel's back: '*I'm shit.*' Since no one comes forward to admit they did it, the entire class has to spend an extra hour at school. Predictably, one of the pupils whispers 'bitch' at Merel. In a group discussion, Merel is asked whether she regards the note as a form of bullying, but she timidly calls it 'teasing'. In a later scene, she raises her finger in class to use the bathroom. Immediately, Martijn, the worst wretch, raises his finger as well. We get a long shot of the bathroom, with a broom blocking the door-latch, and we hear Merel yell. Cut to a shot of Merel who is being interrogated in the room of the principal, but to his great annoyance she refuses to give the name of the suspect. The bathroom scene is exemplary of the film's style, for many shots are handheld and close to the body, but such shots, which have a haptic effect, are alternated with clinical wide shots. This kind of alternation is in sync with the changing moods of Merel. At times she is clearly hurt and in distress: she tries to beautify herself in front of the mirror in her own bedroom; she puts on heavy make-up; she prefers to wait in the car as her mother visits Kasper's institution; she blackens the faces of the pupils on the school picture with a pencil. But there are also redeeming features in her life: she is proud that she has been awarded an encouragement prize for springboard diving; and one boy in class resists participation in the bullying but does not dare to choose her side too obviously to avoid becoming the next scapegoat.

Apart from her tender care for her brother, the most joyful moments are the occasional meetings in a train with Charles, a black man in his thirties with whom she speaks some basic English. He is impressed that she is reading *Anna Karenina*, and after he says that the name 'Merel' is 'Blackbird' in English, he sings this Beatles song for her while she accompanies him to Hoek van Holland. But actually she is not a blackbird, he tells her, for bluebird suits her better. A bluebird is the harbinger of happiness, he explains. During their next encounter, he hands her a book, *L'oiseau bleu* by Maurice Maeterlinck, and signs it '*For my bluebird*'. The book becomes the most concrete sign for Merel that she is seen by the black traveller, who has no ties with her whatsoever, as a bright star rather than a worrisome outcast-teenager. Such symbolic recognition functions as a safety net for the fragile girl.

It is no wonder that Merel, usually reluctant to stand up for herself, behaves as in a game of piggy-in-the-middle to get this book back when it is taken from her. It ends in a struggle, but when all the kids involved have to talk about the incident to the principal, no one spills the beans. BLUEBIRD confronts its viewer with Merel's moral dilemma of how best to protect herself against bullying. Merel realizes that the bullies can perpetuate their behaviour when she does not talk, but she is sufficiently smart to realize that the torments can get worse once she mentions names. Her cowardly choice of refusing to talk to any of the adults seems at the same time the wisest option.

BLUEBIRD is one of those Dutch films in this millennium that 'reinvent realism' in the vein of the art and politics of the Belgian brothers Jean-Pierre and Luc Dardenne. As Emilie Bickerton claims, the Dardenne brothers like to concentrate on a single character, there is little dialogue, and the films have the sparest of narratives, based on the idea that in one's daily life there is hardly any dramatic line (14). If there is music, it is usually diegetic, though BLUEBIRD is an exception with its extradiegetic score. In a Dardenne film, 'we feel and follow the movements of bodies, are conscious of surrounding traffic noises, and notice the little habits and accessories that define the characters' (Bickerton, 14). Their cinema abounds in shots of the back of a head or glimpses of a face rather than regular close-ups. There is a minimal use of establishing shots, and many scenes start in the middle of the action so that viewers do not quite know what is happening (Rushton, 304). Instead of editing a conversation, the handheld camera often goes back and forth between the interlocutors.

On the one hand, the viewer feels sorry for Merel: despite her good heart, this vulnerable girl is being bullied for no particular reason. On the other hand, she is asking for it due to her nerdy behaviour: kids who know the answers to the teacher's questions are hardly ever popular among young teenagers and can easily become a target for bullying. Since it is not hard to identify with Merel, the viewer is invited to wonder what strategic attitude she should take to protect herself against her peers. After BLUEBIRD, De Jong made two more films about 'fragile young girls', and it increasingly becomes more difficult to identify with them. In HET ZUSJE VAN KATIA [KATIA'S SISTER] (2008), a teenage girl of Russian descent is so introverted that she doesn't even have a name until her older sister Katia, who has started working as a dancer in nightclubs, calls her 'Lucia' at the very end. The eighteen-year-old title heroine in JOY (2010) with her 'fuck you' mentality is scarred by the fact that she was a foundling as a baby. She has a life of quarrels and shoplifting and tries to make some money playing the accordion in the subway. She thinks she has successfully discovered the identity of her biological mother and her sister, and she secretly enters their middle-class home. Later, when she is invited for an official meeting with her real mother, she walks away in frustration when the mother turns out to be someone other than she had expected. JOY is an exercise in identification, for the viewer has to make an effort to appreciate a film with such an obstinate main character.[10] The film obviously had a small audience, but it nonetheless won a Golden Calf for Best Dutch Picture, a decision that raised some controversy because opponents argued that JOY was too much of a niche to be awarded such a prestigious prize.

HAPTIC EFFECTS (WITH A PROVISO)

Those Dutch films that have adopted the stylistic traits of the Dardennes are structured around confusing and/or traumatic experiences. One example is KAN DOOR HUID HEEN [CAN GO THROUGH SKIN] (Esther Rots, 2009) where a woman becomes confused after being raped by a pizza delivery boy and starts her life anew in a run-down building in the countryside. RETROSPEKT (2019), another film by Rots, constantly alternates between scenes of the young mother Mette before and after the brutal assault that is about to take place as the film ends and that will turn her into a handicapped woman.[11] In WALDSTILLE (Martijn Maria Smits, 2017), a father is frustrated that his parents-in-law are keeping his child from him after he served in prison for causing an accident while drunk that killed his wife (their daughter). Few films have as many close-ups of a protagonist's eyes, mouth, hands as DIEP [Deep] (Simone van Dusseldorp, 2005), in which fifteen-year-old Heleen wants to discover the meaning of sex and love in the 1970s. Her hippie mother, who is about to separate from her cheating father, is disillusioned: sex is no more than 'eating a sandwich'. But the mysterious punk-musician Steve, who is too doped to perform the act himself, teaches her that sex is 'a voyage to the sublime'. Heleen is as uncertain as she is determined, and she decides to lose her virginity on New Year's Eve, even if she does not really love the boy she has selected.

The close-ups in ZURICH (Sacha Polak, 2015), however, are even more relentless, for this film, with many handheld scenes, features the deeply scarred Nina, who is a singer in a choir. It starts with Nina beside her car in a canal, and then we jump to the intertitle—'Part 2: Hund' (German for 'dog'). During the first 50 minutes, we cannot really make head or tails of the story: first Nina is just traveling and hitchhiking; then she is playing with the dog Hund in the woods; then she is visiting an art exhibition. She starts an affair with the German truck driver Matthias, the father of two children. Her moods change quickly, but to the frustration of Matthias she never reveals what is troubling her. During a struggle between the two, Hund runs away and is hit by a truck. Nina starts crying her eyes out, but then we have suddenly a black screen whereupon 'Part 1: Boris' starts, which chronologically precedes everything we have seen so far. The last half an hour shows why Nina has become such an impenetrable woman. Her lover Boris, father of her five-year-old daughter Pien, died in an accident with his truck. Apparently unbeknownst to Nina, Boris was a married man, father of three boys, and we learn that Hund was his dog. Since the affair was a secret to his family, Nina is excluded from the official funeral: she only visits Boris's corpse after opening hours, when she removes his marriage ring with the name 'Anne' engraved in it. Paco, one of Boris's sons, discusses with two friends the possibility that his father's death might be a suicide, but in that case one often takes one's shoes off. Nina is so traumatized that she leaves Pien behind in the garden of Boris's family, and she starts driving her car with her pumps on the passenger's seat and her eyes closed. The end of the film is then followed by the opening shot of the car in the canal.

The five films mentioned—KAN DOOR HUID HEEN; RETROSPEKT; WALDSTILLE; DIEP; and ZURICH—do not visually orient the viewer but instead revel in so-called 'haptic visuality', a term coined by Laura Marks: close-to-the-body camera positions and panning across the surface of objects; changing of focus; images that appeal to the senses (touch, smell, hearing). These films use these devices to address a register of emotions, from joy to sadness, from relief to pain. But the haptic effect of these films comes with a proviso. Let me refer to LA HOLANDESA [MESSI AND MAUD] (Marleen Jonkman, 2017), a road movie about a woman in distress.

Maud and her boyfriend Frank, in their early forties, are trying to reset their relationship on holidays in Chile, but he gets angry that she has not given up the hope of having a child together after many fruitless attempts. Annoyed, she runs away from him and starts hitchhiking around the country. One day she steps into a truck, encouraged by the young boy Diego who calls himself 'Messi'. The kid's father is not only an alcoholic but also a male-chauvinist pig, and when he tries to sexually harass Maud, she escapes from the truck and 'Messi' accompanies her. After a night in a hotel together, she encourages the eight-year-old to go back to his mother and puts him on a bus. When she wakes up herself, in a bus on the way to Valparaiso, he is sitting next to her. From this moment onwards, Maud, still regretting her motherless existence, apparently feels justified in travelling with the boy. She suggests that he call her 'mama', also for practical reasons. Meeting a couple of Chilean hippies on a beach, she learns to say 'fuck it' in Spanish to her child's wish, and after reading a news item in a paper about the disappearance of the boy, she decides to bring him to his mother's place. Dressed in a Barcelona shirt with Messi's name on it, which she had stolen at a gas station, Diego reunites with his mother, a scene that brings tears to Maud's eyes, looking on from a distance. All in all, Jonkman's film never really colours outside the lines, except maybe for the brief sex scene with a young Chilean father during a nocturnal intermission of a bus trip. Given the fact that she has a strong desire to have children, the choices Maud makes are understandable, and the film presents her running away with 'Messi' as a form of protection of the boy's safety rather than an abduction. But precisely by avoiding the risk of losing the viewer's sympathy for the main protagonist, the emotions in LA HOLANDESA are too quickly exhausted.

Similar to my criticism of Jonkman's film, Sasja Koetsier, in her review of COBAIN (Nanouk Leopold, 2018), mentions the paradox that this sixth feature by Leopold made her feel indifferent towards the characters and their fate while the presentation of this film is much less aloof and detached than her previous cold and meticulously stylized work. The fifteen-year-old boy Cobain, portrayed as someone who is as impenetrable as a Dardenne kid, has been abandoned by his mother Mia at a young age. The mother is not only addicted but also heavily pregnant, and once he has tracked her down, Cobain decides that he has to help her because, well, she is his mother. In its 'fly-on-the-wall realism', however, Leopold's film never poses questions that are really confrontational. Perhaps the most intriguing question is whether it is perhaps not his mother that is the actual subject of devotion for Cobain but the unborn sibling she carries, as Ben Croll observes in his review.

The 'problem', if that is not too big a word for these titles, is that films such as LA HOLANDESA or COBAIN focus on an emotional range rather than a moral dilemma, as is always the case with the very best of the Dardenne films. And though I consider ZURICH and the two pictures by Rots as stylistically daring pictures about tormented protagonists, these films lack compelling moral issues which, I guess, explains why the reputation of these directors is not on a par with the Dardennes. There is a clear moral issue in ZURICH, for Nina leaves behind her young daughter Pien as a reaction to her impossibility to mourn the death of her lover, but this act is presented in the margins. Polak has decided not to give it much emphasis on screen, which is a defendable choice, but a Dardenne film owes its strength, as one can gather from the many positive reviews, to the ways it puts moral issues centre stage. Due to their impoverished circumstances, which are never romanticized, characters in a Dardenne film make awkward decisions and have to amend their most unfortunate actions, resulting in misery again. For example, an adolescent in L'ENFANT [THE CHILD] (2005) sells his baby without informing his girlfriend, buys it back, but has to steal money to satisfy his aggressive creditors. Or they are put to a morality test, as with the boy in LA PROMESSE [THE PROMISE] (1996) who promises a dying immigrant who works illegally at his father's place to take care of the man's wife and kid while the boy's father wants to keep the death a secret. Of all the film's mentioned in this chapter so far I think BLUEBIRD comes closest to the profound moral questions of a Dardenne film. In such a film, a 'realist' depiction is combined with the didacticism of a 'Brechtian fable' (Rancière), inviting the viewer to ponder the question: What would you do if you were in the shoes of that character? Are his or her actions good or bad, or are these qualifications simply not applicable?

Apart from this combination of handheld 'realism' and Brechtian reflection, a Dardenne film derives its poignancy from the fact that, despite the proximity of the camera to bodies, the faces of the characters lack 'expressive depth'. The point, however, is not that they are unemotional but, as Rushton claims, 'they must be so *overcome with emotion* that they cannot outwardly express it' (310, emphasis in original). In her article on the 'spiritual style' in the films of Robert Bresson, Susan Sontag takes the view that his rigid form is designed 'to discipline the emotions at the same time that it arouses them' (180). Paradoxically, an anti-dramatic style that works to hold back one's emotions is an appropriate way to intensify them, according to Sontag (181). In general, the Dutch films mentioned in this 'haptic visuality' section prefer a dramatic over an anti-dramatic approach, whereas the very best Dutch films on traumatic experiences do take Sontag's guideline to heart and favour detached distanciation over emotional sympathy in viewers.

ASCETIC STYLES: *GUERNSEY* AND *BROWNIAN MOVEMENT*

In contrast to the 'fly-on-the-wall realism' of COBAIN, Nanouk Leopold's sublime film GUERNSEY (2005) has an ascetic style that translates into no camera movements, coldly framed images, and deadpan editing. Olaf Möller describes her framing as 'schizophrenic', for Leopold favours 'strong graphic tensions on vast canvasses, reflecting her love of more monochromatic styles of 20th-century painting' (15). The net result of such rigid formalism is that the viewer lacks any clues or guidance as to how to respond emotionally to the scenes. In the end, Leopold's anti-dramatic style—inspired by the cinema of Robert Bresson, Bruno Dumont, and/or Tsai Ming-liang—only succeeds in eroding any sympathy for the characters because identification with them, if possible at all, requires an effort.

Because of the stylistic consistency, the events hardly influence how the scene is shot. Whether characters are shopping in a supermarket or taking a bath or making love is irrelevant to the mise-en-scène. When her characters speak, they 'say only what needs to be said, in a strangely matter-of-fact tone' (Möller, 15). Since an emotional articulation is lacking, the characters in GUERNSEY are presented as an empty canvas (Koetsier): the viewer has to fill in their motivations, for the film consists of a series of relatively loosely connected scenes, often shot from a distance or with objects partly blocking our view. Because she prefers 'light with an opaque quality', GUERNSEY seems at times 'shot from behind a pane of frosted glass' (Möller, 15).

Main protagonist Anna is regularly shown at the edge of the frame to emphasize that she is displaced. She travels to Egypt to set up an irrigation project to grow seedless grapes but regularly returns home to her husband Sebastiaan and their son Kees in a typically modern suburb. Back in Egypt she is on inspection with a colleague, Patricia, who tells Anna about her child. A bit later we see Anna in the bathroom, but when she turns around, she gets the fright of her life. It takes a while before we see the off-screen space: Patricia has hung herself in the shower. Thereafter, the camera is fixated on Anna for a while. She has a conversation with Patricia's husband Paul, a Flemish doctor in Africa, but he can do no more than express his surprise: he claims she was a balanced woman, and he had presumed his wife was happy.

Back home, Anna looks in the mirror, but her face is fragmented from our perspective. She seems to wonder whether we can judge someone's mood from one's appearance. If even Paul could not guess that his wife was sad, she was apparently good at hiding her unhappiness. The look in the mirror can be taken as Anna asking herself: What does my face reveal? Can someone read what is beneath its surface? The ascetic style of Leopold's GUERNSEY makes sense because it gives us the bodily expressions of the characters but not their inner motivations. Characters tend to be closed books, except maybe Anna's talkative sister Bobby with her cynical wisecracks. When their father considers migrating to the island of Guernsey with Mimi, his young Latin-American woman, Bobby's response is off-the-cuff: 'You're moving to a fiscal paradise to get even richer. Ridiculous.' Since Bobby is loose-tongued and extravert, we know she holds a grudge against her sister. With Bobby in the backseat of the car, it becomes clear that Anna's husband Sebastiaan used to be her lover but that 'luckily, Anna got your life back on track'. And in a slightly vicious tone, she adds: 'If I knew you would become this cute, I would never have let you go.'

This remark indicates that Bobby had misjudged her then boyfriend and current brother-in-law. Whether there is a causal connection or not, from this moment onwards, Anna starts to spy on her husband. She secretly peeps at him from a distance when he is watching birds, his favourite leisure activity, or when he takes their son Kees to the playground, or when he is eating french fries in town. One day she looks on as he enters a house, and to her amazement, a woman with an umbrella arrives as well. She cannot hear the conversation, but from a distance, it seems her husband comforts and kisses her. Later when he comes home, he says that the principal wants him to work extra hours. When she tells her sister about Sebastiaan's affair, Bobby says: 'Well, he cheats, we all do something.' Anna: 'So, you knew.' Bobby: 'Yes, he needed some advice. It's not all about you; you are not the centre of the universe.'

If Anna does something unpredictable when she is back in Egypt, this could be related to her realization that Sebastiaan is leading a double life. After she had paid the widower Paul a surprise visit in his home country in Belgium just to see how he was doing, she meets him again in Egypt. He tells her that the promising relation with 'the new mother of his son' was short-lived—another misjudgement. We get a long scene, quite awkward: when Paul takes Anna's lock of hair, she looks surly; when she seems to give herself over to him, he pulls back; after some silence, he starts to cry; framed through a window, he takes off his shirt; they lie next to each other, and after a while, they kiss. Cut to the next morning, which ends with her taking a shower. There is no reason why she might have been intimate with Paul—for he is not particularly attractive—except that they both share, or shared, a partner who holds, or held, a mystery. And this way, Anna responds to Sebastiaan's unpredictability by doing something that is at odds with her own personality.

There is a sudden transition to a family gathering in Guernsey: everyone is anxiously awaiting Bobby's arrival, who ultimately enters with the usual fanfare. Anna is as taciturn as ever and as observant as well. In the new villa of her father, Anna looks on as Bobby kisses Juan the gardener, and when Bobby turns her head, she asks her sister: 'Hey, are you peeping again? Beautiful man, isn't he? You want to have him, too? Go ahead.' Stunned by this frankness, Anna can only reply: 'You can't be mad at me your entire life.' Bobby: 'Oh yes, I can.' The two sisters seem to make up together. The camera is focused on the pensive Anna during a long stroll over the rocky island, without a reverse shot. When she sees Bobby uphill, Anna quickens her pace, slips, and starts to cry. Bobby walks in her direction and embraces her, while Anna's weeping continues gently in a long take. As Anna recuperates, they remain seated for a while without saying a word. On leaving Guernsey by boat, Anna is seated next to Sebastiaan, and after a long silence she says: 'That woman at work with whom you have an affair ... I would like you to end it.' Sebastiaan does not utter a word. Back at the airport, they encounter Paul who is just passing by. Anna tells her husband: 'His wife just passed away.' Sebastiaan: 'How?' After Anna's 'I don't know', we see them leave the frame.

Though we guess that Patricia's suicide has made her aware of the extent to which appearances can be deceptive, Anna pretends as if everything is normal and as if she is still her old self by denying that she knows the cause of death. That old self presumes that she is the trustworthy counterpart to her capricious sister. She is a mother, Bobby is not; she has influence with her father according to Bobby; unlike Bobby, she was able to turn the undisciplined Sebastiaan into a man with a teaching job. Anna fulfils the role of a mediator in the family, holding social ties together. She was supposed to guarantee familial harmony, especially since Bobby has the tendency to create an awkward atmosphere. Anna prospered as the binding agent until she is confronted with the fact that there is a discord between one's social appearance and one's actions. At one point, Anna's father reminds his daughter that mother always had difficulty waking her up, which here is an indication that Anna was quite oblivious to this discord. Since her own symbolic identity is so fixed and stable, the gap between one's appearance and actions alienates her to such an extent that she herself starts to act against character. This time, she plays the game of deceit herself, thus confirming that in Leopold's cinema 'good and evil are equally possible options, both easily within reach', as Möller puts succinctly (14).

Anna's actions are not at the expense of her symbolic consistency, at least not yet, but GUERNSEY seems to prepare the viewers for the even more radical BROWNIAN MOVEMENT (2010),[12] in which the medical researcher Charlotte von Ribeck, mother of a son and married to the handsome Max, transgresses professional and moral boundaries by having sex with unappealing—obese, hairy—male patients in a sterile, rented apartment. Charlotte's nymphomaniac behaviour seems motivated by putting her symbolic position at risk, as if she, the widely respected doctor, wants to be condemned for her outrageous debauchery. It is not even clear whether she enjoys the sex, for she usually has a blank expression, also during her daily activities.[13] But when one of the men, working at a construction site, asks her whether she recognizes him, she starts to scream out loud and hits him in the face with a fist before she collapses. After this incident, she undergoes therapy, but she has no words for her emotions: '*I really don't know what I'm supposed to feel.*' She describes her husband as a good, tender, and attractive lover and touching him is '*almost automatic*', but she can say no more except that it is only a '*completely different sort of touching*' with the other men.

Brownian movement refers to the irregular motion of microscopic particles suspended in a liquid or a gas, and Leopold adopted this term from physics to indicate that we humans can also be led by invisible, and thus inexplicable, forces (Op den Velde, 100). Partly unable to verbalize the reasons for her behaviour and partly unwilling to do so in the presence of Max, for that will only make '*things worse*', we can only guess that she challenged her good reputation just for the sake of putting things at stake. She is subjected to motives that prevent her from taking control over her own life, or rather, she seems to derive a certain satisfaction from this lack of control. After a psychiatric assessment in which her moral conscience is qualified as underdeveloped, her name is removed from the medical register. In the third and final part, the couple moves to India, but even after two new-born children, Max remains suspicious of Charlotte's whereabouts and keeps on spying on her. Her reassurance that, despite everything, she is still the '*same person*' cannot fully satisfy him.

LEAVE NO TRACE: *CODE BLUE* AND *NOTHING PERSONAL*

Both critics and the audience had a difficult time appreciating such excessive, apparently unmotivated steps by a female protagonist.[14] To quote from *Variety*'s review: the widescreen tableaux are again 'exquisitely lit', but the development of characters is too impenetrable (Van Hoeij). This pattern of a benevolent attitude and enthusiasm for GUERNSEY to only a lukewarm response and even dejection for BROWNIAN MOVEMENT repeated itself with two successive films by Urszula Antoniak, more or less on the same grounds. After a successful debut feature, her CODE BLUE (2011), as stylistically austere as Leopold's work, did not get a favourable reception because it was considered too ghastly.

The middle-aged control freak Marian lives in an apartment with a great view. She keeps everything clean and tidy, and the scene in which she publicly embarrasses a cashier who has made a mistake shows that she is unforgiving to anyone who commits errors. Working as a nurse, the perfectionist Marian takes good care of her helpless patients, but at times this borders on illicit intimacy. Moreover, she even occasionally 'saves' the terminally ill among them by giving them deadly injections. The role she takes upon herself to decide over life and death seems to illustrate on the one hand that she does not doubt her own estimations, but on the other hand it is a token of her coldness. The shot in which we see her out of focus in the foreground in a crowded bus while all the other passengers are in sharp focus is emblematic of her awkwardness in social contacts. When she witnesses how a man is gruesomely raped in the night outside her apartment, she goes out to find the condom and spreads the sperm over her self-mutilated upper leg. After this incident, she starts to lose control. A neighbour, Konrad, rings her bell, saying: 'Let me in, you little piggy.' A male patient violently rejects her attempt to inject him, but while hurt herself, she disconnects him from oxygen. When she tells a night-nurse that she feels a bit weird lately, her colleague advises her to go to a party and to fuck. At the party, she is introduced to Konrad and they discover that they both consider DR. ZHIVAGO (David Lean, 1965) their favourite movie. Back at her place, Konrad does not want to touch her and while jerking off, gets angry at her attempts to say sweet words. He beats her face until it bleeds. After Konrad is gone, she mutilates herself again, before we see in a slow motion scene how she takes a shower against an entirely black background, accompanied by Hildegard von Bingen's 'O Viridissima virga'.

Antoniak deliberately set out to make an uncompromising arthouse picture. She delivered, but it was considered too uncompromising by many. The film was selected for the Quinzaine des réalisateurs section in Cannes, but outside the venue there was even an announcement that CODE BLUE might hurt the audience's feelings, a warning aimed at the final scene of ugly/explicit sex and ugly/explicit violence. In response to the controversy, Antoniak said in an interview with Pauline Kleijer that some critics can only deal with depressing themes on the condition that there is a glimpse of a utopian solution. Rather than address the question whether death can be comforting, Antoniak considers one's passing away as a most intimate moment in a person's life, and a nurse happens to be an inherent part of that world of intimacy. According to her, a nurse lives 'above our life, above our reality'. Her Code Blue reverses the commonplace that death is a cruel conclusion to one's life; in her film, death is depicted as 'tender' and even anthropomorphized. Viewers have difficulty identifying with Marian who is, in the words of Antoniak, afforded the status of 'death incarnate'. The predecessor to Code Blue, the lyrical Nothing Personal (2009), was much easier to digest, especially since there is a suggestion of hope at the end, but 'unpleasant movies have a right to exist as well' (Antoniak, qtd. in Kleijer).

Nothing Personal catapulted Antoniak's career, for it won many awards, including the Golden Calf for Best Film and the FIPRESCI prize at the Locarno film festival. In its first fifteen minutes, Antoniak's debut feature clearly pays tribute to Agnès Varda's uncompromising Sans toit ni loi [Vagabond] (1985) about a hitchhiking young woman who has deliberately chosen a solitary existence ('being alone is good'). In Nothing Personal, we see that a young woman takes up hitchhiking after she takes off her ring in an empty apartment. At night, she sleeps near a rocky coast, which is followed by the intertitle '*Loneliness*'. Like the protagonist in Sans toit ni loi, she is not interested in social interaction and can respond brusquely to people's questions. When she is seeking food among garbage and a family asks her whether she needs help, she replies: '*No. Do you?*' A main distinction between the two films is that Varda's film is explicitly told in retrospect, whereas Antoniak's film is chronological, apart from one remarkable crosscutting scene. This difference has an almost opposite effect, though.

Four minutes into Sans toit ni loi, a voice-over mentions that she wants to reconstruct the last weeks in the life of the girl whose corpse has been found in a ditch. She had no papers on her, and she had apparently frozen to death. The narrator will meet the people she has encountered but will neither disclose to them her presumed identity—Mona Bergeron—nor the fact that she has died. Varda's film seems simple, with characters narrating about the female vagrant. The film's structure is actually quite complicated, since their flashbacks can have flashforwards or they are interrupted by other flashbacks and then picked up again at some later juncture (Hayward, 290). I am not so much interested here in the exact nature of the narrative structure or in the composition of the lengthy tracking shots which go from right to left against the Western reading order, but rather in the vain attempts to fix Mona's identity. Varda's film illustrates that the young woman becomes the equation of a myriad of interpretations, but because of the divergence of opinions, the sum total is unfixable. For one person, she is just a filthy girl, for another a sexual object, for a third a symbol of independence, for a fourth a naïve dreamer, and the young man who had a brief affair with her even believed her to be a 'homebody' at heart. In short, Mona 'refuses to be coopted into any image' (Hayward, 286), even to the extent that her name is a mystery. To the Tunisian Assoun, she says: 'My name is Simone, but they call me Mona.'

SANS TOIT NI LOI is shot as a quasi-documentary with the explicit aim of sketching a portrait of a vagabond as a young woman, while exposing the limitations of such an endeavour. Mona functions as a screen of projection for those who talk about her, and since she refused to comply with symbolic codes, the film turns into an 'assertion of her *altérité* (her otherness)' (Hayward, 286). The efforts to attribute meanings to this independent woman offer too refracted impressions, or to quote Varda's voice-over: 'This death leaves no trace.' Whereas the French film highlights the futility of understanding the young woman, Antoniak's NOTHING PERSONAL precludes such an attempt at understanding the protagonist, for she does not share anything personal with anyone. After her hitchhiking adventures during which she even jumps out of a jeep when she suspects the driver might have groping hands, she ends up in the vicinity of an Irish cottage in the region of Connemara, inhabited by the widower Martin. She continues to sleep in her tent but stays at the spot because she can work on his land in exchange for food. She answers any attempt by Martin to be cordial ('*I'm only being polite*') in a snappy tone: '*I'm not.*' When he says: '*Since my wife died*', she interrupts him: '*I'm not interested in your life stories.*' As she is about to depart, he goes after her and proposes: '*I won't ask anything, and I won't talk about myself. Only one question: What is your name?*' She replies: '*You can just call me "you".*' At one point, Martin inadvertently asks her '*Do you like opera?*' which she regards as a violation of the deal. He quickly suggests that every time he asks her a question, he has to sing a song for compensation.

In spite of her rigid attitude, there are some developments. He asks her to sleep in one of the empty rooms when the weather is too bad; he asks her to watch over him when he is not feeling well; they attend a pub together, where she dances cheerfully to folk music; she cooks him a special meal with potato, the '*spirit of the earth*'. And NOTHING PERSONAL has, apart from '*Loneliness*', four randomly inserted intertitles: '*The end of a relationship*', '*Marriage*', '*The beginning of a relationship*' and '*Alone*', as if the film responds to a classic five-act structure. When she asks him about his favourite colour, he says: '*Hey you, that sounds suspiciously like a personal question.*' She sings a song as '*punishment*', after which Martin asks, '*What kind of zodiac are you?*' But before she has even the chance to answer, he starts singing a country gothic number.

One day Martin secretly looks into 'you's' stuff. On her passport he reads her name 'Anne' and an address in Amsterdam. We see him visit Anne's empty apartment, which is alternated with some shots of her playing the piano in his cottage, and then they are back together again at his cottage. It is a puzzling scene: did he really make the trip? The visit is never mentioned, his absence is never mentioned, it is as if it never took place. One morning, just after their hands have intimately touched each other, Martin does not wake up. 'You' finds a suicide note, containing among others the lines: *'Dear You, sorry to leave you like this. ... The place is yours. ... I love you.'* She folds the deceased Martin in sheets, and lies besides him, naked. Then she is back at sea, as we see her from the back. She walks the stairs in a town somewhere before checking into a small hotel—in Spain.

The film's title NOTHING PERSONAL defies any notion of understanding you's character: she presents herself as a young woman without a background, and we only know a few snippets about her because Martin cannot resist searching for anything personal. When Martin asks what she wants, she responds: *'I want to be like you. Nobody looks at you. Nobody talks.'* So she is seeking total anonymity and wants to be cut loose from any past concerns and future prospects. Despite its one-time digression from chronology (Martin visiting Amsterdam), Antoniak's film displayed, in its sheer present-ness, an undeniably visceral quality. The camera focuses on her hands feeling the vegetables and plants in the garden, enjoying the texture of seaweed; we see how she covers herself in blue plastic to shelter against heavy rain; her endless tossing and turning in the bed of a deserted place, and pulling one of her lengthy hairs to leave it behind for the owner. Since a rational understanding is sacrificed, the viewers are alerted to the aesthetic of the audio-visual images as such. The film opens with sound on a black screen, but when we see 'you' in her empty apartment, there is only static noise. When she is on the coast close to the sea, she puts her hands on and off her ears. This is the best indication that the audio-track is often subjectivized, consisting of a mixture of ambient music and diegetic sounds.

In one of the early scenes, she is asleep, but in the meantime 'the noise of cars rushing by has imperceptibly turned into the sound of waves on the shore' (111), Katharina Schmid remarks in her analysis of the film, as if we experience her projection of her journey. It is obvious that she attempts to rediscover her sensuality by going from an urban dystopia to Ireland, often associated with 'rurality, a pre-industrial lifestyle, spiritual values' (106), while the pub scenes with their dancing and excessive drinking posit a 'vision of an ideal community' (107). If this de-peopled and 'uncultivated landscape under an overcast sky' (ibid.) functions as an overtly conventional antidote to modern society, Schmid adds to this that Antoniak's film also undermines the images of Ireland. In THE QUIET MAN (John Ford, 1952), stock signifiers of Irishness are identified with the young native woman, the red-haired Colleen, but in NOTHING PERSONAL, Anne, the red-haired foreign visitor, displays them: she is outside most of the time; she works in an unspoilt landscape; she claims that her breath can animate the landscape (110). We are not shown Ireland as it is, but this Ireland is produced as a projection of Anne's spiritual needs onto the empty countryside (111). Schmid points out a remarkable transition: when she is walking on a small path in the forest, she is followed by Martin. The dripping wet leaves of the trees have 'dark shades of green and brown, establishing a rather gloomy' atmosphere. As soon as she is on her own and enters a clearing in a next scene, the atmosphere is reversed: the colours have become much brighter and the clearing is full of sunlight, as if she is entering a 'parallel world all of her own making' (111).

NOTHING PERSONAL portrays a young woman at a low point in her life: she is no longer attached to anything and keeps her name and past a secret. We also see that she is trying to re-attune to the physical world in the barren landscape of Ireland. She can only bear Martin as company on the condition that he accepts that they do not share anything personal. She is about to reset her senses: she has undergone aphanisis, and in order to recover from her subjective destitution, she has to feel anew, to hear anew, to touch anew. Antoniak's film requires its viewers to start from zero as well: we should resist the temptation to know anything about 'you' and let ourselves be affected by the sound design, by the close-ups of hands and white sheets, by the long shots of landscapes and sea, by the hard wind and heavy rain. In its repression of narrativity, both the excellent cinematography and soundtrack of NOTHING PERSONAL encourage its viewers to enjoy it as a sensory experience.

WINTER SONATA: *VERDWIJNEN*

The audio design is at least as important, if not more so, in VERDWIJNEN [DISAPPEARANCE] (Boudewijn Koole, 2017). The film starts with the sound of restrained but heavy breathing, and once we have visuals, we see a little girl on stage next to a piano. She gets a round of applause, and when she is seated, we see her arms in close-up, followed by a shot of the back of her head with the piano keys out of focus. Once again we hear the breathing, which can be related to the girl's nerves. There is a transition to the 30-something Roos on her way by car to the snow-covered regions of Norway, accompanied by piano sounds (which could be the melody the girl is playing). Roos's half-brother Bengt is about to celebrate his thirteenth birthday, and she is welcomed by her mother's sledge dogs. She has not been to her mother's place for a long time: her mother Louise has had one dog already for one-and-a-half year, while she thought it was new. Moreover, Bengt is still a bit sore that Roos had left last time without saying goodbye to him. He makes her swear not to quarrel with their mother during this visit. Roos gives him a recording device as a birthday present, and while she is asleep, he tapes her breathing. It sounds like a bjørk, a white tree, according to Bengt who has a musical ear. He has made a gigantic ice sculpture, and the icicles produce specific notes: accidently, Roos breaks one icicle, and now the 'A' sounds false.

Bengt has inherited his musicality from his mother, who still teaches piano to twelve pupils and practices every day. Louise has a recital at home, but Roos keeps herself at a distance. The mother-daughter relationship is difficult; their conversations are scarce. 'I forgive you for what happened last year', Roos tells her, but mother's reply is snappish: 'Roos, you are no longer a child. Water under the bridge.' To which Roos adds: 'Until we drown.' In an attempt to improve their contact, Roos joins her mother at the piano and they play Franz Schubert's 'Fantasia in F minor for piano four-hands, D.940'. Mother sounds like a bitch when she remarks: 'Schubert is merciless. You never ever play piano anymore?' We then have three inserts of the girl playing the piano that we already saw at the opening. The first time is right after Roos has had sex with her old fling Johnny in his car and tells him that she is dying. As Roos smokes outside the car in the snowy landscape, we see the neatly dressed girl at the piano. The second time is after she finally tells her mother that she is seriously ill. A close-up of Roos who sees her mother walk away, speechless, is followed by a flashback. And the third time is the very final shot: stared at by her mother and her sledge dogs, Roos walks towards the horizon into an all-white landscape. Separated by a black screen, we then have an extremely long shot of a girl who has finished her piano recital. So the shots of the girl at the piano are identified with either an announcement of her death or her final disappearance into 'nothing'.[15] Playing the piano is apparently so traumatic for Roos that she has become competent in the particularly silent art of photography: she shows her mother some of her published pictures in a magazine, but Louise is too busy rolling dough.

The root of the conflict in VERDWIJNEN seems obvious, certainly for everyone who has seen the film with which Koole's film has been compared, HÖSTSONATEN [AUTUMN SONATA] (Ingmar Bergman, 1978).[16] Mother Louise pushed her young daughter into a career as a concert pianist, but the latter could not cope with the pressure. In one of the few talks they have, Louise still reproaches her for deciding at the age of eight to live with her father. Mother then describes her own upbringing with a minimum of words, apparently meant to explain her callousness and her lack of emotion: at the age of eight, she was sent to boarding school and she had to practice six hours a day; she never saw her parents; from the age of ten onwards, she gave performances in concert halls all over the world; at the age of eleven, her parents had her fingers insured. So how could she ever miss her parents, how could she be attached to someone?

This insensibility not only explains how Roos's mother can live in such a remote place, hardly populated, it also determines Roos's independent stance: she works as a freelance photographer; she has no relationships, only about 'some hundred flings': and when Johnny's girlfriend Astrid shows her pregnant belly, she asks: 'Is it scary?' This indicates that Roos associates motherhood with a suffocating bond. Roos is a woman set adrift who has been trying to escape from symbolic bonds ever since she stopped playing the piano. Significantly, the shots of the little girl are always isolated from an audience. There is only a spotlight on her and the instrument, but the rest is entirely dark. There is applause at the beginning, but no applause at the end. She has finally reconciled with her mother, as best they could, but only by revealing her forthcoming death. As a daughter of a famous pianist, Roos could never gain her mother's approval due to her failed career: she did not live up to Louise's expectations. The recurrent flashbacks of the piano performance illustrate that Roos is marred by this lack of acceptance and the fact that her mother never acknowledged her as a full-fledged 'I'. The advance of her death implies at least that this non-I has become part of 'us', best signified by the fact that Bengt has produced a sound that is a mixture of three heartbeats.

DANCING IN THE DARK: *LENA*

Several characters in this chapter have a problem with names, significantly expressed in NOTHING PERSONAL, for the young woman only wants to be called 'you'.[17] They have lost their name (temporarily or otherwise) or wish to ignore it as a result of some traumatic experience: war crimes; a planned accident; being bullied; a break-up.[18] It may then seem illogical to analyze the film LENA (Christophe Van Rompaey, 2011), for it bears the name of the main protagonist, a seventeen-year-old girl. But the speech-act of saying her name as the final word of this unduly underrated film by Flemish-born director Van Rompaey is precisely related to moments of self-obliteration.

LENA is shot in a 4:3 ratio, which makes it intimate, but it also indicates that her existence is burdensome. She lives in a cramped apartment with her young and skinny Polish mother Danka, who calls her a 'hippopotamus' because her build is plump. At the very beginning, her face is in close-up and when the camera zooms out, we see her having sex with a boy in a dark corner. While zipping his pants, the boy asks her name. 'Lena', she says, and he replies, just before leaving: 'Oh, I've never had a Lena before.' Later she is having another quickie, but when the boy's name is called out in the indoor swimming pool, he immediately runs off to his mates, not wishing to be seen with an overweight girl. Lena offers her body in the hope of winning affection, but this never happens. She uses her sexual experiences to tell her more popular blonde girlfriend Hanneke about the good times she has had: it was great fun in the swimming pool (but, as we know, it was not). The two have country line dancing as a common hobby. The repetitions are a red thread in LENA, and it is only during those moments that we hear a voice-over, and though her comments are restricted to the art of dancing itself, they also have the status of encouraging life lessons. In these intermezzos, the camera is attached to Lena herself, but while her upper body remains stable, all the rest becomes a blur because of her movements: 'I used to think I would never learn the moves: *strap*, *rock*, *touch*, *hook*, *kick*, *shuffle* all by heart. But once you practice enough, you manage. You can get used to anything.' Or, 'When something goes wrong, make sure no one sees it ... always go on', or '... always count properly'.

One evening on her moped through her hometown Rotterdam, she sees a guy running on the pavement and after their eyes meet and she greets him ('hey'), he jumps on her backseat as we hear the sirens of police cars. It was all a misunderstanding, he explains, the police erroneously believed he had robbed an old lady. They keep in touch, and the handsome charmer Daan invites her to his place, a detached house with only his widowed father Tom, an absent-minded jazz musician, as the other inhabitant. She is even allowed to stay over for an indefinite duration, so she picks up her things from home, to the chagrin of her Polish mother. Although she criticizes her daughter, she is also in need of her when there does not happen to be a man around. Daan gives her presents now and then, but the alarm bell only starts ringing when police show up at the door. She discovers that her boyfriend steals stuff, that his fake gun is a real one, and that he has only been pretending to attend school. She goes back to her mother, but her return is ill-timed, for Danka has male company; Hanneke cannot accommodate her either, since she has a boy as well. Daan's father happens to be at the dancing school, for he has heard about her departure, and due to her limited options, she accepts Tom's suggestion to go back to his house.

During one of the dinners at their home, Lena is adamantly outspoken and speaks to Daan like a stern mother. She is only prepared to stay on the condition that Daan stops with his lies and his illegal activities, like the possession of a gun and driving around without a licence. She addresses Daan's father as well: she tells him his lack of authority is pathetic and that he has to act normal. Surprisingly, her words do not fall on deaf ears, for father and son take her advice to heart. When Lena is rehearsing some dance steps in the living room, they even take delight in joining in. After Tom visits her line dancing repetitions one evening, he tries to kiss her in his car. Since she does not give in, Tom tells her the day after that he is ashamed of his behaviour but that she had better leave, for her presence embarrasses him: 'I hear you, I smell you ... it is a compliment.' So far, some 85 minutes into Van Rompaey's film, Lena's behaviour is shown as pragmatic, but now she takes her pragmatism to another level. Since she has nowhere else to go, she puts on make-up and seduces the father of her boyfriend. To articulate the gravity of this step, we do not hear any sound at all, while she sits atop on him. She will have sex with him a second time, after both she and Tom have told Daan to fulfil his duty. She tries to contact her mother, who works as a bus driver, but when Lena recommends Tom as a nice and rich man, Danka closes the door of her bus on her daughter. That the entire situation has derailed Lena becomes clear during a dance rehearsal on her own. The sequence starts entirely out of focus, but once her face is sharp, her energetic movements are shown in jump cuts. Her hair goes in her face; the camera circles around her; one of the inserted shots is out of focus, again. Lena is trying to count properly, for that is the basis of a well-executed dance, but she fails: '1, 2, 4 ... no, 1, 2, 5, 4.' The blurred shots and the jump cuts now function to accentuate the fact that she is off balance: she has overstepped a limit by sleeping with Tom. She requests a pill from Daan though she is not in favour of drugs. Thereupon she has sex with him in the bathtub, witnessed by Tom who enters the bathroom inadvertently and excuses himself. The situation takes a turn for the worse when, in an attempt to set things straight, she tells Daan that his father touched her indecently. She runs after Daan who starts yelling at his father in a menacing manner. It was not like that, Tom says, and he wants her to say that she was the one who took the initiative. Lena only asks the father to show the tattoo to the son: 'Lena' is written on Tom's upper left arm. Because Daan is still furious, Lena has taken the gun from him, but she fires it by accident, hitting Daan's father. In the final scene, she enters her mother's apartment, but soon the police ring the bell. When Danka opens the door, they ask whether she is 'Lena ...'. Lena then comes forward and says her name, in close-up, in a firm fashion: 'I'm Lena.' She has not only recuperated from her temporary loss of self, but this final shot also implies that she is prepared to take the consequence for her mishap. The 'I'm Lena' indicates that she is able to count properly, once again.[19]

CONCLUSION: THE DISCOMFORT OF STRANGERS

The protagonists in the films in this chapter were traumatized for various reasons, which most of the time resulted in a crisis (temporary or otherwise) of their names. Aaron is registered as Mr. X after he fails to utter anything other than the name of his enemy Krenn (The Rose Garden); consumed by guilt, Alex in Amnesia does not mind being called 'Theo', the name of his father; Mériora Gillibrand had to go in hiding under another gender name, as 'Monsieur Hawarden'; Roos in KRACHT collapsed, for she felt she had turned into the 'second Mrs. Bollens'; 'Boris' is one of only two chapter titles in ZURICH, but Boris is an absent character, for the film shows how his mistress Nina tries to cope with his death as well as with the posthumous discovery of his deceit; the unhappy Merel is more than delighted with the fact that the black man calls her 'Bluebird'; the protagonist in NOTHING PERSONAL refused to share any particularities with the Irish widower, not even her own name. All these characters try to come to terms with traumatic events in their own ways. They break with old habits, such as those female characters who go to the countryside (in KRACHT; in KAN DOOR HUID HEEN; and in NOTHING PERSONAL), or hope to reconcile with an overly strict mother (VERDWIJNEN), or aim to create a pseudo-family (LENA).

A film that goes one step beyond this is BROZER [FRAILER] (Mijke de Jong, 2014), the successor to BROOS [FRAIL] (1997), because the viewer is implicated here in a most uncanny manner. In BROOS, the main actresses play five sisters who have gathered in a summer house to make a videotape for the 40th wedding anniversary of their parents. As becomes clear, the marriage has gone through a difficult phase, when their father was away for about one and a half year. This is the source of many a discussion—about secrecy, about responsibilities, about false integrity. Whereas the sisters utter their minor and major mutual irritations, they also have a good laugh together. At the end of the film, pregnant Ted's water breaks, and they all join her on the way to the hospital.

Seventeen years later, the four sisters reunite for the sequel BROZER, this time because one of them, Muis, is suffering from cancer. They are preparing for her upcoming death: there are four coffins so she can rehearse the lying pose with her sisters besides her. But the drama, largely improvised, quite imperceptibly transforms into a docudrama: the actress playing Muis, Leonoor Pauw, has cancer for real, and the characters turn into the actresses; the fictional sisters become the real-life friends. From this moment onwards, Pauw's husband and daughter feature in BROZER as well, and the viewer is suddenly witness to an actual deathbed. Even though the camera is never particularly obtrusive, the viewer is made privy to something that seems too private. De Jong's film becomes a memorial video for family and close relatives, but what about the average viewer: Is she/he excluded, or not? Strictly speaking, the staging of the foretold death of the character Muis may exactly resemble the registration of the last days of the life of the actress Leonoor Pauw, but not quite. The reverent registration will probably function as comforting to her beloved ones for whom her passing away is truly sad, but it provokes a sense of discomfort among the viewer who does not belong to the inner circle: 'Do I feel like a welcome guest in this intimate setting?' But such puzzling discomfort can be a most productive affect: the film viewer is usually positioned as a voyeur in a darkened auditorium, but confronted with a death on screen in the case of BROZER, this relatively safe position becomes one of slight embarrassment.[20]

NOTES

1 THE ROSE GARDEN was 'een echte opdrachtfilm, efficiënt gemaakt maar niet echt interessant'.

2 Rademakers' sarcasm about the use of the English language was justified nonetheless because (the first half of) THE ROSE GARDEN is about the difficulty of speaking (one's) language, like few other films are.

3 A photo of the rescue operation is later published in a newspaper, with the unknown man in the left frame.

4 The wounded accomplice could be taken as a reference to Bobby Eerhart's WILDSCHUT (1985), a nouvelle violence B picture avant la lettre, discussed in chapter three. AMNESIA is also inspired by the British production CUL-DE-SAC (Roman Polanski, 1966). Like Wouter, the gangster Albie in Polanski's thriller is seriously injured in the stomach after a botched robbery. His accomplice finds an old castle near the sea and meets the two occupants, a bald Englishman and his much younger, French wife. The two gangsters are waiting for Mr. Katelbach, but this man never shows up. In the course of the film, after Albie's death, the confrontation between Dickie and the married couple gets increasingly absurd.

5 When Wouter sees Alex for the first time, he mentions that he fits the description: he has a 'loser's look on his face', indeed.

6 See for a brief analysis of ROPE, Žižek *Enjoy*, 13, also mentioned in note 1, chapter four.

7 Because of the ominous and uncanny quality of KRACHT, with its barren landscape, I personally prefer Fokkema's film over Pieter Verhoeff's heritage drama NYNKE, although this latter film was awarded a Golden Calf for Best Picture in 2001. Stylistically, Verhoeff's film is an example of a 'quality film', but for that reason it is also a bit slick and low-risk. The protagonist in NYNKE is Sjoukje Bokma de Boer who founds a magazine with her husband, the lawyer and poet Pieter Jelles Troelstra. So far so good, until he becomes a 'warrior for the people' and betrays the aristocratic class, to the contempt of his father. By becoming a socialist politician, Pieter Jelles obstructs the ambitions of his wife, who gives birth to a second child. Since she becomes cold as ice, Sjoukje burns her hands with hot coal. She is diagnosed as an incurably hysterical woman due to fact that she cannot pursue a career. She is advised to accept her duty as a mother and housewife, but when she becomes chilly again, she chooses to write under the pseudonym of Nynke van Hichtum.

Her best-known novel is *Afke's tiental*, about a poor working-class family with ten children, but thanks to the strength of mother Afke, they persevere. Her husband criticizes Sjoukje/Nynke for romanticizing poverty, but she does not want to write rebellious novels. Despite the fact that she is delighted that her readers send her affectionate letters, she has to return to the health resort. Upon her arrival back home, she finds out that her husband has started an affair with the new maid. She takes the children under her care.

8 I call Roos the 'second Mrs. Bollens' to emphasize the parallel with Alfred Hitchcock's gothic film REBECCA (1940) in which the main protagonist, named the 'second Mrs. de Winter', is constantly reminded of the fact that she is the successor to the late Rebecca, an object of adoration for the entire household, and for Mrs. Danvers in particular. Rebecca is idealized to such an extent that it almost drives the 'second Mrs. de Winter' mad. As she is about to jump to her death, there is news that the body of Rebecca has been found, and this will introduce a new turn of events: the stories of the saint-like deceased were slightly exaggerated.

9 Two other telefilms that stand out in this period were both made by Nicole van Kilsdonk and are based on gimmicks. In OCHTENDZWEMMERS [MORNING SWIMMERS] (2001), crucial dialogues are transformed into the lyrics of (classic) pop songs. In the mosaic film POLONAISE (2002), the characters are caught in a traffic jam.

10 Sacha Polak's DIRTY GOD, the opening film of the International Film Festival Rotterdam in 2019, is another exercise in identification, but the behaviour is here clearly related to a tragic incident. At the beginning, we see Jade Nugent's skin in a series of extreme close-ups. The young mother has been disfigured by her ex-boyfriend due to an acid attack. Her toddler daughter Rae starts to cry when Jade returns from hospital. Ashamed of her look, things go terribly wrong for Jade, for she makes three most unfortunate decisions to compensate for her bad luck. First, she is so angry that Rae has been taken to visit her daddy in prison that she spends a cold and rainy night away from home with her daughter. Therefore, she is no longer permitted to bring up Rae, for she cannot offer her routine. Second, since Jade misses the attention of men, she starts to visit the website Luvbuddies to chat with naked men. She starts to masturbate in front of them, and one day she sees that she is exposed online as an ugly 'UK slut'. Some of her male colleagues are watching the clip, and she starts a fight with one of them. Third, Jade steals money from her mother to pay for plastic surgery at a clinic in Marrakesh that she has contacted online. Predictably, the clinic does not exist: her money is gone. After she has hit rock bottom, DIRTY GOD ends on a slightly positive note. Jade receives the news that her own mother has been arrested for shoplifting, but this means she can get back to her daughter Rae. With the trophy of 'Employee of the month' in her hand, she realizes she has not been destroyed, despite all the drawbacks. In the final shot, we see Jade walk together with her mother and her daughter.

11 When RETROSPEKT premiered at the Berlin Film Festival, Jessica Kiang wrote a spot-on review for *Variety*. She described Rots's film as a 'raw-nerve drama' that constantly dislocates its viewers. It is an unsentimental, sometimes even humorous portrait of Mette, in which 'fragmentary images, nonlinear editing, and the deliberate rupture of the past into the present [are used] to evoke the smash-and-grab effect of deep shock'. The film is not an 'easy watch', according to Kiang, especially since the seriousness of themes contrasts with a 'wacky soundtrack', but this peculiar juxtaposition turns RETROSPEKT into a 'fascinating experience of cinematic dysphasia'.

12 Between GUERNSEY and BROWNIAN MOVEMENT, Leopold directed WOLFSBERGEN (2007), another excellent film, with superb cinematography quite like GUERNSEY.

13 An exception to her detached demeanour is the scene in which she has to laugh because the sci-fi ringtone of a mobile phone disrupts her lecture.

14 Despite the less enthusiastic response, BROWNIAN MOVEMENT won two Golden Calves, one for best screenplay and another for best director.

15 According to the end credits, the girl at the piano is young Louise, although the inserts are consistently embedded in relation to Roos.

16 Whereas VERDWIJNEN begs comparison with Bergman's film, Koole's debut fiction feature KAUWBOY (2012) is clearly indebted to the splendid film KES (Ken Loach, 1969). Loach's film is about a young working-class boy, abused at home, who starts to train a pet falcon. In the terrific KAUWBOY, the ten-year-old Jojo finds a young jackdaw that has fallen from its nest. Jojo lives together with his volatile father, for his mother is a famous singer on tour in America. His father orders him to bring the little bird back, but Jojo secretly continues to take care of the jackdaw. We gradually realize the reason behind the father's ever-changing mood: the mother is not temporarily absent, rather the father is mourning the death of his wife. Jojo finds comfort in the close bond with the jackdaw until the bird flies fatally between the spokes of his bike.

17 ROMEO (Rita Horst, 1990) is a counterexample: a woman becomes angry when the name of her child is not mentioned. Anne and Matthijs are expecting their first child. The gynaecologist tells them that their baby will be born dead since his kidneys do not function. The film registers the sadness of the parents-to-be, and especially Anne is in mourning. To her fury, the autopsy report, which her husband had kept hidden, calls the baby 'foetus' instead of Romeo.

18 The best example of losing one's name is when one becomes the suspect of a most serious crime, as in the case of LUCIA DE B. [ACCUSED] (Paula van der Oest, 2014). Based upon a real-life case, which also inspired Antoniak's CODE BLUE, Lucia de Berk was a nurse accused of seven murders of either babies or elderly people. What is key is the prosecutor's conviction that she poisoned the baby Timo Visser with digoxin, and on the principle that 'if one murder is proven, the other murders are plausible', Lucia is sentenced to life imprisonment. Her lawyer considers it a

'strange mass hysteria', for the evidence is based on a series of unsolid assumptions: her bad childhood, her fondness for crime novels, the grudge against her mother, her weird and private behaviour (according to colleagues), the fact that she speaks of a 'compulsion' in her diary make up the idea that she has all the characteristics of a psychopath. Van der Oest's Lucia de B. takes the perspective of the unjustly accused woman and registers her alienation via formal means, such as slow motion, wide-angle lenses, spaces with low ceilings and hardly any windows, drowned-out surrounding noise, and the out-of-focus close-up of the man who has sex with her as a teenager, with her mother's consent, in a yellow-tinted flashback. Just before she is arrested, the face of the assistant prosecutor is reflected in the glass of a window and partly eclipses Lucia's face. This is the moment of her loss of self, for it punctuates the transition from De Berk into De B., who is nicknamed the 'Angel of Death' in the press. Only her boyfriend Peter and daughter Fabiënne stand by her, as well as her lawyers Theo Bakker and Quirijn Herzberg. At one point she tells Quirijn: 'I have nothing left', and soon thereafter she has a brain haemorrhage, but she survives. After six years, three months and nineteen days in prison, she was fully acquitted of all charges by the Supreme Court in 2010.

19 There is a precise moment in De dirigent [The Conductor] (Maria Peters, 2018) when the female protagonist Willy Wolters, who was adopted as a baby, names herself 'Antonia Brico'. At a young age, she expresses the ambition to become a conductor, but this is considered impossible for a woman—the film is set in the 1920s. She is not on good terms with her foster parents, but even after she has left their house, she keeps calling herself 'Willy'. One day she is sexually assaulted by her piano teacher and bruises the man's hand in self-defence. She wants to file a complaint, but the teacher has anticipated this and accuses Willy of aggressive behaviour. The teacher will only drop the charges if she signs a document that she will leave the school. To underscore that she will not give up her musical ambition, she chooses from this moment on her birth name 'Antonia Brico'. Aand she does eventually triumph as a female 'maestro': first, she successfully starts the New York Women's Symphony Orchestra in 1934, then she becomes the first woman to conduct the New York Philharmonic orchestra, in 1938. Peters' biopic was a Golden Film (more than 100,000 viewers in the Netherlands) but did not receive any Golden Calf nominations. This lack of critical recognition in the Netherlands was more than compensated by considerable attention the film received abroad, including a release in 5,000 theatres in China in 2021. Before De dirigent, another Shooting Star Filmcompany production, Prooi (Dick Maas, 2016), had been exported to China. Maas's biggest failure in his home country (some 30,000 viewers), this film about a lion on the loose in Amsterdam was an unexpectedly big success in Chinese cinemas in 2018.

20 For those readers who may think that I argue against (too much) realism in Dutch films: yes, in the case of pictures that facilitate identification with the characters in

a fairly straightforward fashion, but I make an exception for films which problematize the attitude of the viewer. Such films either confront the viewer with moral issues or they make the viewer's position uncomfortable. This goes for the great majority of titles in this chapter.

BIBLIOGRAPHY

Bernink, Mieke, *Fons Rademakers: Scènes uit leven en werk* (Abcoude: Uniepers, 2003).

Bickerton, Emilie, 'Reinventing Realism: The Art and Politics of the Dardenne Brothers', *Cinéaste* 31, 2 (2006), 14-18.

Croll, Ben, 'COBAIN: Berlin Review', *ScreenDaily* (17 February 2018),https://www.screendaily.com/reviews/cobain-berlin-review/5125718.article [Accessed 15 May 2020].

Graveland, Mariska, Fritz de Jong and Paul Kempers eds., *De broertjes van* ZUSJE*: De nieuwe Nederlandse film 1995-2005* (Amsterdam: International Theatre & Film-Books, 2006).

Hayward, Susan, 'Beyond the gaze and into *femme-filmécriture*: Agnès Varda's SANS TOIT NI LOI (1985)', ed. by Susan Hayward and Ginette Vincendeau, *French Film: Texts and Contexts* (London and New York: Routledge, 1990), 285-296.

Jaehne, Karen, 'ANTONIA'S LINE', *Film Quarterly* 50, 1 (1996): 27-30.

Kiang, Jessica, 'Berlin Film Review: RETROSPEKT', *Variety* (12 February 2019),https://variety.com/2019/film/markets-festivals/retrospekt-review-1203127677/ [Accessed 16 May 2020].

Kleijer, Pauline, 'CODE BLUE: een opzettelijk ongemakkelijke film', *De Volkskrant* (25 September 2011), https://www.volkskrant.nl/nieuws-achtergrond/code-blue-een-opzettelijk-ongemakkelijke-film~b92a6996/ [Accessed 12 May 2020].

Koetsier, Sasja, 'COBAIN: Het is wel mijn moeder', *De Filmkrant* 408 (April 2018), https://filmkrant.nl/recensies/cobain/ [Accessed 13 May 2020].

Lacan, Jacques, *Four Fundamental Concepts of Psycho-analysis*, trans. by Alan Sheridan (New York: Penguin, 1994).

Marks, Laura, *Touch: Sensuous Theory And Multisensory Media* (Minneapolis and London: University Of Minnesota Press, 2002).

Möller, Olaf, 'From the Abyss to Blue Skies', *Film Comment* (July-August 2013), 14-15.

Op den Velde, Minou, 'Dit is Nanouk Leopold', 97-105.http://minouopdenvelde.nl/pdf/interviews/NanoukLeopold.pdf [Accessed 14 May 2020].

Rancière, Jacques, 'The noise of people, the image of art', (1999), trans. by Stoffel Debuysere, *Diagonal Thoughts* (2012), http://www.diagonalthoughts.com/?p=1500 [Accessed 14 May 2020].

Rushton, Richard, 'Empathic Projection in the Films of the Dardenne Brothers', *Screen* 55, 3 (2014): 303-316.

Schmid, Katharina, '"Fremd bin ich eingezogen …" – An Outsider's Vision of Ireland in Urszula Antoniak's NOTHING PERSONAL', *Estudios Irlandeses* 8 (2013), 105-113.
Sontag, Susan, 'Spiritual Style in the Films of Robert Bresson', 1964, *Against Interpretation and Other Essays* (London and New York: Penguin Classics, 2009), 177-195.
Van Hoeij, Boyd, 'BROWNIAN MOVEMENT', *Variety* (26-09-2010), https://variety.com/2010/film/markets-festivals/brownian-movement-1117943707/ [Accessed 17 May 2020].
Van Gelder, Henk, *Hollands Hollywood: Alle Nederlandse speelfilms van de afgelopen zestig jaar* (Amsterdam: Luitingh – Sijthoff, 1995).
Žižek, Slavoj, *Enjoy Your Symptom! Jacques Lacan In and Out of Hollywood*, 1992 (Revised Edition. New York and London: Routledge, 2001).
—, *How to Read Lacan* (New York: W.W. Norton and Company, 2007).

CHAPTER 9

Hysteria, Neurosis, Perversion

Verstraten, P., *Dutch Post-War Fiction Film Through a Lens of Psycho-analysis*. Taylor & Francis Group, 2021
DOI 10.5117/9789463725330_CH09

ABSTRACT

In analyzing the dénouement of DE AANSLAG, chapter nine introduces the notion of 'identification with the symptom'. This usually concerns a ciphered message addressed to the big Other. For an obsessive neurotic, such a message can be sent to wipe out a certain guilt, as in DE AANSLAG or MYSTERIES. The hysteric in ELINE VERE as well as in BLACK BUTTERFLIES is haunted by the question: 'Who I am for the desire of the Other?' whereas in the case of perversion, secret contracts and private rituals are at the core of the matter. Perversion manifests itself in many forms in as many types of films, including avant-garde pictures by Zwartjes, a rape revenge comedy (ELLE), a medieval blockbuster (FLESH + BLOOD), and an 'Edam' western (BRIMSTONE).

KEYWORDS
Identification with the symptom – Ciphered messages to the big Other – Neurosis and Hysteria – Perversion: Secret contracts

At the end of Rademakers' DE AANSLAG (1986), already partially discussed in chapter seven, Anton Steenwijk suffers from a terrible toothache. It is 1983, so it is 38 years after the film's titular incident. A befriended dentist is prepared to relieve him from his pain on condition that Anton joins the mass demonstration against nuclear weapons that is taking place in Amsterdam. Among the crowd, a 60-year-old woman tries to attract his attention, but he does not immediately recognize his former neighbour Karin Korteweg. As soon as she mentions her name, Anton immediately recalls an early erotic memory: in the first minutes of the film, the then twelve-year-old boy was at her place and Karin pulled up a leg so she could put on a long stocking, giving him the opportunity to almost peep between her thighs. Back in the present, people dressed as skeletons carrying a coffin with the word 'humanity' on it pass by them in the demonstration. Amidst the protesters, Karin tells Anton that his older brother Peter had threatened her and her father with a gun on that evening of the assault, January 1945: he was angry that the Kortewegs had moved the dead body of Fake Ploeg in front of the house of the Steenwijks. Before he can pull the trigger—shown to us in flashback—the Germans surround the house and shoot Peter in the head. When Karin's father sees the next day that the house of the Steenwijks had been burned down, he is so afraid that Anton would want revenge for all the misery that he and Karin decided to emigrate to the other end of the world to New Zealand. In 1948, Mr. Korteweg committed suicide, to which Karin adds: 'Ultimately he didn't need you to kill him, you were there inside his head all along.'

Karin's interpretation presupposes that Anton has materialized into Mr. Korteweg's superego, an imaginary voice inducing him with a sense of guilt that can never be redeemed. This makes sense, but this is not the entire story, for there is another flashback by Karin, which could also be a hypothetical reconstruction by Anton visualizing her words. Realizing that Fake Ploeg has been shot, Mr. Korteweg reacts, looking outside the window: 'Oh God' and as he turns around, we get an eyeline match of the man's collection: 'My lizards.' We then see relatively long close-ups of two of his lizards.[1] Out of fear that the Germans might destroy his collection, he removes the corpse of the collaborator (causing the Steenwijks to become the dupes because the grumpy old couple Aarts had a Jewish family in hiding—a revelation reserved for the final minutes of Rademakers' film). After Korteweg's wife had died two years earlier,

Karin explains, 'those creatures meant something like eternity or immortality to him. In the war, they became his only reason for living. He was so unhappy.' But the day after the assault, when he knows that the Steenwijks have been liquidated, he tramples all his beloved lizards: they had become 'ordinary lizards again, just a set of animals'.

Mr. Korteweg has the characteristics of a neurotic suffering from a compulsive disorder. Because of a strongly developed ego, an obsessive neurotic aspires to keep control and hardly discusses his feelings. Since Mr. Korteweg has been confronted with a most tragic loss—his wife's demise—he has become strongly attached to his collection of lizards. If they are symbols of eternity as he believes, these reptiles enable him to regain control: presuming their immortality, he only has to take care of them properly and his duty is fulfilled. If everything runs smoothly, the obsessive neurotic can display an air of inviolability. Once a situation becomes uncontrollable, however, he can retort to so-called acting out, which is defined as 'an identification with the symptom' (Žižek *Looking*, 139). The symptom can be considered a ciphered message that requires interpretation: trying to cope with human mortality, the lizards function as a substitute for his wife's death. She has passed away, but these animals will live, forever.

The status of the reptiles as the ideal alternative shifts after the assault, for his concern for them has indirectly caused the horrific fate met by the Steenwijks. Mr. Korteweg is confronted with an unbearable burden of guilt, and his act of destruction is an attempt to get rid of this burden. Of course, the attempt is in vain, and he undoubtedly knows this, but his act is basically to confess his guilt complex to the big Other, this abstract anonymous collective. In killing the symbols of eternity, he hopes to honour a certain debt to the unfortunate Steenwijks. Mr. Korteweg sacrifices his lizards, which have lost their sublime value and have turned into ordinary reptiles, to acknowledge his irrecoverable guilt. His acting out does not solve anything but only aggravates his despair. A man with a compulsive disorder typically asks himself: Am I alive or am I dead? (Schokker and Schokker, 240), but the answer to this question here can only tip in favour of the latter. The moral obligation to destroy his beloved animals signifies Mr. Korteweg's symbolic death: the aftermath of the assault has made him a dead man walking. His official, biological death by suicide is in fact no more than a formality.[2]

An obsessive neurotic does not necessarily meet an unfortunate fate. Take butler Haneveld from De laatste dagen van Emma Blank [The Last Days of Emma Blank] (Alex van Warmerdam, 2010), discussed in my previous study on Dutch film (289-290). Van Warmerdam's films usually have a slightly bizarre starting point, and though every new development follows logically from this first act, the situation remains slightly odd throughout. Haneveld is an utterly docile character, strictly obeying Madame's orders. If Emma wants him to wear a moustache, he buys some fake exemplars and expects her to pick the most suitable one. But then there is a bizarre twist, for it turns out that Haneveld is actually Madame's husband, merely playing the role of butler. Other family members are also acting a part: Emma's sister is the cook; Emma's daughter plays the maid, and Emma's brother is the dog. Since they presume that Emma, quite a drama queen, is on the verge of dying and has a large heritage to share, the family members have voluntarily decided to role-play, for they think it pleases her. Then Emma reveals that there is hardly any capital left and she is not ill either. The family members are not pleasantly surprised by the good news about Emma's physical condition, but they become angry due to their wrong assumptions. And since they had translated these assumptions into a demand of the Other—'we think that Emma wants us to act these stupid roles, so let's do her this favour in her last days'—they take revenge on her for this demand she never made herself but which sprang from their own imagination.

Probably, Haneveld had had to endure the capricious commands of his wife during his many years of marriage. As a husband, he was always already her butler in a sense, but a limit was transgressed when he has deliberately agreed to the submissive role as butler: he cannot take it anymore. Emma made demands upon him since he was her husband, but it is an entirely different thing that his choice to play butler accrued from the demand of the Other: Emma did not ask them anything, but Haneveld as well as the other family members believed they were paying her due respect by apparently misreading signs regarding her health. One can either obey or resist a concrete injunction, but an inadequate interpretation of a demand of the Other can only result in acting out. When Emma falls to the ground, she is nailed to the floor and is only given a few sips of water to prevent her from dying of dehydration. When she eventually dies, the husband-butler yells at her that they gave her water 'out of goodness'. As an obsessive neurotic, Haneveld was perfect in fulfilling his 'job' as husband, acting according to precise instructions. But when he turns this 'job' into an obvious charade, the submissive role becomes a role of submission that unleashes repressed anger: his meek behaviour gives way to violent acting out.

Elaborating on this aforementioned notion of an identification with the symptom, this chapter will examine a series of obsessive neurotic, hysteric, perverse characters, covering a variety of titles from ELINE VERE (Harry Kümel, 1991) and BLACK BUTTERFLIES (Paula van der Oest, 2011) to PENTIMENTO (Frans Zwartjes, 1979) and BRIMSTONE (Martin Koolhoven, 2016).

PORTRAIT OF A LADY: *ELINE VERE*

Eline Vere, the title heroine in Harry Kümel's 1991 adaptation of Louis Couperus's 1990 literary classic, can be considered the best-known hysteric in Dutch literature.[3] A female hysteric wonders about the desire of the Other and asks herself questions such as: Who am I for the gaze of the Other? and more specifically, What does it mean to be a woman? (Schokker and Schokker, 240). In Kümel's excellent film—though most critics were not enthusiastic—Eline is torn between the strict conventions of the upper-class bourgeoisie in The Hague and her inarticulate longings. A hysteric requires the presence of a 'master' who tells her what kind of object she is for the desire of the Other. Is Eline in search of such a 'master', and if so, who is a likely candidate?

Eline, in her early twenties, lives in the residence of her older sister Betsy who is an impeccable representative of the local high society. In these circles, in which French terms are used frequently, Betsy attends the many *soirées* (evening party's), visits the theatre with *tableaux vivant* performances, and is fond of looking for the perfect crockery, as the ultimate sign that a woman has settled down successfully. In the eyes of her sister, Eline is a capricious woman and her regular headaches are an excuse for missing important events. In one of the earliest scenes, Eline asks Henk van Raat, married to her sister: 'Do you also dislike me?' On the one hand, this question is a clear hint that she knows that Betsy is not fond of her. On the other hand, it indicates that she thinks it is important that she is liked, although, as is typical for the hysteric's ambivalence, she does not make efforts to become popular. Many people expect the ravishing Eline to find a husband soon, including Henk's old mother, Mrs. van Raat, who has a huge photo collection of all her relatives in which Eline occupies a central place. Eline has set her eyes on Fabrice, a brilliant baritone from Brussels. She has a series of photographs of him in which he is dressed up as an exotic man, and she has seen him in The Hague with his hat and his red shawl for his face. She visits the opera, albeit much too late, and after the performance, Fabrice throws her a rose. She is so thrilled that she loses her fan. Later she receives a phonograph for her birthday and can listen to Fabrice's beautiful voice, which further triggers her desire for the artist.

While she comes under the spell of the singer, Eline's nephew Vincent, a true globetrotter, has shown up in The Hague unannounced. In a conversation with Henk's brother Paul, Eline is annoyed that he calls Vincent a 'peculiar fellow' simply because he does not abide by their rules of decency. In the opera, Vincent is talked about as a 'bête noire', a black sheep in the community, but Eline has a problem with their prejudices. Vincent tells her that he is not an expert on Fabrice's music, but 'as a man he is a medicine for love', meaning that the man is ugly. When he takes Eline to another opera evening, he lends her his binoculars and she is shocked: Fabrice is 'unprepossessing', according to her. Vincent helps her to recover by using her new fan, which she had received anonymously. It was a present from Otto van Erlevoort, Vincent reveals, for it is obvious that he adores Eline. Encouraged by these words, Otto soon becomes Eline's fiancé, for by now Vincent has taken the place of her 'master', in spite of—or perhaps thanks to—the many warnings against him. Whereas everyone is pleased with her choice for the punctual Otto, Vincent tells her that he doubts her happiness: you do not really want him, but you think it is preordained. And indeed, after some time, Eline complains that Otto's perpetual calmness suffocates her. Her despair is shown via a written letter, alternated with dissolves of photos of the couple, a zoom-in of her open mouth that initially is silent but becomes a long scream, and a mirror shot that multiplies her appearance.

Later, the pattern repeats itself when she is sent to Aunt Elise in Brussels. She not only meets Vincent again but also his American friend, Lawrence St. Clare, a lover of Walt Whitman poetry. Vincent praises Lawrence as noble and masculine, and Eline guesses that her nephew knows the way to her heart: the American might be the man for her. The three of them visit the Temple of Human Passions. In separate shots, we see that the black gloves of both Vincent and Lawrence grope the great white sculptures. The men have plans to go to Russia, but when they postpone their trip, Eline presumes that Lawrence might fancy her. Vincent tells Eline that Lawrence is not her ticket to happiness, but it only dawns on her when she overhears Uncle Daniel in a conversation with his wife Elise: 'I do not want my niece misused to mask their decadent games', a clear allusion to homoerotic desires.

In ELINE VERE, the title heroine turns her back on the rules and regulations of society. Her tendency to defend the outcast Vincent against scornful remarks affirms her isolation. She starts to depend upon her nephew to teach how and what to desire, but his advices function as a smokescreen for her. She has put him in the position of an authority on love. She wants him to give a verbal sketch of a potential lover, but he then downplays the selected man to such an extent that he becomes liable to the accusation that Vincent is jealous of any candidate with whom she associates herself. Thus, whereas she is expecting him to articulate her desires, Vincent as 'master' disappoints her time and again. If Vincent is her guide to help her answer the question what kind of object she is for the desire of the Other, he only gives evidence of his incapacity. While Eline was always prepared to defend her nephew against nasty chitchat, he in fact contributes to her confusion. She expels him from her life and returns to The Hague, addicted to morphine. She goes to the opera once more, but when she is in her box, all eyes are transfixed upon her—or she hallucinates that everyone is watching her, which is a more likely scenario. If a hysteric typically asks 'who am I for the desire of the Other?', the looks of the audience provide a concrete answer. In the beginning of the film, Eline asks Henk whether he disliked her as her sister did, and now it has definitely entered her mind that everyone casts a glance of contempt at her. She can no longer hide behind her fan and runs away from the opera, while the music continues to 'haunt' her. Back home, she overdoses herself and puts a small photograph of Otto in her mouth.

On the one hand, Kümel's ELINE VERE is shot like a classic melodrama, with its opera music (as performance on a stage and on the soundtrack), its lush cinematography, and its grandiose shot compositions—the copious hunting meal or the fancy *soirées* with the dressed-up guests—that function as a substitute for the subdued emotions. On the other hand, details stand out that exceed this bourgeois environment in which people keep up appearances. It can be taken as an act of resistance that Eline dies, very unceremoniously, with her mouth slightly agape and a tiny portrait of Otto on her tongue. Moreover, in general, the camera movements are smooth, but sometimes they seem deliberately unstable as if in support of the idea that a strict adherence to decorum is stifling: in one scene, Vincent is scrutinizing one of Eline's photo albums and a jerky camera tilts up towards a white curtain and then suddenly down to a collection of books. Outstanding are the film's many mirror shots, and to accentuate Eline's confusion, her face is sometimes multiplied in more than one mirror. But in a moment of despair, she falls on the ground in bad weather, and we then see Vincent's face mirrored in a puddle. The fact that his face is reflected in a dirty pool of water functions as a commentary upon Eline's choice for Vincent as her 'ideal master'. He was an outcast to the decadent circles in which Eline's older sister, the mothering Betsy, feels very much at ease. Instead of teaching her how to desire, Vincent's often ironic words of praise, taken by her as recommendations, lead her astray.

RUNAWAY 'MOTHER': *NADINE*

A typical hysterical scenario has it that a woman wants a trustworthy male guide as a reaction to a strong identification with her mother. She has heard the many grievances of her mother repetitively: contrary to her expectations, her husband has embarrassing weaknesses. Rather than a man who was supposed to be the symbolic bearer of authority, the father postpones repairing the kitchen, he does not take decisions, he spends too much time in a bar with friends, et cetera. A daughter's bond with her father is not without compassion: she dearly hopes he will improve his skills or at least cover his flaws so that mother no longer has any reason to complain about him. A daughter can choose to excel at one of her father's weaknesses: she can learn how to repair the kitchen or she can develop the habit of acting decisively. And in order not to become a complainant herself, she can either try to find a man without weaknesses—good luck with that—or she can sacrifice herself by taking up a 'masculine' role herself so that her partner is relieved from that duty. In the drama / road movie NADINE (Erik de Bruyn, 2007), the title heroine seems on the brink of a white-picket-fence life, but this does not pan out.

NADINE is shot in an atemporal fashion, with the main character played by three different actresses to underscore some pivotal ruptures in her life. In the beginning, Nadine, in her early forties, meets her ex-lover Daniel in a supermarket, with his child Sam in a Maxi-Cosi. She secretly steals the baby, and we follow her on her trip by car all the way to Portugal. The journey is intercut with earlier episodes in the life of Nadine which have the status of her reminiscences. One scene concerns a farewell after her parents have visited her. Her mother is lecturing Nadine: 'You know Chantal, she's starting another company and she's getting married, too. So, that's also a possibility. But then again, you will probably do it all your own way, like always, right?' This one quote neatly summarizes the mother-daughter relationship. We know Nadine has a career as a graphic designer, so what principally piques the mother is that Nadine has no partner yet—and that she herself has no prospect of becoming a grandmother soon. But the addition of the words 'like always' reveals that Nadine is never ever able to satisfy her mother. While the mother is already close to the parked car, father halts to give his daughter a present. Probably the mother had been so dominant during their visit that he did not have the chance to offer it to her at an earlier and more convenient moment. As the mother remains in the background positioned between father and daughter, both in the foreground, to emphasize that she is an obstacle in the father-daughter bond, Nadine unpacks the gift, *The Meditations of Marcus Aurelius*. He points her to the following quote: 'The unripe grape, the ripe bunch, the dried grape, all are changes, not into nothing, but into something which exists not yet.'

Whereas Nadine's mother opts for solidity and permanence—marriage, everlasting conventions—the father teaches her the value of constant transitions. After the mother has expressed her impatience at her husband—'why do you give this present outside, and not inside'—the father steps into the car and drives away at a reckless speed. His frustration has fatal consequences, as a later reminiscence reveals: mother dies in the car accident, father ends up in a rehabilitation centre, but can barely speak anymore. Upon hearing of his passing away eventually, she has a flashback of her father teaching her how to shoot—his favourite masculine pastime—but despite this tough hobby, it was clear that Nadine's mother wore the pants in the family and that he was the weakling. The death of her parents ends the phase of Nadine as an 'unripe grape': she has had a one-night stand with a rock singer, but when she realizes he is a narcissist, she decides to have an abortion. When Nadine is about to turn 37, a different, blonde-haired actress will play her part. Never having met the right guy—which is no wonder with her mother complaining constantly about her husband—she wants to be artificially inseminated. And right then, she is in the chair of her dentist Daniel, who suggests he wants to see her again, next week, which is the beginning of their relationship. As she phones him that it is the perfect time of the month, he is in a bar and has set his eyes on a lascivious woman singing in French. Long story short: Nadine does not get pregnant, and we then realize what the frequently repeated out-of-focus shot of Daniel means: she has just witnessed her boyfriend kissing Aimee, with a pregnant belly, on the street. She ends the relationship on the spot, with a hysterical bolt of anger, which is also the end of Nadine as a 'ripe bunch'.

The perfect man did not turn out to be the perfect man for her, and Nadine, a 'dried grape' by now, played by a third actress, takes revenge upon Daniel. On the run with his baby Sam, whom she renames Bobby, she has left the parents in despair. When they declare a missing child, the police tell them that they are making a grave accusation, since there is nothing to see on the security cameras. When Nadine eventually returns from Portugal to the Netherlands, she brings back the baby to the very same spot in the supermarket where she had taken the child, without anyone addressing her. It is a likely option that she has only imagined the entire trip with the child, which she made in order to feel like a woman, for once in her life.

It seems as if Nadine has gone to great pains to make up for her 'sweet' father's flaws in order to protect him against her mother's criticism. She has sacrificed herself to act as a masculine supplement to her daddy, as a classic hysteric, but after the death of her parents, she has set her mind on becoming a mother herself, a single mum if need be. To refer to *The Meditations by Marcus Aurelius*, this means that the ripe bunch turned into a dried raisin. If that were all, it would be a perspective adopted by Nadine's mother: marry and raise kids before it is too late. But the quote, as the father teaches his daughter, continues with stating that every phase entails a productive change, so that also the dried raisin is not a failure but has the promise of something that has yet to come into existence. If Nadine is able to put this wisdom into practice, she might overcome hysteria.

CALL ME BY MY—NOT YOUR—NAME: *BLACK BUTTERFLIES*

If a classic case of hysteria is the consequence of a daughter trying to mask the father's flaws for a dissatisfied mother, a too strong and authoritative father is a burden as well. In BLACK BUTTERFLIES (Paula van der Oest, 2011), a loose adaptation of the biography of the South-African poet Ingrid Jonker (1933-1965), the poet craves for the recognition of her father Abraham Jonker, an established writer and right-wing politician. Before the opening credits, a car arrives after Anna has told her younger sister Ingrid that grandma has died in her sleep. A man steps out of the car and tells the two girls: '*Just call me pa.*' After the prologue, we move seventeen years forward to Cape Town in 1960. BLACK BUTTERFLIES covers the last years in Ingrid's life, chronicling her bouts of depression, her love affairs, her stance against apartheid, the publication of her volume *Smoke and Ochre* with the help of some good friends, and her tour in Europe. Her experiences result in a number of poems, some written on the walls of her room, and we hear them recited regularly in Van der Oest's film.[4] Most relevant for selecting this film here is Ingrid's problematic relationship with her father who also happened to be the head of the censorship board in South Africa and responsible for the banning of the work of the black writer Nkosi Shosani, whom Ingrid befriends before he exiles himself to Paris.

Ingrid has many a quarrel with her dad, for she does not share his views, neither on a political level nor on a personal. Her father wants her to continue her marriage to the 'good man' Pieter, father of Ingrid's daughter Simone, but she is adamant on separating her husband. She had only married him at the time, she discloses at one point, to '*get out of my father's house*'. Meanwhile Ingrid has met the writer Jack Cope who had saved her from drowning. Jack is also in the process of a '*messy divorce*' but invites Ingrid and Simone to live at his place. Ingrid's father is scornful of Jack when he comes to dinner at his place: '*For some reason I thought you would be younger*', hinting at the difference in age between the two lovers. Moreover, he thinks Jack's latest story about a black man coming to the rescue of a white boy '*quite manipulative*', and adds to this: '*Fortunately for us, blacks cannot grasp allegorical writing.*' After a few more embarrassing remarks by her father, Ingrid goes to her old room. As her father enters, she says: '*You take pleasure in upsetting me*', to which he replies: '*It's mutual.*' Ingrid says that she dedicated her book to him, but he did not say anything about it. '*It's me in those words, pa. Don't you want to know who I am?*' He calmly answers: '*I know who you are. You are your mother.*'

Ingrid is in a permanent competition with her father—'*he does not write novels, he writes books*', she sneers—and she dearly wants to be acknowledged by him as a serious writer herself. But he only makes contemptuous remarks in return: the only reason why *The Sunday Times* had an interview with you, slanting me, is because you are my daughter. Ingrid asks him to read aloud a first draft of the poem *Die Kind* that will eventually gain her a place in history, but he cannot even finish it and tears the piece of paper in small pieces. '*Don't worry, pa*', she says, for she has it all inside her head. After the publication of *Smoke and Ochre*, she is ecstatic that she is awarded an important literary prize in Johannesburg. She guesses she will finally gain her father's respect and requests him to fly with her, but his response is scathing:

> *I wanted to ban the book, but my colleagues convinced me otherwise, not because they believed it had any artistic value, but because of the scandal it would have caused, considering I'm your father. 'My blood child lies in the gutter.' That's disgusting. 'I am with those who abuse sex?' You can say that again. According to my sources, you are having sexual relations with everyone and anyone. (...) I'm the laughingstock of parliament because of you. You're a slut. I never want to see you again.*

The problem with Ingrid's father is that he never admits the slightest bit of weakness: he takes a position as if he is the representative of symbolic law, but he does not acknowledge the impossibility of this position. Her father suffocates her because he ignores the necessary split between father and symbolic patriarch, which is at the heart of Freud's well-known fable of the primal horde in *Totem and Taboo*. To briefly recapitulate (from chapter 2): there is the primordial, narcissistic father who is so authoritative that his sons murder him, but they construct a symbolic position in memory of the dead patriarch. They agree to it that no individual can embody this position, so that the dead-symbolic father becomes a new and impregnable obstacle. Any father gains authority 'insofar as he accepts that it is not himself, but the big Other who speaks through him, in his words' (Žižek *Interrogating*, 289). He is not strong himself, but he derives his strength and authority from 'his identification with the "dead letter" of the symbolic mandate' (ibid.).

Since the place of symbolic law is constitutively unoccupied, a man at best acts as a representative of this law, as a supreme ventriloquist. This is precisely the problem with Abraham Jonker: he is not just like the primordial father who leaves no breathing space for others, but in addition to that, he also pretends to speak from the empty place of authority. He is nothing less than a pretentious impostor, but despite all Ingrid's attempts to make him recognize her achievements, he can only humiliate her time and again. In his eyes, she is only his daughter, doomed to remain in his shadow. Upon her death by drowning, the newspaper headline confirms his paternal authority, since it describes Ingrid as '*daughter of M.P.*' (member of parliament).

Thus, in the case of Nadine, she disavowed the gap between her actual father, who was always under her mother's thumb, and his guise as the dead-symbolic authority. This gap is part of a 'normal' trajectory, though a classic hysteric cannot accept it. By contrast, in the case of Ingrid Jonker, she undergoes her most severe crises every time her father refuses to acknowledge the gap: he does not speak on behalf of the law, he pretends to be the law. Many people respect Ingrid because of her tireless efforts to speak out in poetic lines; and she is even deeply loved by colleague writers. With a father like Abraham Jonker, who considers himself infallible, she apparently deems it impossible to gain any self-esteem, and her continuous dedication to making him proud only frustrates her. To compensate for this frustration, she puts increasing demands upon her lovers. Both Jack Cope and Eugene Maritz will give up on her with the very same phrase: '*You drain me*.' Since no one can help her break her father's pretentious stance, she has Jack read Walt Whitman's poem *Good-bye My Fancy* as a note of farewell. The two of them had met when

Jack saved her from drowning, but this time, she can no longer be saved and drowns herself.

In BLACK BUTTERFLIES, the shadow of Ingrid's father looms large over the daughter to such an extent that she is eclipsed permanently despite her repetitive calls to him: 'I want you to see me. Is it not your desire to see your daughter prosper?' A hysteric wants to make her/his desire compatible with the 'desire of the Other'. This requires that the hysteric discovers the weak spot in the Other so she/he can take the attitude: 'I am prepared to satisfy this desire of the Other.' The problem for Ingrid is that her father assumes the position of the Great Pretender, as if any desire is fulfilled already. He refuses to admit any weakness, since he takes the false pose of embodying the symbolic law: 'I want nothing from you, since I am an incontestable patriarch, period.'

A WALKING CONTRADICTION WITH PRUSSIAN SOUR: *MYSTERIES*

A hysteric suffers from a lack of symbolic recognition, as if she is One-Too-Many. Because her father treats Ingrid like thin air, as if everything she does is worthless, she turns to other men she admires. Despite the fact that they both admire and love her, she asks too much of them—she drains them—so that once again, she is One-Too-Many. The self-doubt of the hysteric usually expresses itself in ambivalent and confused feelings ('What does she want?'), whereas the neurotic is in permanent doubt whether his/her decisions are right or not.

One of the oddest films in the history of Dutch cinema is the unduly neglected MYSTERIES (Paul de Lussanet, 1978), which is almost a textbook case of a male neurotic. It is weird, but for that very reason, it is also fascinating. To start with, MYSTERIES, shot on the Isle of Man, has a most promising cast—Rutger Hauer and Sylvia Kristel in the main roles, substantial roles for David Rappaport as the midget Minuut, and for Rita Tushingham, best known for the British kitchen-sink classic A TASTE OF HONEY (Tony Richardson, 1961), as well as a fine cameo by French actress Andréa Ferréol, known for among others LA GRANDE BOUFFE [THE BIG FEAST] (Marco Ferreri, 1973) and DESPAIR (Rainer Werner Fassbinder, 1978). Moreover, the famous Dutch singer Liesbeth List has a rare acting part, performing Händel's 'Lascia ch'io pianga'. But like the novel it is based upon, *Mysterier* [*Mysteries*] (1892) by Norwegian writer Knut Hamsun, De Lussanet's film is incomprehensible, in spite of the fact that its storytelling is conventional. There is extensive voice-over narration by the dwarf Minuut, who tells us that the arrival of Johan Nagel in the winter of 1891 in a sleepy provincial town on an island brought about a chain of remarkable events. But Minuut immediately raises a number of questions: was Nagel's presence related to the death of Karlsen? And if so, had he come to take vengeance upon his death? No one, the voice-over continues, will be able to give an answer to these questions. In the opening scene we had seen this man Karlsen—a cameo by Peter Faber—running around in despair in an open field. He falls flat on his face in the mud, accompanied by Minuut's voice-over: 'his wrists cut, that ninny, because he was rejected by Dany, the reverend's beautiful daughter.'

In his *The Roots of Modernist Narrative*, Martin Humpal points out that critics have often misread Hamsun's novel because they refuse to accept that it is deliberately incoherent. According to him, *Mysterier* can best be regarded as a decoy: the novel is presented as a realist narrative with an omniscient narrator and the features of a detective mystery. When there are riddles regarding the motivations and behaviour of the characters, the enigmas are usually solved, as befits a detective. There is nothing of the kind, however, in *Mysterier*. Hamsun's book is puzzling from the start and remains so until the very end. According to Humpal, *Mysterier* was Hamsun's reaction to the then widespread 'belief in scientific positivism' (124). Nonetheless, contemporary critics started to fill in the plentiful gaps in an attempt to read the text as an organic unity, ignoring the absence of a clear dénouement and its transgression of a consistent psychology. The novel's incoherence, Humpal argues, was meant to present man as an 'incomprehensible question mark' (116). Its disjointedness serves to indicate that the human mind works in complex and mysterious ways.

If fidelity usually works as a recommendation for an adaptation, De Lussanet's film is so odd because, paradoxically, it is quite faithful to Hamsun's novel, except for the ending. And that means that the film looks like a fairly realistic period drama about the newcomer in this settlement with a pier and a rough sea, the man who calls himself 'Johan Nagel, agronomist'. He moves into the local hotel and explores the town accurately, 'as if he discovered details that we had always neglected carelessly', according to Minuut's voice-over. But the midget continues: 'Whatever he was searching for, he did not find it. Was he suffering from an incurable disease and had he picked our insignificant town to die, intoxicated by an all-consuming love? He had a small bottle of Prussian sour with him, of 90 per cent.'

This voice-over is exemplary of the film: its tone is explanatory, but in the end, Minuut hardly conveys any substantial information. He quotes the innkeeper who mentions the strange light in Nagel's eyes, and the dwarf already announces that the man's mysterious disappearance had an impact upon the community, 'as if a devilish spirit had taken us'. It is not very consistent that Minuut goes on to say that 'the events' had practically been forgotten by the townspeople, 'except for the two women who have so shamefully deceived him'. First, how does Minuut know that these women keep thinking about him? Do they tell him this? Is it legitimate to claim that the women have shamefully deceived him? And is Minuut himself among the townspeople who can no longer remember the events, but if so, how can he tell the story of the couple of months that Nagel was around? These questions may seem a trifle, but it captures in a nutshell the oddity of MYSTERIES as such: the film is not even slightly experimental, but the slices of information, both visually and by voice-over commentary, are enigmatic rather than instructive.

The main protagonist Nagel is a highly eccentric character. He wears the same yellow suit every day, he carries a violin case, but it only contains soiled clothes. He claims he cannot play the instrument, but when he borrows a violin during a fancy fair, the audience admires his musicality, though Minuut comments in voice-over that 'his friend's injured soul' resonated in the melody. Nagel started to play the violin to impress the ravishing, grey-green-eyed Dany Kielland, who often wears a red parasol. A piece of paper found in the mouth of the dead Karlsen referred to her reluctance towards men: 'May the blade of your knife cut as sharp as your final no.' Nagel is fascinated by the quote and has come under the spell of Dany. His frequent attempts to contact her embarrass her, though she tries to remain polite.

In the best of scenes in MYSTERIES, shot by 'master of light' Robby Müller,[5] the characters are dwarfed against the forested hills and the rough sea. In combination, such mise-en-scène suggests both the impenetrability of their psyche and their emotional turmoil. The latter is clear, for it is obvious that he is infatuated with Dany. The incessant barking of her dog indicates that he is even around her place at night. At one point, we see Nagel stare back at the dog, and it is easy to make the calculation afterwards: he brags that he has tested his Prussian sour at an animal successfully; he has been bitten in his hand; Dany comes to the hotel to complain that her dog has been poisoned.

On the one hand, Nagel seems every inch a gentleman. He is pleasant company for the ladies who invite him for social events. He is most kind to Minuut whom he prefers to call by his actual name, Mr. Grogaard: when the midget is bullied in the local bar, he stands up for him and he orders a tailored suit for him. Minuut will confirm in one of his voice-overs that no one has ever been that kind to him. On the other hand, Nagel is a 'walking contradiction', as he himself confesses. Madly in love with Dany, he is capable of vile acts, as the death of the dog illustrates. 'Pardon me', he explains Dany, 'but this race has such a disgusting, human expression. It looks at you as if you are to blame for the suffering of mankind.' Moreover, he speaks ill of Dany, but he says, it is out of pure love. Since he cannot have her, he degrades her in order to comfort himself. And later he will also turn against Minuut. The dwarf had replaced Nagel's Prussian sour with water, and thus the man's attempt at suicide fails. In public, he starts to insult Minuut—'you detest me with your goodness; you are a cheat'—and accuses him of having murdered Karlsen.

Even more peculiar is Nagel's behaviour towards Martha Gude, who lives as a hermit in a small cottage by the sea. Minuut describes her as his only female friend but will not disclose what grief has turned her hair so white. Nagel murmurs to himself that he wants to help her, but as the voice-over adds: he did not know how. When he visits her cottage, he introduces himself as an antique collector. He wants to buy an old chair with broken legs and offers her 200 guilders. Martha wants to give him the chair for free, but he insists on paying her the sum. Since there is no 'deal', there is a cooling-off period of two days, but she has to promise him that she will not sell the treasure to anyone else.

When an old flame visits Nagel in the hotel, he tells this Kamma, an 'elegant lady from the city' according to Minuut, that he will give her money on the condition that she pays a visit to Martha Gude to purchase the chair for 400 guilders. If the '*timidly looking*' woman, with '*eyes like glowing coal*' (Nagel's description) refuses, Kamma will have to ask the captain on her return journey to sound the boat's horn five times. When Nagel hears the horn, he whispers 'little devil', and during his subsequent visit, Martha once again offers her the chair for free. 'Miss Gude, do you want to anger me? Soon you will be asking 500 guilders. What kind of game are you playing?' She then agrees that he pay her three guilders, and when he leaves the cottage with the chair, she runs after him, since he has given her way too much money. But, Nagel replies, now she has sufficient money to buy a dress for the fancy fair: 'A little bit of joy will do you good.'

Nagel's reasons are unfathomable, however: Does he need female company to attend the fancy fair? Is Martha only an excuse to see Dany who performs as a goddess in a *tableau vivant*? After Dany humiliates him by telling everyone that he had poisoned the dog and that Nagel's real name is 'Simonsen, plain Si-mon-sen', he proposes marriage to Martha that evening. 'It does not matter that you are a bit older.' She hesitates and in the end she accepts the proposal, but the next day she reconsiders her decision: 'I am afraid it is not possible ... I am not that much in love with you.' Nagel is convinced that Dany has advised her against the marriage, but he assures Martha that he does not want to deceive her.

In the next scene, we see Nagel climbing uphill and he jumps over a rock, while Dany passes by on a path that is higher than Nagel's position. While he sees that Dany loses a white handkerchief, we hear Minuut's voice-over, accompanied by one of the compositions by Laurens van Rooyen, which walk the middle ground between 'light' and classical music. 'The cruel manner she rejected him, chilled Nagel to the bone ... It was Dany, that snake, who had been spewing her venom in his gullible heart. Nagel's final chance to happiness and calmness had gone.' Dany's handkerchief in his hand, Nagel lies down in the grass and after screaming 'Dany, I hate you', he empties the bottle of Prussian sour. There is a cut to the landscape and then the camera starts to pan to the left. First, we see the handkerchief and then Nagel who realizes he is not dead: 'Goddammit, who has been messing with my bottle? Who?' (We may remember that Minuut had brought him back the bottle a couple of scenes earlier). Nagel starts to laugh out loud and goes back to Martha's cottage: it is completely abandoned.

Back in town, he approaches Dany and asks her to give a letter to Martha, for he thinks she knows her whereabouts. After insulting Minuut and accusing him of killing Karlsen, the midget runs away: 'Grogaard, come back, I do not know what I am saying.' Nagel locks himself in his hotel room and starts to suffer from delirium. In his frenzy, he also sees Dany as a goddess in the lantern light at his hotel. One night, Nagel jumps into the water, never to be seen again. Minuut's voice-over: 'I had to do something. For the first time in his life, Minuut, the ridiculous dwarf, decided to act.' When Dany passes by on a path in the forest, he throws Prussian sour in her face. Minuut will be sentenced to three years in prison, but 'I have not regretted my act for one minute. Sometimes I see the two women walk in town, the two who are guilty at his death; the white-haired out of gullibility, the other out of sheer dissipation.' In the final shot, both Martha and Dany walk towards the pier, the latter with a black veil to cover her disfigured face.

MYSTERIES makes extensive use of voice-over, usually taken as a flaw, since extradiegetic words are a superfluous supplement to the images and sounds. The voice-over in MYSTERIES, however, is not by a detached observer giving an overview of situations—the narrator is a marginal but nonetheless crucial character. As is often the case in a melodrama, the actions are restrained and the emotions by characters are not externalized. Dany is most of the time striking a pose rather than acting, and even when her dog is poisoned, her voice is soft rather than harsh. Nagel pays social visits, attends the cemetery where Karlsen is buried, tries to make a deal with Martha, and attempts to seduce Dany, among others by impressing the audience with a violin. Insofar as there are actions, they are subdued, except for Nagel's quarrel with the Chief Constable and Minuut's late attack on Dany. In a melodrama, the mise-en-scène works as a substitute: a tense situation is indicated by a shelf of china in the room or an excessive use of the colour red; a discord between characters is expressed by positioning a character in the dark, behind the bannister of a staircase or framed between a doorpost. The viewer has to take the shot compositions into account in order to read the inner conflicts of characters. By contrast, in MYSTERIES, Minuut mediates all the seminal scenes, but his words are a clearly biased interpretation of the events. He describes Dany as a 'devil' and a 'snake', although we never see any visual or other evidence of Dany's malign side. Moreover, Minuut never talks about his own personal background; his voice-over only addresses the sorry fate of Nagel, who in the eyes of Minuut is the victim of two conspiring women.

MYSTERIES is a forgotten movie in Dutch history, and it is easy to understand why. De Lussanet's film looks like a melodramatic costume drama, but it does not conform to the rules of classic causality. If one is not familiar with Hamsun's deliberately incoherent novel, it seems as if De Lussanet, a painter by profession, has not heard of the basics of cinematic storytelling. On top of that, it may be tempting to disqualify the film as misogynistic, for its internal narrator can only describe women as serpents, bent on destructing men. Two caveats have to made, though. First, due to his extreme short stature, Minuut, who also acts as the local fool for money, is not a love interest for women. Neglected by the other sex, he may hold a grudge against them. Second, Minuut totally identifies with the sensibilities of Nagel, who acts as his benefactor. The focus of the midget is selective, however: he hardly mentions that most women in the community regard Nagel as a charming albeit peculiar man, but he emphasizes that Dany, and to a minor extent Martha, are femme fatales. It is striking that the midget claims time and again that no one, including himself, could fathom Nagel's motivations for coming to this town. Nonetheless, Minuut is certain of one thing: Nagel will meet the same poor destiny as the unfortunate Karlsen, for a woman like Dany will lead any man to the brink of lunacy.

Because of its partisan narrator, MYSTERIES is to be seen through a grid of misogyny, but in order to appreciate De Lussanet's film as a little gem, we have to take this grid as a smokescreen. MYSTERIES displays a conspicuous discord between its auditive track (the voice-over presenting Dany as a cunning creature) and the visual track: we see how Dany tolerates Nagel's intrusive behaviour and calmly points out that she already has a fiancé. Minuut calls her a 'snake', but this is not punctuated by any of the scenes: in fact, her more than justified complaint about her poisoned dog is a token of her politeness. My main point, however, is that this discord between an auditive track and a visual track has an analogy with a discord between the symbolic and the imaginary that characterizes an obsessive compulsive disorder like the neurotic Nagel.

A neurotic presumes that the Other is enjoying the fact that he has had to make the sacrifice of his 'being'. The question 'what does the Other want from me?' has a disconcerting answer for the neurotic: nothing, for in the fantasy of the neurotic, everything is already available to the Other (Schokker and Schokker, 240). A neurotic will think that he is suffering, and the Other is enjoying the best of lives. He does not see the lack in the Other, and it piques him that the Other has no reason to desire anything from him, that he cannot be of any value to the Other. In the perception of the neurotic, the Other wants to suck him dry just for the sake of it. The Other makes demands, but the neurotic believes the Other can get no satisfaction, since it is not in need of anything. Any gift is a vain and empty gesture, and as a consequence, the neurotic feels himself superfluous. Due to his redundancy, he cannot get rooted in the symbolic order: if it is impossible for him to contribute anything substantial to a social network, he compensates this with imaginary scenarios. Insofar as the townspeople think of Nagel as a bit deranged, his fantastic depictions, including his delirium near the end, are even more grandiose.

Walking with Dany in the forest, he starts to tell her an adventure that he has recently experienced. We then get a fantastic story about a sun-lit environment, a voice that calls his name, the sight of a beautiful young woman in a white dress (Dany), the sighs of a 'little monster' (Minuut), and a tower peopled with many angels without eyes. In another scene, in the company of the town's most important people, Dany encourages Nagel to tell a story, for 'we like to hear you chat; out here in the provinces, we are not used to a lot'. When Nagel mentions that he saw a rocky landscape, and the suspenseful music grows louder, everyone starts staring at a painting on the wall, as if they all know that it triggered Nagel's imagination. We see that Minuut is caught in bushel britches and Nagel liberates him from his awkward position, though it looks very much like a struggle between the two. Minuut spits on the ground and says that he was careful not to dirty Nagel's shoes with the blood dripping from his mouth. Why not? Nagel asks him, 'after all the harm I have done to you'. 'Thank you, for not hurting me more', Minuut says. The Chief Constable starts laughing in Nagel's face: 'Ha ha, what a pompous nonsense.' Doctor Stenersen immediately draws a parallel between Nagel and Karlsen, concluding that the latter's sensibility caused his death.

If MYSTERIES is an uneven and incoherent film, this is due to the fact that all narrative developments are based upon dubious assumptions. It is one thing that Nagel, as a neurotic, privileges his deranged scenarios over any attempt to secure for himself a place in the symbolic circuit, but on top of that, the narrator Minuut, telling the events in retrospect, totally identifies with the figments of Nagel's imagination. So, the one who is supposed to guide us through the story is at least as prejudiced towards women as the protagonist: maltreated as the local fool, Minuut is more ill-disposed towards his fellow citizens than his attitude suggests. And the midget holds a particular grudge against Dany; he thinks she sows the seeds of any man's downfall. This unshakeable conviction leads Minuut into avenging Nagel's fate.

A film set in the nineteenth century is usually concerned with social etiquette: characters are trying to keep up appearances. If a man is cheating on his wife, as in THE AGE OF INNOCENCE (Martin Scorsese, 1993), the wife pretends she is ignorant of the adultery. Hence, the story highlights the importance of keeping the symbolic order running smoothly, at all costs. By contrast, MYSTERIES is based upon a discrepancy between setting and story: apart from the incident that causes Dany's disfigured face, the social order in town continues as usual, but on the level of the story, the figments of imagination of both Nagel and his 'faithful' Minuut have taken precedence. Because the hierarchy between symbolic and imaginary is reversed, De Lussanet's MYSTERIES with its neurotic protagonist has become such a peculiar film.

MOTHER AND SON WITH CHAMPAGNE AND MOZART: *DE WITTE WAAN*

Let me compare the disguised strangeness of MYSTERIES to the deliberate oddity of Adriaan Ditvoorst's last feature DE WITTE WAAN [WHITE MADNESS] (1984), in which all main characters are slightly deranged. Lazlo is a painter who uses heroin regularly. He lives in an abandoned factory complex, with an old man acting as the 'porter' to the area. This man has been trying to invent a machine that should produce such a gigantic noise that silence will set in afterwards, or at least, 'my silence', he says. The beginning of DE WITTE WAAN stands out for its associative editing—with its zoom-ins on eyes; its frequent shots of eagles (on Lazlo's canvas, in the sky, as a stuffed animal); footage of cute white seals clubbed to death—and the film has a remarkable sound pattern as well. Lazlo has the habit of recording environmental noises, and we see Lazlo's mother on a theatre stage, but there is no applause. In a postponed reverse shot, we see that the auditorium is empty, however. In a later scene, mother is talking to a junkie staring at the sky, but we do not hear her voice. Shortly thereafter, we hear her speak to a visitor off-screen: 'You want coffee? With a liqueur?' It turns out she is talking to all kinds of objects in her house.

It is obvious in these first fifteen minutes that none of these three characters are rooted in 'reality'. Symptomatically, Lazlo asks his heroin dealer to recount his latest dream. Ditvoorst's style of editing and his sound design undergird the fact that an imaginary dimension presides over a symbolic one. All three—the mother, the son, the 'porter'—live isolated lives, though the mother has written a letter to Lazlo to establish contact. When she is on her way to put the letter in a mailbox, the camera pans to the right to show us some clean clothes on a washing line, while we hear the sounds of a terrible crash. A car has hit the mother on her bike. Lazlo's aunt, a half-sister of her mother, comes to warn him, but he chases her away disdainfully. Thanks to the porter's book that contains the name of only one other visitor, the aunt contacts Jasja, a former girlfriend of Lazlo. She goes to his place and says: 'Your mother is in pain.' His curt response is: 'At last.' Jasja concludes surprised: 'You really love her.' In the next shot, we see that she accompanies him in a cab to the hospital, but with a mean trick he steals the taxi and gets rid of Jasja. His mother has undergone surgery, and when he arrives at the hospital she hands him the letter. He is shocked to read its content.

In the remainder of DE WITTE WAAN, the bond between mother and son becomes gradually closer. He moves into her house, and while she is talking to herself in a mirror, he hangs over her. The two do everything to exclude the aunt who had set her mind on taking care of her half-sister. The car driver who caused the crash wants to visit the victim, but Lazlo does not permit him to enter. The most important intruder, however, is Lazlo's father whose authoritarian voice we hear at times, either in the son's mind or imitated by mother and son. Visually, the father is present as an enthusiastic jogger, as a figment of Lazlo's imagination, until he strangles his old man after the latter entered the house through an open window. After the father has been removed as an obstacle (most likely mental), Lazlo and his mother are ready for her final act. Dressed and made-up as a theatre diva, mother lies in a bed with satin sheets, surrounded by candles and flowers, and, according to the instructions in the letter, which we can partly read at the very end of the film, she has 'champagne and Mozart, on my birthday'.

Mother and son have cut all ties with a social network as if to reunite their former umbilical cord. Lazlo has found out his heroin dealer and the porter have died, the aunt and the car driver are out of sight, and his father has been 'strangled'. So without anybody left, it is all about mother and son. Adorned with symbolic accoutrements—candles, flowers, champagne, and Mozart—the son has created an imaginary scene according to her instructions. The viewer will remember that Lazlo was shocked when he read the letter, for it contains a clear demand to him, as her ultimate love object, in a reversal of a 'normal' mother-child relationship. Usually, a young child has innumerable requests to the mother—another present, another candy, another bedtime story, et cetera—and its ultimate aim is for the mother to fulfil them in order to prove her love to the child. In DE WITTE WAAN, however, the mother has written down a specific and nearly impossible request to the son containing the conditions for her suicide scene with the pills Lazlo has bought for her, and she ends her letter with the statement that she loves her son 'too much'. Strictly speaking, the mother's demand is so transgressive that by fulfilling it, the son proves the correctness of Jasja's conclusion: He must really love his mother to assist her in her 'love of dying'.[6]

As I argued, MYSTERIES, just like Hamsun's source text, displayed all the signs of a classic story and a conventional dénouement, but it did so to lead the reader/viewer astray. Those who find it hard to accept the deliberate incoherence despite its apparent psychological realism will be tempted to fill in narrative gaps. By contrast, the viewer of DE WITTE WAAN will expect an alienated perspective on account of a number of clues either at the start of the film or early in the movie: the director's reputation, the title ('waan' means delusion), Lazlo's use of heroin, the associative montage, the sound design. It will hardly surprise the viewer of Ditvoorst's film that conventional symbolic codes are marginalized at the expense of an imaginary scenario in which a son supports his mother to die out of love.

The mother in the film has no name, she is just 'mother', even in the credits, as if to accentuate her place in a symbolic network: her existence is entirely determined by her relation to Lazlo. The son has a name, but his father tended to simply call him 'Junior', as we can gather from the scenes in which the old man pops up as a spectral jogger or when Lazlo imitates his way of speaking. Hence, the son carries the name of the father, but the narrative trajectory of DE WITTE WAAN is to expel the father from their bond in order to create a pre-symbolic arena in which the suicide can take place. Such a pre-symbolic arena is, of course, an anomaly, for after one has entered the symbolic order, a point of no return has passed. DE WITTE WAAN is nonetheless motivated by the attempt to negate the Name-of-the-Father, and this implies a choice between *le père ou le pire*, or between 'I' and '*a*'. The foreclosure of the paternal metaphor triggers psychosis, as Lacan explained—though a psychosis can also be induced by Lazlo's use of heroin, to which the title 'white madness' seems to allude.[7]

UNRULY BEHAVIOUR: *PENTIMENTO* VERSUS *SPETTERS* AND *SHOWGIRLS*

The fate of much experimental cinema is that it only speaks to a small audience—Ditvoorst's DE WITTE WAAN attracted less than 2,000 filmgoers. The advantage of the limited number of spectators is that it is a self-selected group of viewers who, in general, can appreciate an unorthodox approach as 'poetic' or politically relevant. It is only on a rare occasion that viewers go to great pains to express their frustration and anger at marginal, experimental cinema. One such occasion was the release of PENTIMENTO (1979) by Frans Zwartjes, and in an interview he recalled the vehemence of the response, especially among feminists. When the film was screened in Rotterdam, some women shouted at Zwartjes that he should be forbidden by law from receiving a subsidy. And 'wherever that film was shown, they stormed the projection room in groups of ten, grabbed the projector and pitched it into the street, film and all. That

happened a couple of times' (qtd. in Abrahams, 206-207).

Practically any article or leaflet that mentions Zwartjes, no matter how brief, includes Susan Sontag's recommendation that he 'was the most important experimental filmmaker of his time'. Zwartjes had an incredible output between 1968 and 1974, when he made about thirty short films, and he counts SPARE BEDROOM (1969) and LIVING (1971) as his two best works. Moreover, LIVING had the distinguished honour of being selected for the Canon of Dutch Cinema in September 2007, a list that is restricted to only sixteen titles in total.[8] In LIVING, a fifteen-minute short, the filmmaker and his wife Trix, who have their faces painted white, explore a large empty apartment. In the most prominent shots, the camera, with its wide-angle lens, is close to the man's face, while his woman is visible over one of his shoulders. There are hardly any static shots; the majority of shots is jerky, for Zwartjes operated the camera himself. It has sudden low as well as high angles, and sometimes the camera goes upside down, which contributes to an overall distorted perspective. Given the fact that the short LIVING is part of the series HOME, SWEET HOME, it is ironic that there is never a moment of joy or excitement on the faces of the couple but rather amazement, anxiety, and panic. A few moments of extremely fast cutting add to the impression of alienation.

In the documentary DE GROTE TOVENAAR [THE GREAT MAGICIAN] (Ruud Monster, 2005), Zwartjes mentions that he was much inspired by the behaviour of psychiatric patients whom he had met when he worked a year as a male nurse at a clinic. They frankly spoke their mind, they urinated in a corridor, they heard noises no one else registered, or a former professor claimed he saw spirochetes in the nurse's eyes. Moreover, this professor told him that he was declared mad by a psychiatrist who had an affair with his wife and that the declaration was a convenient means to get rid of a rival. Zwartjes did not believe the story, but he also asked himself: why would it not be true? Intrigued by patients like this professor, Zwartjes chronicled so-called 'unruly behaviour' and 'deranged minds' in his films, provoking questions but leaving them unanswered: Could a weird phenomenon not be an audio-visual expression of a higher wisdom? Are what we describe as uninhibited acts or irregular patterns not products of repression?

The title of his controversial feature-length fiction PENTIMENTO refers to an art-historical process when an underlying image that had been painted over reappears. The title does not address anything specific in the film but is just an overall reading guide, for the series of scenes defy causality. PENTIMENTO has no dialogue, but it has electronic music on the soundtrack as well as a few unidentifiable off-screen voices, also via intercom. The film presents an uncanny world in which women are stripped naked and tortured in a ramshackle art deco spa by lab scientists, led by an Asian surgeon who perhaps, as some incoherent flashbacks suggest, was himself a victim of torture during World War II; this surgeon attacks stiletto shoes with a hockey stick; wearing a bowler hat, this doctor guards a woman in swimsuit who has to walk on all fours, with a thick rope tied to her neck; a man hunts for fish in shallow water while we hear ocean waves on the soundtrack; men and women are having an orgy with food and urine. Many of the episodes are intercut with one another, encouraging the viewer to establish connections, which, however, are far from obvious.

My aim with this brief description of PENTIMENTO is not to make sense of the provocative accumulation of scenes. The shooting was improvised, as is vintage Zwartjes, and the maker himself admitted that his editing was intuitive and not based on rational grounds. PENTIMENTO has to be taken as a sensory experience, emphasized by the grainy and gritty quality of the film's scenes and the use of an icy-blue filter. The film, 'infused with a grim atmosphere of claustrophobia' (Gocić), is an attempt to explore what lurks beneath the surface of a visible world. In that sense, PENTIMENTO is an 'underground' film that offers glimpses from the underground: it is no wonder that most scenes were not shot in broad daylight but at dusk or twilight. It is a commonly held opinion that the film is raw, dirty, nightmarish, and perverse, but how to qualify its dirty and perverse nature is open to debate. Such experimental cinema often straddles the thin line between radical politics and exploitation, and for those who ignore the form—its defiance of narrative coherence; its unorthodox alternation of scenes and style; its grainy and poorly lit images; the nerve-wrecking combination of sound and image—the 'perverse' shots of mistreated women may come across as despicable exploitation. Moreover, the term 'pentimento' does not indicate the world as it is or as it should be, but rather a world that has been hidden from sight. In the eyes of Zwartjes,

Western culture equals a veneer of social varnish, supposed to cover over dark impulses, and his cinema is meant to address the latter.[9]

For those feminists who believed that Zwartjes endorsed a misogynist worldview instead of offering a cultural critique, it was but a small step to SPETTERS (Paul Verhoeven, 1980), released a few months after PENTIMENTO. Verhoeven 's film was from their perspective probably equally perverse. The reception for this film was extremely hostile, as has been elaborately discussed in my previous study (*Humour and Irony*, 203-210), but I reiterate the case to compare SPETTERS with PENTIMENTO. His critics had judged SPETTERS as 'decadent, perverted, and sleazy', to quote Verhoeven's own words, and similar terms could be applied to Zwartjes' feature film. Despite this common denominator, their approaches differ significantly for three reasons. First, Zwartjes had the tendency to look at the world awry. Vincent van Gogh, he explained, painted wheat fields but always transformed them. Similarly, a filmmaker should not just record reality, he/she should also address the process of distortion somehow. A visual image gains its impact owing to the way it has been transformed. The 'unrealistic' image has to enable the viewer to see reality askew, with the piercing eyes of a psychiatric patient so to speak. By contrast, Verhoeven defended himself against the accusations that SPETTERS revelled in anti-feminist and homophobic sentiments by claiming that he had put himself in the position of the rural adolescents. Verhoeven's response was as follows: Why call him a cynic when he had basically given a realist depiction of the lives of his protagonists in the countryside? He may have dramatized the rudeness of the three friends a bit, but the main problem was that the critics were not used to representations of low-class teenagers in Dutch cinema and in art in general. Seen this way, the judgement that SPETTERS was sleazy and perverted backfired: familiar with middle-class life in the city, the critics were too far removed from the coarse mentality in small-town Holland to recognize the gritty realism of Verhoeven's film.

Second, in Monster's documentary DE GROTE TOVENAAR, when Zwartjes recalled that feminists had thrown red paint onto a film screen to punish the theatre for showing PENTIMENTO, he did not criticize them for the act as such but instead humorously blamed them for not seeing the aesthetic quality of the red onto the white. For a filmmaker like Zwartjes, the option to identify with characters, as in narrative cinema, has to be sacrificed in order to better experience the sensation that audio-visual images can provoke. Rather than a nuisance, a screen spilled with red paint can have a particular aesthetic impact. Like Zwartjes, Verhoeven is also known for taking delight in shock effects but for an entirely different purpose. If characters are making love, or if there is a violent scene, or if a character is bleeding like a pig, Verhoeven will not cut away as other directors who follow conventions of decency tend to do.

To legitimize his fondness for graphically detailed depiction in his films, Verhoeven uses 'realism' as his excuse: because life is that way, he would say. That this can be taken as an ironic pretext seems evident to both his opponents and his admirers.

To elaborate upon this ironic pretext, let me mention a third difference between Zwartjes and Verhoeven. Experimental filmmakers choose the strategy of dis-identifying with conventional procedures: e.g. long takes, a refusal of reverse shots, apparently random inserts, fast zooms, a short-circuit between audio and imagery. Verhoeven, however, magnifies the slick visual imagery of commercial cinema, but the effectiveness of his exaggeration is a matter of debate throughout. Alexandra Heller-Nicholas poignantly states that Verhoeven revels in cinematic codes 'to the point that critics and audiences are sometimes not wholly clear on if he is *de*constructing, *re*constructing or outright beatifying the things we suspect he might initially set out to critique'. His opponents will argue that his sensationalist approach caters to the taste of a mainstream audience (hence, he is reconstructing and beatifying): the sceptics will regard him as a dime-a-dozen director who offers violent and/or erotic spectacles for the cheap thrills of his audience.[10] His enthusiasts claim that overdoing the practical rules of cinema is an attempt to undermine filmic conventions from within (deconstructing). For the British scholar and 'fanboy' I.Q. Hunter, the eccentric Verhoeven is a 'bewitched tourist in American excess' (31). In his defence of SHOWGIRLS (1995), Hunter argues that Verhoeven, this 'unapologetic "bad-boy" of flash-trash cinema', frolics in the clichés of Hollywood blockbusters (31). Verhoeven presents these clichés, in the words of Jeffrey Sconce, as 'more vulgar than vulgar': the ludicrous overinvestment in stereotypes is then greeted as a case of subversive satire. Critique is articulated in a style that seems to mimic the sort of cinema Verhoeven criticizes. Akira Mizuta Lippit argued that SHOWGIRLS defies 'a consistent standard of judgment, since about this film, every claim and its opposite can be made'.

The problem of readability has remained a moot point in the case of several Verhoeven films. Those of his films that have become the objects of dispute seem to endorse politically incorrect stances, be it the presumed anti-feminist and homophobic sentiments in SPETTERS (1980) or the noisy militarism of STARSHIP TROOPERS (1997). Because clear markers that these films are taking an ironic distance towards their respective subjects are almost entirely absent if not missing altogether, the appreciation of such films depends upon one's interpretive attitude. One reviewer on IMDb.com aptly described STARSHIP TROOPERS as a 'pro/anti'-war movie. This bombastic science-fiction action movie adopted its iconography from Leni Riefenstahl's documentaries of the 1930s, and hence several scenes look like the propaganda pictures said to have prepared the Germans for war under the Nazis. At the same time, STARSHIP

TROOPERS is 'anti-war' if one regards the film as a persiflage of this fascist iconography: a specific feature is imitated that the reader/viewer has to recognise as too deliberate an imitation (the vain are exposed in their vanity; the trivial in its pettiness; the ugly in its ugliness). There is a thin line between imitation (i.e.: adhering to the conventions of action-packed movies) and deliberate imitation (the over-the-top depiction of graphic gore is then regarded as consciously and explicitly overplaying those conventions), but this makes all the difference in appreciating STARSHIP TROOPERS. If one watches a film with nasty violence in an experimental or arthouse film—by Zwartjes, Michael Haneke, or Pier Paolo Pasolini—the viewer is inclined to accept it as a 'necessary evil'[11] intended to make a critical point about society. But Verhoeven produces commercial fare, and that means that the signpost of 'critical commentary' is not automatically attached to it. In fact, his cinema provides a bigger challenge to the viewer, for it is up to him/her to decide what viewing attitude one adopts: a brutal spectacle to entertain the audience or a subversive picture because of its overt brutality.

KARMA CHAMELEON: *ELLE*

Expectations for a picture that might outdo even SHOWGIRLS or STARSHIP TROOPERS in defiance were stirred up when Verhoeven mentioned in a press release that his film ELLE—selected for the main competition of the 2016 Cannes film festival—had become a French production starring Isabelle Huppert because 'no American actress would take on such an amoral movie'. This time, however, praise for the film was almost unanimous: the collective score of the fifty critics participating in the *Todas Las Criticas* poll gave it no less than an 8.92, the highest of all the films screened at Cannes in 2016. Critics remained largely unshocked by ELLE, apparently because Verhoeven's film does not surpass the risqué nature of post-millennial European hardcore art films like Patrice Chéreau's INTIMACY (2001); LA PIANISTE [THE PIANO TEACHER] (Michael Haneke, 2001); Gaspar Noé's IRRÉVERSIBLE (2002); Michael Winterbottom's 9 SONGS (2004); Lars von Trier's ANTICHRIST (2009). In comparison with these, ELLE is effectively 'amorality lite'.

But even if ELLE did not seem to disturb critics in terms of its moral values—it was a 'dangerous delight', according to Xan Brooks, critic of *The Guardian*—there still remained that familiar challenge for Verhoeven's audience: how is it to be classified in terms of genre? How does one read its tone? ELLE has a rape at its core, but it does not follow the usual rape-revenge cycle of films depicting rape, since the female victim—the middle-aged Parisian Michèle Leblanc—is not driven by vengeful motivations and has not lost her taste for witty retorts. A rape (without revenge) comedy, however apt a characterization of the film, seems like an oxymoron.

The opening scene, in which the first rape is presented obliquely, is a chilling one. The screen is black and we hear the sound of breaking tableware, a slap in the face, and abrasive grunts. The first shot of the film is a close-up of Michèle's cat Marty looking off-screen, who after a few seconds turns around and calmly walks away. While witnessing a rape would assume an empathetic reaction by an onlooker, here the black humour is immediate as Verhoeven highlights the cat's apparent indifference.[12] Remarkably, however, Michèle herself seems also quite unmoved by the incident. When she casually mentions the assault at dinner with three friends, she says simply 'at least, I suppose I have been raped'. When the waiter arrives with champagne at that moment, Robert—her secret lover but also the husband of her business partner and best friend Anna—asks him to wait five minutes. Apparently, Robert knows that in less than five minutes Michèle will get a grip on herself again. And she does: 'Let's order food', she says.

Because Michèle regains her composure remarkably quickly, it seems as if the rape is like a minor nuisance but no grave matter. Her attitude seems related to her controversial reputation as the 'psychopath girl'. Her father has been in prison since 1976, for he was a notorious serial killer responsible for 27 murders. With her father appealing for clemency, a documentary about the case is broadcast again on television, featuring footage of the then ten-year-old Michèle, appearing on the screen with a blank look that makes her susceptible to the accusation that she is indirectly culpable. When the story is back in the news almost 40 years later, a woman in a self-service restaurant throws her food in Michèle's lap, hissing at her that she's 'scum'. On the one hand, it affirms that Michèle is regarded as a despicable creature simply because she is the daughter of a 'monster'; yet on the other hand the scene illustrates that she is able to keep her temper under control.

The scene is emblematic of Michèle. At a very young age she was stigmatized, but she acts as if her dark past has not demoralized her. She apparently copes with her traumatic childhood memories by being pragmatic, adapting to situations like a chameleon. That she has mastered these continual readjustments is also proven by her professional standing: once working in the domain of literature, she switched to the more profitable business of computer games. One of the brusque editing transitions within ELLE suddenly confronts the audience with an animated game where a huge orc brutally assaults a female figure. Michèle does not express shock (as we might assume her to do in the context of her own rape) but dryly comments that the interaction is still too 'timid', signifying both her calculating nature and her commercially oriented attitude.

It is implied that the once so-called 'psychopathic girl' has been able to integrate herself into society by being both opportunistic and by rejecting contact with her father. Her life is structured around her repression of his existence, resulting in a refusal to make real commitments to people. Tellingly, Anna is on much closer terms with Michèle's son Vincent than Michèle herself. As she tells a nurse, she met Anna when they were in the same hospital giving birth to their babies. When Anna's child died, she asked Michèle if she could breastfeed her newborn. Favouring pragmatism over motherly principles, Michèle agreed. Whether it be towards her son or anyone else, she does not have highly developed affections for others.

But her shallow relationships do not contradict the fact that Michèle is embedded in a broad social network, in which she considers herself a hub. Though Peter de Bruijn (a critic from the influential Dutch newspaper *NRC Handelsblad*) complained that this film is crammed with developments as if 'more is more' had been its guiding principle, the large number of characters makes sense from the perspective of Michèle's character. Rather than investing time in relationships, she wants to simply oversee them. When her ex-husband Richard talks about his new flame Hélène, she immediately calls her son for information about the woman, Googles her, enters the yoga centre where she practices and invites her for Christmas dinner, leaving Hélène flabbergasted. To complicate matters further, Michèle does not shy away from nasty tricks: she puts a toothpick in Hélène's food, and she deliberately plays the role of clumsy car driver and ruins the front of her ex's car.

Michèle's pragmatism is visually underscored by an often slightly mobile camera and by the specific placement of Michèle in space: in many shots, either Michèle or her environment is not in sharp focus and, frequently, the focus changes within shots. It feels at times as if the camera in ELLE has to be ready to adapt to new, unexpected changes in mise-en-scène, reflecting Michèle's life after her father's arrest and how it also consisted of a chain of readjustments. Because of this, being raped appears to have little effect on Michèle, encapsulated precisely through how the rape scenes are represented. Whereas the first rape was represented obliquely to signify that the attack was too much of a shock for Michèle to recall it directly, the second rape is much more explicit but contains its own shock. While she vehemently resists the attack, she discovers that her handsome neighbour Patrick—the man whom she fancies, of all people—is the balaclava-wearing assailant. It brings to memory the terrible discovery from decades ago that her father is a killer.

Despite knowing the identity of her rapist, Michèle continues to socialize with him. When she has tried to contact two of her friends in vain after her car has hit a tree, she phones Patrick who not only releases her from her awkward position but even takes care of her leg injury. Michèle asks him, 'Did you like it?' to which he has nothing more to say than 'It was necessary.' His answer does not contain the personal pronoun 'I', an indication that he wants to give the impression as if this urge is beyond his control.

Once Michèle knows that Patrick is a ticking time bomb, she takes the conscious risk of descending into his cellar at home. She is willing to offer herself as pliant prey, but Patrick says this does not work for him. He can get excited only if she resists (or at least pretends to) so that he feels he has no other option than to violently hit her. She then hits him to provoke him to rape her. She has tears rolling over her cheeks, but it is not clear whether she is devastated or perhaps relieved. In a later scene, after the two have attended a party to launch a new game, Patrick rapes her in the living room, but probably again with the silent consent of Michèle. When her son Vincent enters, he only recognizes the violence, not her enjoyment, and he then strikes Patrick fatally.

Michèle is already erotically attracted to her new neighbour the first time he sets foot in her house. Before she was aware of his dark side, she had been masturbating while secretly looking at him during outdoor activities, and she daringly touched his genitals with her foot during a Christmas dinner she has organized. But why does she seem even more attracted to him after the revelation? The traumatized Michele, Sandra E. Cohen argues, is split between an 'often harsh pseudo self-sufficiency' and a 'terrified, child self' which is 'pushed aside by an internal bully'. Such a bully bombards her with accusations like 'How could you be so stupid?' Deliberately offering herself to her perpetrator, as Michèle does, is a masochistic step, meant to 'prevent further trauma by re-enacting the original trauma' (Stoller, 124). This return of the unbearable leads to a hard-shelled attitude on the part of the 'victim' and instigates the need to become 'master of the script': Michèle must decide for herself 'when to suffer pain' (Stoller, 124), and she takes this step when she dares to go down in the basement. Her brief 'do it' does not suffice, so she hits him to provoke his violent reaction. She is left behind on the floor, 'in pain, orgasmic—both' (Cohen). She plays this twisted game as part of her 'perverse defense'. She takes the lead in the trajectory of her own humiliation, required to ward off unwanted feelings.

Michèle's symbolic position is determined by the crimes of her father. Even though she avoids any contact, she will be pinpointed as his daughter, the 'psychopathic girl'. In his study *Het Münchhausenparadigma*, Marc De Kesel claims that the rapist is a reenactor of her father but with a crucial difference. In the case of her father, Michèle is the object of some general gossip or public humiliation, but she refuses this position afforded to her by her environment. In the case of her neighbour, she becomes the direct object of his macabre necessity (De Kesel, 228), and this relationship is exclusive in the sense that the outside world is excluded from it.

For Patrick, the exclusivity is seminal, which is why he was wearing the balaclava in the first place. He is a socially successful man in every regard who wants to keep up the appearance of an extremely polite stockbroker with an attractive wife. For Michèle, the exclusivity is seminal as well, and though she may appear to be the abused object of Patrick's lustfulness, he is also the object of her dark desires. This is not only because she was sexually attracted to him before his unmasking, but she is also in the position to create a setting that works for him. He can only rape her under the specific condition that she violently resists his attempts. Thanks to this condition, Michèle, reduced to an object of his macabre necessity, has some control over Patrick, who is in turn reduced to the role of assailant: she can decide to trigger his aggressive impulses. Such a mutual agreement is a basis of their perverse delights, which can only take place outside the constraints of the paternal law. Son Vincent has no clue that they both function as an instrument for the other's enjoyment and beats Patrick to death; the police detectives have no idea either. In their eyes, Vincent was justified in defending his mother against her rapist. Wisely, Michèle keeps her mouth shut about the brutal intimacy she experienced with Patrick.

Verhoeven's ELLE has a surprise ending in store for Michèle, however, when the fresh widow Rebecca addresses her as she is about to move to another place. So far, we have known her as a righteous woman who presents a friendly façade. Together with Michèle's mother Irene, the pious Rebecca sits on the couch watching the Pope's midnight church service during Christmas. Their shared religious interest suggests a bond. They both believe that people should be forgiven, as befits good Catholics. Irene wants her daughter to visit her father in prison, but Michèle refuses this request. In her eyes, her father is a 'monster', but Irene insists that she should acknowledge him as a 'man'. When Irene repeats her request on her way to the hospital after a stroke, Michèle does not change her mind. A similar question to see a 'monster' as a 'man' is key to the final dénouement of the film. Out of the blue, Rebecca tells Michèle that her late husband had a good nature, but he was a 'tormented soul'. And, after a brief pause, she adds: 'Thanks that you have been able to help him in his bad moments, for a while at least.' Michèle appears too perplexed to be able to reply promptly. Rebecca, she realizes, was not only aware of her husband's impulses but knew that Michèle was his victim. But Michèle was never comforted by Rebecca: no doubt Rebecca knew (just like Patrick) that Michèle would not go to the police due to her reputation as a 'psychopathic girl'. Hence Michèle was left to her own devices by Rebecca, out of consideration for a 'tormented soul'.

Whereas Michèle presumed she might have some silent contract with her rapist, it was ultimately embedded in a secret agreement Rebecca had with her husband. She was conscious of Patrick's anguish, but she kept aloof. Apparently, she took to heart the Catholic dictum of 'love thy neighbour' but did so at the expense of her very own neighbour whose life she literally jeopardized. Rebecca's unconditional readiness to forgive Patrick's vile behaviour is risky business, for as Slavoj Žižek observes in relation to DEAD MAN WALKING (Tim Robbins, 1996), 'when we trespass a certain limit of compassion, we enter a shadowy domain in which compassion turns into perversion, in which the concern for the criminal overshadows the suffering of his victim' ('Death and the Maiden, 209).

Michèle has proven herself an unscrupulous woman. She had an affair with the husband of her best friend, simply 'because she felt like fucking'. Michèle is prepared to tell little white lies insofar as it helps her to play her part in keeping the social order running. When she stops lying (which only takes place after both her parents have died), and tells Anna the truth about her affair with Robert, there is an immediate symbolic short-circuit. Due to their marital crisis, Anna expels Robert from their house and he starts drinking. Whereas Michèle lies and/or withholds information when it suits her, according to Verhoeven's film, Catholics like Rebecca have elevated lying and/or strategic secrecy into principles, if it accords with the idea of 'love thy neighbour'. Rebecca's silent understanding of her husband's 'basic instincts', however, indirectly determined Michèle's victimhood. And, thus, Rebecca's piety, affirmed by her blind adhesion to Catholic principles, can be considered a kind of perversion too—or rather, it is an even more disruptive perversion than Michèle's sexual escapades.[13]

ENJOYING IT LIKE A VIRGIN: *FLESH + BLOOD*

In comparison to other mainstream medieval adventure stories from the 1980s such as EXCALIBUR (John Boorman, 1981) and LADYHAWKE (Richard Donner, 1985), Verhoeven's FLESH + BLOOD (1985), his first international production—shot in Spain, but still with many Dutch among cast and crew[14]—is the most cynical and erotic. According to Verhoeven, the 'dark' Middle Ages were everything but romantic: in those centuries, many people died of poverty, diseases and silly accidents, as the opening scene will reveal. The film starts with the siege of a nameless city, and the young man Steven Arnolfini introduces a smart strategy to conquer the place: someone is appointed to roll a barrel with a very long fuse around it towards the city walls, but, alas, the fuse is lit too soon, and the volunteer is blown to pieces before he has reached the city. Enter Martin who heads a motley crew that will help Sir John Hawkwood's army to invade the city in the name of Steven's father, Lord Arnolfini, but in the end this Lord withholds any reward for Martin's band of mercenaries. This setback is followed by the scene in which the whore Celine delivers a stillborn child. While some men dig a grave in heavy rain, they find the gigantic statue 'Charity of St. Martin'. It is a near life-sized sculpture of the young St. Martin of Tours. The chaplain among the war band, simply called the 'Cardinal', explains that this saint had a sword to slice a piece from his cloak to give it to the naked beggar who grasps the saint's robe. Only one hand of the beggar is still part of the statue, and according to one mercenary, the hand '*looks like a piece of shit*'. Upon hearing this story, Martin immediately says that this is '*my patron saint: I was named after him*'. The 'Cardinal' yells that he regards the discovery as the '*hand of God*'. He adds to this: Consider it a prediction that Martin will get rich one day and that the statue is a sign he will share his fortune with his crew. When Martin says that the Cardinal is right, one member says that this is '*horseshit*', but without further ado, the Cardinal pierces the dissident in his chest with his sword. Thereupon Martin takes the lead by declaring: '*The bastards who cheated us will pay. We'll grab them by the balls and squeeze out every penny they've got.*'

If Martin's leadership is determined by the superstition that the statue is a meaningful sign, the very next scene is its polar opposite, for it exposes Steven's dedication to scientific knowledge. He is building a replica device based on his study of Roman fortifications. His father asks him whether it is of any practical use, and the son answers: '*Not yet.*' Lord Arnolfini wants him to focus on current business: his son is supposed to marry Agnes, the daughter of Prince Niccolo. She is a '*guaranteed virgin*' and is already on her way with an '*enormous dowry*'. Agnes is a virgin, indeed, but very much intrigued by sex: she orders her maid Kathleen to make love in open air with her '*brave soldier*' so she can watch and learn. It is clear that Kathleen enjoys getting laid, shouting '*I'll take you*' repetitively, and Agnes can only make her stop by hitting her. But then Steven happens to arrive with a bunch of his father's men: '*I have longed for this meeting, sir; I have counted the hours*', Agnes says. Steven gets angry, for he thinks his father has arranged this accidental encounter. In the conversation between the two, he tells her that her sight pleases him but he fears that marriage might distract him from his scholarly ambition to investigate nature and to invent new things.[15] She answers that she has her own idea of investigating nature. She starts digging the earth under the body of a hanged man and shows him a mandrake. She has read in a book that if man and woman eat from this magic root together, they will love each other forever. Of course, Steven does not believe this '*nonsense*', but he takes a bite and then concludes it is a '*plain old turnip*'. She replies it cannot be, for she is tingling all over her body.

Dressed as monks on a pilgrimage, Martin's band ambushes Arnolfini's caravan soon thereafter. The group is supposed to share all the acquired goods,

for there is '*no mine and thine anymore*', says the Cardinal. As a token of that, Martin orders everyone to wear red clothes. It is only then that he discovers Agnes, hidden under blankets. He shows her to his troupe, declaring: '*St. Martin has sent us a little angel to play with.*' Summer, one of the supreme fighters, is about to rape her, but Agnes reaches for a piece of wood from the fire and burns his backside. Martin then requests to hold her real tight and gives his crew precise instructions: move her; show me her face. When he is on top of her, there is a role reversal when she says: '*If you think you're hurting me, you're wrong. I like it. I like it. I'll take you. I'll take you!*' in a repetition of the example set by her maid. Except for Celine, Martin's former mistress, the group laughs at the idea that, instead of Martin raping the prince's daughter, he is being raped. She then asks '*my brave soldier*' to go on, another copycat phrase taken from Kathleen. When Martin is finished, he can only order, according to the group's principles of sharing and share alike: '*Next!*' But he secretly sets one of the tents on fire, and thus Summer's rape of Agnes is interrupted a second
time. Under pressure from the flames, the statue inadvertently moves its position, and Martin reads this as a sign: the group has to move in the direction pointed out by the saint. The Cardinal backs him up by yelling that this order has to be obeyed.

As Martin observes that Summer wants to force Agnes into sex again behind his back, he makes the lead wagon stop abruptly. The statue, which was mounted at the head of the wagon as the group's totem, moves again. The Cardinal interprets this as another prophecy: the sword points at a castle, which they will have to conquer. After a ruthless but successful raid, Martin takes some privileges: he and he alone will share the hot tub with Agnes; the couple shows up in white the next morning, another violation of the egalitarian principles. When Steven arrives at the castle with Hawkwood's men, he tells Martin's motley crew that they may keep the spoils but that he wants the girl. They throw oranges at them, but Agnes hides Steven's medallion into it and the young boy catches it. Martin realizes that she fancies him, whereupon she replies that she will not make a choice, but that the choice will be made for her: '*The winner takes it all.*'

Steven outsmarts the occupants of the castle by building a war machine inspired by the theoretical writings of Da Vinci. The Cardinal thinks they can ask for God's assistance by putting Saint Martin's statue on the wall, but Martin says '*Oh, fuck St. Martin.*' The Cardinal is shocked by this blasphemy, but Martin successfully defends the castle by rolling a barrel with a long fuse into the war machine, blowing it to pieces. After the victory, the Cardinal bows his head when he sees Martin with a burning wagon wheel behind his head like a vibrant halo. As a bonus, Steven is made captive. He is humiliated like a '*mad dog*', and Martin orders Agnes to shoot the young Arnolfini. But he is saved by dead dog meat that is catapulted by Hawkwood onto the courtyard. Steven warns them that the dog licked unclean blood and suffers from the plague, but Martin thinks it is a trick. No one is permitted to leave the castle; they must burn the meat and their clothes. Martin then makes love to Agnes behind a screen, and it is presented to the chained Steven as a shadow play. He gets so angry that he throws a forgotten piece of dog meat into the water well. Agnes has witnessed it, but the next morning she hesitates whether or not to warn the members of the band. She only intervenes when Martin is about to drink a cup of water, but by then Celine has already started throwing up. Everyone gets angry at Martin, for he referred to the oracle of Saint Martin to prevent them from leaving the castle. '*I am only led*', Martin defends himself, but Miel says: '*Led by your cock, prancing around in white clothes.*' Martin is thrown into the poisonous well, and the Cardinal starts to punish himself for misinterpreting the sign.

Steven assists Martin in getting out of the well, in the hope of a favour in return. Just as he is about to unchain Steven, Martin hears horses outside the castle and runs away to watch the arrival of Steven's father with his men. Steven is freed after all thanks to a lightning bolt that breaks his chains. In the culminating battle, many of Martin's men die, pierced by swords, but in an appropriate twist the Cardinal is killed when the statue of Saint Martin tumbles down and its pointed sword hits him. Seeing that a loss is unavoidable, Martin starts to choke Agnes, for he does not want her to belong to anyone else. Steven intervenes, and Agnes intervenes in turn, hitting Martin hard, though her hesitance indicates that she still has feelings for Martin, too. The young couple gets away with the remaining troops, while the castle is burning. No one except for Agnes sees that Martin climbs out of the chimney, and Martin W. Walsh describes this 'sole survivor of his scruffy war band' in Verhoeven's 'disturbing, anarchic' medieval 'action flick' as the re-embodiment of the beggar that was missing from the statue found in the mud.[16]

In FLESH + BLOOD, Steven and Martin are antagonists and rivals, but in the eyes of Agnes, their difference is minimal. She tells Martin: '*He is you, only younger.*' And she adds to this: '*You are him, only older.*' To some extent this is true, but there is a fundamental difference: Steven always has an eye on the future and is interested in scientific inventions; Martin only yearns for immediate satisfactions. He acts as if he is really led by the prophetic qualities of his namesake statue, but he is just piggybacking on the Cardinal's questionable authority. Martin himself does not attach any value to the 'signs' but simply uses the Cardinal's interpretations to his own advantage. If necessary, he manipulates the statue in such a manner that the deluded Cardinal reads a sign in it that suits his strategy. Martin has the ability to make his crew believe that they are part of a meaningful universe. The statue is a totem and an oracle for the majority, but for Martin it is just an ordinary, exploitable object.

Whereas Steven is after empirically grounded wisdom, there is a discrepancy between belief and knowledge in the case of Martin. He uses the genuine belief of the Cardinal, though he knows it is '*horseshit*', as the blasphemous band member called it who was killed for speaking out loud. He has some silent contract with the Cardinal: I will act according to your interpretations of signs, and everyone will obey my orders. By taking the statue as a guide, Martin succeeds in affirming his role as the first among others. And thanks to his secure position, backed up by the Cardinal, he overpowers Agnes. She appeals to Martin first and foremost for the simple fact that his enemy Arnolfini is her future father-in-law and her deflowering would be a most serious insult to his rival. Second, he seems all the more erotically attracted to this young virgin when she turns out to be everything but tame. She clearly enjoys being overpowered and begs him: '*Please, only you. I only want to be yours, please.*' Initially, the hierarchy was clear: he was the master and she the spineless prey. But she reverses roles when she suggests that she depends upon him for her own enjoyment. The majority of the groups laughs at this reversal, but it also triggers Martin's perverse desire.

Officially, Martin has a deal with his group: they get along with each other according to egalitarian principles. So he announces '*Next*', giving Summer the opportunity to get laid, but at the same time he is about to seal a silent contract with Agnes, as if it turned him on that she used him as an instrument for her enjoyment. Strictly speaking, anyone is entitled to have sex with Prince Niccolo's daughter, but he makes sure he is the only one who puts it into practice. The contract can also be established if Agnes contributes as well. During dinner, every member of the war band eats the meat with his or her hands, but Agnes uses knife and fork. She makes eye contact with Martin who then tries to copy her good manners. Everyone starts to laugh at his clumsy attempt, so he gives up, but then Agnes massages his crotch with a bare foot under the table. Martin gives it another try, and with success. He orders everyone from now on to eat with a knife and fork. Martin and Agnes share intimacies under the nose of others, but their acts are basically hidden from their eyes. Increasingly, however, they want their liaison to be witnessed. In the bathtub there is space for two, but when Summer claims he would like to join Agnes, he is aggressively put into place by Martin. While two members of the group use forks to pin Summer to the table, the Cardinal asks him some rhetorical questions: '*Who led you to this castle?*' '*Saint Martin.*' '*Who opened up the gates to this castle?*' '*Martin.*' '*So, who gets the girl?*' And of course, Summer can only answer once more: '*Martin.*'

Backed by the Cardinal, Martin has been able to set new rules: the statue should be considered their totemic signpost. On the one hand, Martin will make sure that the statue will lead the way he himself prefers. On the other hand, despite the moral standards imposed upon everyone, Martin avoids them and even violates them. This becomes increasingly visible in the course of FLESH + BLOOD. It contributes to Martin and Agnes's perverse enjoyment of distinguishing themselves from the group as a pair. Their white clothes are a transgression of the agreement they made to all wear red. When Steven is chained, they start making love behind a screen, and the young Arnolfini can witness their sexual act as shadow play. In turn, Agnes witnesses Steven's vile trick of throwing the infected dog meat into the well, probably committed out of frustration over this exhibitionistic behaviour. He knows she has seen it, and it is unclear where her loyalty resides. Since she does not reveal that the well has been infected, she has a kind of contract not only with Martin but with Steven, too. She apparently thinks that Steven deserves his revenge. Whereas Martin restricts himself to a particular kind of perverse desire—'to what extent can I exceed the limits set by my namesake-statue'—Agnes oscillates between two kinds of 'contract', which both defy authority. The war band can only cherish the statue as a totem, affirmed by the vocal readings of the Cardinal, by becoming all equal but, in the 'contract' she has with Martin, the two lovers enjoy creating a special position among the group. At the same time, she jeopardizes the safety of the group when, in a 'pact' of solidarity with Steven, she does not warn the members of Martin's group about the contaminated well: her facial expression shows a mixture of fear and excitement. She only prevents Martin himself from drinking the lethal water. This intervention does not mean she chooses him as the 'older' version of Steven, but first, she prolongs the existence of the double contract: by being brutal, Martin acts as an instrument of her enjoyment, whereas the smart and 'younger' Steven is the object of her desire. Second, she seems to derive excitement from the fact that the two men are vying for her, so the rivalry as such is a source of pleasure for her. She hits Martin on his head near the end of Verhoeven's film, but only to ensure that Steven is not killed. Significantly, she is the only one to observe that Martin leaves the castle alive, but she does not mention this. The film ends, but the rivalry is to be continued, and thus also her perverse enjoyment.

A CALVINIST PERVERT: *BRIMSTONE*

In Rob van Scheers' 2017 study *Paul Verhoeven: Een filmersleven*—an update of the authorized biography (first edition from 1996)—Martin Koolhoven was asked to write a preface to emphasize the fact that he could be regarded as a successor to Paul Verhoeven. After eight feature films in the Netherlands between 1999 and 2008, it took some years before Koolhoven's long-awaited BRIMSTONE premiered in the Competition at the Venice film festival in 2016.

The production history has some analogies with Verhoeven's first international co-production. The shooting of FLESH + BLOOD had been sheer agony for him due to terrible weather conditions, non-flexible technicians, mutiny on the set by the American actors, and permanent quarrels with lead actor Hauer. BRIMSTONE also had its setbacks due to postponed shooting schedules and the cancelled availability of some lead actors.[17] One crucial difference is that Verhoeven had agreed at the time to the condition imposed by Orion Pictures for Agnes to have a bigger role, something he later regretted. Koolhoven, by contrast, had always insisted on the final cut, no matter what, and that non-negotiable condition had jeopardized the project, for it had displeased the financers. But he got what he wanted, and thus the film title is officially MARTIN KOOLHOVEN'S BRIMSTONE.

As a self-acclaimed aficionado of westerns and spaghetti westerns in particular, Koolhoven rewrote this genre, bearing in mind his dictum that despite the American origin of westerns, they should necessarily be steeped in one's own culture. It is an often-overlooked historical fact that many settlers in America in that particular era were of Dutch descent, and BRIMSTONE chronicles the influence of their Calvinist mentality upon the building of the American nation. The point of the film is that the Calvinist strict adherence to scripture as the Word of God can be abused to the perverse desires of BRIMSTONE's evil character, The Reverend.

The narrative of Koolhoven's 'Edam' western is sandwiched between two voice-over commentaries; the one in the epilogue is the extended version of the prologue. The opening scene, preceding the first of four chapters, is entirely enigmatic, all the more so because the depicted event, which takes place partly underwater, lacks clear contours. At the end, we understand that a grown-up version of Sam remembers how her mother, living under the name of Liz Brundy, jumped into the water from a raft with her hands tied. Liz thus determined her own fate, for she was about to be executed by a sheriff who had tracked her down after finding an old wanted poster. The sheriff persists in firing shots at the drowning woman, but a final underwater shot of a smiling Liz suggests that none of the bullets have struck her.

From a narratological as well as a generic perspective, it is remarkable that the film begins with a scene that is strictly speaking a flashback, but the event depicted in the flashback postdates all developments in the four subsequent chapters. Chronologically, the third chapter, called 'Genesis', comes first, the second chapter 'Exodus' second, the first chapter 'Revelation' third, and the fourth chapter 'Retribution' last, followed by the prologue, which largely overlaps with the epilogue. A gradual unfolding of events in reverse order is in itself not something new, but for a western it is highly uncommon. In BRIMSTONE, we are introduced to a female character, described in the voice-over by her daughter as a '*warrior, always in control*' and the four chapters of the film, which span some fifteen years, explain why this qualification is correct. Step by step, by moving backwards in time, we come to realize why the woman changed her name from Joanna to Liz, why she has no tongue, and why the arrival in the small community of The Reverend, introduced to us via heavy footsteps, gives her the creeps. The denouement at the end of chapter three reveals that Joanna lost her virginity at the age of thirteen to The Reverend, who is also her father. A tracking shot forward that shows us stains of blood on the bedsheets suffices to expose this key moment.

Ever since The Reverend had committed incest, he is persecuting Joanna. In chapter two, Joanna works in a whorehouse, called Frank's Inferno, when an anonymous man pays a large sum of money. Every prostitute is supposed to present herself to the customer. Joanna sees the man from above and is shocked to recognize The Reverend. She is the last to step down from the stairs, blindfolded, but The Reverend feels the birthmarks at the back of her neck and then decides he only wants this one. In her room, when he takes out his whip, she screams for help, and Joanna's best friend Elizabeth immediately comes to her aid and cuts the man's face with a knife, which explains The Reverend's giant facial scar in chapter one. The Reverend overpowers Elizabeth and kills her. Thereupon Joanna takes the knife from Elizabeth's breast, slits The Reverend's throat and sets Elizabeth's corpse on fire. Elizabeth had been about to leave the brothel, for she had had her tongue cut off by the owner of the brothel-saloon as punishment for harassing a male client, and she was not only robbed of speech but was also no longer able to give blow jobs. Since a marriage broker had given Elizabeth a photograph of a widower and his young son, Joanna uses this picture for a strategy of escape. Joanna cuts off her own tongue after the doctor refuses to do it for her, in order to appropriate Elizabeth's identity, and she will marry the widower under the name of 'Liz'. The ultimate drawback of this change of identity is, story-wise, that Joanna/'Liz' will be held responsible for the murder of the owner of the saloon-brothel, presumably committed by Elizabeth. That will be fatal to her in the epilogue.

After she has left her identity as Joanna behind, Liz never seems to look back. The story itself moves backwards in time, but Liz does not. In none of the chapters is there a mental image that can be attributed to her: she herself never reflects upon anything that has taken place in previous years. The past can only come to haunt her in the form of an external force, embodied by The Reverend. By withholding any flashbacks focalized by Liz, Koolhoven's film suggests that she can function properly ('*always in control*') as the local midwife because she has successfully repressed her horrendous past. Though her husband Eli realizes that something has piqued Liz when The Reverend arrives (which coincides with the failed delivery of a baby boy), he is not particularly worried. But he should have been, for soon thereafter The Reverend kills the unsuspecting Eli for the simple reason that she loves her husband instead of him, her father.

The Reverend in Koolhoven's BRIMSTONE equals the spaghetti western protagonists in ruthlessness, but his justification for violence is informed by his faith. When his wife refuses him sexual favours in the third chapter, he considers it his right to torture her; he then turns to his daughter, using a quote from the Apostle Paul on the passing of '*the flower of her age*' to claim possession over her. If only the rites of the ceremony of matrimony are fulfilled, their sexual union, which The Reverend defines as '*pure love*', will be granted permission. The ceremony is interrupted by the wounded cowboy Samuel, to whom Joanna had given shelter in the barn. For Joanna, who fancies this cowboy, this interruption is a blessing, signified by the excessive cascade of light that falls upon her, shown in a reverse shot as coming from behind Samuel, turning him into an angelic figure. The cowboy fails to pull the trigger, however, and to Joanna's despair ends up dead. The Reverend, so enraged that his daughter was about to choose 'lust' over 'love', commits incest before the marriage rites were performed.

As a Calvinist, The Reverend adheres to the doctrine of predestination. Calvinist culture provokes a collective feeling of guilt, for it regards the human race as totally depraved, but even though everyone is a sinner, God has always-already decided that some are among the elect, while others are doomed to damnation. One's life path is determined in advance, and one cannot influence its course. Since God's judgement is inscrutable by definition, the logic of who is chosen and who will be condemned is inexplicable. Due to this determinism, it is 'rather absurd to feel guilty about trespasses one has made' (De Kesel, 'The Brain', 15). The Reverend is the pastor of a group of settlers who hang on to the idea that their coming to the pristine country of America can only mean that they are God's 'chosen people'. Every churchgoer who has received a calling from an angelic figure has been given a revelatory sign that salvation will befall him or her. It is part of the duty of The Reverend to chastise those who as yet have had no visitation.[18]

The point in BRIMSTONE is that The Reverend claims that he has lost the right to heaven and that instead of an elect, he has become a doomed man, due to the sheer gravity of his violation. Things can be amended, however, but that requires the voluntary cooperation of his daughter Joanna. In the brothel he tells her: '*Only you can save me, so that I can save you.*' According to him, she has to yield her body to him as his wife. The Reverend is a pervert par excellence in the sense that he wants to set up a contract with his daughter. She is supposed to believe that incest is permissible on specific conditions. Since these conditions are not met, due to the interruption by the cowboy, The Reverend has transgressed symbolic law, but he knows a way to undo his infringement: the 'gift' of her body. If she refuses to do so, he will be an outlaw who roams the earth without rules or contract. When he has tracked her down in chapter one, several years after the incident at Frank's Inferno, he tells Liz's daughter Sam that he has come to take her mother to where he has come from, meaning hell. Since he has nothing more to lose, he takes up the role of the Lord's sheepdog to punish those lambs who have strayed from the path. Liz will persevere, however, and while she has turned The Reverend literally into a burning man, she listens to his final soliloquy, in which he claims that it is not the flames that make hell so terrible, but the '*absence of love*'. Since daughter Joanna/'Liz' has declined the secret marriage proposal, which only requires a few ritual gestures, The Reverend's fantasy to be the instrument of her enjoyment cannot be materialized.

CONCLUSION: CIPHERED MESSAGES AND SILENT CONTRACTS

Briefly recapitulating, this chapter has covered various forms of 'identification with the symptom'. This identification presumes an act, albeit often a 'crazy' one, addressed to the big Other. That means that the act 'still functions as the bearer of some ciphered message', e.g. to honour a 'certain debt, to wipe out a certain guilt, to embody a certain reproach to the Other, etc.' (Žižek *Looking*, 139). The obsessive neurotic Mr Korteweg first killed his lizards and then himself to come to terms with the terrible fate of his neighbours: this message is first sent to the Other and then arrives at its proper destination when his daughter Karin informs Anton. The hysteric Eline Vere who sees how she is constantly being watched, is so fed up with the looks cast upon her that her suicide is addressed to those who despised her lack of decorum, and the photograph of Otto in her mouth is its proper punctuation. Nadine kidnapped the baby (or imagined the abduction of Sam) so that Daniel would realize the pain his deceit had caused her. Ingrid Jonker yearned for attention from several men, but the real addressee of her frenetic attempts to be noted was her authoritative father. Minuut gives a not entirely coherent account of the mysterious ways of the male neurotic Nagel in order to justify his own share in the tale.

As explained above, in the scenarios of hysteria and neurosis, some ciphered message is sent to the big Other. This means, as Lacan has asserted, that a letter always arrives at its destination, regardless of whether the intended addressee understands it (for example, Anton Steenwijk) or not (Abraham Jonker). By contrast, in the cases of perversion, a secret contract was the pinnacle of the matter: the private ritual of mother and son in DE WITTE WAAN; the silent agreement Zwartjes had with his viewer to depict a world of deranged behaviour and dark impulses (a 'contract' violated by the feminists who loudly protested against his 1979 film PENTIMENTO); the contract between Michèle and her rapist in ELLE, which has some parallel with the twisted games played between princess Agnes and her rapist Martin in FLESH + BLOOD; and, finally, the contract that the Reverend failed to establish between him and his daughter Joanna, who had taken up a new identity as Liz, in BRIMSTONE. Overlooking this latter series of titles, one can say that perversion manifests itself in many forms in as many types of films: avant-garde pictures, a rape revenge comedy, a medieval blockbuster, an 'Edam' western. It is meant to give credibility to the idea that anachronistic readings can reveal surprising analogies.

NOTES

1 We have seen these lizards before, though the film does not make a reference to that earlier scene. In the very first scene of DE AANSLAG, the twelve-year-old Anton is collecting worms from the snow-covered ground. There is a cut to a lizard in its terrarium, and then Anton's head appears in the background, behind the glass. It results in a change of focus: the lizard is out of focus, and Anton's face is sharp. Gathering from his fascinated look, he has a great liking for these animals. He gives the lizard one of the worms from his jar.

2 A film that illustrates that you can die twice is the low-budget, drily comic DE NOBELPRIJSWINNAAR [THE NOBEL PRIZE WINNER] (Timo Veltkamp, 2010), shot in black and white. Joachim West is a writer with little confidence. He has published a volume of short stories, but that was ten years ago. He asks the new director of the publishing company for an advance, but this Lea is not willing to give money to this 'in-house Dostoevsky', as she calls him contemptuously. Unable to pay the rent, his landlord has him evicted and the bailiff finds an envelope that contains Joachim's manuscript. Since it already has stamps, he sends it to the address written on the envelope. After the publisher has received the lengthy manuscript, she starts searching for Joachim. But when she visits the Salvation Army, he hides himself and asks a hobo to tell her that he is not there. The hobo invents a story that Joachim has committed suicide by jumping from the roof of a hotel, but that the police kept it silent. Joachim decides to start his life anew under the name 'Fjodor Schilder'. Since the most successful author of the publishing house, Fabian Remarque, is suffering from serious writer's block, Lea concocts a plan to publish Joachim's manuscript *Zonder allure* [*Without Airs*] as *Verloren stad* [*A City Depraved*]. Because Fabian is a celebrity, there is an enormous advertisement campaign, but the more his new novel is praised, even by those who always disliked the conceited author, the more fearful he becomes that the deceit will be discovered. When the

former director of the publishing house detects similarities to one of the stories from Joachim's volume, the net result of a number of complicating developments is that Fabian kills Joachim by saying: 'Your talent is too great. It's you or me.' By sheer coincidence, in this film full of humorous coincidences, Joachim/Fjodor had just written a message to his daughter which, given the situation of his death, is taken as a farewell note. As Joachim's death is interpreted as a suicide, Fabian has every reason to laugh out loud, especially when the daughter hands to the publisher a novella he had recently finished, but she did not make the effort to read the stuff. The film ends with the news that Fabian, born Jan Kramer, has received the Nobel Prize for Literature. A journalist who interviews Fabian (only audible during the end credits) suggests that not only his masterpiece *Verloren stad* but above all the recently published 'painfully honest novella', called *De Nobelprijskandidaat* [*The Nobel Prize Candidate*], tipped the balance for the honour. Thus, Veltkamp's film shows that Fabian owes his symbolic recognition to Joachim's symbolic death (affirmed by his new name Fjodor), so that Fabian can gain a reputation as a sort of present-day Dostoevsky. When Fabian then traces Joachim down, the latter dies a second time. His biological death is under the name of Fjodor, however, as we can read on the coffin.

3 *Eline Vere* was originally published as a feuilleton and the title heroine can be regarded as the Dutch equivalent of Gustave Flaubert's *Emma Bovary* and Theodor Fontane's *Effi Briest*.

4 Jonker's most celebrated poem is 'Die Kind' [The Child], conceived after she was a witness to police brutality against blacks, and at the end of BLACK BUTTERFLIES, we hear Nelson Mandela's voice, reciting the poem at the opening of the first democratically chosen parliament in South Africa in 1994.

5 Credited as Robbie Müller.

6 Ditvoorst had chosen as a motto for his film the last two lines from Malcolm Lowry's poem 'For the Love of Dying': 'If death can fly, just for the love of flying, what might not life do, for the love of dying?'

7 HET ZUIDEN [SOUTH] (Martin Koolhoven, 2004) was inspired by the Dogme 95 movement, and most striking are the jump cuts and the use of a handheld camera, which often shoots the female protagonist Martje Portegies close to her skin. The formal brusqueness in this film is functional, since her life is in disarray. On the surface, everything seems fine, for she is the boss of a blossoming laundry and dry-cleaning service, and she is popular among her staff which consists of women of Russian, Turkish, and Surinamese descent. The one male employee is the truck driver, and when Guus goes into retirement, he is replaced by Loe de Koning, who shows he is a 'great dancer' during a party. Martje who is single ends up with Loe in an office at work, but suddenly he jumps backwards when he discovers that Martje has a breast prosthesis. She is deeply hurt although she has experienced this response before. Loe defends himself by saying that his response was one of

surprise rather than shock: he does not mind that she has a fake breast. Once Loe has left, Galina, one of her most devoted workers, enters the office and sees Martje in tears: the Russian thinks Loe has assaulted her, and Martje does not contradict this. Loyal to their boss, the women put Loe in the boiler room the next day to teach him that they cannot be played around with. Martje congratulates them: 'Your action gave him a good fright.' The women do not know that Martje keeps him locked up in the incredibly hot boiler room, and she will keep him there for days. She turns on a machine during working hours so that no one will hear Loe scream. One day, Loe's wife Dorien comes by, to Martje's surprise, for she thought that Loe was single. She says she does not know about her husband's whereabouts but later pays Dorien a return visit. The married couple wanted to have a baby, Dorien tells, and maybe their childless marriage had started to bore him. Martje replies that she has a son, an 'unexpected gift from heaven', and what seems like a lie will turn out to be the start of a psychosis. From this point onwards, she starts making preparations for Loe's release: she asks for an adhesive prosthesis with nipple at the pharmacy; she takes care of the nameless baby boy of the teenage Russian mother Zoya; she buys a sexy dress. She wants his release to be a warm welcome. 'You won't be startled by me again', she yells at him in the boiler room, for she has turned herself into a sexy woman with 'real' breasts and with a child as a bonus. Martje tells him about her plans to go south with him—Loe used to drive to Spain and Morocco in previous years. But when she opens the door of the boiler room and brings grilled chicken and whisky, there is no reaction from Loe. Zoya returns late in the evening to pick up her son, whom Martje has called 'Jan'. The young Russian immediately sees that Loe is dead and wants to help her '*good boss*'. She proposes making a small fire in a container to burn the corpse, but Martje cannot face reality: she tries to imprison Zoya who just barely escapes. She runs away from the laundry service with the baby in her arms. In the final scene, Martje whispers about her dream voyage with Loe, her 'Royal Highness' in a blue uniform, to the sea.

8 The other experimental short on the list happened to be Ditvoorst's black-and-white debut IK KOM WAT LATER NAAR MADRA [THAT WAY TO MADRA] (1965).

9 One year after PENTIMENTO, De la Parra made DIRTY PICTURE (1980), which features several naked and scantily dressed women, similar to Zwartjes' controversial film. A few years earlier, De la Parra had just realized his dream project WAN PIPEL (1976), the very first feature film shot in an independent Suriname. In his native country, the film was regarded as 'the anthem of our new nation' (De la Parra, qtd. in Martens, 88), but it was such a box-office failure in the Netherlands that De la Parra's subsequent projects did not receive funding. Then he got the chance to make a film on a shoestring budget, so he decided to shoot DIRTY PICTURE as if it were 1927: no sound, no zoom lenses, no intertitles, and according to the poster, 'no comedy'. As is written on a mirror, we can read that Dr. Ignacio Cosso, an

optometrist from Colombia, is visiting Amsterdam, '*the Venice of the North*'. Soon the film, '*dedicated to Warren Beatty*', as we can read on a window, turns into a male fantasy scenario: after he has seen a leaflet of '*Tonight ... Rubia*', he encounters a great variety of women: a girl on roller skates, a dominatrix, a disco dancer, a woman who rides him in her rickshaw through the city of Amsterdam. And though DIRTY PICTURE is 'no comedy', there are funny moments: the doctor is nude on a rocking horse; when dressed in a white suit, he slips over dog poop on the street; there is a woman dressed as a giant bottle of beer who is disoriented throughout. When he puts a coin in a parking meter, he sees a view-master exposition of women in erotic poses.

10 Verhoeven himself referred to this kind of response when his American film SHOWGIRLS (1995) won no less than seven 'Razzies' (mock Academy Awards for the worst achievements of the year, among others for Worst Picture and Worst Director), and in truly sportsmanlike fashion, he gave an acceptance speech in person upon receiving the Golden Raspberry Award for Worst Picture. Alluding to the biblical quote that a prophet has no honour in his own country, he also said during the speech: 'When I was making movies in Holland, my films were judged by critics as decadent, perverted and sleazy. So I moved to the United States ten years ago. Now my movies are criticized as being perverted, decadent and sleazy in this country ... This means the United States has become my own country.' This quote is a fine example of Verhoeven's self-mockery, in which he turns the derogatory reviews into his favour: the derision aimed at my picture makes me feel at home in America.

11 The angered reception of PENTIMENTO by feminists is the proverbial exception.

12 Later we get a clearer depiction of the first rape scene in ELLE, when the cat's presence prompts Michèle to recall the scene. This flashback makes it evident that Marty's hesitation when called inside gave the perpetrator time to violently enter the house.

13 In her reading of UTZ (George Sluizer, 1992), based on the eponymous novella by Bruce Chatwin, Anita Weinreb Katz challenges the tendency to see perversion as negative and proposes how it can be used as a comfort. Sluizer's film, she argues, teaches us how perversion may make existence bearable (950). UTZ goes back and forth in time, presenting us flashbacks and flashforwards. Utz bears the title of Baron, but he has had a life of little affection: his father died prematurely, his mother is never mentioned, and in a crucial flashback we see that an anxious grandmother forbids the young kid the porcelain figure of a harlequin, displayed in her vitrine. Since he has difficulty building lasting relationships with people, Utz starts to collect Meissen porcelain, and when he is already quite old of age, as we see at the beginning of the film, set in Prague in 1985, he has finally completed the set of twenty-one monkey musicians. Moreover, as a lover of operas, he seduces female singers and sopranos, but once he has made love to them, he loses

interest. Meanwhile, he has married his servant Marta, who also has a complicated background, but they do not consummate their love, though she expresses her jealousy at his affairs with barely disguised rage. The figurines in his collections are 'erotic equivalents' of his one-night divas, for he can exercise absolute control over these porcelain objects. As such, Katz claims, the collection offers him the perverse compromise, which 'can protect and enable passion when the powerful ambivalences of erotic love are too overwhelming to be risked' (962). Since Utz knows that the communist regime will confiscate his collection after his death, he encourages Marta on his sickbed (in 1989) to destroy his collection. His frustrated wife and servant is more than delighted to shatter the priceless Meissen figurines piece by piece, starting with the harlequin itself.

14 FLESH + BLOOD, also the name of a Roxy Music album from 1980, was sufficiently 'Dutch' to compete at the Netherlands Film Festival. It won a Golden Calf for Best Picture and one for Best Director, although it was explicitly mentioned that the jury was not unanimous. The day after the premiere in Utrecht, Verhoeven went to America to continue his career with ROBOCOP.

15 Later, when Hawkwood suffers from bubonic plague, Steven advises the stubborn doctor to try a new remedy and to lance the swellings. The doctor refuses to listen to the '*un-Christian*' lessons of an '*Arab quack*', but at the very end of FLESH + BLOOD he puts this new method into practice nonetheless.

16 Walsh mentions that there was a consensus that the film was well made and well-acted but bordered on bad taste. He adds that European reviewers took the film more seriously than the American critics, and rightly so, for his central argument is that FLESH + BLOOD may seem 'over the top', but that nonetheless Verhoeven and his scriptwriter Soeteman can be considered honorary medievalists. There are many secular manifestations of the cult of Saint Martin, and the painters Jeronimus Bosch and Pieter Brueghel, in particular, have emphasized the 'wild, violent, even demonic images of the celebration of the Feast of St. Martin'. The excessive and carnivalesque elements in their paintings are a 'close match' to the cynical depiction in Verhoeven's feature, which thus 'manages to tap into a genuine vein of medieval popular mentalite [sic] (...) of the Christian inheritance'.

17 Koolhoven's film had been close to failure after first Mia Wasikowska and then Robert Pattinson dropped out of the project. BRIMSTONE would not have been made—and Koolhoven's production company N279 Entertainment would have gone bankrupt—had it not been for Guy Pearce's confirmation that he would participate which reassured some sceptical film producers. Pearce was enthralled by BRIMSTONE's screenplay, and he believed that Koolhoven's film would allow him to relive his fond memories of his contribution to the Australian western THE PROPOSITION (John Hillcoat, 2005). Wasikowska was replaced by Dakota Fanning who had always been on Koolhoven's wish list but initially had been unavailable, whereas Kit Harington agreed to play Pattinson's vacated role.

18 See my article 'Fortunate Sinners: Martin Koolhoven's BRIMSTONE as an 'Edam' Western' for a lengthier discussion of how the film responds to a Calvinist distrust of images by three formal devices: first, most of the gruesome violence is off-screen; second, Koolhoven uses out-of-focus shots and overhead shots frequently; and third, his use of intertextuality is indeterminate, except for one direct visual quote from THE NIGHT OF THE HUNTER (Charles Laughton, 1955). Whereas Calvinists adhere to textuality in the pretence that it helps them to control meaning, these three devices have the effect of pushing the viewer's imagination beyond our control.

BIBLIOGRAPHY

Abrahams, Anna, 'Not knowing but doing: Frans Zwartjes on Rules', ed. by Anna Abrahams, Mariska Graveland, Erwin van 't Hart and Peter van Hoof, *mm2: Experimental Film in the Netherlands Since 1960*, trans. by Kate Simms and Martin Cleaver (Amsterdam: Filmbank/uitgeverij de Balie, 2004), 197-207.

Brooks, Xan, 'ELLE Review: Paul Verhoeven's Brazen Rape Revenge Comedy is a Dangerous Delight', *The Guardian* (21 May 2016).

Cohen, Sandra E., 'ELLE: Trauma and Perversion: What Does Triumph Have To Do With It?' https://charactersonthecouch.com/film/elle-trauma-perversion-triumph/ [Accessed 12 May 2020].

De Bruijn, Peter, 'Verhoevens ELLE is technisch briljant, maar soms ook tikkeltje saai', *NRC Handelsblad* (31 May 2016).

De Kesel, Marc, *Het Münchhausenparadigma: Waarom Freud en Lacan ertoe doen* (Nijmegen: Vantilt, 2019).

—, 'The Brain: A Nostalgic Dream: Some Notes on Neuroscience and the Problem of Modern Knowledge', ed. by Jan De Vos & Ed Pluth, *Neuroscience and Critique: Exploring the Limits of the Neurological Turn* (London, New York: Routledge, 2016), 11-21.

Freud, Sigmund, 'Totem and Taboo', *The Standard Edition of the Complete Psychological Works of Sigmund Freud. Vol. XIII (1913-1914): Totem and Taboo and Other Works*, 24 vols. (London: Vintage, 2001), 1-161.

Gocić, Nikola, 'PENTIMENTO (Frans Zwartjes, 1979)', *NGboo Art* (12 January 2017), http://ngbooart.blogspot.com/2017/01/pentimento-frans-zwartjes-1979.html [Accessed 14 May 2020].

Heller-Nicholas, Alexandra, 'Cinema as Sex on Cocaine: BASIC INSTINCT (Paul Verhoeven, 1992)', *Senses of Cinema* 83 (June 2017), http://sensesofcinema.com/2017/cteq/basic-instinct/ [Accessed 7 April 2020].

Humpal, Martin, *The Roots of Modernist Narrative: Knut Hamsun's Novels Hunger, Mysteries, and Pan* (Oslo: Solum Forlag, 1998).

Hunter, I.Q., *Cult Film as a Guide to Life: Fandom, Adaptation, and Identity* (New York: Bloomsbury, 2016).

Katz, Anita Weinreb, 'Perversion, Fetish, and Creativity: The Fate of Desire in UTZ', *Psychoanalytic Review* 94, 6 (2007): 943-966.

Lippit, Akira Mizuta, 'Half-Star: Showgirls & Sexbombs.' *Film Quarterly* 56, 3 (2003), p. 34.

Martens, Emiel, 'A Parradox in Caribbean Cinema? An Interview with Minimal Movie Filmmaker Pim de la Parra, Pragmatic Dreamer from Suriname', *Imaginations: Journal of Cross-Cultural Image Studies* 6, 2 (2015): 84-97.https://doi.org/10.17742/IMAGE.CCN.6-2.8

Schokker, Johan and Tim Schokker, *Extimiteit: Jacques Lacans terugkeer naar Freud* (Amsterdam: Boom, 2000).

Sconce, Jeffrey, 'I Have Grown Weary of Your Tiresome Cinema', *Film Quarterly* 56.3 (2003), p. 45.

Stoller, Robert, *Sexual Excitement: Dynamics of Erotic Life* (New York: Pantheon Books, 1979).

Van Scheers, Rob, *Paul Verhoeven: Een filmersleven* (Amsterdam: Podium, 2017).

Walsh, Martin W., 'Sex, Violence, and Saints' Images: Paul Verhoeven's 1985 Film FLESH + BLOOD', *Michigan Academician* 38, 3 (Fall 2008): 175-184.

Žižek, Slavoj, *Enjoy Your Symptom! Jacques Lacan In and Out of Hollywood*, 1992 (Revised Edition. New York and London: Routledge, 2001).

—, *Interrogating the Real*, ed. by Rex Butler and Scott Stephens (London: Bloomsbury, 2013).

—, *Looking Awry: An Introduction to Jacques Lacan through Popular Culture* (Cambridge, Mass.: The MIT Press, 1991).

Epilogue

Verstraten, P., *Dutch Post-War Fiction Film Through a Lens of Psycho-analysis*. Taylor & Francis Group, 2021
DOI 10.5117/9789463725330_EPI

ABSTRACT

Referring to two films by Lili Rademakers and the so-called 'Manifesto for the Imagination', I argue why the oft-mentioned 'realism' of Dutch cinema has contributed to a lack of appreciation for Dutch fiction features. There are good reasons to read Dutch cinema 'anew' and to privilege fantasy over realism, as brief re-readings of SOLDAAT VAN ORANJE, TURKS FRUIT, and BORGMAN illustrate. Some recent films are promising, for they seem to breathe new life into that repressed history of Dutch art cinema from the late 1960s, discussed in the introduction.

KEYWORDS
Manifesto for the Imagination – Reading 'anew' – Fantasy rather than realism – Foreign influences

MENUET [MINUET] (1982), one of only two films directed by Lili Rademakers, has a realistic setting with three protagonists: the taciturn worker at a brewery Pol, his wife Mariëtte, and their young maid Eva.[1] There are only a few developments, shot in a non-spectacular and matter-of-fact style: Mariëtte receives regular visits from her brother-in-law André, who obviously fancies her. Pol is not aware of this flirt, too busy collecting romantic images of wildflowers as well as cutting out gruesome reports from newspapers. Eva has detected the obtrusive behaviour of André, although she has not been witness to the fact that Mariëtte, tired of his persistence, has permitted him to have sex with her in the back of the garden. Pol is surprised to hear that his wife is pregnant, for during the three years of marriage he has been very cautious, he claims. Since Eva makes some insinuating remarks, Mariëtte fires her, but after the baby is born, she is allowed to return. A few days later, Pol falls from a staircase in the cold-storage cellars of the brewery. In the final scenes we hear voice-overs by the three main characters. Mariëtte thinks that Pol knows about her affair with André and that his accident at work is a veiled suicide attempt. Recovering at home from the fall, Pol muses on his unexpressed love for the pretty young maid and the sheer beauty of the hand Eva does not use while cleaning the house. Eva recognizes his sexual excitement; she kneels by his side and puts her hand in his coveralls, whispering: that child is not yours. At that moment, Mariëtte is watching everything from the outside through the window. Since it starts to rain, the baby is handed to Pol, as Eva and Mariëtte take down the laundry to bring it inside.[2]

I have chosen to discuss MENUET by Lili Rademakers—married to Fons from 1960 until his death in 2007—because the narrative is time and again interrupted by peculiar scenes: a farmer finds a naked woman tied to a tree; a middle-aged woman steals a teddy bear and is being caught by the security guard and promptly falls to the ground; the face of a scantily dressed woman on a couch is covered with concrete by two naked men; a retarded boy is shot by his father at his mother's grave. The light in these intermezzos seems a bit softer and the movements slightly protracted. Thus the brusquely inserted scenes, which do not seem to have any bearing on the main story whatsoever, have a surreal quality. At one point, however, we can read the headline of one of the newspaper clippings on his desk: 'widower kills retarded son', and only much later do we see how this killing took place. Hence, we can surmise that the bizarre mini-narratives are the visualizations of the news items Pol cuts out from his paper.

Rademakers' MENUET seems realistic in style and narrative, but her film is interlaced with fantastic scenes. Insofar as these short digressions can be regarded as 'real', they follow the adage that sometimes truth is stranger than fiction. And because of the dark intermezzos, probably an indication of Pol's dark and cynical worldview, the realistic story itself becomes all the more sinister in atmosphere. In the successor to MENUET, DAGBOEK VAN EEN OUDE DWAAS [DIARY OF A MAD, OLD MAN][3] (Lili Rademakers, 1987), fantastic scenes are embedded once more in a realistic scenario. The wealthy Marcel Hamelinck has to retire from work after contracting a chronic muscle disease. He does not give anything to his daughter Karin, for he wants to spend all his money on Simone, the wife of his son Philippe, though the old man knows she is cheating on her husband with his nephew Harry. Marcel wants to build a swimming pool so he can see Simone rehearse her water ballets. In a later scene, she asks for an expensive gem, and in exchange he may caress and suck her red-polished toes. Marcel makes a quick calculation: this will cost him 40,000 francs for each toe. On another occasion, Simone allows him to kiss her lower leg while she is taking a shower, or is this part of his reveries? Even when he is about to die, the end scene shows us Simone swimming under water—his final fantasy, perhaps?

The idea that Dutch fiction cinema tends to privilege 'realism' was at the core of the so-called 'Manifest voor de verbeelding' [Manifesto for the Imagination], presented during the Netherlands Film Festival in 1999.[4] A prejudice reigns, the subscribers claimed, that a scenario has social importance when based upon actual affairs and news items, but when it features goblins, aliens, and/or monsters, it is only fantasy—and thus superficial. Due to this assumption, Dutch cinema is rooted in realism, and, as a corollary, the Netherlands has built a 'great documentary tradition', apparently at the expense of genre films ('Manifest'). In the introduction, I have mentioned that Dutch films that reek of theatricality, including stylized dialogues, risk an unfavourable box-office result, and it is one of the reasons that genre films in the Netherlands have been restricted to movies with a quite 'realistic' angle: pictures about World War II or about the country's Calvinist tradition. Significantly, when the Manifest addresses the possibility of a 'Dutch EXISTENZ' (David Cronenberg's 1999 sci-fi-horror about a virtual reality game), it immediately denies the option by stating that 'bio-ports and Calvinists seem incompatible'. It is usually assumed that the Manifest had little impact, for there are still many biopics (films inspired by true events), and documentaries have neither diminished in quantity nor, fortunately, in quality. And while the output of fantasy films and genre films may have increased, their growth has regrettably not been considerable. There is a different way of looking at the matter, nonetheless.

Steven Jay Schneider mentions in his discussion of SPOORLOOS that 'British and American reviewers (as well as scholars) have consistently, even insistently, analysed [the film - pv] in generic terms, if only to highlight Sluizer's innovative "take" on mainstream/Hollywood horror, thriller and suspense conventions' ('SPOORLOOS', 179). He suggests, by contrast, that Dutch critics and viewers prefer to qualify SPOORLOOS as a 'realistic' film, for they resist the idea that a genre 'associated with cheap American mass-produced fiction (...) can lead to a quality product' (Joke Hermes, qtd. in Schneider, 180). From this angle, I would argue, any report that Dutch fiction features are deeply rooted in realism must be put into perspective. One can claim that MENUET and DAGBOEK VAN EEN OUDE DWAAS are 'realistic' pictures—because of the setting, the 'normal' family relations, the conventional editing—but the fantastic interruptions or erotic daydreams are at least as important, if not more so.

As in these two films by Lili Rademakers, I became struck, during my research, by the imaginative approach of many other Dutch films, even in the cases of biopics, true-event films, or movies motivated by psychological realism: hallucinatory scenes in VAN GOD LOS and BEYOND SLEEP, in LEEDVERMAAK and DE VLIEGENDE HOLLANDER; the remarkable camera angles in AMNESIA and MONSIEUR HAWARDEN, in MYSTERIES and GEBROKEN SPIEGELS; theatrical acting in KARAKTER and VAN DE KOELE MEREN DES DOODS, in HOOGSTE TIJD and ELINE VERE; the suspense in SPOORLOOS and HET ZWIJGEN, in AMSTERDAMNED and ZWART WATER; poetic sequences in BOVEN IS HET STIL and PARANOIA, in PENTIMENTO and 170HZ; the elliptical storytelling in GUERNSEY and ONDER ONS, in GLUCKAUF and NOTHING PERSONAL; and of course, the 'middle-of-the-road absurdism' of Alex van Warmerdam, who was the key reference in my previous study.

Perhaps the oft-mentioned 'realism' of Dutch cinema is a persistent myth that has worked to the disadvantage of the fiction features. The idea of 'realism' was grist to the mill of those critics who said that Dutch filmmakers are better in making documentaries; of those who said it was proof that there is no real film culture; and of those who claimed that the Manifest had not even thrown the tiniest of pebbles in the pond of Dutch film funding. One of my aims by reading the selected films through a psychoanalytic lens was to dissociate Dutch cinema from the presumed standard of 'realism' and to call for a benevolent stance towards Dutch cinema: look at them 'anew' and dare to privilege fantasy over realism. Let me illustrate this point by briefly recapitulating a few of the very best pictures in Dutch film history.

AWAKENINGS: *SOLDAAT VAN ORANJE, TURKS FRUIT,* AND *BORGMAN*

There are good reasons to read SOLDAAT VAN ORANJE as a historical account of the Dutch resistance against the Nazis, especially since it starts with black-and-white newsreel footage. Though the colour film places the actors convincingly in the world depicted in the newsreel, as J.P. Telotte asserts (6), he adds to this that the narrative 'develops into a play of visual deceptions or subterfuges' (9). A laundry line is also the antenna for a clandestine radio; Esther strips in front of a window to divert a Gestapo agent so Erik can meet Robbie; Erik wears a British naval uniform which, he is told, looks just like a German naval uniform '*from a distance*'; before going on board a ship, a group of sailors, including Erik, pretend to be drunk to avoid control by Nazi officers; Guus is in the boiler room of a ship, disguised as a sailor, and even Erik does not recognize him; the British 'allies' send Guus and others back to Holland to make the Germans believe that the invasion will be planned through the Netherlands (Telotte, 9-11). SOLDAAT VAN ORANJE teaches us 'that in a constantly deceptive world one need not see very well to prosper' (12). Erik suffers from poor eyesight, but in order to become a pilot, he cheats during the examination. Susan advises him to secretly use a tiny piece of his broken glasses to read aloud the required letters. Having fooled the examining officer who casually declares his eyes are excellent, Erik is permitted to fly as a pilot, which earns him the title of 'soldier of Orange'. In a world mediated by imageries—from newsreels to advertisements and propaganda[5]—it can be more beneficial not to trust one's eyes but to gradually awaken oneself to 'the power of the imagination' (Telotte, 13).

Another Erik, the bohemian-artist in Verhoeven's crowd-puller TURKS FRUIT, has a series of bed partners in the beginning (see also the introduction). It soon becomes clear, however, that this is not so much the result of sexual appetite but of melancholy. He brings a young woman inside his unlit home, and his eyes catch a silhouette. He is mesmerized, something that is affirmed by the soundtrack. He sees the contours of Olga, posing with her chin up. When he switches on the light, he returns to 'reality': Olga has not come back, but the woman near the window is one of his sculptures. Though regarded as a realistic picture, this 'hallucinatory' vision in TURKS FRUIT is a crucial one, for it sets in motion the lengthy flashback that explains why Erik became spellbound by Olga.

In my previous book with the American poster of Van Warmerdam's BORGMAN (2013) on its cover, I described this film as a 'black horror-pastiche'. BORGMAN was about the disintegration of the marriage between Richard and Marina after the vagrant Camiel Borgman has invaded their house. Initially, Marina felt guilty about the aggressive way her husband had treated the hobo, who had only asked to take a bath. She keeps him out of sight of her husband,

and when he walks inside the house, he is like a ghost: he seems invisible to Richard. Later, a clean-shaven Borgman is accepted by Richard as the new gardener, and in the vein of a true vampire, he says that he never enters a house uninvited. Whether Borgman is a vampire, an angel, a devil, a magician, or a virus[6] remains an enigma, but in the end he causes the death of the married couple. Since the identity of the title character is so elusive, I argued in *Humour and Irony*, Van Warmerdam's film escapes categorization, oscillating between horror and hilarity, between irony and seriousness (288).

Though I still stand by this analysis, I would like to use BORGMAN as a brief example of my idea of reading 'anew'. At the end of the film, Borgman and his offbeat company leave the ruined residence. We see the three docile children of Richard and Marina plus the Danish au-pair joining them. Unlike her siblings, the middle child Isolde had been perceptive of the presence of Borgman from the very start, and she seemed most hospitable to the vagrant. Thus, one can also read the film according to Freud's theory of the neurotic's family romance. According to a young child, the father is the noblest and strongest of men and the mother the dearest and loveliest of women. As the kid grows up, she/he learns that the parents do not have the unique qualities attributed to them and starts to fantasize that she/he is an adopted child, born of parents with a higher social standing. In the child's fantasy, 'both parents are replaced by others of better birth' (Freud 'Family', 239). In a second sexual stage of the family romance, a child can fantasize that he/she is the product of a secret love affair the mother has had with someone of nobler origin than the kid's own father. The perverted pseudo-family of Borgman lives up to this fantasy of Isolde, who herself displays some dark impulses, as in the scene when she hits a wounded man on the head with a tile. BORGMAN is then staged according to Isolde's fantasy that she wants a more intriguing family tree. In her eyes, the enigmatic Borgman is a valid substitute for her father with his short fuse.[7]

In all fairness, most Dutch film critics do take a generous attitude towards Dutch arthouse pictures, realizing their vulnerability, but despite quite favourable reviews, this usually does not result into well-attended movies.[8] Critics Dana Linssen and Jan Pieter Ekker initiated in 2015 the so-called 'Forum van de Regisseurs' ('Forum of the Directors') with the aim of putting Dutch art films in the limelight. Many of the key films in this section of the Netherlands Film Festival seem to downplay their Dutch background. Let's consider the consecutive winners of the editions until 2020, with the exception of the year 2019 when a documentary was awarded instead of a fiction feature: the poetic docudrama THOSE WHO FEEL THE FIRE BURNING (Morgan Knibbe, 2014) had seven languages spoken but no Dutch; FULL CONTACT (David Verbeek, 2015) had English, French, and Arabic spoken, but no Dutch; QUALITY TIME (Daan Bakker, 2017) was in Dutch but also in Norwegian; LIGHT AS FEATHERS

(Rosanne Pel, 2018) was entirely in Polish,[9] whereas the main prize in 2020 was for Janis Rafa's Greek-spoken KALA AZAR. Several talented Dutch directors have opted for non-Dutch spoken films, such as REGAINED MEMORY (Stijn Bouma, 2017) in Bosnian; TAKE ME SOMEWHERE NICE (Ena Sendijarević, 2018) in Bosnian, English, and Dutch; DIRTY GOD (Sacha Polak, 2018), Polak's first feature film in English; THE BEAST IN THE JUNGLE (Clara van Gool, 2018) in English; PARADISE DRIFTERS (Mees Peijnenburg, 2020) in Dutch, English, French, and Spanish, whereas the winner of the Golden Calf Best Feature Film BULADÓ (Eché Janga, 2020), is predominantly in Papiamento, for its story is set on the island of Curaçao.

More important than the fact that other languages than Dutch are being used is that the majority of these recent films, though small-scale productions, try to explore the rules of cinema. THE BEAST IN THE JUNGLE stands out for its choreographed scenes and ravishing cinematography. NOCTURNE (Victor van der Valk, 2019) is like a visual stream-of-consciousness, portraying the doubts and musings of a filmmaker about both a problematic relationship and a creative crisis: 'art is at odds with compromises', protagonist Alex claims. Van der Valk's 'Brechtian film noir' describes itself as an 'attempt at cinema', thereby alluding not only to an early Godard picture such as À BOUT DE SOUFFLE but also to Weisz's HET GANGSTERMEISJE. And the aforementioned TAKE ME SOMEWHERE NICE could be classified as a hyper styled version of Jim Jarmusch's nomadic road movie STRANGER THAN PARADISE (1984). Though Sendijarević's film is shot in a cramped 4:3 aspect ratio and is dominated by the colours candy pink and mint green, it has a similar ensemble as Jarmusch's picture: a girl visits her nephew's place in another country and meets the latter's friend. In both films, hanging about is their main occupation. The Dutch Alma goes to Bosnia to visit her father in hospital. To prove to Denis that she is Emir's niece, she shows him that she has similar dogteeth. Emir is supposed to bring her to the hospital, but despite not having a job, he is always too busy, or so he says. Alma decides to take a bus, but she fails to board the bus in time after a break, and her suitcase is gone. After several more detours, she finally arrives at the hospital in the company of both Emir and Denis, who displays a romantic interest in Alma. She hears that her father has already died the other day, and the three thereupon spend a night in the old man's empty house. When they are about to bury the deceased, two policemen want to control the content of the coffin in the back of the car. They end up at the sea where Denis becomes the victim of senseless violence. Heavily bruised in his face and only half-conscious, Alma makes love to him.

Apart from its dreamy and bright colours, the quirky TAKE ME SOMEWHERE NICE stands out for its odd framing, especially its many high angles, which invite the viewer to detect geometric patterns. The film also has amplified sounds to emphasize the quirkiness: the noise of a neighbour's electric hedge trimmer forces Alma and her mother to converse in louder voices when sitting in their garden. In an interview in *De Filmkrant*, Sendijarević said that she does not want to 'just' document the world or add humour to it, for the only way a filmmaker can hope to encourage viewers to change the world is by exposing it as an 'absurd construction' (qtd. in Rovers). If filmmakers adopt a mentality of traveling the road of their imagination,[10] then an upcoming generation of directors might be able to produce 'fantastic' pictures—from wayward exercises in identification in the vein of GUERNSEY to genre rewrites such as BRIMSTONE; from new takes on the tradition of war pictures depicting a moral grey area, established since ALS TWEE DRUPPELS WATER to challenging perspectives on Dutch colonial practices that shed further light on what the cover-up in DE SCHORPIOEN was all about.

NOTES

1 MENUET was a Belgian production, with the Netherlands as minority co-production partner. The Flemish Film Committee considered this project so typically Flemish that the board objected to the Dutch Lili Rademakers as director. Her husband Fons intervened by contacting the Belgian minister of culture. In the end, the Film Committee approved the project in the hope that it might give a new impetus to Flemish-Dutch co-productions (Willems *Subsidie*, 96).

2 Rademakers' debut feature is an adaptation of the modernist novella *Menuet* (1955) written by the well-known Flemish writer Louis Paul Boon. The novella is divided into three parts: 'The cold-storage cellars', told in the first person by the husband; 'My planet', told by the maid; and 'The Island', told by the wife. The structure and the significant chapter titles imply that the characters are isolated from one another. Since the three talk about the same events, it becomes clear that an interpretation of a scene depends on the eye of the beholder. In addition, each page has eight lines at the top, printed in small caps, that describe an endless stream of often gruesome news item reports. The screenplay was by Hugo Claus, who had written the scenarios of five films by Lili's husband.

3 The film is based upon a novel by Jun'ichirô Tanizaki; Claus wrote the script once again, but this time with Claudine Bouvier.

4 Originally an initiative by Elbert van Strien, Guido van Gennep, and Djie Han Thung, the manifesto was signed by 46 filmmakers who supported the demand for more funding for projects that were not rooted in (daily) reality.

5 Verhoeven's American films in particular, such as ROBOCOP, TOTAL RECALL, and STARSHIP TROOPERS, are pervaded with commercial spots, television news, and

propaganda clips. Such imagery has an almost irresistible power upon the characters in these movies. Verhoeven's films beg the question whether strategies are possible for resisting the visual attraction of modern mediated culture (Telotte, 3).

6 In ABEL [VOYEUR] (Alex van Warmerdam, 1986), the main protagonist asks a theatre actress whether she is able to play the role of a potato. As Jan Maarten Dalmeijer once suggested, the film BORGMAN tries to answer the question whether it is possible to play the role of a virus.

7 This was suggested by Willem Heuves during his introductory lecture to the film in the Louis Hartlooper Complex in Utrecht on 25 October 2017.

8 There were about 115,000 moviegoers for BORGMAN in the Netherlands and almost 200,000 for BRIMSTONE. But it is quite rare for a Dutch arthouse film to gain the status of 'Gouden Film' [Golden Film], meaning that it has attracted more than 100,000 viewers in the Dutch theatres.

9 LIGHT AS FEATHERS had to share the VEVAM Fonds prize of the Forum van de Regisseurs with the VR documentary DE STOEL VAN DE LAATSTE JAREN [THE LAST CHAIR] (Anke Teunissen and Jessie van Vreden, 2018), which has an English voice-over by Rutger Hauer.

10 An example of a recent Dutch film that had a commercial release in a great many theatres and nonetheless travels the road of imagination is DE BELOFTE VAN PISA [THE PROMISE] (Norbert ter Hall, 2019), based on Mano Bouzamour's eponymous novel. In the film, the Moroccan teenager Samir, raised in a traditional Islamic family, is permitted to attend a high-class, all-white music school thanks to his talents as an aspiring trumpet player. Apart from convincing acting, the film stands out for its mobile camera including overhead shots, its changes of focus, slowed-down movements, and jump cuts. Rather than a multi-cultural drama set in Amsterdam, these formal choices turn DE BELOFTE VAN PISA into a 'big city blues', and the use of George Gershwin's 'Rhapsody in Blue' as one of its musical themes, just as in Woody Allen's MANHATTAN (1979) is the icing on the cake.

BIBLIOGRAPHY

De Fantasten, 'Manifest voor de Verbeelding / Manifesto for the Imagination', https://dht.home.xs4all.nl/fantasten/manifesto.html [Accessed 10 May 2020].

Freud, Sigmund. 'Family Romances', *The Standard Edition of the Complete Psychological Works of Sigmund Freud, Volume IX (1906-1908): Jensen's 'Gradiva' and Other Works*, 24 vols. (London: Vintage, 2001), 235-241.

Reinsma, Janna, 'TAKE ME SOMEWHERE NICE: Zuurstokroze zwerfmovie door godverlaten Bosnië', *De Filmkrant* 420 (May 2019): 7.

Rovers, Ronald, 'Ena Sendijarević over TAKE ME SOMEWHERE NICE: "Dat denk ik dus niet dat we sowieso richting de dood gaan"', *De Filmkrant* 420 (May 2019): 6-7.

Schneider, Steven Jay, 'SPOORLOOS / THE VANISHING', ed. by Mathijs, *The Cinema of the Low Countries*, 177-185.

Telotte, J.P., 'Narratives of Resistance: Verhoeven's SOLDIER OF ORANGE', *Film Criticism* 30, 3 (2006): 3-16.

Verstraten, Peter, *Humour and Irony in Dutch Post-war Fiction Film* (Amsterdam: Amsterdam University Press, 2016).

Willems, Gertjan, *Subsidie, Camera, Actie! Filmbeleid in Vlaanderen* (1964-2002) (Gent: Academia Press, 2017).

BIBLIOGRAPHY

Abrahams, Anna, 'Not Knowing but Doing: Frans Zwartjes on Rules', ed. by Anna Abrahams, Mariska Graveland, Erwin van 't Hart and Peter van Hoof, *mm2: Experimental Film in the Netherlands Since 1960*, trans. by Kate Simms and Martin Cleaver (Amsterdam: Filmbank/uitgeverij de Balie, 2004), 97-207.

Anonymous, 'Nouchka van Brakel over het kleine opdondertje', *Vrij Nederland* (16 September 1995), https://www.vn.nl/nouchka-van-brakel-over-het-kleine-opdondertje/ [Accessed 17 May 2020].

Balakian, Anna, *Surrealism: The Road to the Absolute*, 1959, revised and enlarged (London: Unwin Books, 1972).

Barten, Egbert, 'Toenemende vrijheid: De verwerking van de Tweede Wereldoorlog in de Nederlandse speelfilm', ed. by D.H. Schram and C. Geljon, *Overal sporen: De verwerking van de Tweede Wereldoorlog in literatuur en kunst* (Amsterdam: VU Uitgeverij, 1990), 213-251.

Baudry, Jean-Louis, 'Ideological Effects of the Basic Cinematographic Apparatus', 1970, *Film Quarterly* Vol. 28, No. 2 (Winter, 1974-1975): 39-47.

Beekman, Bor, 'Met Koolhoven de grens over', *de Volkskrant*, 30 December 2015, V4-6.

—, 'We hébben al een neger', kreeg Jack Monkau te horen. De acteur kan er nog om lachen', *de Volkskrant* (4 March 2020), https://www.volkskrant.nl/cultuur-media/we-hebben-al-een-neger-kreeg-jack-monkau-te-horen-de-acteur-kan-er-nog-om-lachen~b09d0427/ [Accessed 16 May 2020].

Beerekamp, Hans, 'ALS TWEE DRUPPELS WATER', *NRC Handelsblad*, 21 August 1996.

Bellour, Raymond, 'Symbolic Blockage (on NORTH BY NORTHWEST)', *The Analysis of Film* (Bloomington and Indianapolis: Indiana University Press, 2000), 77-192.

Bernink, Mieke, *Fons Rademakers: Scènes uit leven en werk* (Abcoude: Uniepers, 2003).

Bickerton, Emilie, 'Reinventing Realism: The Art and Politics of the Dardenne Brothers', *Cinéaste* 31, 2 (2006): 14-18.

Boon, Louis Paul, *Menuet* (Amsterdam: Arbeiderspers, 1955).

Bouineau, Jean-Marc, *Paul Verhoeven: Beyond Flesh and Blood* (Paris: Cinephage, 2001).

Bordwell, David, and Noël Carroll, *Post-Theory: Reconstructing Film Studies* (Madison, Wisconsin: University of Wisconsin Press, 1996).

Bovekerk, Henk, 'Waarom kijken mensen naar films vol ellende?' *Vice*, 11 December 2015, http://www.henkbovekerk.nl/waarom-kijken-mensen-naar-films-vol-ellende/ [Accessed 3 February 2020]

Broeren, Joost, 'BEYOND SLEEP: Dwalen in een slapeloos moeras', *De Filmkrant* 384 (February 2016), https://filmkrant.nl/recensies/beyond-sleep/ [Accessed 10 October 2019]

Brooks, Xan, 'ELLE Review: Paul Verhoeven's Brazen Rape Revenge Comedy is a Dangerous Delight', *The Guardian*, 21 May 2016.

Burke, Wendy, *Images of Occupation in Dutch Film: Memory, Myth and the Cultural Legacy of War* (Amsterdam: Amsterdam University Press, 2017).

Casey, Kieron, 'BIFF Film Review: 170 Hz', *The Totality*, http://www.wondrouskennel.com/2013/04/film-review-170hz.html [Accessed 17 May 2020]

Choe, Steve, *Sovereign Violence: Ethics and South Korean Cinema in the New Millennium* (Amsterdam: Amsterdam University Press, 2016).

Claus, Hugo, *De dans van de reiger: Een nare komedie in twee delen*, 1962 (Amsterdam: De Bezige Bij, 1965).

Clover, Carol J., 'Her Body, Himself: Gender in the Slasher Film', 1993, ed. by Mark Jancovich, *Horror: The Film Reader* (London and New York: Routledge, 2002), 77-89.

Cohen, Sandra E., 'ELLE: Trauma and Perversion: What Does Triumph Have To Do With It?' https://charactersonthecouch.com/film/elle-trauma-perversion-triumph/ [Accessed 12 May 2020].

Cowie, Peter, *Dutch Cinema* (London: Tantivy Press, 1979).

Croll, Ben, 'COBAIN: Berlin Review', *ScreenDaily* (17 February 2018), https://www.screendaily.com/reviews/cobain-berlin-review/5125718.article [Accessed 15 May 2020].

De Bruijn, Peter, 'Verhoevens ELLE is technisch briljant, maar soms ook tikkeltje saai', *NRC Handelsblad*, 31 May 2016.

De Fantasten, 'Manifest voor de Verbeelding / Manifesto for the Imagination', https://dht.home.xs4all.nl/fantasten/manifesto.html [Accessed 10 May 2020].

De Kesel, Marc, *Het Münchhausenparadigma: Waarom Freud en Lacan ertoe doen* (Nijmegen: Vantilt, 2019).

—, 'The Brain: A Nostalgic Dream: Some Notes on Neuroscience and the Problem of Modern Knowledge', ed. by Jan De Vos and Ed Pluth, *Neuroscience and Critique: Exploring the Limits of the Neurological Turn* (London, New York: Routledge, 2016), 11-21.

Den Drijver, Ruud, *Circus Bloteman: Biografie van Wim Verstappen, Filmpionier uit de West* (Amsterdam: Stichting Wim Verstappen Scorpio Films, 2015).

DiPiero, Thomas, 'The Patriarch Is Not (Just) a Man', *Camera Obscura* 25-26 (1991): 101-24.

Doane, Mary Ann, *The Desire to Desire: The Woman's Film of the 1940s* (Bloomington and Indianapolis: Indiana University Press, 1987).

Elsaesser, Thomas, 'Specularity and Engulfment: Francis Ford Coppola's and BRAM STOKER'S DRACULA', ed. by Steve Neale and Murray Smith, *Contemporary Hollywood Cinema* (London and New York: Routledge, 1998), 191-208.

Foundas, Scott, 'THE VANISHING: The End of the Road', *The Criterion Collection* (29 October 2014), https://www.criterion.com/current/posts/3340-the-vanishing-the-end-of-the-road [Accessed 12 May 2020].

Freedman, Ariela, 'Charlotte Salomon, Degenerate Art and Modernism as Resistance', *Journal of Modern Literature* 41, 1 (2017): 3-18.

Freud, Sigmund. 'Family Romances', *The Standard Edition of the Complete Psychological Works of Sigmund Freud, Volume IX (1906-1908): Jensen's 'Gradiva' and Other Works*, 24 vols. (London: Vintage, 2001), 235-241.

—, 'The Interpretation of Dreams', *The Standard Edition of the Complete Psychological Works of Sigmund Freud, Volume V (1900-1901): The Interpretation of Dreams (Second Part) and On Dreams*, 24 vols. (London: Vintage, 2001), 339-622.

—, 'Moses and Monotheism', *The Standard Edition of the Complete Psychological Works of Sigmund Freud, Volume XXIII (1937-1939): Moses and Monotheism, An Outline of Psycho-analysis and Other Works*, 24 vols. (London: Vintage, 2001), 3-137.

—, 'Neurosis and Psychosis', *The Standard Edition of the Complete Psychological Works of Sigmund Freud, Volume XIX (1923-1925): The Ego and the Id and Other Works*, 24 vols. (London: Vintage, 2001), 147-154.

—, 'On Narcissism: An Introduction', *The Standard Edition of the Complete Psychological Works of Sigmund Freud, Volume XIV (1914-1916): On the History of the Psycho-analytic Movement, Papers on Metapsychology and Other Works*, 24 vols. (London: Vintage, 2001), 67-102.

—, 'Psycho-analytic Notes on an Autobiographical Account of a Case of Paranoia (Dementia Paranoides)', *The Standard Edition of the Complete Psychological Works of Sigmund Freud. Vol. XII (1911-1913): The Case of Schreber, Papers on Technique and Other Works*, 24 vols. (London: Vintage, 2001), 9-79.

—, 'Totem and Taboo', *The Standard Edition of the Complete Psychological Works of Sigmund Freud. Vol. XIII (1913-1914): Totem and Taboo and Other Works*, 24 vols. (London: Vintage, 2001), 1-161.

Gallop, Jane, *Reading Lacan* (Ithaca: Cornell University Press, 1985).

Geske, Colleen, *You Know That You're Dutch When ...* (Amsterdam, Edenfrost VOF, 2017).

Gocić, Nikola, 'PENTIMENTO (Frans Zwartjes, 1979)', *NGboo Art* (12 January 2017), http://ngbooart.blogspot.com/2017/01/pentimento-frans-zwartjes-1979.html [Accessed 14 May 2020].

Graveland, Mariska, '"Er knaagt iets": David Verbeek over R U THERE', *De Filmkrant* 382 (December 2015): http://filmkrant.nl/interview/david-verbeek-over-r-u-there/ [Accessed 14 May 2020].

—, Fritz de Jong and Paul Kempers eds., *De broertjes van* ZUSJE: *De nieuwe Nederlandse film 1995-2005* (Amsterdam: International Theatre & Film Books, 2006).

Hassler-Forest, Dan, *Capitalist Superheroes: Caped Crusaders in the Neoliberal Age* (Alresford: Zero Books, 2012).

Hayward, Susan, 'Beyond the gaze and into *femme-filmécriture*: Agnès Varda's SANS TOIT NI LOI (1985)', ed. by Susan Hayward and Ginette Vincendeau, *French Film: Texts and Contexts* (London and New York: Routledge, 1990), 285-296.

Heller-Nicholas, Alexandra, 'Cinema as Sex on Cocaine: BASIC INSTINCT (Paul Verhoeven, 1992)', *Senses of Cinema* 83 (June 2017), http://sensesofcinema.com/2017/cteq/basic-instinct/ [Accessed 7 April 2020].

Hermans, Willem Frederik, 'Blokker en Bommel', *Podium* 18, 1 (October 1963): 38-48.

—, *De donkere kamer van Damokles*, 1958 (Amsterdam: G.A. van Oorschot, 1997, 34e ed.).

—, 'Paranoia', *Paranoia*, 1953 (Amsterdam: G.A. van Oorschot, 1985).

Hewitson, Owen, 'What Does Lacan Say About ... Acting Out?' *Lacanonline.com*,https://www.lacanonline.com/2010/12/what-does-lacan-say-about-acting-out/ [Accessed 13 March 2020].

Hinson, Hal, 'Tracks in the Snow', *Washington Post*, 24 August 1987.

Hofstede, Bart, *Nederlandse cinema wereldwijd: De internationale positie van de Nederlandse film* (Amsterdam: Boekmanstudies, 2000).

Hoogendoorn, Maurice, 'Religie in films is nu exotische folklore', *Nederlands Dagblad*, 19 February 2016.

Hughes, Judith M., *From Freud's Consulting Room: The Unconscious in a Scientific Age* (Cambridge, Mass.: Harvard University Press, 1994).

Humpal, Martin, *The Roots of Modernist Narrative: Knut Hamsun's Novels* Hunger, Mysteries, *and* Pan (Oslo: Solum Forlag, 1998).

Hunter, I.Q., *Cult Film as a Guide to Life: Fandom, Adaptation, and Identity* (New York: Bloomsbury, 2016).

IMAGO, ed., *Making Pictures: A Century of European Cinematography* (New York: Harry N. Abrams, Inc., 2003).

Jaehne, Karen, 'ANTONIA'S LINE', *Film Quarterly* 50, 1 (1996): 27-30.

Juttmann, Bart, *Op zoek naar* SOLDAAT VAN ORANJE*: De geschiedenis van de Nederlandse filmklassieker* (Amsterdam: International Theatre & Film Books, 2020).

Katz, Anita Weinreb, 'Perversion, Fetish, and Creativity: The Fate of Desire in UTZ', *Psychoanalytic Review* 94, 6 (2007): 943-966.

Keulemans, Chris, 'Karim Traïdia: een Algerijnse dromer die meer wil weten dan er te weten valt', ed. by Wim Willems, *Cultuur en migratie in Nederland: De kunst van het overleven* (The Hague: Sdu Uitgevers, 2004), 247-275.

Kiang, Jessica, 'Berlin Film Review: RETROSPEKT', *Variety* (12 February 2019), https://variety.com/2019/film/markets-festivals/retrospekt-review-1203127677/ [Accessed 16 May 2020].

Kleijer, Pauline, 'CODE BLUE: een opzettelijk ongemakkelijke film', *De Volkskrant*, 25 September 2011, https://www.volkskrant.nl/nieuws-achtergrond/code-blue-een-opzettelijk-ongemakkelijke-film~b92a6996/ [Accessed 12 May 2020].

Koetsier, Sasja, 'COBAIN: Het is wel mijn moeder', *De Filmkrant* 408 (April 2018), https://filmkrant.nl/recensies/cobain/ [Accessed 13 May 2020].

Kovács, András Bálint, *Screening Modernism: European Art Cinema, 1950-1980* (Chicago: University of Chicago Press, 2007).

Koven, Mikel J., '*Twee koffers vol* / LEFT LUGGAGE', ed. by Mathijs, 231-237.

Lacan, Jacques, 'Desire and the Interpretation of Desire in *Hamlet*', *Yale French Studies* 55/56 (1977): 11-52.

—, *Écrits: A Selection*, trans. by Alan Sheridan, 1977 (London: Routledge, 2001).

—, *Encore: Book XX, 1972-1973*, trans. by Cormac Gallagher, 1994 (Eastbourne, Antony Rowe Ltd., 2004).

—, *The Ethics of Psychoanalysis: Book VII, 1959-1960*, trans. by Dennis Porter (London: Routledge, 1991).

—, *Four Fundamental Concepts of Psycho-analysis*, trans. by Alan Sheridan (New York: Penguin, 1994).

—, *The Psychoses: Book III, 1955-1956*, trans. by Russell Grigg (London: Routledge, 1993).

—, *Television: A Challenge to the Psychoanalytic Establishment*, trans. by Denis Hollier, Rosalind Krauss, and Annette Michelson (New York: W.W. Norton and Company, 1990).

Linssen, Dana, 'Jim Taihuttu in zwart-wit: Checklist tegen politiekcorrect filmmaken', *De Filmkrant* (August 2013), https://filmkrant.nl/interview/jim-taihuttu-in-zwart-wit/ [Accessed 13 May 2020].

Lippit, Akira Mizuta, 'Half-Star: Showgirls & Sexbombs', *Film Quarterly* 56, 3 (2003): 34.

Maas, Dick, *Buurman, wat doet u nu? Films maken in Nederland: Tips, trucs, anekdotes, roddel & achterklap* (Amsterdam: Parachute Pictures, 2017).

Marks, Laura, *Touch: Sensuous Theory And Multisensory Media* (Minneapolis and London: University Of Minnesota Press, 2002).

Martens, Emiel, 'A Parradox in Caribbean Cinema? An Interview with Minimal Movie Filmmaker Pim de la Parra, Pragmatic Dreamer from Suriname', *Imaginations: Journal of Cross-Cultural Image Studies* 6, 2 (2015): 84-97. https://doi.org/10.17742/IMAGE.CCN.6-2.8

Martin, Adrian, *Mise en Scene and Film Style: From Classical Hollywood to New Media Art* (New York: Palgrave MacMillan, 2014).

Mathijs, Ernest, 'LES LÈVRES ROUGES / DAUGHTERS OF DARKNESS', ed. by Mathijs, 97-106.

—, ed. *The Cinema of the Low Countries* (London and New York: Wallflower Press, 2004).

McCrea, Christian, 'Fascism for Liberals: ROBOCOP (Paul Verhoeven, 1987)', *Senses of Cinema* 83 (June 2017): http://sensesofcinema.com/2017/cteq/robocop/ [Accessed 17 May 2020].

McGowan, Todd, *Psychoanalytic Film Theory and* THE RULES OF THE GAME (New York: Bloomsbury, 2015).

McGrath, Alistair E., *A Life of John Calvin: A Study in the Shaping of Western Culture* (Oxford: Basil Blackwell, 1990).

Metz, Christian, *The Imaginary Signifier: Psychoanalysis and Cinema*, trans. by Celia Britton, Annwyl Williams, Ben Brewster, and Alfred Guzzetti (Bloomington and Indianapolis: Indiana University Press, 1982).

Möller, Olaf, 'From the Abyss to Blue Skies', *Film Comment* (July-August 2013): 14-15.

Mooij, Antoine, *Taal en verlangen: Lacans theorie van de psychoanalyse* (Meppel: Boom, 1975).

Mosley, Philip, 'DE MAN DIE ZIJN HAAR KORT LIET KNIPPEN / THE MAN WHO HAD HIS HAIR CUT SHORT', ed. by Mathijs, 76-85.

Mulvey, Laura. 'Visual Pleasure and Narrative Cinema.' *Screen* 16, no. 3 (1975): 6-18.

Op den Kamp, Claudy, *The Greatest Films Never Seen: The Film Archive and the Copyright Smokescreen* (Amsterdam: Amsterdam University Press, 2018).

Op den Velde, Minou, 'Dit is Nanouk Leopold', 97-105. http://minouopdenvelde.nl/pdf/interviews/NanoukLeopold.pdf [Accessed 14 May 2020].

Pattynama, Pamela, '*Max Havelaar*, of de invloed van de populaire media op de herinnering aan Indië.' *Indische Letteren* 21, 3 (2006): 169-185.

Pirandello, Luigi, *One, No One and a Hundred Thousand* http://gutenberg.net.au/ebooks16/1600681h.html [Accessed 14 May 2020].

Pisters, Patricia, 'Lili and Rachel: Hollywood, History, and Women in Fassbinder and Verhoeven', ed. by Jaap Kooijman, Patricia Pisters, and Wanda Strauven, *Mind the Screen: Media Concepts According to Thomas Elsaesser* (Amsterdam: Amsterdam University Press, 2008), 177-187.

Pollock, Griselda, 'Crimes, Confession, and the Everyday: Challenges in Reading Charlotte Salomon's *Leben? oder Theater?* 1941-1942', *Journal of Visual Culture* 13, 2 (2014): 200-235.

Rancière, Jacques, 'The noise of people, the image of art', (1999), trans. by Stoffel Debuysere, *Diagonal Thoughts* (2012), http://www.diagonalthoughts.com/?p=1500 [Accessed 14 May 2020].

Reinsma, Janna, 'TAKE ME SOMEWHERE NICE: Zuurstokroze zwerfmovie door godverlaten Bosnië', *De Filmkrant* 420 (May 2019): 7.

Rovers, Ronald, 'Ena Sendijarević over TAKE ME SOMEWHERE NICE: "Dat denk ik dus niet dat we sowieso richting de dood gaan"', *De Filmkrant* 420 (May 2019): 6-7.

Rushton, Richard, 'Empathic Projection in the Films of the Dardenne Brothers', *Screen* 55, 3 (2014): 303-316.

Scheffer, Paul, 'Het multiculturele drama', *NRC Handelsblad*, 29 January 2000, https://www.nrc.nl/nieuws/2000/01/29/het-multiculturele-drama-a3987586 [Accessed 12 May 2020].

Schmid, Katharina, '"Fremd bin ich eingezogen ..." – An Outsider's Vision of Ireland in Urszula Antoniak's NOTHING PERSONAL', *Estudios Irlandeses* 8 (2013): 105-113.

Schneider, Steven Jay, 'Repackaging Rage: THE VANISHING and NIGHTWATCH', *Kinema: A Journal for Film and Audiovisual Media* 17 (1 April 2002): 47-66.

—, 'SPOORLOOS / THE VANISHING', ed. by Mathijs, 177-185.

Schokker, Johan and Tim Schokker, *Extimiteit: Jacques Lacans terugkeer naar Freud* (Amsterdam: Boom, 2000).

Schoots, Hans, *Bert Haanstra: Filmer van Nederland* (Amsterdam: Mets en Schilt, 2009).

—, *Van* FANFARE *tot* SPETTERS: *Een cultuurgeschiedenis van de jaren zestig en zeventig* (Amsterdam: Lubberhuizen, 2004).

Sconce, Jeffrey, 'I Have Grown Weary of Your Tiresome Cinema', *Film Quarterly* 56.3 (2003): 45.

Silverman, Kaja, *Male Subjectivity at the Margins* (New York: Routledge, 1992).

Smelik, Anneke, 'And the Mirror Cracked: Metaphors of Violence in the Films of Marleen Gorris', *Women's Studies International Forum* 16, 4 (1993): 349-363.

Sontag, Susan, 'Notes on "Camp"', 1964, *Against Interpretation and Other Essays* (London and New York: Penguin Classics, 2009), 275-292.

—, 'Spiritual Style in the Films of Robert Bresson', 1964, *Against Interpretation and Other Essays* (London and New York: Penguin Classics, 2009), 177-195.

Stewart, Garrett, *Framed Time: Toward a Postfilmic Cinema* (Chicago and London: University of Chicago Press, 2007).

Stoller, Robert, *Sexual Excitement: Dynamics of Erotic Life* (New York: Pantheon Books, 1979).

Telotte, J.P., 'Narratives of Resistance: Verhoeven's SOLDIER OF ORANGE', *Film Criticism* 30, 3 (2006): 3-16.

Todorov, Tzvetan, *The Fantastic: A Structural Approach to a Literary Genre* (Ithaca, New York: Cornell University Press, 1975).

Truffaut, François, 'Une certaine tendance du cinéma français', *Cahiers du cinéma* 31 (1954): 13-17.

Turkle, Sherry, *Alone Together: Why We Expect More From Technology and Less From Each Other* (New York: Basic Books, 2011).

Van Alphen, Ernst, 'On the Possibility and Impossibility of Modernist Cinema: Peter Forgács' OWN DEATH', *Filozofski vestnik* 35, 2 (2014): 255-269.

Van Bueren, Peter, 'Absurd en kluchtig spektakel van een gevoelig fantast', *de Volkskrant*, 11 May 1995, https://www.volkskrant.nl/nieuws-achtergrond/absurd-en-kluchtig-spektakel-van-een-gevoelig-fantast~b6c1bb1b/ [Accessed 12 May 2020].

Van den Tempel, Mark, 'Dutch Treat: De opkomst en ondergang van Cannon', *De Filmkrant* 379 (September 2015), https://filmkrant.nl/artikel/filmslot-de-opkomst-en-ondergang-van-cannon/ [Accessed 12 May 2020].

Van der Burg, Jos, 'De stront wordt duur betaald: De vliegende Hollander', *De Filmkrant* 156 (May 1995), https://filmkrant.nl/recensies/de-vliegende-hollander/ [Accessed 12 May 2020].

—, '"Ik neem het op voor de brave burger: Lodewijk Crijns over Bumperkleef"', *De Filmkrant* 425 (November 2019), https://filmkrant.nl/interview/lodewijk-crijns-bumperkleef/ [Accessed 12 May 2020].

Van Gelder, Henk, *Hollands Hollywood: Alle Nederlandse speelfilms van de afgelopen zestig jaar* (Amsterdam: Luitingh – Sijthoff, 1995).

Van Hoeij, Boyd, 'Brownian Movement', *Variety* (26 September 2010), https://variety.com/2010/film/markets-festivals/brownian-movement-1117943707/ [Accessed 17 May 2020].

Van Scheers, Rob, *Paul Verhoeven: Een filmersleven* (Amsterdam: Podium, 2017).

Van Uffelen, René. 'Op de montagetafel: Als twee druppels water', *Skrien* (April 2001): 28-30.

Verdaasdonk, Dorothée, 'Interview met WFH: Een fantasie waar geen romancier tegenop kan', ed. by Dorothée Verdaasdonk, *Fons Rademakers: Literatuur en film* (Utrecht: Uitgeverij Cambium, 1984), 8-21.

Verhaeghe, Paul, *Identiteit* (Amsterdam: De Bezige Bij, 2012).

—, *Love in a Time of Loneliness: Three Essays on Drive and Desire* (London: Karnac Books, 2011).

Verstraten, Peter, *Humour and Irony in Dutch Post-war Fiction Film* (Amsterdam: Amsterdam University Press, 2016).

—, '"My Very Own Citizen Kane", Inspired by Godard and Fellini: Frans Weisz's Adaptation of Remco Campert's *Het gangstermeisje*', *Journal of Dutch Literature* 8, 1 (2017): 60-74.

—, 'Theatrical Films and Cinematic Novels: De dans van de reiger and L'Année dernière à Marienbad', *Image [&] Narrative* 17, 2 (2016): 61-73.

Walsh, Martin W., 'Sex, Violence, and Saints' Images: Paul Verhoeven's 1985 Film Flesh + Blood', *Michigan Academician* 38, 3 (Fall 2008): 175-184.

White, Colin and Laurie Boucke, *The UnDutchables: An Observation of the Netherlands, Its Culture, and Its Inhabitants*, 8th edition (Lafayette, Colo.: White Boucke Pub., 2017).

Willemen, Paul, 'Through the Glass Darkly: Cinephilia Reconsidered', *Looks and Frictions: Essays in Cultural Studies and Film Theory*, London: BFI, 1994, 223-257.

Willems, Gertjan, 'Hugo Claus, de snelste en goedkoopste filmer van Europa: De totstandkoming van *De Vijanden*', *Zacht Lawijd*, 17, 1 (2018): 68-85.

—, *Subsidie, Camera, Actie! Filmbeleid in Vlaanderen (1964-2002)* (Gent: Academia Press, 2017).

Williams, Linda Ruth, *The Erotic Thriller in Contemporary Cinema* (Bloomington and Indianapolis: Indiana University Press, 2005).
Žižek, Slavoj, 'Cyberspace, or, How to Traverse the Fantasy in the Age of the Retreat of the Big Other', *Public Culture* 10, 3 (1998): 483-513.
—, 'Death and the Maiden', ed. by Elizabeth Wright and Edmond Wright, *The Žižek Reader* (Oxford: Blackwell Publishers, 1999), 206-221.
—, *Enjoy Your Symptom! Jacques Lacan In and Out of Hollywood*, 1992 (Revised Edition. New York and London: Routledge, 2001).
—, ed. *Everything You Always Wanted to Know about Lacan (But Were Afraid to Ask Hitchcock)* (London: Verso, 1992).
—, *How to Read Lacan* (New York: W.W. Norton and Company, 2007).
—, *Interrogating the Real*, ed. by Rex Butler and Scott Stephens (London: Bloomsbury, 2013).
—, *Looking Awry: An Introduction to Jacques Lacan through Popular Culture* (Cambridge, Mass.: The MIT Press, 1991).
—, 'The Act and Its Vicissitudes', *The Symptom* (2005): http://www.lacan.com/symptom6_articles/zizek.html [Accessed 17 May 2020].
—, *The Art of the Ridiculous Sublime:* LOST HIGHWAY (Seattle: Walter Chapin Simpson Center for the Humanities, University of Washington Press, 2000).
—, 'The Big Other Doesn't Exist', *Journal of European Psychoanalysis*, Spring – Fall (1997), http://www.lacan.com/zizekother.htm [Accessed 17 May 2020].
—, *The Fright of Real Tears: Krzysztof Kieślowski Between Theory and Post-Theory* (London: BFI, 2001).
—, *The Parallax View* (Cambridge, Mass.: The MIT Press , 2006).
—, *The Plague of Fantasies* (London and New York: Verso, 1997).
—, *The Sublime Object of Ideology* (London: Verso, 1989).
—, *Violence: Six Sideways Reflections* (London: Profile Books, 2009).

FILMOGRAPHY

Including information on the projection copies available in the Collection Centre of Eye Filmmuseum, Amsterdam

170 Hz. Dir. Joost van Ginkel. Sc. Joost van Ginkel. Cin. Rogier den Boer. Perf. Gaite Jansen, Michael Muller. Column Film, 2011. [L: Dutch | playable rendition | 720x576, graded YUV | 1'22''41]

Als twee druppels water. Dir. Fons Rademakers. Sc. Willem Frederik Hermans (novel), Fons Rademakers. Cin. Raoul Coutard. Perf. Lex Schoorel, Nan Los. Cineurope, 1963. [bw | L: Dutch, German | positive, acetate, 35mm | 3228,50mtr., 1'57''00 | preservation in 2003]

Amnesia. Dir. Martin Koolhoven. Sc. Martin Koolhoven. Cin. Menno Westendorp. Perf. Fedja van Huêt, Sacha Bulthuis, Carice van Houten. Motel Films, 2001. [L: Dutch | positive, polyester, 35mm | 2438,90mtr., 1'28''00]

Antonia. Dir. Marleen Gorris. Sc. Marleen Gorris. Cin. Willy Stassen. Perf. Willeke van Ammelrooy, Jan Decleir, Els Dottermans. Bergen, Prime Time, 1995. [L: Dutch | positive, acetate, 35mm | 2802,50mtr., 1'41''00]

Because of the Cats. Dir. Fons Rademakers. Sc. Nicolas Freeling (novel), Hugo Claus. Cin. Eduard van der Enden. Perf. Bryan Marshall, Alexandra Stewart. Fons Rademakers Produktie, 1973. [L: English | positive, acetate, 35mm | 2675,80mtr., 1'37''00 | preservation 1999]

Beyond Sleep. Dir. Boudewijn Koole. Sc. Willem Frederik Hermans (novel), Boudewijn Koole. Cin. Melle van Essen. Perf. Reinout Scholten van Aschat, Pål Sverre Hagen. FilmCamp, KeyFilm, 2016. [L: Dutch, English | CPL; 2048x858, graded XYZ | 1'47''17]

Black Butterflies. Dir. Paula van der Oest. Sc. Greg Latter. Cin. Giulio Biccari. Perf. Carice van Houten, Liam Cunningham, Rutger Hauer. IDTV Film, 2011. [L: English, Dutch | positive, polyester, 35mm | 2727,00mtr., 1'38''00]

Bloed, zweet & tranen. Dir. Diederick Koopal. Sc. Frank Ketelaar, Diederick Koopal. Cin. Bert Pot. Perf. Martijn Fischer, Hadewych Minis, Fedja van Huêt. Lemming Film, 2015. [L: Dutch | CPL; 2048x858, graded XYZ | 1'52"05]

Bluebird. Dir. Mijke de Jong. Sc. Helena van der Meulen. Cin. Goert Giltay. Perf. Elske Rotteveel, Kees Scholten. Egmond Film & Television, 2004. [L: Dutch | negative, polyester, 35mm | 2170,00mtr., 1'18"02 | playable rendition | 720x576, graded YUV]

Boven is het stil. Dir. Nanouk Leopold. Sc. Gerbrand Bakker (novel), Nanouk Leopold. Cin. Frank van den Eeden. Perf. Jeroen Willems, Henri Garcin, Wim Opbrouck. Circe Films, N279 Entertainment, 2013. [L: Dutch | CPL; 1998x1080, graded RGB | 1'30"56]

Brimstone. Dir. Martin Koolhoven. Sc. Martin Koolhoven. Cin. Rogier Stoffers. Perf. Dakota Fanning, Guy Pearce, Carice van Houten. N279 Entertainment, 2016. [L: English, Dutch | CPL; 2048x858, graded XYZ | 2'28"48]

Broos. Dir. Mijke de Jong. Sc. Jolein Laarman, Mijke de Jong. Cin. Joost van Starrenburg. Perf. Adelheid Roosen, Leonoor Pauw, Lieneke le Roux. SNG Film, 1997. [L: Dutch | positive, acetate, 35mm | 2198,00mtr., 1'19"00]

Brownian Movement. Dir. Nanouk Leopold. Sc. Nanouk Leopold. Cin. Frank van den Eeden. Perf. Sandra Hüller, Dragan Bakema. Circe Films, 2010. [L: English | positive, polyester, 35mm | 2757,00mtr., 1'40"00]

Brozer. Dir. Mijke de Jong. Sc. Jolein Laarman, Mijke de Jong. Cin. Ton Peters. Perf. Adelheid Roosen, Leonoor Pauw, Lieneke le Roux. Topkapi Films, PRPL, 2014. [L: Dutch | CPL; 1998x1080, graded XYZ | 1'19"47]

Charlotte. Dir. Frans Weisz. Sc. Judith Herzberg, Frans Weisz. Cin. Jerzy Lipman, Theo van de Sande. Perf. Birgit Doll, Derek Jacobi, Elisabeth Trissenaar. Concorde Film, Cineteam Features, 1981. [L: English | positive, acetate, 35mm | 2594,00mtr., 1'34"00]

Code Blue. Dir. Urszula Antoniak. Sc. Urszula Antoniak. Cin. Jasper Wolf. Perf. Bien de Moor, Lars Eidinger. IDTV Film, Family Affair Films, 2011. [L: Dutch | positive, polyester, 35mm | 2200,00mtr., 1'19"00]

Dagboek van een oude dwaas. Dir. Lili Rademakers. Sc. Jun'ichirô Tanizaki (novel), Claudine Bouvier, Hugo Claus. Cin. Paul van den Bos. Perf. Ralph Michael, Beatie Edney, Suzanne Flon, Derek de Lint. Fons Rademakers Produktie, Iblis Films, 1987. [L: English | positive, answerprint, polyester, 35mm | 2541,00mtr., 1'32"00 | preservation 2010]

De aanslag. Dir. Fons Rademakers. Sc. Harry Mulisch (novel), Gerard Soeteman. Cin. Theo van de Sande. Perf. Derek de Lint, Marc van Uchelen, Monique van de Ven, Johnny Kraaykamp. Fons Rademakers Produktie, 1986. [L: Dutch | positive, acetate, 35mm | 4034,70, 2'26"00]

De avonden. Dir. Rudolf van den Berg. Sc. Gerard Reve (novel), Rudolf van den Berg, Jean Ummels. Cin. Willy Stassen. Perf. Thom Hoffman, Rijk de Gooyer, Viviane de Muynck. Concorde Film, 1989. [L: Dutch | positive, polyester, 35mm | 3304,00mtr., 1'59''00 | preservation 2008]

De bende van Oss. Dir. André van Duren. Sc. Paul Jan Nelissen, André van Duren. Cin. Piotr Kukla. Perf. Sylvia Hoeks, Frank Lammers, Matthias Schoenaerts. Sigma Film Productions, 2011. [L: Dutch | positive, polyester, 35mm | 3050,00mtr., 1'50''08]

De Boskampi's. Dir. Arne Toonen. Sc. Marjon Hoffman (novel), Lotte Tabbers. Cin. Rutger Storm, Alex Wuijts. Perf. Thor Braun, Henry van Loon, Meral Polat. Shooting Star Filmcompany BV, Hazazah Pictures, 2015. [L: Dutch | CPL; 2048x858, graded XYZ | 1'45''44]

De dans van de reiger. Dir. Fons Rademakers. Sc. Hugo Claus. Cin. Sacha Vierny. Perf. Jean Desailly, Gunnel Lindblom, Van Doude. Atlas Film, Rademakers Productie B.V., 1966. [bw | L: Dutch | positive, answerprint, acetate, 35mm | 2476,00mtr., 1'29''00 | preservation 1999]

De grot. Dir. Martin Koolhoven. Sc. Tim Krabbé. Cin. Philip Van Volsem. Perf. Fedja van Huêt, Marcel Hensema, Kim Huffman. Get Reel Productions, 2001. [L: Dutch, English | positive, polyester, 35mm | 2502,00mtr., 1'30''00]

De IJssalon. Dir. Dimitri Frenkel Frank. Sc. Dimitri Frenkel Frank. Cin. Theo van de Sande. Perf. Gerard Thoolen, Bruno Ganz, Renée Soutendijk. Roeland Kerbosch Filmproduktie B.V., 1985. [L: Dutch, German | positive, acetate, 35mm | 2720,00 mtr; 1'38''00]

De Johnsons. Dir. Rudolf van den Berg. Sc. Leon de Winter, Rocco Simonelli, Roy Frumkes, Linda Bogers. Cin. Theo Bierkens. Perf. Esmée de la Bretonnière, Monique van de Ven, Kenneth Herdigein. Movies Film Productions, 1992. [L: Dutch, English | positive, acetate, 35mm | 2805,60mtr., 1'41''19]

De lift. Dir. Dick Maas. Sc. Dick Maas. Cin. Marc Felperlaan. Perf. Huub Stapel, Willeke van Ammelrooy. First Floor Features, Sigma Film Productions, 1983. [L: Dutch | positive, acetate, 35mm | 2700,20mtr., 1'37''30 | digitization 2016 by Dick Maas]

De marionettenwereld. Dir. Elbert van Strien. Sc. Elbert van Strien. Cin. Chiel van Dongen. Perf. Bart Klever, Daan Hogendoorn. Netherlands Film Academy, 1993. [L: Dutch | positive, acetate, 16mm | 360,00mtr., 0'33''00]

De poel. Dir. Chris W. Mitchell. Sc. Chris W. Mitchell, Gijs Scholten van Aschat. Cin. Gábor Deák. Perf. Gijs Scholten van Aschat, Carine Crutzen, Bart Klever. Fu Works, 2014. [L: Dutch | CPL; 2048x858, graded XYZ | 1'16''14]

De Poolse bruid. Dir. Karim Traïdia. Sc. Kees van der Hulst. Cin. Jacques Laureys. Perf. Jaap Spijkers, Monic Hendrickx. IJswater Films, Motel Films, 1998. [L: Dutch, Polish | positive, polyester, 35mm | 2440,00mtr., 1'25''00]

De schorpioen. Dir. Ben Verbong. Sc. Ben Verbong, Pieter de Vos. Cin. Theo van de Sande. Perf. Peter Tuinman, Adrian Brine, Monique van de Ven. Movies Film Productions, 1984. [L: Dutch | no copy available, 1'38''00]

De vijanden. Dir. Hugo Claus. Sc. Hugo Claus. Cin. Herman Wuyts. Perf. Robbe De Hert, Del Negro, Fons Rademakers. Jan Vrijman Cineproduktie, 1968. [bw | L: French, English | positive, acetate, 35mm | 2495,00mtr., 1'30''06 | preservation 1999]

De vliegende Hollander. Dir. Jos Stelling. Sc. Hans Heesen, Jos Stelling. Cin. Goert Giltay. Perf. René Groothof, Veerle Dobbelaere, Gene Bervoets. Black Forest Films, 1995. [L: Dutch, French, Italian | positive, answerprint, acetate, 35mm | 3539,50mtr., 2'08''00]

De witte waan. Dir. Adriaan Ditvoorst. Sc. Adriaan Ditvoorst. Cin. Albert van der Wildt. Perf. Thom Hoffman, Pim Labeau. Cineproductie, 1984. [L: Dutch | positive, answerprint, polyester, 35mm | 2876,00mtr., 1'44''00]

Diep. Dir. Simone van Dusseldorp. Sc. Hendrickje Spoor (novel), Tamara Bos. Cin. Ton Peters. Perf. Melody Klaver, Damien Hope, Monic Hendrickx. IJswater Films, 2005. [L: Dutch, English | positive, polyester, 35mm | 2368,00mtr., 1'26''00]

Dokter Pulder zaait papavers. Dir. Bert Haanstra. Sc. Anton Koolhaas. Cin. Anton van Munster. Perf. Kees Brusse, Ton Lensink, Dora van der Groen. Bert Haanstra Films, 1975. [L: Dutch | positive, answerprint, acetate, 35mm | 2884,00mtr., 1'44''00]

Dorp aan de rivier. Dir. Fons Rademakers. Sc. Antoon Coolen (novel), Hugo Claus, Fons Rademakers. Cin. Eduard van der Enden. Perf. Max Croiset, Mary Dresselhuys, Jan Teulings, Bernard Droog. Nationale Film Productie Maatschappij, 1958. [bw | L: Dutch | positive, answerprint, acetate, 35mm | 2522,00mtr., 1'31''00 | preservation 1999]

Een maand later. Dir. Nouchka van Brakel. Sc. Jan Donkers, Ate de Jong, Nouchka van Brakel. Cin. Peter De Bont. Perf. Renée Soutendijk, Monique van de Ven, Edwin de Vries. Sigma Film Productions, 1987. [L: Dutch, English | positive, answerprint, polyester, 35mm | 2838,00mtr., 1'42''00 | preservation 2010]

Een ochtend van zes weken. Dir. Nikolai van der Heyde. Sc. Nikolai van der Heyde. Cin. Gérard Vandenberg. Perf. Hans Culeman, Anne Collette. Cineurope, 1966. [bw | L: Dutch, French | positive, acetate, 35mm | 2218,50mtr., 1'20''08 | preservation 2010]

Een vrouw als Eva. Dir. Nouchka van Brakel. Sc. Judith Herzberg, Nouchka van Brakel, Carel Donck. Cin. Nurith Aviv. Perf. Monique van de Ven, Maria Schneider. Sigma Film Productions, 1979. [L: Dutch, French, English | positive, answerprint, polyester, 35mm | 2818,00mtr., 1'42''00 | preservation 2011]

Eline Vere. Dir. Harry Kümel. Sc. Louis Couperus (novel), Jan Blokker, Patrick Pesnot. Cin. Eduard van der Enden. Perf. Marianne Basler, Thom Hoffman, Monique van de Ven. Sigma Film Productions, 1991. [L: Dutch, French, English | positive, answerprint, polyester, 35mm | 3645,00mtr., 2'12''00]

Elle. Dir. Paul Verhoeven. Sc. Philippe Djian (novel), David Birke. Cin. Stéphane Fontaine. Perf. Isabella Huppert, Laurent Lafitte. SBS Productions, 2016. [L: French | no copy available | 2'10''00]

Flanagan. Dir. Adriaan Ditvoorst. Sc. Tim Krabbé (novel), Adriaan Ditvoorst, Antón Quintana. Cin. Eduard van der Enden. Perf. Guido de Moor, Eric Schneider, Petra Laseur, Josée Ruiter. Sigma Film Productions, 1975. [L: Dutch | positive, polyester, 35mm | 2907,00mtr., 1'45''00 | preservation 2010]

Flesh + Blood. Dir. Paul Verhoeven. Sc. Gerard Soeteman, Paul Verhoeven. Cin. Jan de Bont. Perf. Rutger Hauer, Jennifer Jason Leigh, Tom Burlinson. Riverside Pictures, 1985. [L: English | positive, polyester, 35mm | 3535,00mtr., 2'08''00]

Gebroken spiegels. Dir. Marleen Gorris. Sc. Marleen Gorris. Cin. Frans Bromet. Perf. Lineke Rijxman, Henriëtte Tol, Eddy Brugman. Sigma Film Productions. [L: Dutch | positive, answerprint, polyester, 35mm | 3050,00mtr., 1'50''00 | preservation 2011]

Gluckauf. Dir. Remy van Heugten. Sc. Gustaaf Peek, Remy van Heugten. Cin. Mark van Aller. Perf. Bart Slegers, Vincent van der Valk, Johan Leysen. BIND, 2015. [L: Dutch (dialect) | CPL; 1998x1080, graded XYZ | 1'41''37]

Guernsey. Dir. Nanouk Leopold. Sc. Nanouk Leopold. Cin. Richard van Oosterhout. Perf. Maria Kraakman, Fedja van Huêt, Johanna ter Steege. Circe Films, 2005. [L: Dutch, English | positive, answerprint, polyester, 35mm |2469,00mtr., 1'26''00]

Havinck. Dir. Frans Weisz. Sc. Marja Brouwers (novel), Ger Thijs. Cin. Giuseppe Lanci. Perf. Willem Nijholt, Anne Martien Lousberg, Will van Kralingen. Riverside Pictures, 1987. [L: Dutch | positive, acetate, 35mm | 2706,00mtr., 1'37''43]

Hemel. Dir. Sacha Polak. Sc. Helena van der Meulen. Cin. Daniël Bouquet. Perf. Hannah Hoekstra, Hans Dagelet. Circe Films, 2012. [L: Dutch | playable rendition | 1920x1080, graded YUV | 1'17''40]

Het gangstermeisje. Dir. Frans Weisz. Sc. Remco Campert (novel), Jan Blokker, Frans Weisz. Cin. Gérard Vandenberg. Perf. Paolo Graziosi, Kitty Courbois, Gian Maria Volontè. Jan Vrijman Cineproduktie, 1966. [bw | L: Dutch, Italian | positive, volgprint, acetate, 35mm | 3017,00mtr., 1'48''57 | preservation 1999]

Het meisje en de dood. Dir. Jos Stelling. Sc. Jos Stelling, Bert Rijkelijkhuizen. Cin. Goert Giltay. Perf. Sylvia Hoeks, Leonid Bichevin, Sergey Makovetskiy, Dieter Hallervorden. Jos Stelling Filmprodukties, 2012. [L: Russian, German | CPL; 2048x858, graded XYZ | 2'07''08]

Het meisje met het rode haar. Dir. Ben Verbong. Sc. Theun de Vries (novel), Ben Verbong, Pieter de Vos. Cin. Theo van de Sande. Perf. Renée Soutendijk, Peter Tuinman, Loes Luca. Meteor Film Productions, 1981. [L: Dutch, German | positive, acetate, 35mm | 3106,00mtr., 1'52''11]

Het mes. Dir. Fons Rademakers. Sc. Hugo Claus. Cin. Eduard van der Enden. Perf. Reitze van der Linden, Marie-Louise Videc, Ellen Vogel. NFM, 1961. [bw | L: Dutch | positive, answerprint, acetate, 35mm | 2426,60mtr., 1'28''00 | preservation 2000]

Het teken van het beest. Dir. Pieter Verhoeff. Sc. Anton Haakman, Jurriën Rood, Pieter Verhoeff, Cherry Duyns. Cin. Mat van Hensbergen. Concorde Film, 1980. [L: Dutch | positive, acetate, 35mm | 2582,50mtr., 1'33''00 | preservation 2010]

Het zwijgen. Dir. Adri Schrover and André van der Hout. Sc. Adri Schrover, André van der Hout. Cin. Adri Schrover. Perf. Vincent Croiset, Rosa Reuten, Huib Broos. The Film Kitchen, Waterland Film & TV, 2006. [L: Dutch | positive, polyester, 35mm | 2717,00mtr., 1'38''00]

In de schaduw van de overwinning. Dir. Ate de Jong. Sc. Ate de Jong, Edwin de Vries. Cin. Eduard van der Enden. Perf. Jeroen Krabbé, Edwin de Vries, Tom Jansen. Sigma Film Productions, 1986. [L: Dutch, German | positive, answerprint, acetate, 35mm | 3070,00mtr., 1'51''00 | preservation 2010]

Instinct. Dir. Halina Reijn. Sc. Esther Gerritsen, Halina Reijn. Cin. Jasper Wolf. Perf. Carice van Houten, Marwan Kenzari. Topkapi Films, 2019. [L: Dutch | CPL; 2048x858, graded XYZ | 1'38''17]

João en het mes. Dir. George Sluizer. Sc. Odylo Costa Filho (novel), George Sluizer. Cin. Jan de Bont. Perf. Joffre Soares, Ana Maria Miranda. Sluizer Films, 1972. [L: Portuguese | positive, polyester, 35mm | 2585,00mtr., 1'33''00 – restoration in 2018]

Joy. Dir. Mijke de Jong. Sc. Helena van der Meulen. Cin. Ton Peters. Perf. Samira Maas, Coosje Smid. IDTV Film, 2010. [L: Dutch | positive, polyester, 35mm | 2116,00mtr., 1'13''00]

Karakter. Dir. Mike van Diem. Sc. Ferdinand Bordewijk (novel), Laurens Geels, Mike van Diem, Ruud van Megen. Cin. Rogier Stoffers. Perf. Fedja van Huêt, Jan Decleir, Victor Löw. First Floor Features, 1997. [L: Dutch, English | positive, acetate, 35mm | 3419,00mtr., 2'03''00 – digital restoration 2020: CPL; 3996x2160, graded XYZ | 2'04''38]

Keetje Tippel. Dir. Paul Verhoeven. Sc. Neel Doff (novel), Gerard Soeteman. Cin. Jan de Bont. Perf. Monique van de Ven, Andrea Domburg, Rutger Hauer. Rob Houwer Productions, 1975. [L: Dutch | positive, volgprint, acetate, 35mm | 2923,00mtr., 1'46''03]

Kracht. Dir. Frouke Fokkema. Sc. Frouke Fokkema. Cin. Theo Bierkens. Perf. Theu Boermans, Anneke Blok. Sigma Film Productions, 1990. [L: Dutch (dialect) | positive, acetate, 35mm | 2887,00mtr., 1'43''00 | preservation 2010]

Layla M. Dir. Mijke de Jong. Sc. Jan Eilander, Mijke de Jong. Cin. Danny Elsen. Perf. Nora El Koussour, Ilias Addab. Topkapi Films, 2016. [L: Dutch, English, Arabic | CPL; 2048x858, graded XYZ | 1'38''12]

Leedvermaak. Dir. Frans Weisz. Sc. Judith Herzberg (play), Frans Weisz. Cin. Goert Giltay. Perf. Kitty Courbois, Peter Oosthoek, Catherine ten Bruggencate. Riverside Pictures, 1989. [L: Dutch | positive, acetate, 35mm | 2416,00mtr., 1'27''00]

Lek. Dir. Jean van de Velde. Sc. Jan van Daalen (novel), Simon de Waal, Jean van de Velde. Cin. Jules van den Steenhoven. Perf. Cas Jansen, Ricky Koole, Victor Löw, Thomas Acda. M & B Film BV, 2000. [L: Dutch | positive, polyester, 35mm | 2964,50mtr., 1'47''00]

Lena. Dir. Christophe Van Rompaey. Sc. Mieke de Jong. Cin. Menno Westendorp. Perf. Emma Levie, Niels Gomperts, Jeroen Willems. Isabella Films, 2011. [L: Dutch, Polish | positive, polyester, 35mm | 3237,00mtr., 1'56''54]

Les lèvres rouges / la rouge aux lèvres. Dir. Harry Kümel. Perf. Pierre Drouot, Harry Kümel. Cin. Eduard van der Enden. Perf. John Karlen, Danielle Ouiemet, Delphine Seyrig. Showking Films, Maya Films, 1971. [L: English, German, French | positive, acetate, 35mm | 2617,50mtr., 1'35''00]

Liefdesbekentenissen. Dir. Wim Verstappen. Sc. Wim Verstappen, Pim de la Parra. Cin. Mat van Hensbergen. Perf. Ramses Shaffy, Kitty Courbois, Shireen Strooker, Michael York. Scorpio Production, 1967. [bw | L: Dutch, English | positive, answerprint, polyester, 35mm | 2248,50mtr., 1'21''00 | preservation 2008]

Loos. Dir. Theo van Gogh. Sc. Guus Luijters, Theo van Gogh. Cin. Tom Erisman. Perf. Tom Jansen, Renée Fokker, Max Pam. Shooting Star Filmcompany BV, 1989. [L: Dutch | positive, acetate, 35mm | 2816,00mtr., 1'42''00]

Max Havelaar of de koffieveilingen der Nederlandsche Handelsmaatschappij. Dir. Fons Rademakers. Sc. Multatuli (novel), Gerard Soeteman. Perf. Peter Faber, Sacha Bulthuis, Adendu Soesilaningrat. P.T. Mondial Motion Pictures, Rademakers Productie, Jakarta Film, 1976. [L: Dutch, Malay | positive, answerprint, polyester, 35mm | 4596,00mtr., 2'45''58 | preservation 2002 and 2008]

Menuet. Dir. Lili Rademakers. Sc. Louis Paul Boon (novel), Hugo Claus. Cin. Paul van den Bos. Perf. Hubert Fermin, Carla Hardy, Akkemay. Fons Rademakers Produktie, Iblis Films, 1982. [L | Dutch | positive, answerprint, polyester, 35mm | 2380,00mtr., 1'26''00 | preservation 2010]

Mijn vriend of het verborgen leven van Jules Depraeter. Dir. Fons Rademakers. Sc. Gerard Soeteman. Cin. Theo van de Sande. Perf. Peter Faber, André van den Heuvel, Pleuni Touw. Cinemagna, Fons Rademakers Productie, 1979. [L: Dutch, French | positive, answerprint, polyester, 35mm | 3499,60mtr., 2'06''00 | preservation 1997]

Milo. Dir. Berend Boorsma, Roel Boorsma. Sc. Berend Boorsma, Roel Boorsma, Heather Imani. Cin. Frank van den Eeden. Perf. Lorcan Bonner, Laura Vasiliu, Stuart Graham, Jer O'Leary. Samson Films, A Private View, Fu Works, 2012. [L: English | analogue video, tape, digibeta | 1'34''00]

Monsieur Hawarden. Dir. Harry Kümel. Sc. Filip De Pillecyn (novel), Jan Blokker. Cin. Eduard van der Enden. Perf. Ellen Vogel, Hilde Uitterlinden, Xander Fisher. Parkfilm, 1968. [bw | L: Dutch | positive, acetate, 35mm | 2797,00mtr., 1'40''32]

Mysteries. Dir. Paul de Lussanet. Sc. Knut Hamsun (novel), Paul de Lussanet. Cin. Robby Müller. Perf. Rutger Hauer, Sylvia Kristel, Rita Tushingham, David Rappaport. Sigma Film Productions, 1975. [L: Dutch, English | positive, polyester, 35mm | 2801,30mtr., 1'41''58 | preservation 2010]

Nachtrit. Dir. Dana Nechushtan. Sc. Franky Ribbens. Cin. Bert Pot. Perf. Frank Lammers, Fedja van Huêt, Henk Poort. The Film Kitchen, Waterland Film & TV, 2006. [L: Dutch | positive, polyester, 35mm | 2843,00mtr., 1'43''00]

Nothing Personal. Dir. Urszula Antoniak. Sc. Urszula Antoniak. Cin. Daniël Bouquet. Perf. Lotte Verbeek, Stephen Rea. Rinkel Film, Family Affair Films, 2009. [L: English | positive, polyester, 35mm | 2345,00mtr., 1'25''00]

Obsessions. Dir. Pim de la Parra. Sc. Pim de la Parra, Martin Scorsese, Wim Verstappen. Cin. Frans Bromet, Hubertus Hagen. Perf. Dieter Geissler, Alexandra Stewart, Tom van Beek. Scorpio Films, 1969. [L: English | positive, acetate, 35mm | 2700,00mtr., 1'38''00 | digital restoration 2015: CPL; 1998x1080; graded XYZ; 1'30''37]

Onder ons. Dir. Marco van Geffen. Sc. Jolein Laarman, Marco van Geffen. Cin. Ton Peters. Perf. Dagmara Bak, Natalia Rybicka, Rifka Lodeizen, Reinout Bussemaker. Lemming Film, 2011. [L: Dutch, English, Polish | positive, polyester, 35mm | 2303,00mtr., 1'23''00]

Oorlogswinter. Dir. Martin Koolhoven. Sc. Jan Terlouw (novel), Martin Koolhoven, Paul Jan Nelissen, Mieke de Jong. Cin. Guido van Gennep. Perf. Martijn Lakemeier, Yorick van Wageningen, Jamie Campbell Bower. Fu Works, Isabella Films, 2008. [L: Dutch, German, English | positive, polyester, 35mm | 2820,00mtr., 1'42''00]

Out of Love. Dir. Paloma Aguilera Valdebenito. Sc. Paloma Aguilera Valdebenito. Cin. Jasper Wolf. Perf. Naomi Velissariu, Daniil Vorobyov. Topkapi Films, 2016. [L: Dutch, English | CPL; 1998x1080, graded XYZ | 1'40''25]

Paranoia. Dir. Adriaan Ditvoorst. Sc. Willem Frederik Hermans (novel), Adriaan Ditvoorst. Cin. Jan de Bont. Perf. Kees van Eyck, Pamela Koevoets. Parnasse Produkties, 1967. [bw | L: Dutch | positive, answerprint, polyester, 35mm | 2773,00mtr., 1'40''06 | preservation 1999]

Pastorale 1943. Dir. Wim Verstappen. Sc. Simon Vestdijk (novel), Wim Verstappen. Cin. Marc Felperlaan. Perf. Frederik de Groot, Bram van der Vlugt, Bernard Droog, Sylvia Kristel. Spieghel Productiemaatschappij, 1978. [L: Dutch, German | positive, polyester, 35mm | 3507,00mtr., 2'02''00 | preservation 2009]

Pentimento. Dir. Frans Zwartjes. Sc. Frans Zwartjes. Cin. Frans Zwartjes. Perf. Helen Hedy, Ronald Beer, Moniek Toebosch, Trix Zwartjes. Fugitive Cinema Holland, 1979. [L: none | positive, polyester, 16mm | 821,00mtr., 1'14''00 | preservation 2006]

Pervola, sporen in de sneeuw. Dir. Orlow Seunke. Sc. Dirk Ayelt Kooiman, Maarten Koopman, Orlow Seunke, Gerard Thoolen. Cin. Theo Bierkens. Perf. Gerard Thoolen, Bram van der Vlugt. Maya Filmproduktie, 1985. [L: Dutch, English | positive, answerprint, polyester, 35mm | 2765,00mtr., 1'40''00 | preservation 2010 | digital restoration 2019: CPL; 1998x1080, graded XYZ | 1'41''17]

R U THERE. Dir. David Verbeek. Sc. Rogier de Blok. Cin. Lennert Hillege. Perf. Stijn Koomen, Huan-Ru Ke. IDTV Film, 2010. [L: Dutch, English, Min Nan, Mandarin | positive, polyester, 35mm | 2372,00mtr., 1'26"00]

RIPHAGEN. Dir. Pieter Kuijpers. Sc. Thomas van der Ree, Paul Jan Nelissen. Cin. Bert Pot. Perf. Jeroen van Koningsbrugge, Kay Greidanus. Pupkin Film, 2016. [L: Dutch, German | CPL; 2048x858, graded XYZ | 2'11"08]

ROBOCOP. Dir. Paul Verhoeven. Sc. Edward Neumeier, Michael Miner. Cin. Jost Vacano. Perf. Peter Weller, Nancy Allen, Ronny Cox. Orion Pictures, 1987. [L: English | positive, acetate, 35mm | 2803,00mtr., 1'41"13]

ROOIE SIEN. Dir. Frans Weisz. Sc. Judith Herzberg, Rob du Mee, Beppie Nooij, jr., Richard Nooij, Marius Spree, Frans Weisz. Cin. Ferenc Kálmán-Gáll. Perf. Willeke Alberti, Jules Hamel, Kees Brusse. Actueel Film, Rob du Mee Park Film, 1975. [L: Dutch | positive, acetate, 35mm | 2950,20mtr., 1'47"00]

SCHEMER. Dir. Hanro Smitsman. Sc. Anjet Daanje. Cin. Joost Rietdijk. Perf. Matthijs van de Sande Bakhuyzen, Gaite Jansen, Robert de Hoog. Corrino Studios, 2010. [L: Dutch | positive, polyester, 35mm | 2522,00mtr., 1'31"04]

SHOCK HEAD SOUL. Dir. Simon Pummell. Sc. Simon Pummell. Cin. Reinier van Brummelen. Perf. Hugo Koolschijn, Anniek Pheifer. Hot Property Films, Submarine, 2011. [L: English | playable rendition, master file | 1920x1080, graded YUV | 1'22"07]

SOLDAAT VAN ORANJE. Dir. Paul Verhoeven. Sc. Erik Hazelhoff Roelfzema (novel), Gerard Soeteman, Kees Holierhoek, Paul Verhoeven. Cin. Jost Vacano. Perf. Rutger Hauer, Jeroen Krabbé, Susan Penhaligon. Rob Houwer Productions, 1977. [L: Dutch, English, German | positive, Volgprint, acetate, 35mm | 4062,00mtr., 2'25"40]

SPOORLOOS. Dir. George Sluizer. Sc. Tim Krabbé (novel), George Sluizer. Cin. Toni Kuhn. Perf. Gene Bervoets, Bernard-Pierre Donnadieu, Johanna ter Steege. Argos Films, Golden Egg. 1988. [L: Dutch, French | positive, answerprint, polyester, 35mm | 2893,00mtr., 1'44"00 – digital restoration 2017]

SÜSKIND. Dir. Rudolf van den Berg. Sc. Chris W. Mitchell, Rudolf van den Berg. Cin. Guido van Gennep. Perf. Jeroen Spitzenberger, Karl Markovics, Nyncke Beekhuyzen. Fu Works, Rinkel Film, 2012. [L: Dutch, German | no copy available | 1'58"00]

TAKE ME SOMEWHERE NICE. Dir. Ena Sendijarević. Sc. Ena Sendijarević. Cin. Emo Weemhoff. Perf. Sara Luna Zoric, Lazar Dragojevic, Ernad Prnjavorac. Pupkin Film, 2018. [L: Bosnian | CPL; 1998x1080, graded XYZ | 1'31"33]

TERUG NAAR OEGSTGEEST. Dir. Theo van Gogh. Sc. Jan Wolkers (novel), Theo van Gogh. Sc. Marc Felperlaan. Perf. Tom Jansen, Hidde Kuiper, Casper de Boer. Movies Film Productions, 1987. [L: Dutch | positive | acetate, 35mm | 2563,00mtr., 1'33"00]

THE PARADISE SUITE. Dir. Joost van Ginkel. Sc. Joost van Ginkel. Cin. Andréas Lennartsson. Perf. Angela Nedyalkova, Boris Isakovic, Issaka Sawadogo. PRPL, 2015. [L: Dutch, English | CPL; 2048x858, graded XYZ | 2'03"11]

Tirza. Dir. Rudolf van den Berg. Sc. Arnon Grunberg (novel), Rudolf van den Berg. Cin. Gábor Szabó. Perf. Gijs Scholten van Aschat, Sylvia Hoeks, Nasrdin Dchar, 2010. [L: Dutch, English | positive, polyester, 35mm | 2862,00mtr., 1'43''21]

Van de koele meren des doods. Dir. Nouchka van Brakel. Sc. Frederik van Eeden (novel), Ton Vorstenbosch, Nouchka van Brakel. Cin. Theo van de Sande. Perf. Renée Soutendijk, Derek de Lint, Adriaan Olree. Sigma Film Productions, 1982. [L: Dutch, English, French | positive, polyester, 35mm | 3395,00mtr. 2'03''00 | digital restoration 2020 | CPL; 3996x2160, graded XYZ | 2'04''23]

Van God los. Dir. Pieter Kuijpers. Sc. Pieter Kuijpers, Paul Jan Nelissen. Cin. Bert Pot. Perf. Tygo Gernandt, Egbert Jan Weeber. IDTV Films, Rinkel Film & TV Productions BV, 2003. [L: Dutch | positive, polyester, 35mm | 2378,40mtr. | 1'26''00]

Verdwijnen. Dir. Boudewijn Koole. Sc. Jolein Laarman. Cin. Melle van Essen. Perf. Rifka Lodeizen, Elsie de Brauw. The Film Kitchen, Sweet Films, 2017. [L: Dutch, English, Norwegian | CPL; 2048x858, graded XYZ | 1'31''33]

Wereld van stilstand. Dir. Elbert van Strien. Sc. Elbert van Strien, Paulo van Vliet. Cin. Guido van Gennep. Perf. Fedja van Huêt. Accento Films, 2005. [bw | L: Dutch | positive, Polyester, 35mm | 817,00mtr., 0'3000]

Wildschut. Dir. Bobby Eerhart. Sc. Felix Thijssen (novel). Cin. Paul van den Bos. Perf. Hidde Maas, Jack Monkau, Annick Christiaens. Cine/Vista, 1985. [L: Dutch | positive | 2584,00mtr., 1'33''00 | preservation 2010]

Wolf. Dir. Jim Taihuttu. Sc. Jim Taihuttu. Cin. Lennart Verstegen. Perf. Marwan Kenzari, Chems Eddine Amar. Habbekrats, New Amsterdam Film Company, 2013. [bw | L: Dutch, Arabic, Turkish, English, French | CPL; 1998x1080, graded XYZ | 2'02''38]

Zurich. Dir. Sacha Polak. Sc. Helena van der Meulen. Cin. Frank van den Eeden. Perf. Wende Snijders, Sascha Alexander Gersak. Viking Film, 2015. [L: English, Dutch | CPL; 1998x1080, graded XYZ | 1'28''30]

Zwart water. Dir. Elbert van Strien. Sc. Elbert van Strien, Paulo van Vliet. Cin. Guido van Gennep. Perf. Hadewych Minis, Isabelle Stokkel, Barry Atsma. Accento Films, 2010. [L: Dutch | positive, polyester, 35mm | 3062,00mtr., 1'51''00]

Zwartboek. Dir. Paul Verhoeven. Sc. Gerard Soeteman, Paul Verhoeven. Cin. Karl Walter Lindenlaub. Perf. Carice van Houten, Sebastian Koch, Thom Hoffman. Fu Works, 2016. [L: Dutch, English, German | positive, polyester, 35 mm | 3982,00mtr., 2'23''48]

INDEX OF CONCEPTS

INDEX OF FILMS

E

X

Z

INDEX OF NAMES

W

Z

For Product Safety Concerns and Information please contact our EU representative GPSR@taylorandfrancis.com Taylor & Francis Verlag GmbH, Kaufingerstraße 24, 80331 München, Germany

Batch number: 10722100

Printed by Printforce, the Netherlands